a **LANGE** clini

Poisoning & Drug Overdose

by the faculty and staff of the San Francisco Bay
Area Regional Poison Control Center

Second Edition

Edited by
Kent R. Olson, MD, FACEP
Medical Director
SF Bay Area Regional Poison Control Center
San Francisco General Hospital
Attending Emergency Physician
Eden Hospital Medical Center
Associate Clinical Professor of Medicine and Lecturer in Pharmacy
University of California, San Francisco

Associate Editors

Ilene B. Anderson, PharmD
Poison Information Specialist
SF Bay Area Regional Poison Control Center
Assistant Clinical Professor of Pharmacy
University of California, San Francisco

Paul D. Blanc, MD, MSPH
Attending Toxicologist
SF Bay Area Regional Poison Control Center
Chief, Division of Occupational Medicine
Assistant Professor of Medicine
University of California, San Francisco

Neal L. Benowitz, MD
Attending Toxicologist
SF Bay Area Regional Poison Control Center
Chief, Division of Clinical Pharmacology
Professor of Medicine
University of California, San Francisco

Thomas E. Kearney, PharmD
Managing Director
SF Bay Area Regional Poison Control Center
Associate Clinical Professor of Pharmacy
University of California, San Francisco

John D. Osterloh, MD
Attending Toxicologist
SF Bay Area Regional Poison Control Center
Director, Toxicology Laboratory
San Francisco General Hospital
Associate Professor of Laboratory Medicine
University of California, San Francisco

Olga F. Woo, PharmD
Poison Information Specialist
SF Bay Area Regional Poison Control Center
Assistant Clinical Professor of Pharmacy
University of California, San Francisco

APPLETON & LANGE
Norwalk, Connecticut

Notice: The authors and the publisher of this volume have taken care to make certain that the doses of drugs and schedules of treatment are correct and compatible with the standards generally accepted at the time of publication. Nevertheless, as new information becomes available, changes in treatment and the use of drugs become necessary. The reader is advised to carefully consult the instruction and information material included in the package insert of each drug or therapeutic agent before administration. This advice is especially important when using new or infrequently used drugs. The publisher disclaims any liability, loss, injury, or damage incurred as a consequence, directly or indirectly, of the use and application of any of the contents of this volume.

Copyright © 1994 by Appleton & Lange
Paramount Publishing Business and Professional Group

All rights reserved. This book, or any parts thereof, may not be used or reproduced in any manner without written permission. For information, address Appleton & Lange, 25 Van Zant Street, East Norwalk, Connecticut 06855.

94 95 96 97 98 / 10 9 8 7 6 5 4 3

Prentice Hall International (UK) Limited, *London*
Prentice Hall of Australia Pty. Limited, *Sydney*
Prentice Hall of Canada, Inc., *Toronto*
Prentice Hall Hispanoamericana, S.A., *Mexico*
Prentice Hall of India Private Limited, *New Delhi*
Prentice Hall of Japan, Inc., *Tokyo*
Simon & Schuster Asia Pte. Ltd., *Singapore*
Editora Prentice Hall do Brasil Ltda., *Rio de Janeiro*
Prentice Hall, *Englewood Cliffs, New Jersey*

ISBN 0-8385-1108-2
90000
9 780838 511084

ISSN 1048-8847

Acquisitions Editor: Shelley Reinhardt
Production Editor: Christine Langan

PRINTED IN THE UNITED STATES OF AMERICA

Contents

Preface

Poisoning & Drug Overdose provides practical advice for the management of poisoning and drug overdose and essential information about industrial chemicals and occupational illness.

This manual outlines a comprehensive approach to management, including essential advice on how to diagnose and treat poisoning and how to recognize and treat common complications.

This manual is divided into 4 sections and an index, each one identified by black tabs in the right margins. **Section I** guides the user through initial emergency steps to physical diagnosis, laboratory tests, and methods of decontamination. **Section II** provides information on diagnosis and treatment of approximately 150 common drugs and poisons. Icons at the beginning of each topic provide a quick reference on the availability of antidotes and the advisability of various decontamination methods. **Section III** describes the use and side effects of about 60 common antidotes and therapeutic drugs. **Section IV** describes the urgent medical evaluation and management of occupational illness and the medical management of industrial accidents. This section includes a table of common industrial chemicals. The **Index** is comprehensive and extensively cross-referenced.

The manual allows the reader to move quickly from section to section to obtain needed information from each. For example, in managing a patient with theophylline intoxication, the reader will find specific information about theophylline toxicity in Section II, practical advice for management and complications such as seizures or hypotension in Section I, and detailed information about dosing and potential side effects of esmolol in Section III. In this way, a complete discussion of each complication, each toxin, and each antidote is provided in a consistent manner, but without repetition.

Acknowledgments

The first and now second editions of this manual would not have been possible without the combined efforts of the staff, fellows and faculty of the San Francisco Bay Area Regional Poison Control Center, to whom I am deeply indebted. From its inception, this book has been a project by and for our poison control center; as a result, all royalties from its sale go to our center's operating fund and not to any individual.

On behalf of the authors and editors of the second edition, my sincere thanks to all those who assisted with the first edition but who are no longer affiliated with the SF Poison Control Center. We are also grateful for the numerous comments and suggestions received from colleagues, students, and the editorial staff at Appleton & Lange, which helped us to make the second edition even better.

Finally, a special thanks to Donna, Bradley, Marlene, and Gregory, for their patience and support during these past several months.

Kent R. Olson, MD
San Francisco
September 1993

Contributors

Contributors to the 2nd Edition

All contributing editors and authors were staff, faculty or fellows affiliated with the San Francisco Bay Area Regional Poison Control Center at the time of their contributions.

Ilene Brewer Anderson, PharmD
John Balmes, M.D.
Charles E. Becker, MD
Neil L. Benowitz, MD
Paul D. Blanc, MD
Christopher R. Brown, MD
Delia Dempsey, MD
Jo Ellen Dyer, PharmD
Mark J. Galbo, MS
Patricia H. Hiatt, BS
Gerald Joe, PharmD
Thomas E. Kearney, PharmD
Kathryn H. Keller, PharmD

Susan Kim, PharmD
Michael Kosnett, MD
Diane Liu, MD, MPH
Timothy D. McCarthy, PharmD
Kathryn H. Meier, PharmD
Frank Mycroft, PhD, MPH
Kent R. Olson, MD
John D. Osterloh, MD, MS
Karl A. Sporer, MD
S. Alan Tani, PharmD
Olga F. Woo, PharmD
Evan Wythe, MD

Contributors to the 1st Edition (1990)

We also recognize and appreciate the contributions of the following editors and authors to the first edition of this book. Because the book was conceived as and remains a product of the Poison Control Center, some contributors to the first edition may have been replaced as their affiliation with the center changed.

Ilene Brewer Anderson, PharmD
Margaret Atterbury, MD
Georgeanne M. Backman
Charles E. Becker, MD
Neal L. Benowitz, MD
Bruce Bernard, MD
Paul D. Blanc, MD
Christopher R. Brown, MD
James F. Buchanan, PharmD
Chris Dutra, MD
Donna E. Foliart, MD, MPH
Gail M. Gullickson, MD
Patricia Hess Hiatt, BS
Jeffrey R. Jones, MPH, CIH
Kathryn H. Keller, PharmD

Michael T. Kelley, MD
Susan Kim, PharmD
Belle L. Lee, PharmD
Timothy McCarthy, PharmD
Howard E. McKinney, PharmD
Frank J. Mycroft, PhD, MPH
Kent R. Olson, MD
John D. Osterloh, MD, MS
Gary Pasternak, MD
Mary Tweig, MD
Peter H. Wald, MD, MPH
Olga F. Woo, PharmD
Evan T. Wythe, MD
Peter Yip, MD

SECTION I. Comprehensive Evaluation and Treatment of Poisoning and Drug Overdose

Kent R. Olson, MD

EMERGENCY EVALUATION AND TREATMENT

Even though they may not appear acutely ill, all poisoned patients should be treated as if they have a potentially life-threatening intoxication. Below is a checklist (Fig I–1) of emergency evaluation and treatment procedures. More detailed information on diagnosis and treatment for each emergency step is referenced by page and presented immediately following the checklist.

Quickly review the checklist to determine the scope of appropriate interventions and **begin needed life-saving treatment.** If further information is required for any step, turn to the cited pages for detailed discussion of each topic. Although the checklist is presented in a **sequential format,** many steps may be performed **simultaneously** (eg, airway management, naloxone and dextrose administration, gastric lavage).

AIRWAY

I. **Assessment.** The greatest contributor to death from drug overdose or poisoning is loss of airway protective reflexes with subsequent airway obstruction by the flaccid tongue, pulmonary aspiration of gastric contents, or respiratory arrest. All patients should be suspected of having a potentially compromised airway.

   A. **Patients who are awake** and talking are likely to have intact airway reflexes, but should be monitored closely because worsening intoxication can result in rapid loss of airway control.

   B. **In lethargic or obtunded patients,** the gag or cough reflex may give an indirect estimation of the patient's ability to protect the airway. If there is any doubt, it is best to perform endotracheal intubation (see below).

II. **Treatment.** Optimize airway position and perform endotracheal intubation, if necessary. Early use of naloxone, (see pp 19 and 355) or flumazenil (see pp 19 and 340) may awaken a patient intoxicated with opiates or benzodiazepines, respectively, and obviate the need for endotracheal intubation.

   A. **Position the patient and clear the airway** (see Fig I–2).

      1. **Optimize airway position** to force the flaccid tongue forward and to maxi-

mize the airway opening. The following techniques are useful. ***Caution:*** Do ***not*** perform neck manipulation if there is a suspicion of neck injury.

    a. Place the neck and head in the **"sniffing" position,** with the neck flexed forward and the head extended (Fig I–2b).

    b. Apply the **"jaw thrust"** to create forward movement of the tongue without flexing or extending the neck. Pull the jaw forward by placing the fingers of each hand on the angle of the mandible just below the ears (Fig I–2c). (This motion also provides a painful stimulus to the angle of the jaw, the response to which gives an estimate of the patient's depth of coma.)

    c. Place the patient in a **head-down, left-sided position** that allows the tongue to fall forward and secretions or vomitus to drain out of the mouth (Fig I–2d).

  2. If the airway is still not patent, examine the oropharynx and **remove any obstruction or secretions** by suction, by a sweep with the finger, or with Magill forceps.

  3. The airway can also be maintained with **artificial oropharyngeal or nasopharyngeal airway devices.** These are placed in the mouth or nose to lift the tongue and push it forward. They are only temporary measures. A patient who can tolerate an artificial airway without complaint probably needs an endotracheal tube.

B. Perform endotracheal intubation if personnel trained in the procedure are available. Intubation of the trachea provides the most reliable protection of the airway, preventing aspiration and obstruction and allowing for mechanically assisted ventilation. However, it is not a simple procedure and *should be attempted only by those with training and experience.* Complications include local trauma to the oropharynx, nasopharynx, and larynx; inadvertent intubation of the esophagus or a main stem bronchus; and failure to intubate the patient after respiratory arrest has been induced by a neuromuscular blocker. There are 2 routes for endotracheal intubation: nasotracheal and orotracheal.

  1. Nasotracheal intubation. In nasotracheal intubation, a soft flexible tube is passed through the nose and into the trachea using a "blind" technique (Fig I–3a).

    a. Technique

      (1) Instill local anesthetic and vasoconstrictor into the nose before the procedure to limit pain and bleeding. Use phenylephrine spray and 2% lidocaine jelly or 3–4 mL of a 5% cocaine solution.

      (2) Pass the nasotracheal tube gently through the nose and into the nasopharynx. As the patient inspires, gently but firmly push the tube into the trachea. Success is usually marked by abrupt coughing.

      (3) Check breath sounds to rule out accidental esophageal intubation or intubation of the right main stem bronchus.

      (4) Secure the tube and fill the cuff balloon. (Tubes used for children do not have inflatable cuffs.)

      (5) Obtain a chest x-ray to confirm appropriate tube placement.

    b. Advantages

      (1) May be performed in a conscious patient without requiring neuromuscular paralysis.

      (2) Once placed, it is better tolerated than orotracheal tube.

    c. Disadvantages

      (1) Perforation of the nasal mucosa, with epistaxis.

      (2) Stimulation of vomiting in an obtunded patient.

      (3) Patient must be breathing spontaneously.

      (4) Anatomically more difficult in infants because of anterior epiglottis.

  2. Orotracheal intubation. In orotracheal intubation, the tube is passed through the mouth into the trachea under direct vision (Fig I–3b).

    a. Technique

      (1) If the patient is not fully relaxed (eg, flaccid jaw and unrestricted neck

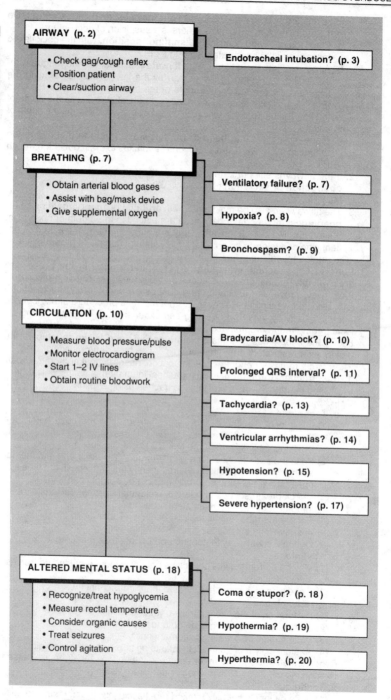

AIRWAY (p. 2)

- Check gag/cough reflex
- Position patient
- Clear/suction airway

Endotracheal intubation? (p. 3)

BREATHING (p. 7)

- Obtain arterial blood gases
- Assist with bag/mask device
- Give supplemental oxygen

Ventilatory failure? (p. 7)

Hypoxia? (p. 8)

Bronchospasm? (p. 9)

CIRCULATION (p. 10)

- Measure blood pressure/pulse
- Monitor electrocardiogram
- Start 1–2 IV lines
- Obtain routine bloodwork

Bradycardia/AV block? (p. 10)

Prolonged QRS interval? (p. 11)

Tachycardia? (p. 13)

Ventricular arrhythmias? (p. 14)

Hypotension? (p. 15)

Severe hypertension? (p. 17)

ALTERED MENTAL STATUS (p. 18)

- Recognize/treat hypoglycemia
- Measure rectal temperature
- Consider organic causes
- Treat seizures
- Control agitation

Coma or stupor? (p. 18)

Hypothermia? (p. 19)

Hyperthermia? (p. 20)

FIGURE I–1. Checklist of emergency evaluation and treatment procedures.

FIGURE I–2. Airway positioning. **A:** Normal position. **B:** "Sniffing" position. **C:** "Jaw thrust" maneuver. **D:** Left-side, head-down position, showing nasal and oral airway.

mobility), induce neuromuscular paralysis with succinylcholine, 1–1.5 mg/kg IV, pancuronium, 0.1 mg/kg IV, or other neuromuscular blocking agent (see p 357). *Caution:* In children, succinylcholine may induce excessive vagal tone, resulting in bradycardia or asystole. Pretreat with atropine, 0.01 mg/kg IV, or use pancuronium for paralysis.

(2) Ventilate the patient manually with 100% oxygen while awaiting full paralysis (1 minute for succinylcholine, 2–3 minutes for pancuronium).

(3) Using a lighted laryngoscope, visualize the larynx and pass the endotracheal tube into the trachea under direct vision.

(4) Check breath sounds to rule out accidental esophageal intubation or intubation of the right main stem bronchus.

FIGURE I–3. Two routes for endotracheal intubation. **A:** Nasotracheal intubation. **B:** Orotracheal intubation.

(5) Secure the tube and inflate the cuff balloon. (Tubes used for children do not have inflatable cuffs.)
(6) Obtain a chest x-ray to confirm appropriate tube position.
b. Advantages
(1) Performed under direct vision, making accidental esophageal intubation unlikely.
(2) Insignificant risk of bleeding.
(3) Patient need not be breathing spontaneously.
(4) Higher success rate than that with nasotracheal route.
c. Disadvantages
(1) Frequently requires neuromuscular paralysis, creating risk of fatal respiratory arrest if intubation is unsuccessful.
(2) Requires neck manipulation, which may cause spinal cord injury after neck trauma.

BREATHING

Along with airway problems, breathing difficulties are the major cause of morbidity and death in patients with poisoning or drug overdose. Patients may have one or more of the following complications: ventilatory failure, hypoxia, or bronchospasm.

I. Ventilatory failure
A. Assessment. Ventilatory failure has multiple causes, including failure of the ventilatory muscles, central depression of respiratory drive, and severe pneumonia or pulmonary edema. Examples of drugs and toxins that cause ventilatory failure and the causative mechanisms are listed in Table I–1.
B. Complications. Ventilatory failure is the most common cause of death in poisoned patients.

TABLE I–1. SELECTED DRUGS AND TOXINS CAUSING VENTILATORY FAILURE[a]

Paralysis of ventilatory muscles	Depression of central respiratory drive
Botulin toxin	Barbiturates
Neuromuscular blockers	Clonidine and other sympatholytic agents
Organophosphates and carbamates	Cyclic antidepressants
Snakebite	Ethanol and alcohols
Strychnine	Opiates
Tetanus	Sedative-hypnotics

[a]Adapted, with permission, from Olson KR, Pentel PR, Kelly MT: Physical assessment and differential diagnosis of the poisoned patient. *Med Toxicol* 1987;**2**:52.

   1. Hypoxia may result in brain damage, cardiac arrhythmias, and cardiac arrest.
   2. Hypercarbia results in acidosis, which may contribute to arrhythmias, especially in patients with cyclic antidepressant overdose.
C. **Differential diagnosis.** Rule out:
   1. Bacterial or viral pneumonia.
   2. Viral encephalitis or myelitis (eg, polio).
   3. Traumatic or ischemic spinal cord or central nervous system injury.
   4. Tetanus, causing chest wall muscle rigidity.
D. **Treatment.** Obtain arterial blood gases. The adequacy of ventilation is quickly estimated from the P_{CO2}; obtundation with an elevated or rising P_{CO2} (eg, > 60 mm Hg) indicates a need for assisted ventilation. Do **not** wait until the patient is apneic or until the P_{CO2} is above 60 mm to begin assisted ventilation.
   1. **Assist breathing manually** with a bag-valve-mask device or bag-valve-endotracheal tube device until the mechanical ventilator is ready for use.
   2. If not already accomplished, **perform endotracheal intubation.**
   3. **Program the ventilator** for tidal volume (usually 15 mL/kg), rate (usually 12–15 breaths/min), and oxygen concentration (usually 30–35% to start). Monitor the patient's response to ventilator settings frequently by obtaining arterial blood gas values.
      a. If the patient has some spontaneous ventilations, the machine can be set to allow the patient to breathe spontaneously with only intermittent mandatory ventilation (usually 10–12 breaths/min).
      b. If the endotracheal tube was placed only for airway protection, the patient can be left to breathe entirely spontaneously with blow-by oxygen mist (T-piece).

II. **Hypoxia**
   A. **Assessment.** Examples of drugs or toxins causing hypoxia are listed in Table I–2. Hypoxia can be caused by the following conditions:
      1. **Insufficient oxygen** in ambient air (eg, displacement of oxygen by inert gases).
      2. **Disruption of oxygen absorption** by the lung (eg, resulting from pneumonia or pulmonary edema).
         a. **Pneumonia.** The most common cause of pneumonia in overdosed patients is pulmonary aspiration of gastric contents. Pneumonia may also be caused by intravenous injection of foreign material or bacteria, aspiration of petroleum distillates, or inhalation of irritant gases.
         b. **Pulmonary edema.** All the agents that can cause chemical pneumonia

TABLE I–2. SELECTED CAUSES OF HYPOXIA

Inert gases	**Pneumonia or noncardiogenic pulmonary edema**
Carbon dioxide	Aspiration of gastric contents
Methane and propane	Aspiration of hydrocarbons
Nitrogen	Chlorine and other irritant gases
Cardiogenic pulmonary edema	Cocaine
Beta blockers	Ethchlorvynol (IV and oral)
Cyclic antidepressants	Ethylene glycol
Quinidine, procainamide,	Mercury vapor
and disopyramide	Metal fumes ("metal fumes fever")
Verapamil	Nitrogen dioxide
Cellular hypoxia	Opiates
Carbon monoxide	Paraquat
Cyanide	Phosgene
Hydrogen sulfide	Salicylates
Methemoglobinemia	Sedative-hypnotic drugs
Sulfhemoglobinemia	Smoke inhalation

(eg, irritant gases, hydrocarbons) may also cause pulmonary edema. This usually involves alteration of pulmonary capillary permeability, resulting in **noncardiogenic** pulmonary edema (adult respiratory distress syndrome, ARDS). In noncardiogenic pulmonary edema, the pulmonary capillary wedge pressure (reflecting left ventricular filling pressure) is usually normal or low. In contrast, **cardiogenic** pulmonary edema caused by cardiac-depressant drugs is characterized by low cardiac output with elevated pulmonary wedge pressure.

3. **Cellular hypoxia,** which may be present despite a normal arterial blood gas value.

   a. Carbon monoxide poisoning (see p 121) and methemoglobinemia (p 217) may severely limit oxygen binding to hemoglobin (and, therefore, oxygen-carrying capacity) without altering the P_{O_2}, because the routine blood gas determination measures dissolved oxygen in the plasma but does not measure actual oxygen content. In such cases, direct measurement of the oxygen saturation will reveal decreased oxyhemoglobin saturation. *Note:* Pulse oximetry gives falsely normal or near-normal results and is not reliable.

   b. Cyanide poisoning (p 145) and hydrogen sulfide poisoning (p 182) interfere with cellular oxygen utilization, resulting in decreased oxygen uptake by the tissues, and may cause the venous oxygen saturation to be abnormally high.

B. **Complications.** Significant or sustained hypoxia may result in brain damage and cardiac arrhythmias.

C. **Differential diagnosis.** Rule out:

   1. Erroneous sampling (eg, inadvertent venous blood gas).
   2. Bacterial or viral pneumonia.
   3. Pulmonary contusion caused by trauma.
   4. Acute myocardial infarction with pump failure.

D. **Treatment**

   1. **Correct hypoxia.** Administer supplemental oxygen as indicated based on arterial P_{O_2}. Intubation and assisted ventilation may be required.

      a. If carbon monoxide poisoning is suspected, give 100% oxygen (see p 364).

      b. See also treatment guides for cyanide (p 145), hydrogen sulfide (p 182), and methemoglobinemia (p 121).

   2. **Treat pneumonia.** Obtain frequent sputum samples and initiate appropriate antibiotic therapy when there is evidence of infection.

      a. There is no basis for prophylactic antibiotic treatment of aspiration- or chemical-induced pneumonia.

      b. Although some physicians recommend corticosteroids for chemical-induced pneumonia, there is little evidence of their benefit.

   3. **Treat pulmonary edema**

      a. Avoid excessive fluid administration. Pulmonary artery cannulation and wedge pressure measurements may be necessary to guide fluid therapy.

      b. Administer supplemental oxygen to maintain a P_{O_2} of at least 60–70 mm Hg. Endotracheal intubation and use of positive end-expiratory pressure (PEEP) ventilation may be necessary to maintain adequate oxygenation.

III. **Bronchospasm**

A. **Assessment.** Examples of drugs and toxins that cause bronchospasm are listed in Table I–3. Bronchospasm may result from the following:

   1. **Direct irritant injury** from inhaled gases or pulmonary aspiration of petroleum distillates or stomach contents.
   2. **Pharmacologic effects** of toxins, eg, organophosphate or carbamate insecticides or beta-adrenergic blockers.
   3. **Hypersensitivity** or allergic reactions may also cause bronchospasm.

TABLE I–3. SELECTED DRUGS AND TOXINS CAUSING BRONCHOSPASM

Beta blockers	Metal fumes ("metal fumes fever")
Chlorine and other irritant gases	Organophosphates and other anticholinesterases
Hydrocarbon aspiration	Smoke inhalation

   B. Complications. Severe bronchospasm may result in hypoxia and ventilatory failure.

   C. Differential diagnosis. Rule out:

   1. Asthma or other preexisting bronchospastic disorder.
   2. Stridor caused by upper airway injury and edema (progressive airway edema may result in acute airway obstruction).

   D. Treatment

   1. Administer supplemental oxygen.
   2. Remove the patient from the source of exposure to any irritant gas or other offending agent.
   3. Immediately discontinue any beta-blocker treatment.
   4. Administer bronchodilators:
      a. Aerosolized β_2 stimulant (eg, albuterol 2.5 mg in nebulizer).
      b. If this is not effective, and particularly for beta blocker–induced wheezing, give aminophylline, 6 mg/kg IV over 30 minutes.
   5. For patients with bronchospasm and bronchorrhea caused by organophosphate or other anticholinesterase poisoning, give atropine (see p 315).

CIRCULATION

   I. General assessment and initial treatment

   A. Check blood pressure and pulse rate and rhythm. Perform cardiopulmonary resuscitation (CPR) if there is no pulse and advanced cardiac life support (ACLS) for arrhythmias and shock.

   B. Begin continuous electrocardiographic (ECG) monitoring. Arrhythmias may complicate a variety of drug overdoses, and all patients with potentially cardiotoxic drug poisoning should be monitored in the emergency department or an intensive care unit for at least 6 hours after the ingestion.

   C. Secure venous access. Antecubital or forearm veins are usually easy to cannulate. Alternative sites include femoral, subclavian, internal jugular, or other central veins. Central vein access is technically more difficult but allows measurement of central venous pressure and placement of pacemaker or pulmonary artery lines.

   D. Draw blood for routine studies (see p 29).

   E. Begin intravenous infusion of dextrose 5% in water (D5W) at a keep-open rate; for children, use dextrose 5% in 0.25 normal saline. If the patient is hypotensive (see p 15), use normal saline, or other isotonic crystalloid solution.

   F. In seriously ill patients (eg, hypotensive, obtunded, convulsing, or comatose), **place a Foley catheter** in the bladder, obtain urine for routine and toxicologic testing, and measure hourly urine output.

   II. Bradycardia and atrioventricular (AV) block

   A. Assessment. Examples of drugs and toxins causing bradycardia or AV block and their mechanisms are listed in Table I–4.

   1. Bradycardia and AV block are common features of intoxication with calcium antagonists (see p 113) and drugs that depress sympathetic tone or increase parasympathetic tone. They may also result from severe intoxication with membrane-depressant drugs (eg, cyclic antidepressants, quinidine, other type Ia and type Ic antiarrhythmic agents).
   2. Bradycardia or AV block may also be a reflex response (baroreceptor re-

TABLE I–4. SELECTED DRUGS AND TOXINS CAUSING BRADYCARDIA OR ATRIOVENTRICULAR BLOCK[a]

Cholinergic or vagotonic agents	**Sympatholytic agents**
Carbamate insecticides	Beta blockers
Digitalis glycosides	Clonidine
Organophosphates	Opiates
Physostigmine	**Other**
Membrane-depressant drugs	Calcium antagonists
Beta blockers	Lithium
Cyclic antidepressants	Phenylpropanolamine and other alpha-adrenergic
Encainide and flecainide	agonists
Quinidine, procainamide, and disopyramide	Propoxyphene

[a]Adapted, with permission, from Olson KR et al. *Med Toxicol* 1987;2:71.

flex) to hypertension induced by alpha-adrenergic agents such as phenyl-propanolamine.

    3. In children, bradycardia is commonly caused by respiratory compromise and usually responds to ventilation and oxygenation.

B. Complications. Bradycardia and AV block frequently cause hypotension, which may progress to asystolic cardiac arrest.

C. Differential diagnosis. Rule out:
    1. Hypothermia.
    2. Myocardial ischemia or infarction.
    3. Electrolyte abnormality (eg, hyperkalemia).
    4. Metabolic disturbance (eg, hypothyroidism).
    5. Intrinsic slow rate (common in athletes).
    6. Cushing reflex (caused by severe intracranial hypertension).

D. Treatment. Do *not* treat bradycardia or AV block unless the patient is symptomatic (eg, syncope, hypotension). *Note:* Bradycardia or even AV block may be a protective reflex to lower the blood pressure in a patient with life-threatening hypertension (see **VII**, below).
    1. Maintain the airway and assist ventilation (see p 4) if necessary. Administer supplemental oxygen.
    2. Rewarm hypothermic patients. A sinus bradycardia of 40–50/min is normal when the body temperature is 32–35 °C (90–95 °F).
    3. Administer atropine, 0.01–0.03 mg/kg IV (p 315). If this is not successful, use isoproterenol 1–10 mcg/min IV (p 346), titrated to desired rate, or an emergency transcutaneous or transvenous pacemaker.
    4. Use the following specific antidotes if appropriate:
        a. For beta-blocker overdose, give glucagon (p 342).
        b. For digitalis intoxication, use Fab fragments (p 329).
        c. For cyclic antidepressant or membrane-depressant drug overdose, administer sodium bicarbonate (p 318).
        d. For calcium antagonist overdose, give calcium (p 323).

III. QRS interval prolongation

    A. Assessment. Examples of drugs and toxins causing QRS interval prolongation are listed in Table I–5.
        1. QRS interval prolongation greater than 0.12 seconds in the limb leads (Fig I–4) is highly suggestive of serious poisoning by cyclic antidepressants (see p 147) or other membrane-depressant drugs (eg, propranolol). QRS interval prolongation in this setting reflects inhibition of sodium-dependent depolarization of cardiac tissue and is usually accompanied by QT interval prolongation, AV block, and depressed cardiac contractility. A significant exception is amoxapine (Asendin), which causes serious central nervous system toxicity with normal QRS intervals.
        2. QRS interval prolongation may also result from ventricular escape rhythm in

TABLE I–5. SELECTED DRUGS AND TOXINS CAUSING QRS INTERVAL PROLONGATION[a]

Beta blockers (propranolol)	Hyperkalemia
Cyclic antidepressants	Phenothiazines (thioridazine)
Digitalis glycosides (complete heart block)	Propoxyphene
Diphenhydramine	Quinidine, procainamide, and disopyramide
Encainide and flecainide	

[a]Adapted, with permission, from Olson KR et al. *Med Toxicol* 1987;2:71.

    a patient with complete heart block (eg, from digitalis or calcium antagonist poisoning).

B. Complications. QRS interval widening in cyclic antidepressant or membrane-depressant drug overdose is often accompanied by hypotension, AV block, and seizures.

C. Differential diagnosis. Rule out:

1. Intrinsic conduction system disease (bundle branch block or complete heart block) caused by coronary artery disease. Check an old ECG if available.
2. Hyperkalemia with critical cardiac toxicity may appear as a "sine wave" pattern with markedly wide QRS complexes. These are usually preceded by peaked T waves (Fig I–7, p 36).
3. Hypothermia with a core temperature of less than 32 °C (90 °F) often causes an extra terminal QRS deflection (J wave or Osborne wave), resulting in a widened QRS appearance (Fig I–5).

D. Treatment

1. Maintain the airway and assist ventilation if necessary (see p 4). Administer supplemental oxygen.
2. Treat hyperkalemia (see p 35) and hypothermia (p 19) if they occur.
3. Treat AV block with atropine (p 315), isoproterenol (p 346), and a pacemaker if necessary.
4. For cyclic antidepressant or membrane-depressant drug overdose, give sodium bicarbonate, 1–2 meq/kg IV bolus (p 318); repeat as needed.

FIGURE I–4. Widened QRS interval caused by cyclic antidepressant overdose. **A:** Delayed intraventricular conduction results in prolonged QRS interval (0.18 s). **B** and **C:** Supraventricular tachycardia with progressive widening of QRS complexes mimics ventricular tachycardia. (Reproduced, with permission, from Benowitz NL, Goldschlager N: Cardiac disturbances in the toxicologic patient. (Page 71 in: *Clinical Management of Poisoning and Drug Overdose.* Haddad LM, Winchester JF [editors]. Saunders, 1983.)

FIGURE I–5. Electrocardiogram of patient with hypothermia, showing prominent J waves. (Modified and reproduced, with permission, from Goldschlager N, Goldman MJ: Miscellaneous abnormal electrocardiogram patterns. Page 227 in: *Electrocardiography: Essentials of Interpretation.* Goldschlager N, Goldman MJ [editors]. Lange, 1984.)

    5. Give other antidotes if appropriate:
       a. Digoxin-specific Fab antibodies for complete heart block induced by digitalis (p 329).
       b. Glucagon for beta-blocker intoxication (p 342).
       c. Calcium for calcium antagonist poisoning (p 323).

IV. Tachycardia
  A. Assessment. Examples of drugs and toxins causing tachycardia and their mechanisms are shown in Table I–6.
    1. Sinus tachycardia and supraventricular tachycardia are often caused by excessive sympathetic system stimulation or inhibition of parasympathetic tone. Sinus tachycardia may also be a reflex response to hypotension or hypoxia.
    2. Sinus tachycardia and supraventricular tachycardia accompanied by QRS interval prolongation (eg, with cyclic antidepressant overdose) may have the appearance of ventricular tachycardia (Fig I–4, p 12).
  B. Complications. Simple sinus tachycardia (heart rate < 140/min) is rarely of hemodynamic consequence; children and healthy adults easily tolerate rates up to 160–180/min. However, sustained rapid rates may result in hypotension, chest pain, or syncope.
  C. Differential diagnosis. Rule out:
    1. Occult blood loss (eg, gastrointestinal bleeding, trauma).
    2. Fluid loss (eg, gastritis, gastroenteritis).
    3. Fever and infection.
    4. Myocardial infarction.
    5. Anxiety.
    6. Intrinsic conduction system disease (eg, Wolff-Parkinson-White syndrome).

TABLE I–6. SELECTED DRUGS AND TOXINS CAUSING TACHYCARDIA[a]

Sympathomimetic agents	**Anticholinergic agents**
Amphetamines and derivatives	*Amanita muscaria* mushrooms
Caffeine	Antihistamines
Cocaine	Atropine and other anticholinergics
Ephedrine and pseudoephedrine	Cyclic antidepressants
Phencyclidine (PCP)	Phenothiazines
Theophylline	Plants (many)
Agents causing cellular hypoxia	**Other**
Carbon monoxide	Ethanol or sedative-hypnotic drug
Cyanide	withdrawal
Hydrogen sulfide	Hydralazine and other vasodilators
Oxidizing agents (methemoglobinemia)	Thyroid hormone

[a]Adapted, with permission, from Olson KR et al. *Med Toxicol* 1987;2:71.

D. Treatment. If tachycardia is not associated with hypotension or chest pain, observation and sedation (especially for stimulant intoxication) are usually adequate.

1. For sympathomimetic-induced tachycardia, give propranolol, 0.01–0.03 mg/kg IV (p 373); or esmolol, 25–100 mcg/kg/min IV (p 338).

2. For anticholinergic-induced tachycardia, give physostigmine, 0.01–0.03 mg/kg IV (p 370); or neostigmine, 0.01–0.03 mg/kg IV. **Caution:** Do **not** use these drugs in patients with cyclic antidepressant overdose, because additive depression of conduction may result in asystole.

V. Ventricular arrhythmias

A. Assessment. Examples of drugs and toxins causing ventricular arrhythmias are listed in Table I–7.

1. Ventricular irritability is commonly associated with excessive sympathetic stimulation (eg, cocaine, amphetamines). Patients intoxicated by chlorinated, fluorinated, or aromatic hydrocarbons may have heightened myocardial sensitivity to the arrhythmogenic effects of catecholamines.

2. Ventricular tachycardia may also be a manifestation of cyclic antidepressant or other membrane-depressant drug intoxication, although with these drugs true ventricular tachycardia may be difficult to distinguish from sinus or supraventricular tachycardia accompanied by QRS interval prolongation (Fig I–4, p 12).

3. Agents that cause QT interval prolongation (QTc > 0.42 sec) may produce "atypical" ventricular tachycardia (torsades de pointes). Torsades is characterized by polymorphous ventricular tachycardia that appears to rotate its axis continuously (Fig I–6 p 15). Torsades may also be caused by hypocalcemia or hypomagnesemia.

B. Complications. Ventricular tachycardia with a pulse may be associated with hypotension or may deteriorate into pulseless ventricular tachycardia or ventricular fibrillation.

C. Differential diagnosis. Rule out the following possible causes of ventricular premature beats, ventricular tachycardia, or ventricular fibrillation.

1. Hypoxemia.
2. Hypokalemia.
3. Metabolic acidosis.
4. Myocardial ischemia or infarction.
5. Electrolyte disturbances (eg, hypocalcemia, hypomagnesemia) or congenital disorders that may cause QT prolongation and torsades.

D. Treatment. Perform CPR if necessary, and follow advanced cardiac life support (ACLS) guidelines for management of arrhythmias, with the exception that procainamide and bretylium should **not** be used, especially if cyclic antidepressant or membrane-depressant drug overdose is suspected.

TABLE I–7. SELECTED DRUGS AND TOXINS CAUSING VENTRICULAR ARRHYTHMIAS[a]

Ventricular tachycardia or fibrillation	QT prolongation or torsades de pointes[b]
Amphetamines and other sympathomimetic agents	Amiodarone
Aromatic hydrocarbon solvents	Arsenic
Caffeine	Chloroquine and related agents
Chloral hydrate	Citrate
Chlorinated or fluorinated hydrocarbon solvents	Cyclic antidepressants
Cocaine	Fluoride
Cyclic antidepressants	Organophosphate insecticides
Digitalis glycosides	Quinidine, procainamide, and disopyramide
Fluoride	Quinine
Phenothiazines	Thallium
Theophylline	Thioridazine

[a]Adapted, with permission, from Olson KR et al. *Med Toxicol* 1987;2:71.
[b]These agents can also cause ventricular tachycardia or fibrillation.

FIGURE I–6. Polymorphic ventricular tachycardia (torsades des pointes). (Modified and reproduced, with permission, from Goldschlager N, Goldman MJ: Effect of drugs and electrolytes on the electrocardiogram. Page 197 in: *Electrocardiography: Essentials of Interpretation*. Goldschlager N, Goldman MJ [editors]. Lange, 1984.)

1. Maintain the airway and assist ventilation if necessary (see p 4). Administer supplemental oxygen.
2. Correct acid-base and electrolyte disturbances.
3. **For ventricular fibrillation,** immediately apply direct current countershock at 3–5 J/kg. Repeat once if needed. Continue CPR if patient remains pulseless, and administer epinephrine, repeated countershocks, and lidocaine as recommended in ACLS guidelines.
4. **For ventricular tachycardia without a pulse,** immediately give a precordial thump or apply synchronized direct current countershock at 1–3 J/kg. If not successful, begin CPR and apply countershock at 3–5 J/kg; administer lidocaine and repeated countershocks as recommended in ACLS guidelines.
5. **For ventricular tachycardia with a pulse,** use lidocaine, 1–3 mg/kg IV (p 349); or phenytoin, 5–15 mg/kg IV (p 370). Do *not* use procainamide (Pronestyl) or other type Ia antiarrhythmic agents. For suspected myocardial sensitivity caused by chloral hydrate, or halogenated or aromatic hydrocarbons, use esmolol 25–100 µg/kg/min (see p 338).
6. **For cyclic antidepressant or other membrane-depressant drug overdose,** administer sodium bicarbonate, 1–2 meq/kg IV (p 318), in repeated boluses until QRS interval narrows or serum pH exceeds 7.5.
7. **For "atypical" or polymorphic ventricular tachycardia (torsades):**
   a. Use overdrive pacing or isoproterenol, 1–10 mcg/min IV (p 346), to increase the heart rate (this makes repolarization more homogeneous and abolishes the arrhythmia).
   b. Alternately, administer magnesium sulfate, 1–2 g in adults, followed by infusion at 3–20 mg/min.

VI. Hypotension
A. Assessment. Examples of drugs and toxins causing hypotension and their mechanisms are listed in Table I–8.
1. Physiologic derangements resulting in hypotension include: volume loss because of vomiting, diarrhea, or blood loss; apparent volume depletion caused by venodilation; arteriolar dilation; depression of cardiac contractility; arrhythmias that interfere with cardiac output; and hypothermia.
2. Volume loss, venodilation, and arteriolar dilation are likely to result in hypotension with reflex tachycardia. In contrast, hypotension accompanied by bradycardia should suggest intoxication by sympatholytic agents, membrane-depressant drugs, calcium channel blockers, or cardiac glycosides or the presence of hypothermia.

B. Complications. Severe or prolonged hypotension can cause acute renal tubular necrosis, brain damage, and cardiac ischemia. Metabolic acidosis is a common finding.

TABLE I–8. SELECTED DRUGS AND TOXINS CAUSING HYPOTENSION[a]

HYPOTENSION WITH RELATIVE BRADYCARDIA

Sympatholytic agents
Beta blockers
Bretylium
Clonidine, prazosin, and methyldopa
Hypothermia
Opiates
Reserpine
Tetrahydrozoline

Membrane-depressant drugs
Beta blockers (mainly propranolol)
Cyclic antidepressants
Encainide and flecainide
Quinidine, procainamide, and disopyramide
Propoxyphene

Others
Barbiturates
Calcium antagonists
Cyanide
Fluoride
Organophosphates and carbamates
Sedative-hypnotic agents

HYPOTENSION WITH TACHYCARDIA

Fluid loss or third spacing
Amatoxin-containing mushrooms
Arsenic
Colchicine
Copper sulfate
Hyperthermia
Iron
Rattlesnake envenomation
Sedative-hypnotic agents

Peripheral venous or arteriolar dilation
β_2-stimulants (eg, metaproterenol, terbutaline)
Caffeine
Cyclic antidepressants
Hydralazine
Hyperthermia
Nitrites
Sodium nitroprusside
Phenothiazines
Theophylline

[a]Adapted, with permission, from Olson KR et al. *Med Toxicol* 1987;2:57.

C. Differential diagnosis. Rule out:
  1. Hypothermia, which results in decreased metabolic rate and lowered blood pressure demands.
  2. Hyperthermia, which causes arteriolar and venodilation and direct myocardial depression.
  3. Fluid loss caused by gastroenteritis.
  4. Blood loss (eg, from trauma or gastrointestinal bleeding).
  5. Myocardial infarction.
  6. Sepsis.
  7. Spinal cord injury.
D. Treatment. Fortunately, hypotension usually responds readily to empirical therapy with intravenous fluids and low doses of pressor drugs (eg, dopamine). When hypotension does not resolve after simple measures, a systematic approach should be followed to determine the cause of hypotension and to select the appropriate treatment.
  1. Maintain the airway and assist ventilation if necessary (see p 4). Administer supplemental oxygen.
  2. Treat cardiac arrhythmias that may contribute to hypotension (heart rate < 40–50/min or > 180–200/min [p 4]).
  3. Hypotension associated with hypothermia often will not improve with routine fluid therapy but will rapidly normalize upon rewarming of the patient. A systolic blood pressure of 80–90 mm Hg is expected when the body temperature is 32 °C (90 °F).
  4. Give a fluid challenge using normal saline, 10–20 mL/kg, or other crystalloid solution.
  5. Administer dopamine, 5–15 mcg/kg/min (p 334).
  6. Consider specific antidotes:
      a. Sodium bicarbonate (p 318) for cyclic antidepressant or membrane-depressant drug overdose.
      b. Glucagon (p 342) for beta-blocker overdose.
      c. Calcium (p 323) for calcium antagonist overdose.

      d. Propranolol (p 373) or esmolol (p 338) for theophylline, caffeine, or metaproterenol or other beta agonist overdose.

    7. If the above measures are unsuccessful, insert a central venous pressure (CVP) monitor or pulmonary artery (PA) catheter to determine whether further fluids are needed and to measure the cardiac output (CO) and calculate the systemic vascular resistance (SVR = 80[MAP−CVP]/CO; normal SVR = 770–1500; MAP = mean arterial pressure). Select further therapy based on the results:

      a. If the central venous pressure or pulmonary artery wedge pressure remains low, give more intravenous fluids.

      b. If the cardiac output is low, give more dopamine (p 334) or dobutamine.

      c. If the systemic vascular resistance is low, administer norepinephrine 4–8 μg/min (p 363).

VII. Hypertension

  A. Assessment. Hypertension is frequently overlooked in drug-intoxicated patients and often goes untreated. Many young persons have normal blood pressures in the range of 90/60 mm Hg to 100/70 mm Hg; in such a person an abrupt elevation to 170/100 is much more significant (and potentially catastrophic) than the same blood pressure elevation in an older person with chronic hypertension. Examples of drugs and toxins causing hypertension are listed in Table I–9. Hypertension may be caused by a variety of mechanisms:

    1. Amphetamines and other related drugs cause hypertension and tachycardia through generalized sympathetic stimulation.

    2. Selective alpha-adrenergic agents cause hypertension with reflex (baroreceptor-mediated) bradycardia or even AV block.

    3. Anticholinergic agents cause mild hypertension with tachycardia.

    4. Substances that stimulate nicotinic cholinergic receptors (eg, organophosphates) may initially cause tachycardia and hypertension, followed later by bradycardia and hypotension.

  B. Complications. Severe hypertension can result in intracranial hemorrhage, aortic dissection, myocardial infarction, and congestive heart failure.

  C. Differential diagnosis. Rule out:

    1. Idiopathic hypertension, which is common in the general population. However, without a prior history of hypertension it should not be initially assumed to be the cause of the elevated blood pressure.

    2. Increased intracranial pressure caused by spontaneous hemorrhage, trauma, or other causes. This may result in hypertension with reflex bradycardia (Cushing reflex).

TABLE I–9. SELECTED DRUGS AND TOXINS CAUSING HYPERTENSION[a]

HYPERTENSION WITH TACHYCARDIA

Generalized sympathomimetic agents	Anticholinergic agents
Amphetamines and derivatives	Antihistamines
Cocaine	Atropine and other anticholinergics
Ephedrine	Cyclic antidepressants
Epinephrine	Phenothiazines
Levodopa	**Other**
LSD (lysergic acid diethylamide)	Ethanol and sedative-hypnotic drug withdrawal
Marihuana	Nicotine (early stage)
Monoamine oxidase inhibitors	Organophosphates (early stage)
Phencyclidine	

HYPERTENSION WITH BRADYCARDIA OR ATRIOVENTRICULAR BLOCK

Clonidine	Norepinephrine
Ergot derivatives	Phenylephrine
Methoxamine	Phenylpropanolamine

[a]Adapted, with permission, from Olson KR et al. *Med Toxicol* 1987;2:56.

D. Treatment. Rapid lowering of the blood pressure is desirable as long as it does not result in hypotension, which can potentially cause an ischemic cerebral infarction in older patients with cerebrovascular disease. For a patient with chronic hypertension, lowering the diastolic pressure to 100 mm Hg is acceptable. On the other hand, for a young person whose normal diastolic blood pressure is 60 mm Hg, the diastolic pressure should be lowered to 80 mm Hg.

  1. **For hypertension with little or no tachycardia,** use phentolamine, 0.02–0.1 mg/kg IV (see p 369); nifedipine, 0.1–0.2 mg/kg chewable capsule or liquid form (p 360); or nitroprusside, 2–10 mcg/kg/min IV (p 362).

  2. **For hypertension with tachycardia,** add to the above treatment (see **1** above) propranolol, 0.02–0.1 mg/kg IV (p 373); or esmolol, 25–100 mcg/kg/min IV (p 338); or labetalol, 0.2–0.3 mg/kg IV (p 338). *Caution:* Do **not** use propranolol or esmolol alone to treat hypertensive crisis; beta blockers may paradoxically worsen hypertension if it is caused primarily by alpha stimulation.

  3. **If hypertension is accompanied by a focally abnormal neurologic examination** (eg, hemiparesis), perform a computed tomography (CT) scan as quickly as possible. In a patient with a cerebrovascular accident, hypertension should generally not be treated unless specific complications of the elevated pressure (eg, heart failure, cardiac ischemia) are present. Consult a neurologist.

ALTERED MENTAL STATUS

  I. Coma and stupor
  A. Assessment. Decreased level of consciousness is the most common serious complication of drug overdose or poisoning. Examples of drugs and toxins causing coma are listed in Table I–10.

  1. Coma is most often a result of global depression of the brain's reticular activating system, caused by anticholinergic agents, sympatholytic drugs, generalized CNS depressants, or toxins that result in cellular hypoxia.

  2. Coma sometimes represents a postictal phenomenon after a drug- or toxin-induced seizure.

  3. Coma may also be caused by brain injury associated with infarction or intracranial bleeding. Brain injury is suggested by the presence of focal neurologic deficits and is confirmed by CT scan.

  B. Complications. Coma is frequently accompanied by respiratory depression, which is a major cause of death. Other conditions that may accompany or complicate coma include hypotension (see p 15), hypothermia (p 19), hyperthermia (p 20, and rhabdomyolysis (p 25).

TABLE I–10. SELECTED DRUGS AND TOXINS CAUSING COMA OR STUPOR[a]

General CNS depressants	Cellular hypoxia
Anticholinergics	Carbon monoxide
Antihistamines	Cyanide
Barbiturates	Hydrogen sulfide
Cyclic antidepressants	Methemoglobinemia
Ethanol and other alcohols	**Other or unknown mechanisms**
Phenothiazines	Bromide
Sedative-hypnotic agents	Diquat
Sympatholytic agents	Disulfiram
Clonidine	Hypoglycemic agents
Methyldopa	Lithium
Opiates	Phencyclidine
Tetrahydrozoline	Phenylbutazone and enolic acid derivatives
	Salicylates

[a]Adapted, with permission, from Olson KR et al. *Med Toxicol* 1987;2:61.

C. Differential diagnosis. Rule out:
1. Head trauma or other causes of intracranial bleeding.
2. Abnormal levels of blood glucose, sodium, or other electrolytes.
3. Hypoxia.
4. Hypothyroidism.
5. Liver or renal failure.
6. Environmental hyperthermia or hypothermia.
7. Serious infections such as encephalitis or meningitis.

D. Treatment
1. Maintain the airway and assist ventilation if necessary (see p 4). Administer supplemental oxygen.
2. Give dextrose, thiamine, and naloxone.
   a. **Dextrose.** All patients with depressed consciousness should receive concentrated dextrose unless hypoglycemia is ruled out with an immediate bedside glucose determination. Use a secure vein and avoid extravasation; concentrated dextrose is highly irritating to tissues. Initial doses:
      (1) Adults: 50% dextrose, 50 mL (25 g) IV.
      (2) Children: 25% dextrose, 2 mL/kg IV.
   b. **Thiamine.** Thiamine is given to prevent abrupt precipitation of Wernicke's syndrome resulting from thiamine deficiency in alcoholic patients and others with suspected vitamin deficiencies. It is **not** given routinely to children. Give thiamine, 100 mg, in the IV bottle or intramuscularly (p 375).
   c. **Naloxone.** All patients with respiratory depression should receive naloxone (p 355); if the patient is already intubated and being artificially ventilated, then naloxone is not immediately necessary and can be considered diagnostic rather than therapeutic. **Caution:** Although naloxone has no depressant activity of its own and can normally be given safely in large doses, it may precipitate abrupt opiate withdrawal. If amphetamines or cocaine has been injected along with heroin, reversal of the opiate-induced sedation may unmask stimulant-mediated hypertension, tachycardia, or psychosis. In addition, acute pulmonary edema is sometimes temporally associated with abrupt naloxone reversal of opiate intoxication.
      (1) Give naloxone, 0.4 mg IV (may also be given IM).
      (2) If there is no response within 1–2 minutes, give naloxone, 2 mg IV.
      (3) If there is still no response and opiate overdose is highly suspected by history or clinical presentation (pinpoint pupils, apnea, hypotension), give naloxone, 10–20 mg IV.
   d. Consider **flumazenil** (Romazicon®) if benzodiazepines are suspected cause of coma and there are no contraindications (see p 340).
3. Normalize the body temperature (see hypothermia, p 19, or hyperthermia, p 20).
4. If there is any possibility of central nervous system trauma or cerebrovascular accident, perform a CT scan.
5. If meningitis or encephalitis is suspected, perform a lumbar puncture and treat with appropriate antibiotics.

II. Hypothermia

A. Assessment. Hypothermia may mimic or complicate drug overdose and should be suspected in every comatose patient. Examples of drugs and toxins causing hypothermia are listed in Table I–11.
1. Hypothermia is usually caused by exposure to low ambient temperatures in a patient with blunted thermoregulatory response mechanisms. Drugs and toxins may induce hypothermia by causing vasodilation, inhibiting the shivering response, decreasing metabolic activity, or causing the person to lose consciousness in a cold environment.
2. The patient with a temperature lower than 32 °C (90 °F) may appear to be dead, with barely detectable pulse or blood pressure and with absent re-

TABLE I–11. SELECTED DRUGS AND TOXINS ASSOCIATED WITH HYPOTHERMIA[a]

Barbiturates	Opiates
Cyclic antidepressants	Phenothiazines
Ethanol and other alcohols	Sedative-hypnotic agents
Hypoglycemic agents	

[a]Adapted, with permission, from Olson KR et al. *Med Toxicol* 1987;2:60.

flexes. The ECG may reveal an abnormal terminal deflection (J wave or Osborne wave, Fig I–5, p 13).

B. Complications. Because there is a generalized reduction of metabolic activity and less demand for blood flow, hypothermia is commonly accompanied by hypotension and bradycardia.

1. Mild hypotension (systolic blood pressure of 70–90 mm Hg) in a patient with hypothermia should **not** be aggressively treated; excessive intravenous fluids may cause fluid overload and further lowering of the temperature.
2. Severe hypothermia (temperature < 28–30 °C) may cause intractable ventricular fibrillation and cardiac arrest. This may occur abruptly, such as when the patient is moved or rewarmed too quickly or if CPR is performed.

C. Differential diagnosis. Rule out:

1. Sepsis.
2. Hypoglycemia.
3. Hypothyroidism.
4. Environmental hypothermia, caused by exposure to a cold environment.

D. Treatment

1. Maintain the airway and assist ventilation if necessary (see p 4). Administer supplemental oxygen.
2. Because the pulse rate may be profoundly slow (10/min) and weak, perform careful cardiac evaluation before assuming that the patient is in cardiac arrest. Do **not** treat bradycardia; it will resolve with rewarming.
3. Unless the patient is in cardiac arrest (asystole or ventricular fibrillation), rewarm slowly (using blankets, warm intravenous fluids, and warmed mist inhalation) to prevent rewarming arrhythmias.
4. For patients in cardiac arrest, usual antiarrhythmic agents and direct current countershock are frequently ineffective until the core temperature is above 32–35 °C (90–95 °F). Provide gastric or peritoneal lavage with warmed fluids and perform CPR. For ventricular fibrillation, bretylium, 5–10 mg/kg IV (see p 320), may be effective.
5. Open cardiac massage with direct warm irrigation of the ventricle, or partial cardiopulmonary bypass, may be necessary in hypothermic patients in cardiac arrest who are unresponsive to the above treatment.

III. Hyperthermia

A. Assessment. Hyperthermia (temperature > 40 °C or 104 °F) may be a catastrophic complication of intoxication by a variety of drugs and toxins (Table I–12). Hyperthermia may be caused by excessive heat generation because of sustained seizures, rigidity, or other muscular hyperactivity; increased metabolic rate; impaired dissipation of heat secondary to absent sweating (eg, anticholinergic agents); or hypothalamic disorders.

1. **Neuroleptic malignant syndrome (NMS)** is a hyperthermic disorder seen in patients chronically using antipsychotic agents and is characterized by hyperthermia, muscle rigidity (often "lead-pipe"), metabolic acidosis, and confusion.
2. **Malignant hyperthermia** is an inherited disorder that causes severe hyperthermia, metabolic acidosis, and rigidity after use of certain anesthetic agents (most commonly halothane and succinylcholine).

TABLE I–12. SELECTED DRUGS AND TOXINS ASSOCIATED WITH HYPERTHERMIA*

Excessive muscular hyperactivity, rigidity, or seizures	Impaired heat dissipation or disrupted thermoregulation
Amoxapine	Amoxapine
Amphetamines and derivatives	Anticholinergic agents
Cocaine	Antihistamines
Cyclic antidepressants	Cyclic antidepressants
Lithium	Phenothiazines and other antipsychotic agents
LSD (lysergic acid diethylamide)	**Other**
Maprotiline	Exertional heatstroke
Monoamine oxidase inhibitors	Malignant hyperthermia
Phencyclidine	Metal fumes fever
Increased metabolic rate	Neuroleptic malignant syndrome
Dinitrophenol and pentachlorophenol	Serotonin syndrome
Salicylates	Withdrawal from ethanol or sedative-hypnotic
Thyroid hormone	drugs

*Adapted, with permission, from Olson KR et al. *Med Toxicol* 1987;2:59.

3. **Serotonin syndrome** occurs primarily in patients taking MAO inhibitors (see p 222) who take serotonergic drugs, such as meperidine (Demerol) or fluoxetine (Prozac), and is characterized by irritability, rigidity, myoclonus, diaphoresis, and hyperthermia.

B. **Complications.** Untreated hyperthermia is likely to result in hypotension, rhabdomyolysis, coagulopathy, cardiac and renal failure, brain injury, and death. Survivors often have permanent neurologic sequelae.

C. **Differential diagnosis.** Rule out:
   1. Sedative-hypnotic drug or ethanol withdrawal (delirium tremens).
   2. Exertional or environmental heat stroke.
   3. Thyrotoxicosis.
   4. Meningitis or encephalitis.
   5. Other serious infections.

D. **Treatment.** *Immediate rapid cooling* is essential to prevent death or serious brain damage.
   1. Maintain the airway and assist ventilation if necessary (see p 4). Administer supplemental oxygen.
   2. Administer glucose-containing intravenous fluids, and give concentrated glucose bolus (p 343) if the patient is hypoglycemic.
   3. Rapidly gain control of seizures (p 22), agitation (p 23), or muscular rigidity (p 24).
   4. Begin external cooling with tepid (lukewarm) sponging and fanning. This evaporative method is the most efficient way of cooling. Other methods include iced gastric or colonic lavage or even ice-water immersion.
   5. Shivering often occurs with rapid external cooling, and shivering may generate yet more heat. Some physicians recommend chlorpromazine to abolish shivering, but this agent can lower the seizure threshold and may cause hypotension. It is preferable to use diazepam, 0.1–0.2 mg/kg IV (p 327); midazolam, 0.05–0.1 mg/kg IV (p 353); or neuromuscular paralysis (see below).
   6. The most rapidly effective and reliable means of lowering the temperature is by neuromuscular paralysis. Administer pancuronium, 0.1 mg/kg IV (p 357); or vecuronium, 0.1 mg/kg IV. *Caution:* The patient will stop breathing; be prepared to ventilate and intubate endotracheally.
   7. **Malignant hyperthermia:** If muscle rigidity persists despite administration of neuromuscular blockers, a defect at the muscle cell level (ie, malignant hyperthermia) should be suspected. Give dantrolene, 1–10 mg/kg IV (p 325).

    8. Neuroleptic malignant syndrome: consider bromocriptine (see p 321).

    9. Serotonin syndrome: Anecdotal case reports suggest benefit with methylsergide, 2 mg orally every 6 hours for 3–4 doses, or cyproheptadine (Periactin), 4 mg orally every hour for 3–4 doses.

IV. Seizures

A. Assessment. Seizures are a major cause of morbidity and mortality from drug overdose or poisoning. Seizures may be single and brief or multiple and sustained and may result from a variety of mechanisms (Table I–13).

    1. Generalized seizures usually result in loss of consciousness, often accompanied by tongue biting and fecal and urinary incontinence.

    2. Other causes of muscular hyperactivity or rigidity (see p 24) may be mistaken for seizures, especially if the patient is also unconscious.

B. Complications

    1. Any seizure can cause airway compromise, resulting in apnea or pulmonary aspiration.

    2. Multiple or prolonged seizures may cause severe metabolic acidosis, hyperthermia, rhabdomyolysis, and brain damage.

C. Differential diagnosis. Rule out:

    1. Serious metabolic disturbance (hypoglycemia, hyponatremia, hypocalcemia, hypoxia).

    2. Head trauma with intracranial injury.

    3. Idiopathic epilepsy.

    4. Alcohol or sedative-hypnotic drug withdrawal.

    5. Exertional or environmental hyperthermia.

    6. Central nervous system infection such as meningitis or encephalitis.

D. Treatment

    1. Maintain the airway and assist ventilation if necessary (see p 4). Administer supplemental oxygen.

    2. Administer naloxone (p 355) if seizures are thought to be caused by hypoxia resulting from narcotic-associated respiratory depression.

TABLE I–13. SELECTED DRUGS AND TOXINS CAUSING SEIZURES[a]

Adrenergic-sympathomimetic agents	Antidepressants and antipsychotics
Amphetamines and derivatives	Amoxapine
Caffeine	Cyclic antidepressants
Cocaine	Haloperidol and butyrophenones
Phencyclidine	Loxapine
Phenylpropanolamine	Phenothiazines
Theophylline	
Others	
Antihistamines (diphenhydramine, hydroxyzine)	Fluoride
Beta blockers (primarily propranolol; not reported	Isoniazid
for atenolol, metoprolol, pindolol, or practolol)	Lead and other heavy metals
Boric acid	Lidocaine and other local anesthetics
Camphor	Lithium
Carbamazepine	Mefenamic acid
Cellular hypoxia (eg, carbon monoxide, cyanide,	Meperidine
hydrogen sulfide)	Metaldehyde
Chlorinated hydrocarbon solvents and insecticides	Methanol
Cholinergic agents (carbamates, nicotine, organo-	Phenols
phosphates)	Phenylbutazone
Cicutoxin and other plant toxins	Piroxicam
Citrate	Salicylates
DEET (diethyltoluamide)	Strychnine (opisthotonus and rigidity)
Ethylene glycol	Withdrawal from ethanol or sedative-hypnotic
	drugs

[a]Adapted, with permission, from Olson KR et al. *Med Toxicol* 1987;2:63.

3. Check for hypoglycemia and administer dextrose and thiamine as for coma (p 18).
4. Use one or more of the following anticonvulsants. *Caution:* Anticonvulsants can cause hypotension, cardiac arrest, or respiratory arrest if administered rapidly.
   a. Diazepam, 0.1–0.2 mg/kg IV (p 327).
   b. Midazolam, 0.1–0.2 mg/kg IM (useful when intravenous access is difficult; p 353).
   c. Phenobarbital, 10–15 mg/kg IV, slow infusion over 15–20 minutes (p 368).
   d. Phenytoin, 15–20 mg/kg IV, slow infusion over 25–30 minutes (p 370).
   e. Pentobarbital, 5–6 mg/kg IV, slow infusion over 8–10 minutes, then continuous infusion at 0.5–3 mg/kg/h titrated to effect (p 367).
5. Immediately check the rectal or tympanic temperature and cool the patient rapidly (p 20) if the temperature is above 40 °C (104 °F). The most rapid and reliably effective method of temperature control is neuromuscular paralysis with pancuronium, 0.1 mg/kg IV (p 357). *Caution:* If paralysis is used, the patient must be intubated and ventilated; in addition, monitor the electroencephalogram (EEG) for continued brain seizure activity because peripheral muscular hyperactivity is no longer visible.
6. Use specific antidotes if available:
   a. Pyridoxine for isoniazid (INH; p 192 and 375).
   b. Pralidoxime (2-PAM) or atropine, or both, for organophosphate or carbamate insecticides (p 240 and 118).

V. Agitation, delirium, or psychosis
A. Assessment. Agitation, delirium, or psychosis may be caused by a variety of drugs and toxins (Table I–14). In addition, such symptoms may result from a functional thought disorder or metabolic encephalopathy caused by medical illness.
1. Functional psychosis or stimulant-induced agitation and psychosis are usually associated with an intact sensorium, and hallucinations are predominantly auditory.
2. With metabolic encephalopathy or drug-induced delirium, there is usually alteration of sensorium (confusion, disorientation). Hallucinations, when they occur, are predominantly visual.

B. Complications. Agitation, especially if accompanied by hyperkinetic behavior and struggling, may result in hyperthermia (see p 20) and rhabdomyolysis (see p 25).

C. Differential diagnosis. Rule out:
1. Serious metabolic disturbance (hypoxia, hypoglycemia, hyponatremia).

TABLE I–14. SELECTED DRUGS AND TOXINS CAUSING AGITATION, DELIRIUM, OR CONFUSION[a]

Predominant confusion or delirium	Predominant agitation or psychosis
Amantadine	Amphetamines and derivatives
Anticholinergic agents	Caffeine
Antihistamines	Cocaine
Carbon monoxide	Cycloserine
Cimetidine	LSD (lysergic acid diethylamide)
Disulfiram	Marihuana
Lead and other heavy metals	Phencyclidine (PCP)
Levodopa	Phenylpropanolamine
Lidocaine and other local anesthetics	Procaine
Lithium	Theophylline
Salicylates	
Withdrawal from ethanol or sedative-hypnotic drugs	

[a]Adapted, in part, with permission, from Olson KR et al. *Med Toxicol* 1987;2:62.

      2. Alcohol or sedative-hypnotic drug withdrawal.

      3. Thyrotoxicosis.

      4. Central nervous system infection such as meningitis or encephalitis.

      5. Exertional or environmental hyperthermia.

   D. Treatment. Sometimes the patient can be calmed with reassuring words and by eliminating excessive noise, light, and physical stimulation. If this is not quickly effective, rapidly gain control of the patient in order to determine the rectal or tympanic temperature and to begin rapid cooling and other treatment if needed.

      1. Maintain the airway and assist ventilation if necessary (see p 4). Administer supplemental oxygen.

      2. Treat hypoglycemia (p 32), hypoxia (p 8), or other metabolic disturbances.

      3. Administer one of the following sedatives:

         a. Midazolam, 0.05–0.1 mg/kg IV over 1 minute, or 0.1–0.2 mg/kg IM (p 353).

         b. Diazepam, 0.1–0.2 mg/kg IV over 1 minute (p 327).

         c. Haloperidol, 0.1–0.2 mg/kg IM or IV over 1 minute (p 343). **Note:** Do not give decanoate salt IV.

      4. If hyperthermia occurs as a result of excessive muscular hyperactivity, then skeletal muscle paralysis is indicated: Use pancuronium, 0.1 mg/kg IV (see p 357). **Caution:** Be prepared to ventilate and endotracheally intubate the patient after muscle paralysis.

OTHER COMPLICATIONS

  I. Dystonia, dyskinesia, and rigidity

   A. Assessment. Examples of drugs and toxins causing abnormal movements or rigidity are listed in Table I–15.

      1. Dystonic reactions are common with therapeutic or toxic doses of many antipsychotic agents and with some antiemetics. The mechanism is thought to be related to central dopamine blockade. Dystonias usually consist of forced, involuntary, and often painful neck rotation (torticollis); tongue protrusion; jaw extension; or trismus. Other extrapyramidal or parkinsonian movement disorders (eg, pill rolling, bradykinesia, masked facies) may also be seen with these agents.

      2. In contrast, **dyskinesias** are usually rapid, repetitive body movements that may involve small localized muscle groups (eg, tongue darting, focal myoclonus) or may consist of generalized hyperkinetic activity. The cause is not dopamine blockade but, more commonly, increased dopamine effect or blockade of central cholinergic effect.

TABLE I–15. SELECTED DRUGS AND TOXINS CAUSING DYSTONIAS, DYSKINESIAS, AND RIGIDITY[a]

Dystonia	Dyskinesias
Haloperidol and butyrophenones	Amphetamines
Metoclopramide	Anticholinergic agents
Phenothiazines	Antihistamines
Rigidity	Caffeine
Black widow spider bite	Cocaine
Lithium	Cyclic antidepressants
Malignant hyperthermia	Ketamine
Methaqualone	Levodopa
Monoamine oxidase inhibitors	Lithium
Neuroleptic malignant syndrome	Phencyclidine (PCP)
Phencyclidine (PCP)	
Strychnine	

[a] Adapted, with permission, from Olson KR et al. *Med Toxicol* 1987;2:64.

       3. Rigidity may also be seen with a number of toxins and may be caused by central nervous system effects or spinal cord stimulation. Neuroleptic malignant syndrome and serotonin syndrome (see p 20) are characterized by rigidity, hyperthermia, metabolic acidosis, and altered mental status. Rigidity seen with malignant hyperthermia (see p 20) is caused by a defect at the muscle cell level and may not reverse with neuromuscular blockade.

    B. Complications. Sustained muscular rigidity or hyperactivity may result in rhabdomyolysis (see p 25), hyperthermia (p 20), ventilatory failure (p 7), or metabolic acidosis (p 30).

    C. Differential diagnosis. Rule out:
       1. Catatonic rigidity caused by functional thought disorder.
       2. Tetanus.
       3. Cerebrovascular accident.
       4. Postanoxic encephalopathy.
       5. Idiopathic parkinsonism.

    D. Treatment
       1. Maintain the airway and assist ventilation if necessary (see p 4). Administer supplemental oxygen.
       2. Check the rectal or tympanic temperature, and treat hyperthermia (p 20) rapidly if the temperature is above 39 °C (102.2 °F).
       3. Dystonia. Administer an anticholinergic agent such as diphenhydramine (Benadryl; p 331), 0.5–1 mg/kg IM or IV; or benztropine (Cogentin; p 318), 1–4 mg IM in adults. Follow with oral therapy for 2–3 days.
       4. Dyskinesia. Do *not* treat with anticholinergic agents. Instead, administer a sedative such as diazepam, 0.1–0.2 mg/kg IV (p 327); or midazolam, 0.05–0.1 mg/kg IV or 0.1–0.2 mg/kg IM (p 353).
       5. Rigidity. Do *not* treat with anticholinergic agents. Instead, administer a sedative (see **4,** above) or provide specific pharmacologic therapy:
          a. Intravenous calcium (p 323) for black widow spider bite (p 288).
          b. Dantrolene (p 325) for malignant hyperthermia (p 20).
          c. Bromocriptine (p 321) for neuroleptic malignant syndrome (p 20).

II. Rhabdomyolysis
    A. Assessment. Muscle cell necrosis is a common complication of poisoning. Examples of drugs and toxins causing rhabdomyolysis are listed in Table I–16.
       1. Mechanisms of rhabdomyolysis include prolonged immobilization on a hard surface, excessive seizures or muscular hyperactivity, hyperthermia, or direct cytotoxic effects of the drug or toxin (eg, carbon monoxide, colchicine, *Amanita phalloides* mushrooms).
       2. The diagnosis is made by finding hematest-positive urine with few or no intact red blood cells or an elevated serum creatinine phosphokinase (CPK) level.
    B. Complications. Myoglobin released by damaged muscle cells may precipitate in the kidneys, causing acute tubular necrosis and renal failure. This usually

TABLE I–16. SELECTED DRUGS AND TOXINS ASSOCIATED WITH RHABDOMYOLYSIS

Excessive muscular hyperactivity, rigidity, or seizures	Direct cellular toxicity
Amphetamines and derivatives	Amatoxin-containing mushrooms
Cocaine	Carbon monoxide
Cyclic antidepressants	Colchicine
Lithium	Ethylene glycol
Monoamine oxidase inhibitors	**Other or unknown mechanisms**
Phencyclidine (PCP)	Barbiturates (prolonged immobility)
Seizures caused by a variety of agents	Ethanol
Strychnine	Hyperthermia caused by a variety of agents
Tetanus	Sedative-hypnotic agents (prolonged immobility)
	Trauma

occurs only when the serum CPK level exceeds 10,000 units. With severe rhabdomyolysis, hyperkalemia, hyperphosphatemia, and hypocalcemia may also occur.

C. Differential diagnosis. Hemolysis with hemoglobinuria may also produce hematest-positive urine.

D. Treatment

1. Establish a steady urine flow rate (2–3 mL/kg/h) with intravenous fluids. For massive rhabdomyolysis accompanied by oliguria, administer mannitol, 0.5 g/kg IV.
2. Alkalinize the urine by adding 100 meq of sodium bicarbonate to each L of 5% dextrose. (Acidic urine promotes deposition of myoglobin in the tubules.)
3. Provide intensive supportive care, including hemodialysis if needed, for acute renal failure. Kidney function is usually regained in 2–3 weeks.

III. Anaphylactic and anaphylactoid reactions

A. Assessment. Examples of drugs and toxins causing anaphylactic or anaphylactoid reactions are listed in Table I–17. These reactions are characterized by bronchospasm and increased vascular permeability that may lead to laryngeal edema, skin rash, and hypotension.

1. **Anaphylaxis** occurs when a patient with antigen-specific immunoglobulin E (IgE) bound to the surface of mast cells and basophils is exposed to the antigen, triggering the release of histamine and various other vasoactive compounds.
2. **Anaphylactoid reactions** are also caused by release of active compounds from mast cells but do not involve prior sensitization or mediation through IgE.

B. Complications. Severe anaphylactic or anaphylactoid reactions can result in laryngeal obstruction, respiratory arrest, hypotension, and death.

C. Differential diagnosis. Rule out:

1. Anxiety, with vasodepressor syncope or hyperventilation.
2. Pharmacologic effects of the drug or toxin (eg, procaine reaction with procaine penicillin).
3. Bronchospasm or laryngeal edema from irritant gas exposure.

D. Treatment

1. Maintain the airway and assist ventilation if necessary (see p 4). Endotracheal intubation may be needed if laryngeal swelling is severe. Administer supplemental oxygen.
2. Treat hypotension with intravenous crystalloid fluids (eg, normal saline) and place patient in supine position.
3. Administer epinephrine (p 337):
   a. Mild to moderate reactions: 0.3–0.5 mg SC (children, 0.01 mg/kg; maximum 0.5 mg).

TABLE I–17. EXAMPLES OF DRUGS AND TOXINS CAUSING ANAPHYLACTIC OR ANAPHYLACTOID REACTIONS

Anaphylactic reactions (IgE-mediated)	Anaphylactoid reactions (not IgE-mediated)
Antisera (antivenins)	Acetylcysteine
Foods (nuts, fish, shellfish)	Blood products
Hymenoptera and other insect stings	Iodinated contrast media
Immunotherapy allergen extracts	Opiates
Penicillins and other antibiotics	Scombroid
Vaccines	Tubocurarine
Other or unclassified	
Exercise	
Sulfites	

    b. Severe reactions: 0.05–0.1 mg IV bolus every 5 minutes, or an infusion of 1–4 mcg/min.

  4. Administer diphenhydramine (Benadryl; p 331), 0.5–1 mg/kg IV over 1 minute. Follow with oral therapy for 2–3 days. Cimetidine (Tagamet), 300 mg IV every 8 hours, is also helpful.

  5. Administer corticosteroid such as hydrocortisone, 200–300 mg IV; or methylprednisolone, 40–80 mg IV.

DIAGNOSIS OF POISONING

Diagnosis and treatment of poisoning often must proceed rapidly without the results of extensive toxicologic screening. Fortunately, in most cases the correct diagnosis can be made by using carefully collected data from the history, a directed physical examination, and commonly available laboratory tests.

  I. History. Although frequently unreliable or incomplete, the history of ingestion may be very useful if carefully obtained.

    A. Ask the patient about all drugs taken, including nonprescription drugs or vitamins.

    B. Ask family members, friends, and paramedical personnel about any prescriptions or over-the-counter medications known to be used by the patient or others in the house.

    C. Obtain any available drugs or drug paraphernalia for later testing, but handle them very carefully to avoid poisoning by skin contact or inadvertent needle stick with potential for hepatitis B or HIV transmission.

    D. Check with the pharmacy on the label of any medications found with the patient to determine if other prescription drugs have been obtained there.

  II. Physical examination

    A. General findings. Perform a carefully directed examination emphasizing key physical findings that may uncover one of the common **autonomic syndromes;** this may suggest a certain class of drugs or toxins and specific empirical treatment. Important variables in the autonomic physical examination include blood pressure, pulse rate, pupil size, sweating, and peristaltic activity. The autonomic syndromes are summarized in Table I–18.

      1. Alpha-adrenergic syndrome. Hypertension with reflex bradycardia is characteristic. The pupils are usually dilated. (Examples: phenylpropanolamine, phenylephrine, methoxamine.)

      2. Beta-adrenergic syndrome. β_2-mediated vasodilation may cause hypotension. Tachycardia is common. (Examples: terbutaline, metaproterenol, theophylline, caffeine.)

TABLE I–18. AUTONOMIC SYNDROMES[a,b]

	Blood Pressure	Pulse Rate	Pupil Size	Sweating	Peristalsis
Alpha-adrenergic	+	−	+	+	−
Beta-adrenergic	±	+	±	±	±
Mixed adrenergic	+	+	+	+	−
Sympatholytic	−	−	- -	−	−
Nicotinic	+	+	±	+	+
Muscarinic	−	- -	- -	+	+
Mixed cholinergic	±	±	- -	+	+
Anticholinergic	+	+	+	- -	- -

[a]Key to symbols: + = increased; ++ = markedly increased; − = decreased; - - = markedly decreased; ± = mixed effect, no effect, or unpredictable.
[b]Adapted, with permission, from Olson KR et al. *Med Toxicol* 1987;2:54.

3. **Mixed alpha- and beta-adrenergic syndrome.** Hypertension is accompanied by tachycardia. The pupils are dilated. The skin is sweaty, although mucous membranes are dry. (Examples: cocaine, amphetamines, phencyclidine.)

4. **Sympatholytic syndrome.** Blood pressure and pulse rate are both decreased (peripheral alpha blockers such as hydralazine may cause hypotension with reflex tachycardia). The pupils are small, often pinpoint. Peristalsis is often decreased. (Examples: agents that decrease central nervous system sympathetic output, such as centrally acting α_2-agonists [clonidine, methyldopa], opiates, phenothiazines.)

5. **Nicotinic cholinergic syndrome.** Stimulation of nicotinic receptors at autonomic ganglia activates both parasympathetic and sympathetic systems, with unpredictable results. Excessive stimulation frequently causes depolarization blockage. Thus, initial tachycardia may be followed by bradycardia and muscle fasciculations may be followed by paralysis. (Examples: nicotine; in addition, the depolarizing neuromuscular blocker succinylcholine which acts on nicotinic receptors in skeletal muscle.)

6. **Muscarinic cholinergic syndrome.** Muscarinic receptors are located at effector organs of the parasympathetic system. Stimulation causes bradycardia, miosis, sweating, hyperperistalsis, bronchorrhea, wheezing, excessive salivation, and urinary incontinence. (Examples: There are no pure muscarinic drugs.)

7. **Mixed cholinergic syndrome.** Because both nicotinic and muscarinic receptors are stimulated, mixed effects may be seen. The pupils are usually miotic (pinpoint in size). The skin is sweaty, and peristaltic activity is increased. Fasciculations are a manifestation of nicotinic stimulation and may progress to muscle weakness or paralysis. (Examples: organophosphate and carbamate insecticides, physostigmine.)

8. **Anticholinergic syndrome.** Tachycardia with mild hypertension is common. The pupils are widely dilated. The skin is flushed, hot, and dry. Peristalsis is decreased, and urinary retention is common. Patients may have myoclonic jerking or choreoathetoid movements. Agitated delirium is common, and hyperthermia may occur. (Examples: atropine, scopolamine, benztropine, antihistamines, antidepressants; all these drugs are primarily antimuscarinic).

B. **Eye findings**

1. **Pupil size** is affected by a number of drugs acting on the autonomic nervous system. Table I–19 lists common causes of miosis and mydriasis.

2. **Horizontal gaze nystagmus** is common with a variety of drugs and toxins, including barbiturates, ethanol, carbamazepine, phenytoin, and scorpion envenomation. Phencyclidine (PCP) may cause horizontal, vertical, and even rotatory nystagmus.

C. **Abdominal findings.** Peristaltic activity is commonly affected by drugs and toxins (see Table I–18 on autonomic syndromes).

1. Ileus may also be caused by **mechanical factors** such as injury to the gastrointestinal tract with perforation and peritonitis, or mechanical obstruction by a swallowed foreign body.

2. Abdominal distension and ileus may also be a manifestation of acute **bowel infarction,** a rare but catastrophic complication that results from prolonged hypotension or mesenteric artery vasospasm (caused, for example, by ergot or amphetamines). Radiographs or CT scan may reveal air in the intestinal wall, biliary tree, or hepatic vein. The serum phosphorus level is often elevated.

D. **Skin findings**

1. **Sweating** or absence of sweating may provide a clue to one of the autonomic syndromes (Table I–18).

2. **Flushed red skin** may be caused by carbon monoxide poisoning, boric acid intoxication, chemical burns from corrosives or hydrocarbons, or anti-

TABLE I-19. SELECTED CAUSES OF PUPIL SIZE CHANGES[a]

CONSTRICTED PUPILS
  Sympatholytic agents
    Clonidine
    Opiates
    Phenothiazines
    Tetrahydrozoline
  Cholinergic agents
    Carbamate insecticides
    Nicotine
    Organophosphates
    Physostigmine
    Pilocarpine
  Others
    Barbiturates
    Ethanol
    Heatstroke
    Isopropyl alcohol
    Phencyclidine (PCP)
    Pontine hemorrhage
    Sedative-hypnotic agents
    Subarachnoid hemorrhage

DILATED PUPILS
  Sympathomimetic agents
    Amphetamines and derivatives
    Cocaine
    Dopamine
    LSD (lysergic acid diethylamide)
    Monoamine oxidase inhibitors
    Nicotine
  Anticholinergic agents
    Antihistamines
    Atropine and other anticholinergics
    Cyclic antidepressants
    Glutethimide

[a]Adapted, with permission, from Olson KR et al. *Med Toxicol* 1987;2:66.

cholinergic agents. It may also result from vasodilation (eg, phenothiazines or disulfiram-ethanol interaction).

3. **Pale coloration** with diaphoresis is frequently caused by sympathomimetic agents. Severe pallor should suggest possible arterial vasospasm, such as that caused by ergot (see p 158) or amphetamines (p 66).

4. **Cyanosis** may indicate hypoxia, sulfhemoglobinemia, or methemoglobinemia (p 8 and p 217).

E. **Odors.** A number of toxins may have characteristic odors (Table I-20). However, the odor may be subtle and may be obscured by the smell of emesis or other ambient odors. In addition, the ability to smell an odor may vary; for example, only about 50% of the general population can smell the "bitter almond" odor of cyanide. Thus, the absence of an odor does not guarantee the absence of the toxin.

III. **Essential clinical laboratory tests.** Simple, readily available clinical laboratory tests may provide important clues to the diagnosis of poisoning and may guide the investigation toward specific toxicology testing.

A. **Routine tests.** The following tests are recommended for routine screening of the overdose patient:

TABLE I-20. SOME COMMON ODORS CAUSED BY TOXINS AND DRUGS[a]

Odor	Drug or Toxin
Acetone	Acetone, chloroform, isopropyl alcohol
Acrid or pearlike	Chloral hydrate, paraldehyde
Bitter almonds	Cyanide
Carrots	Cicutoxin (water hemlock)
Garlic	Arsenic, organophosphates, selenium, thallium
Mothballs	Naphthalene, paradichlorobenzene
Pungent aromatic	Ethchlorvynol
Wintergreen	Methyl salicylate

[a]Adapted, with permission, from Olson KR et al. *Med Toxicol* 1987;2:67.

1. Serum osmolality and osmolar gap.
2. Electrolytes for determination of sodium, potassium, and anion gap.
3. Serum glucose.
4. Blood urea nitrogen (BUN) and creatinine for evaluation of renal function.
5. Hepatic transaminases and hepatic function tests.
6. Urinalysis to check for crystalluria, hemoglobinuria, or myoglobinuria.
7. Electrocardiogram (ECG).
8. Stat serum acetaminophen level and serum ethanol level.

B. Serum osmolality and osmolar gap. Serum osmolality may be measured in the laboratory with the freezing point depression osmometer or the heat of vaporization osmometer. Under normal circumstances the measured serum osmolality is approximately 290 mosm/L, and can be calculated from the sodium, glucose, and BUN. The difference between the calculated osmolality and the osmolality measured in the laboratory is known as the osmolar gap (Table I–21).

1. **Causes of elevated osmolar gap** (Table I–21)
   a. The osmolar gap may be increased in the presence of low-molecular-weight substances such as ethanol, other alcohols, and glycols that contribute to the measured but not the calculated gap. Table I–22 describes how to estimate alcohol and glycol levels from the osmolar gap.
   b. Osmolar gap accompanied by anion gap acidosis should immediately suggest poisoning by methanol or ethylene glycol.
   Note: A falsely normal osmolar gap despite the presence of alcohols may result from using a heat of vaporization method for measuring osmolality, because the alcohols will boil off before the serum boiling point is reached.

2. **Differential diagnosis**
   a. Patients with chronic renal failure who are not undergoing hemodialysis may have an elevated osmolar gap owing to accumulation of low-molecular-weight solutes.
   b. False elevation of the osmolar gap may be caused by the use of an inappropriate sample tube (lavender top, EDTA; grey top, fluoride-oxalate; blue top, citrate); see Table I–32, p 40.
   c. Falsely elevated gap may occur in patients with severe hyperlipidemia.

3. **Treatment** depends on the cause. If ethylene glycol (p 163) or methanol (p 215) poisoning is suspected, based upon elevated osmolar gap not accounted for by ethanol or other alcohols and the presence of metabolic acidosis, then ethanol infusion therapy and hemodialysis may be indicated.

C. Anion gap metabolic acidosis. The normal anion gap of 8–12 meq/L ac-

---

TABLE I–21. CAUSES OF ELEVATED OSMOLAR GAP[a,b]

Acetone	Mannitol
Ethanol	Methanol
Ethyl ether	Propylene glycol
Ethylene glycol	Renal failure without dialysis
Isopropyl alcohol	Severe alcoholic ketoacidosis or lactic acidosis
Magnesium	

[a] Osmolar gap = measured − calculated osmolality.

Calculated osmolality = $2[NA] + \dfrac{[glucose]}{18} + \dfrac{[BUN]}{2.8} = 290$ mosm/L.

Na (serum sodium) in meq/L; glucose and BUN (urea nitrogen) in mg/dL.

Note: The osmolality may be measured as falsely normal if a vaporization point osmometer is used instead of the freezing point device, because volatile alcohols will be boiled off.
[b] Adapted, with permission, from Olson KR et al. *Med Toxicol* 1987;2:74.

TABLE I–22. ESTIMATION OF ALCOHOL AND GLYCOL LEVELS FROM THE OSMOLAR GAP[a]

Alcohol or Glycol	Molecular Weight (mg/mmol)	Conversion Factor[b]
Acetone	58	5.8
Ethanol	46	4.6
Ethylene glycol	62	6.2
Isopropyl alcohol	60	6
Methanol	32	3.2
Propylene glycol	72	7.2

[a]Adapted, with permission, from *Current Emergency Diagnosis & Treatment*, 3rd ed. Ho MT, Saunders CE (editors). Appleton & Lange, 1990.
[b]To obtain estimated serum level (in mg/dL), multiply osmolar gap by conversion factor.

counts for unmeasured anions (eg, phosphate, sulfate) in the plasma. Metabolic acidosis is usually associated with an elevated anion gap.

1. **Causes of elevated anion gap** (Table I–23)
   a. An elevated anion gap acidosis is usually caused by accumulation of lactic acid but may also be caused by other unmeasured acid anions such as formate (eg, methanol poisoning) or oxalate (eg, ethylene glycol poisoning).
   b. In any patient with an elevated anion gap, also check the osmolar gap; combined anion and osmolar gap suggests poisoning by methanol or ethylene glycol.
   c. A narrow anion gap may occur with overdose by lithium, bromide, or nitrate, all of which will increase the measured serum chloride level.
2. **Differential diagnosis.** Rule out:
   a. Common causes of lactic acidosis such as hypoxia or ischemia.
   b. False depression of the serum bicarbonate and P_{CO_2}, which can occur from incomplete filling of the red-topped Vacutainer blood collection tube.
   c. False depression of the P_{CO_2} and calculated bicarbonate, which can result from excess heparin when obtaining arterial blood gases (0.25 mL heparin and 2 mL blood falsely lowers P_{CO_2} 8 mm and bicarbonate 5 meq/L).
3. **Treatment**
   a. Treat the underlying cause of the acidosis:

TABLE I–23. SELECTED DRUGS AND TOXINS CAUSING ELEVATED ANION GAP ACIDOSIS[a,b]

Lactic acidosis	Other
Beta-adrenergic drugs	Benzyl alcohol
Caffeine	Ethanol (ketoacidosis)
Carbon monoxide	Ethylene glycol
Cyanide	Exogenous organic and mineral acids
Hydrogen sulfide	Formaldehyde
Ibuprofen	Metaldehyde
Iron	Methanol
Isoniazid	
Phenformin	
Salicylates	
Seizures	
Theophylline	

[a]Anion gap = [Na] − [Cl] − [HCO_3] = 8–12 meq/L.
[b]Adapted, with permission, from Olson KR et al. *Med Toxicol* 1987;2:73.

(1) Treat seizures (see p 22) with anticonvulsants or neuromuscular paralysis.

(2) Treat hypoxia (p 8) and hypotension (p 15) if they occur.

(3) Treat methanol (p 215) or ethylene glycol (p 163) poisoning with ethanol and hemodialysis.

(4) Treat salicylate intoxication (p 277) with alkaline diuresis and hemodialysis.

b. Treatment of the acidemia itself is not generally necessary, unless the pH is less than 7–7.1. In fact, mild acidosis may be beneficial by promoting oxygen release to tissues. However, acidemia may be harmful in poisoning by salicylates or cyclic antidepressants.

(1) In salicylate intoxication (p 277), acidemia enhances salicylate entry into the brain and must be prevented. Alkalinization of the urine promotes salicylate elimination.

(2) In cyclic antidepressant overdose (p 147), acidemia enhances cardiotoxicity. Maintain the serum pH at 7.45–7.5 with boluses of sodium bicarbonate.

D. Hyperglycemia and hypoglycemia. A variety of drugs and disease states can cause alterations in the serum glucose level (Table I–24). Blood glucose is determined by nutritional state, endogenous insulin levels, endocrine function, and the presence of various drugs or toxins.

1. Hyperglycemia, especially if severe (> 500 mg/dL) or sustained, may result in dehydration and electrolyte imbalance caused by the osmotic effect of excess glucose in the urine; shift of water from the brain into plasma may result in hyperosmolar coma. More commonly, hyperglycemia in the setting of poisoning or drug overdose is mild and transient. Significant or sustained hyperglycemia should be treated if it is not resolving spontaneously or if the patient is symptomatic.

a. If the patient has altered mental status, maintain the airway, assist ventilation if necessary, and administer supplemental oxygen (see p 4).

b. Replace fluid deficits with intravenous normal saline or other isotonic crystalloid solution.

c. Correct acid-base and electrolyte disturbances.

d. Administer regular insulin, 5–10 units IV initially, followed by infusion of 5–10 units/h, monitoring effects on serum glucose level (children: administer 0.1 unit/kg initially and 0.1 unit/kg/h).

2. Hypoglycemia, if severe (serum glucose < 40 mg/dL) and sustained, can rapidly cause permanent brain injury. For this reason, whenever hypoglycemia is suspected as a cause of seizures, coma, or altered mental status, immediate empirical treatment with dextrose is indicated.

a. If the patient has altered mental status, maintain the airway, assist ventilation if necessary, and administer supplemental oxygen (see p 4).

TABLE I–24. SELECTED CAUSES OF ALTERATIONS IN SERUM GLUCOSE

Hyperglycemia	Hypoglycemia
β_2-adrenergic drugs	Akee fruit
Caffeine intoxication	Endocrine disorders (hypopituitarism, Addison's disease,
Corticosteroids	myxedema)
Dextrose administration	Ethanol intoxication
Diabetes mellitus	Fasting
Diazoxide	Hepatic failure
Excessive circulating epinephrine	Insulin
Glucagon	Oral hypoglycemic agents
Theophylline intoxication	Propranolol intoxication
Thiazide diuretics	Reactive hypoglycemia
Vacor	Renal failure
	Salicylate intoxication

b. If available, perform rapid bedside blood glucose testing (now possible in most emergency departments).

c. If the blood glucose is low (< 70 mg/dL) or if bedside testing is not available, administer concentrated dextrose 50%, 50 mL IV (25 g). In children, give 25% dextrose, 2 mL/kg (see p 343).

d. In malnourished or alcoholic patients, also give thiamine, 100 mg IM or IV, to prevent acute Wernicke's syndrome.

E. Hypernatremia and hyponatremia. Sodium disorders occur infrequently in poisoned patients (see Table I–25). More commonly they are associated with underlying disease states. Antidiuretic hormone (ADH) is responsible for concentrating the urine and preventing excess water loss.

1. Hypernatremia (serum sodium > 145 meq/L) may be caused by excessive sodium intake, excessive free water loss, or impaired renal concentrating ability.

a. Dehydration with normal kidney function. Excessive sweating, hyperventilation, diarrhea, or osmotic diuresis (eg, hyperglycemia, mannitol administration) may cause disproportional water loss. The urine osmolality is usually greater than 400 mosm/kg, and ADH function is normal.

b. Impaired renal concentrating ability. Excess free water is lost in the urine, and urine osmolality is usually less than 250 mosm/L. This may be caused by hypothalamic dysfunction with reduced ADH production **(diabetes insipidus)** or impaired kidney response to ADH **(nephrogenic diabetes insipidus).** Nephrogenic DI has been associated with chronic lithium therapy.

2. Treatment of hypernatremia. Treatment depends on the cause, but in most cases, the patient is hypovolemic and needs fluids. *Caution:* Do **not** reduce the serum sodium too quickly, as osmotic imbalance may cause excessive fluid shift into brain cells, resulting in cerebral edema. The correction should take place over 24–36 hours; the serum sodium should be lowered about 1 meq/L/h.

a. Hypovolemia. Administer normal saline (0.9% saline) to restore fluid balance, then half-normal saline in dextrose (D5W 0.45 saline).

b. Volume overload. Treat with a combination of free water administration (5% dextrose) and a loop diuretic such as furosemide (Lasix), 0.5–1 mg/kg.

c. Lithium-induced nephrogenic diabetes insipidus. Administer fluids (see **a,** above). Discontinue lithium therapy. Partial improvement may be seen with oral administration of indomethacin, 50 mg 3 times a day, and hydrochlorothiazide, 50–100 mg/d.

3. Hyponatremia (serum sodium < 130 meq/L) is a common electrolyte abnormality and may result from a variety of mechanisms. Severe hyponatremia (serum sodium < 110–120 meq/L) can result in seizures and altered mental status.

a. Pseudohyponatremia may result from reduced blood water volume (eg, hyperlipidemia, hyperproteinemia) or shift of water from the extracellular

---

TABLE I–25. SELECTED DRUGS AND TOXINS ASSOCIATED WITH ALTERED SERUM SODIUM

Hypernatremia	Hyponatremia
Cathartic abuse	Beer potomania
Lactulose therapy	Psychogenic polydipsia
Lithium therapy	Syndrome of inappropriate ADH (SIADH):
Mannitol	Amitriptyline
Severe gastroenteritis (many poisons)	Chlorpropamide
Sodium overdose	Clofibrate
	Oxytocin
	Phenothiazines

space (eg, hyperglycemia). Plasma sodium falls by about 1.6 meq/L for each 100 mg/dL rise in glucose.

b. **Hyponatremia with hypovolemia** may be caused by excessive volume loss (sodium and water) that is partially replaced by free water. In order to maintain intravascular volume, the body secretes ADH, which causes water retention. A urine sodium less than 10 meq/L suggests that the kidney is appropriately attempting to compensate for volume losses. An elevated urine sodium (> 20 meq/L) implies renal salt wasting, which can be caused by diuretics, adrenal insufficiency, or nephropathy.

c. **Hyponatremia with volume overload** occurs in conditions such as congestive heart failure and cirrhosis. Although the total body sodium is increased, baroreceptors sense an inadequate circulating volume and stimulate release of ADH. The urine sodium is usually less than 10 meq/L, unless the patient has been on diuretics.

d. **Hyponatremia with normal volume** occurs in a variety of situations. Measurement of the serum and urine osmolalities may help determine the diagnosis.

  (1) **Syndrome of inappropriate ADH secretion (SIADH).** In patients with SIADH, ADH is secreted independent of volume or osmolality. Causes include malignancies, pulmonary disease, and some drugs (see Table I–25). The serum osmolality is low, but the urine osmolality is inappropriately increased (> 300 mosm/L). The serum blood urea nitrogen (BUN) is usually low (< 10 mg/dL).

  (2) **Psychogenic polydipsia,** or compulsive water drinking (generally > 10 L/d), causes reduced serum sodium because of the excessive free water intake and because the kidney excretes sodium to maintain euvolemia. The urine sodium may be elevated, but urine osmolality is appropriately low because the kidney is attempting to excrete the excess water and ADH secretion is suppressed.

  (3) **Beer potomania** may result from chronic daily excessive beer drinking (> 4 L/d). It usually occurs in patients with cirrhosis who already have elevated ADH levels.

  (4) Other causes of euvolemic hyponatremia include hypothyroidism, postoperative state, and idiosyncratic reactions to diuretics (generally thiazides).

4. **Treatment of hyponatremia.** Treatment depends on the cause, the patient's volume status, and most important, the patient's clinical condition. *Caution:* Avoid overly rapid correction of the sodium, as brain damage (central pontine myelinolysis) may occur if the sodium is increased by more than 25 meq/L in the first 24 hours. Obtain frequent measurements of serum and urine sodium and adjust the rate of infusion as needed to increase the serum sodium by no more than 1–1.5 meq/h. Obtain consultation with a nephrologist as soon as possible. **For patients with profound hyponatremia** (serum sodium < 110 meq/L) accompanied by coma or seizures, administer hypertonic (3%) saline, 100–200 mL.

a. **Hyponatremia with hypovolemia.** Replace volume using normal saline. If adrenal insufficiency is suspected, give hydrocortisone, 100 mg every 6–8 hours. Hypertonic saline is rarely indicated.

b. **Hyponatremia with volume overload.** Restrict water (0.5–1 L/d) and treat the underlying condition (eg, congestive heart failure). If diuretics are given, do **not** allow excessive free water intake. Hypertonic saline is dangerous in these patients; if it is used, also administer furosemide, 0.5–1 mg/kg. Consider hemodialysis to reduce volume and restore the sodium level.

c. **Hyponatremia with normal volume.** Asymptomatic patients may be treated conservatively with water restriction (0.5–1 L/d). Psychogenic compulsive water drinkers may have to be restrained or separated from all sources of water, including washbasins and toilets. Demeclocycline (a tetracycline antibiotic that can produce nephrogenic diabetes insipidus), 300–600 mg twice a day, is used to treat mild SIADH. Onset of action may require a week. For patients with coma or seizures, give hypertonic (3%) saline, 100–200 mL, along with furosemide, 0.5–1 mg/kg.

F. Hyperkalemia and hypokalemia. A variety of drugs and toxins can cause serious alterations in the serum potassium level (Table I–26). Potassium levels are dependent upon potassium intake and release (eg, from muscles), diuretic use, proper functioning of the ATPase pump, serum pH, and beta-adrenergic activity. Changes in serum potassium do not always reflect overall body gain or loss but may be caused by intracellular shifts (eg, acidosis drives potassium out of cells; beta-adrenergic stimulation drives it into cells).

1. **Hyperkalemia** (serum K^+ > 5 meq/L) produces muscle weakness and interferes with normal cardiac conduction. Peaked T waves and prolonged PR intervals are the earliest sign of cardiotoxicity. Critical hyperkalemia produces QRS interval widening, AV block, ventricular fibrillation, and cardiac arrest (see Fig I–7).
   a. Hyperkalemia caused by **fluoride intoxication** (see p 168) is usually accompanied by hypocalcemia.
   b. **Digitalis intoxication** associated with hyperkalemia is an indication for administration of digoxin-specific Fab antibodies (p 329).
2. **Treatment of hyperkalemia.** A potassium level higher than 6 meq/L is a medical emergency; greater than 7 meq/L is critical.
   a. Monitor the ECG. QRS prolongation indicates critical cardiac poisoning.
   b. Administer calcium chloride, 10–20 mg/kg IV (p 323), if there are signs of critical cardiac toxicity. *Caution:* Do **not** use calcium in patients with digitalis glycoside poisoning; intractable ventricular fibrillation may result.
   c. Sodium bicarbonate, 1–2 meq/kg IV (p 318), rapidly drives potassium intracellularly.
   d. Glucose plus insulin also promotes intracellular movement of potassium. Give 50% dextrose, 50 mL (25% dextrose, 2 mL/kg in children), plus regular insulin, 0.1 unit/kg IV.
   e. Kayexalate (sodium polystyrene sulfonate), 0.3–0.6 g/kg orally in 2 mL/kg sorbitol 70%, is effective but takes several hours.
   f. Hemodialysis rapidly lowers serum potassium levels.
3. **Hypokalemia** (serum K^+ < 3.5 meq/L) may cause muscle weakness, hyporeflexia, and ileus. Rhabdomyolysis may occur. The ECG shows flattened T waves and prominent U waves. With severe hypokalemia, AV block, ventricular arrhythmias, and cardiac arrest may occur.
   a. **With theophylline, caffeine, or β_2-agonist intoxication,** intracellular shift of potassium may produce a very low serum K^+ level with normal total body stores. Patients usually do not have serious symptoms or ECG signs of hypokalemia, and aggressive potassium therapy is not required.
   b. **With barium poisoning** (p 95), profound hypokalemia may lead to re-

TABLE I–26. SELECTED DRUGS AND TOXINS AND OTHER CAUSES OF ALTERED SERUM POTASSIUM[a]

Hyperkalemia	Hypokalemia
Alpha-adrenergic agents	Barium
Angiotensin converting enzyme inhibitors	Beta-adrenergic drugs
Beta blockers	Caffeine
Digitalis glycosides	Diuretics (chronic)
Fluoride	Epinephrine
Lithium	Theophylline
Potassium	Toluene (chronic)
Renal failure	
Rhabdomyolysis	

[a]Adapted, with permission, from Olson KR et al. *Med Toxicol* 1987;**2**:73.

FIGURE I–7. Electrocardiogram of patient with hyperkalemia. (Modified and reproduced, with permission, from Goldschlager N, Goldman MJ: Effect of drugs and electrolytes on the electrocardiogram. Page 199 in: *Electrocardiography: Essentials of Interpretation.* Goldschlager N, Goldman MJ [editors]. Lange, 1984.)

       spiratory muscle weakness and cardiac and respiratory arrest, and therefore intensive potassium therapy is necessary. Up to 420 meq has been given in 24 hours.

    c. Hypokalemia resulting from diuretic therapy may contribute to ventricular arrhythmias, especially those associated with chronic digitalis glycoside poisoning.

  4. Treatment of hypokalemia. Mild hypokalemia (K^+ = 3–3.5 meq/L) is usually not associated with serious symptoms.

    a. Administer potassium chloride orally or intravenously. Do *not* give more than 10–15 meq/h IV (0.25–0.5 meq/kg/h in children).

    b. Monitor serum potassium and the ECG for signs of hyperkalemia from excessive potassium therapy.

    c. If hypokalemia is caused by diuretic therapy or gastrointestinal fluid losses, measure and replace other ions such as magnesium, sodium, and chloride.

G. Renal failure. Examples of drugs and toxins causing renal failure are listed in Table I–27. Renal failure may be caused by a direct nephrotoxic action of the poison; acute massive tubular precipitation of myoglobin (rhabdomyolysis), hemoglobin (hemolysis), or calcium oxalate crystals (ethylene glycol); or it may be secondary to shock owing to blood or fluid loss or cardiovascular collapse.

  1. Assessment. Renal failure is characterized by progressive rise in the serum creatinine and blood urea nitrogen (BUN) levels, usually accompanied by oliguria or anuria.

    a. The serum creatinine level usually rises about 1 mg/dL/d after total anuric renal failure.

TABLE I–27. EXAMPLES OF DRUGS AND TOXINS AND OTHER CAUSES OF RENAL FAILURE

Direct nephrotoxic effect
  Acetaminophen
  Amanita phalloides mushrooms
  Analgesics (eg, phenacetin)
  Antibiotics (eg, aminoglycosides)
  Chlorinated hydrocarbons
  Cortinarius sp. mushrooms
  Cyclosporin
  Ethylene glycol (oxalate)
  Heavy metals (eg, mercury)

Hemolysis
  Arsine
  Methemoglobinemia
  Naphthalene
  Oxidizing agents (eg, chlorates)

Rhabdomyolysis (see also Table I–16)
  Amphetamines and derivatives
  Carbon monoxide
  Cocaine
  Coma with prolonged immobility
  Hyperthermia
  Phencyclidine (PCP)
  Status epilepticus
  Strychnine

   b. More abrupt rise should suggest rapid muscle breakdown (rhabdomyolysis), which increases the creatinine load and also results in elevated creatinine phosphokinase (CPK) levels that may interfere with the serum creatinine determination.

   c. Oliguria may be seen before renal failure occurs, especially with hypovolemia. In this case, the BUN level is usually elevated out of proportion to the serum creatinine level.

2. Complications. The earliest complication of acute renal failure is hyperkalemia (see p 35); this may be more pronounced if the cause of the renal failure is rhabdomyolysis or hemolysis, both of which release large amounts of intracellular potassium into the circulation. Later complications include metabolic acidosis, delirium, and coma.

3. Treatment

   a. Prevent renal failure, is possible, by administering specific treatment (eg, acetylcysteine for acetaminophen overdose, BAL [dimercaprol] chelation for mercury poisoning, intravenous fluids for rhabdomyolysis or shock).

   b. Monitor the serum potassium frequently and treat hyperkalemia (see p 35) if it occurs.

   c. Do *not* give supplemental potassium, and avoid cathartics or other medications containing magnesium, phosphate, or sodium.

   d. Perform hemodialysis as needed.

H. Hepatic failure. A variety of drugs and toxins may cause hepatic failure (Table I–28). Mechanisms of toxicity include direct hepatocellular damage (eg, *A phalloides*), metabolic creation of a hepatotoxic intermediate (eg, acetaminophen, carbon tetrachloride), or hepatic vein thrombosis (eg, pyrrolizidine alkaloids).

1. Assessment. Laboratory and clinical evidence of hepatitis usually does not become apparent until at least 24–36 hours after exposure to the poison. Then transaminase levels rise sharply and may fall to normal over the next 3–5 days. If hepatic damage is severe, measures of hepatic function (eg, bilirubin, prothrombin time) will continue to worsen after 2–3 days, even as transaminase levels are returning to normal. Metabolic acidosis and hypoglycemia usually indicate a poor prognosis.

2. Complications

   a. Abnormal hepatic function may result in excessive bleeding owing to insufficient production of vitamin K-dependent coagulation factors.

   b. Hepatic encephalopathy may lead to coma and death, usually within 5–7 days of massive hepatic failure.

3. Treatment

   a. Prevent hepatic injury if possible by administering specific treatment (eg, acetylcysteine for acetaminophen overdose).

   b. Obtain baseline and daily transaminase, bilirubin, and glucose levels and prothrombin time.

   c. Provide intensive supportive care for hepatic failure and encephalopathy (eg, glucose for hypoglycemia, fresh-frozen plasma for coagulopathy, lactulose for encephalopathy).

TABLE I–28. EXAMPLES OF DRUGS AND TOXINS CAUSING HEPATIC DAMAGE

Acetaminophen	Insecticides (chlorinated)
Amanita phalloides mushrooms	Iron
Aromatic hydrocarbons	Phosphorus
Arsenic	Polychlorinated biphenyls (PCBs)
Carbon tetrachloride and other chlorinated hydrocarbons	Pyrrolizidine alkaloids
Copper	Thallium
Dimethylformamide	2-Nitropropane
Ethanol (chronic)	Valproic acid
Halothane	

    d. Liver transplant may be the only effective treatment once massive hepatic necrosis has resulted in severe encephalopathy.

IV. Toxicology screening.* To maximize the utility of the toxicology laboratory, it is necessary to understand what the laboratory can and cannot do and how knowledge of the results will affect the patient. The routine "tox screen" is of minimal value in the initial care of the poisoned patient. On the other hand, specific toxicologic analyses and quantitative levels of certain drugs may be extremely helpful. Before ordering any tests, always ask these 2 questions: (1) How will the result of the test alter the approach to treatment? and (2) Can the result of the test be returned in a timely manner to affect therapy positively?

    A. Limitations of toxicology screens. Owing to long turnaround time, lack of availability, reliability factors, and the low risk of serious morbidity with supportive clinical management, toxicology screening is estimated to affect management in less than 15% of all cases of poisoning or drug overdose.

        1. Toxicology screens or panels may look specifically for only 40–50 drugs out of more than 10,000 possible drugs or toxins (or 6 million chemicals). However, these 40–50 drugs (Tables I–29 and I–30) account for more than 80% of overdoses.

        2. To detect many different drugs, screens utilize methods with broad specificity, and sensitivity may be poor for some drugs (analytic false-negatives).

TABLE I–29. DRUGS COMMONLY INCLUDED IN URINE OR GASTRIC SCREEN[a]

Alcohols	**Phenothiazines**
Acetone	Chlorpromazine
Ethanol	Prochlorperazine
Isopropyl alcohol	Promethazine
Methanol	Thioridazine
Analgesics	Trifluoperazine
Acetaminophen	**Sedative-hypnotic drugs**
Salicylates	Barbiturates
Anticonvulsants	Benzodiazepines
Carbamazepine	Carisoprodol
Phenobarbital	Chloral hydrate
Phenytoin	Ethchlorvynol
Primidone	Glutethimide
Antihistamines	Meprobamate
Benztropine	Methaqualone
Chlorpheniramine	**Stimulants**
Diphenhydramine	Amphetamines
Pyrilamine	Caffeine
Trihexylphenidyl	Cocaine and benzoylecgonine
Opiates	Phencyclidine (PCP)
Codeine	Strychnine
Dextromethorphan	**Tricyclic antidepressants**
Hydrocodone	Amitriptyline
Meperidine	Desipramine
Methadone	Doxepin
Morphine	Imipramine
Oxycodone	Nortriptyline
Pentazocine	Protriptyline
Propoxyphene	**Other drugs**
	Lidocaine
	Propranolol
	Quinidine and quinine

[a]Newer drugs in any category may not be included in screening.

*By John Osterloh, MD.

TABLE I–30. DRUGS COMMONLY INCLUDED IN BLOOD TOXICOLOGY SCREEN

Alcohols	**Sedative-hypnotic drugs**
Acetone	Barbiturates
Ethanol	Carisoprodol
Isopropyl alcohol	Chlordiazepoxide
Methanol	Diazepam
Analgesics	Ethchlorvynol
Acetaminophen	Glutethimide
Salicylates	Meprobamate
Anticonvulsants	Methaqualone
Ethosuximide	
Carbamazepine	
Phenobarbital	
Phenytoin	

On the other hand, some drugs present in therapeutic amounts may be detected on the screen even though they are causing no clinical symptoms (clinical false-positives).

3. Because many agents are not sought or detected (Table I–31), a negative toxicology screen does not always rule out poisoning; the negative predictive value of the screen is only about 70%. In contrast, ruling in a drug etiology with a positive screen is better, with a positive predictive value of about 90%.

4. The specificity of toxicologic tests is dependent on the method and the laboratory. The presence of other drugs, drug metabolites, disease states, or incorrect sampling may cause erroneous results (Table I–32).

B. **Uses for toxicology screens**
1. Broad (urine and blood) screening is essential whenever the diagnosis of brain death is being considered, to rule out common depressant drugs that might result in temporary loss of brain activity and mimic brain death.
2. Toxicology screens may be used to confirm clinical impressions during hospitalization and can be inserted in the permanent medicolegal record. This may be important if homicide, assault, or child abuse is suspected.

C. **Approach to toxicology testing**
1. Communicate clinical suspicions to the laboratory.
2. Obtain gastric, blood, and urine specimens on admission and have the laboratory store them temporarily. If the patient rapidly recovers, they can be discarded.

TABLE I–31. DRUGS AND TOXINS *NOT* COMMONLY INCLUDED IN TOXICOLOGIC SCREENING PANELS[a]

Anesthetic gases	Fentanyl and other opiate derivatives
Antiarrhythmic agents	Fluoride
Antibiotics	Formate
Antihypertensives	Hypoglycemic agents
Benzodiazepines (newer generation)	Isoniazid
Beta blockers other than propranolol	Lithium
Borate	LSD (lysergic acid diethylamide)
Bromide	MAO inhibitors
Calcium antagonists	Marihuana
Colchicine	Noxious gases
Cyanide	Plant toxins
Digitalis glycosides	Pressors (eg, dopamine)
Diuretics	Solvents and hydrocarbons
Ergot alkaloids	Theophylline
Ethylene glycol	Vasodilators

[a]Many of these are available as separate specific tests.

TABLE I–32. INTERFERENCES IN TOXICOLOGIC BLOOD TESTS

Drug or Toxin	Method[a]	Causes of Falsely Increased Blood Level
Acetaminophen	SC	Salicylate, salicylamide, methyl salicylate (each will increase acetaminophen level by 10% of their level in mg/L); bilirubin; phenols; renal failure (each 1 mg/dL increase in creatinine = 30 mg/L acetaminophen).
	GC, IA	Phenacetin.
	HPLC	Cephalosporins; sulfonamides.
Amitriptyline	HPLC	Cyclobenzaprine.
Amphetamines	GC[b]	Other volatile stimulant amines (misidentified). GC mass spectrometry cannot distinguish d-methamphetamine from l-methamphetamine (Vicks inhaler).
	IA[b]	Phenylpropanolamine, ephedrine, phenteramine, phenmetrazine, labetalol; many phenylethylamine and amphetamine derivatives.
	TLC[b]	MDA (and several similar amines); labetalol.
Chloride	SC	Bromide (0.8 meq Cl = 1 meq Br).
Creatinine	SC	Ketoacidosis (may increase Cr up to 2–3 mg/dL); cephalosoporins; creatine (eg, with rhabdomyolysis).
Digoxin	IA	Endogenous digoxinlike natriuretic substances in newborns and in patients with renal failure (up to 1 ng/mL); oleander ingestion (other cardiac glycosides identified as digoxin); after digoxin antibody (Fab) administration.
Ethanol	SC[c]	Other alcohols, ketones (by oxidation methods); isopropyl alcohol (by enzymatic methods).
Ethylene glycol	SC	Other glycols; elevated triglycerides.
Iron	SC	Deferoxamine causes 15% lowering of total iron-binding capacity (TIBC). Lavender-top Vacutainer tube contains EDTA, which lowers total iron.
Isopropanol	GC	Skin disinfectant containing isopropyl alcohol used before venipuncture (highly variable, usually trivial, but up to 40 mg/dL).
Lithium	SC	Green-top Vacutainer specimen tube (contains lithium heparin) may cause marked elevation (up to 6–8 meq/L).
Methemoglobin	SC	Sulfhemoglobin (cross-positive ~ 10% by co-oximeter); methylene blue (2 mg/kg dose gives transient false-positive 15% methemoglobin level); hyperlipidemia (triglyceride, 6000 mg/dL, may give false methemoglobin of 28.6%).
		Falsely decreased level with in vitro spontaneous reduction to hemoglobin in Vacutainer tube (~ 10%/h). Analyze within 1 hour.
Morphine/codeine	TLC[b]	Hydromorphone, hydrocodone, oxycodone (misidentification)
	IA[b]	Cross-reactants: hydrocodone, hydromorphone, oxycodone, monoacetylmorphine, morphine from poppy-seed ingestion.
Osmolality	Osm	Lavender-top (EDTA) Vacutainer specimen tube (15 mosm/L); gray-top (fluoride-oxalate) tube (150 mosm/L); blue-top (citrate) tube (10 mosm/L); green-top (lithium heparin) tube (theoretically, up to 6–8 mosm/L).
		Falsely normal if vapor pressure method used (alcohols are volatilized).
Salicylate	SC	Phenothiazines,[b] acetaminophen; diflunisal; ketosis,[b] salicylamide; accumulated salicylate metabolites in patients with renal failure (~ 10% increase).
	IA	Diflunisal.
	SC	**Decreased or altered salicylate level:** bilirubin; phenylketones.
	GC[c]	Methysalicylate; eucalyptol; theophylline.
	HPLC	Theophylline; antibiotics.

Drug or Toxin	Method[a]	Causes of Falsely Increased Blood Level
Theophylline	SC[c]	Diazepam; caffeine; accumulated theophylline metabolites in renal failure.
	HPLC	Acetazolamide; cephalosporins; endogenous xanthines and accumulated theophylline metabolites in renal failure (minor effect).
	GC[c]	Phenobarbital (rare).
	IA	Caffeine; accumulated theophylline metabolites in renal failure.

[a]GC = gas chromatography (interferences primarily with older methods); HPLC = high-pressure liquid chromatography; IA = immunoassay; SC = spectrochemical; TLC = thin-layer chromatography.
[b]More common with urine test.
[c]Uncommon methodology.

3. Urine and gastric specimens are the best samples for broad qualitative screening. Blood samples should be saved for possible quantitative testing, but blood is not a good specimen for screening for many common drugs, including psychotropic agents, opiates, and stimulants.

4. Decide if a specific quantitative blood level may assist in management decisions (eg, use of an antidote or dialysis; Table I–33). Quantitative levels are helpful only if there is a predictable correlation between the serum level and clinical effect.

5. A regional poison control center (see Table I–41) or toxicology consultant may provide assistance in considering certain drug etiologies and in selection of specific tests.

V. Abdominal x-rays. Abdominal x-rays may reveal radiopaque tablets, drug-filled condoms, or other toxic material.

    A. The radiograph is useful only if positive; recent studies suggest that few types of tablets are predictably visible (Table I–34).

    B. Do *not* attempt to determine radiopacity of a tablet by placing it directly on the x-ray plate. This often produces a false-positive result because of an air-contrast effect.

DECONTAMINATION

I. Surface decontamination

    A. Skin. Corrosive agents rapidly injure the skin and must be removed immediately. In addition, many toxins are readily absorbed through the skin and systemic absorption can be prevented only by rapid action. Table II–17 (p 127)

TABLE I–33. SPECIFIC QUANTITATIVE LEVELS AND POTENTIAL INTERVENTIONS[a]

Drug or Toxin	Potential Intervention
Acetaminophen	Acetylcysteine
Carboxyhemoglobin	100% oxygen
Digitalis	Digitalis antibodies
Ethanol	Low level indicates search for other toxins
Ethylene glycol	Ethanol therapy, hemodialysis
Iron	Deferoxamine chelation
Lithium	Hemodialysis
Methanol	Ethanol therapy, hemodialysis
Methemoglobin	Methylene blue
Salicylate	Alkalinization, hemodialysis
Theophylline	Repeat-dose charcoal, hemoperfusion

[a]Adapted from Olson KR: Toxicology screens and asymptomatic poisoning. In: *Current Practice of Emergency Medicine,* 2nd ed. Callaham M (editor). Decker, 1991.

TABLE I–34. RADIOPAQUE DRUGS AND POISONS[a]

Usually visible
    Bismuth subsalicylate (Pepto-Bismol)
    Calcium carbonate (Tums)
    Iron tablets
    Lead and lead-containing paint
    Metallic foreign bodies
    Potassium tablets

Sometimes/weakly visible
    Acetazolamide
    Arsenic
    Brompheniramine and dexbrompheniramine
    Busulfan
    Chloral hydrate
    Enteric-coated or sustained-release preparations (highly variable)
    Meclizine
    Perphenazine with amitriptyline
    Phosphorus
    Prochlorperazine
    Sodium chloride
    Thiamine
    Tranylcypromine
    Trifluoperazine
    Trimeprazine
    Zinc sulfate

[a]Reference: Savitt DL, Hawkins HH, Roberts JR: The radiopacity of ingested medications. *Ann Emerg Med* 1987;**16**:331.

lists several corrosive chemical agents that can have systemic toxicity, and many of them are well absorbed through the skin.

1. Be careful not to expose yourself or other care providers to potentially contaminating substances. Wear protective gear (gloves, gown, goggles) and wash exposed areas promptly. Contact a regional poison center for information about the hazards of the chemicals involved; in the majority of cases, health care providers are not at significant personal risk for secondary contamination, and simple measures such as emergency department gowns and plain latex gloves are sufficient protection. For radiation and other hazardous materials incidents, see also section IV, (p 380).
2. Remove contaminated clothing and flush exposed areas with copious quantities of tepid (lukewarm) water or saline. Wash carefully behind ears, under nails, and in skin folds. Use soap and shampoo for oily substances.
3. There is rarely a need for chemical neutralization of a substance spilled on the skin. In fact, the heat generated by chemical neutralization can potentially create worse injury. Some of the few exceptions to this rule are listed in Table I–35.

B. **Eyes.** The cornea is especially sensitive to corrosive agents and hydrocarbon solvents that may rapidly damage the corneal surface and lead to permanent scarring.

1. Act quickly to prevent serious damage. Flush exposed eyes with copious quantities of tepid tap water or saline. If available, instill local anesthetic drops in the eye first to facilitate irrigation. Remove contact lenses, if present.
2. Place the victim in a supine position under a tap or use intravenous tubing to direct a stream of water across the nasal bridge into the medial aspect of the eye (Fig I–8). Use at least 1 L to irrigate each eye.
3. If the offending substance is an acid or a base, check the pH of the tears after irrigation and continue irrigation if the pH remains abnormal.

TABLE I–35. SOME TOPICAL AGENTS FOR CHEMICAL EXPOSURES TO THE SKIN[a]

Chemical Corrosive Agent	Topical Treatment
Hydrofluoric acid	Calcium soaks
Oxalic acid	Calcium soaks
Phenol	Mineral oil or other oil
Phosphorus (white)	Copper sulfate 1% (colors embedded granules blue, facilitates removal)

[a]Reference: Edelman PA: Chemical and electrical burns. Pages 183–202 in: *Management of the Burned Patient.* Achauer BM (editor). Appleton & Lange, 1987.

4. Do *not* instill any neutralizing solution; there is no evidence that such treatment works, and it may further damage the eye.
5. After irrigation is complete, check the conjunctival and corneal surfaces carefully for evidence of full-thickness injury. Perform a fluorescein examination of the eye using fluorescein dye and a Wood's lamp to reveal corneal injury.
6. Patients with serious conjunctival or corneal injury should be referred to an ophthalmologist immediately.

FIGURE I–8. Irrigation of the eyes after chemical injury, showing technique for irrigating both upper and lower eyelids.

C. Inhalation. Agents that injure the pulmonary system may be acutely irritating gases or fumes and may have good or poor warning properties (see p 176).

1. Be careful not to expose yourself or other care providers to toxic gases or fumes without adequate respiratory protection (see p 384).
2. Remove the victim from exposure and give supplemental humidified oxygen, if available. Assist ventilation if necessary (see p 4).
3. Observe closely for evidence of upper respiratory tract edema, which is heralded by hoarse voice and stridor and may progress rapidly to complete airway obstruction. Endotracheally intubate patients with evidence of progressive airway compromise.
4. Also observe for late-onset noncardiogenic pulmonary edema resulting from slower-acting toxins, which may take several hours to appear. Early signs and symptoms include dyspnea, hypoxemia, and tachypnea (see p 8).

II. Gastrointestinal decontamination. There is still controversy about the roles of emesis, gastric lavage, activated charcoal, and cathartics to decontaminate the gastrointestinal tract. It is now well established that after a delay of 60 minutes or more, very little of the ingested dose is removed by emesis or gastric lavage. Moreover, recent studies suggest that, in the average overdosed patient, simple oral administration of activated charcoal without prior gut emptying may be as effective as the traditional sequence of gut emptying followed by charcoal.

A. Emesis. Syrup of ipecac-induced emesis remains the most convenient way of emptying the stomach and is used mainly for prehospital treatment of many ingestions (eg, in the home, a factory clinic, or private office). It is rarely used in emergency departments because of the availability of activated charcoal and gastric lavage. After syrup of ipecac administration, vomiting usually occurs within 20–30 minutes. Unfortunately, if the ingestion occurred more than 60 minutes before ipecac administration, emesis is not very effective, removing less than half the stomach's contents. Moreover, persistent vomiting after ipecac use frequently delays the administration of activated charcoal (see **C**, below).

1. **Indications**
   a. Early initial management of oral poisonings, particularly in the home immediately following ingestion or in health care facilities without the capacity to perform gastric lavage.
   b. To remove ingested agents not adsorbed by activated charcoal (eg, iron, lithium, potassium; see Table I–36).
   c. To remove sustained-release or enteric-coated tablets.

2. **Contraindications**
   a. Obtunded, comatose, or convulsing patient.
   b. Ingestion of a substance likely to cause rapid or abrupt coma or seizures (eg, cyclic antidepressants, camphor, cocaine, isoniazid, strychnine).
   c. Ingestion of a corrosive agent (eg, acids, alkali, strong oxidizing agents).
   d. Ingestion of a simple aliphatic hydrocarbon (see p 178). These are likely to cause pneumonitis if aspirated, but usually do not cause systemic poisoning once they enter the stomach. For those hydrocarbons that do carry a potential for systemic toxicity, activated charcoal with or without gastric lavage is preferable.

3. **Adverse effects**
   a. Persistent vomiting may delay administration of activated charcoal or oral antidotes (eg, acetylcysteine).
   b. Protracted forceful vomiting may result in hemorrhagic gastritis or Mallory-Weiss tear.
   c. Drowsiness occurs in about 20% and diarrhea in 25% of children.
   d. Repeated daily use (eg, by bulimic patients) may result in cardiac arrhythmias and cardiomyopathy owing to accumulation of cardiotoxic alkaloids.

4. **Technique.** Use only syrup of ipecac, *not* the fluid extract (which contains much higher concentrations of emetic and cardiotoxic alkaloids).

   a. Administer 30 mL of syrup of ipecac orally (15 mL for children under age 5 years; 10 mL for children under age 1 year; not recommended for children under age 6 months). After 10–15 minutes, give 2–3 glasses of water (there is no consensus on the quantity of water or the timing of administration).

   b. If emesis has not occurred after 20 minutes, give a second dose of ipecac. Repeat the fluid administration. Have the patient sit up or move around, as this sometimes stimulates vomiting.

   c. If the second dose of ipecac does not induce vomiting, then gastric lavage (see **B,** below) should be performed if gastric emptying is still desired. However, it is not necessary to empty the stomach to remove the ipecac.

   d. If ipecac is not available and a pharmacy or emergency department is not within a 10- to 15-minute drive, then soapy water solution may be used as an alternate emetic. Use only standard dishwashing liquid or lotion soap, 2 tablespoons in a glass of water. Do *not* use powdered laundry or dishwasher detergent or liquid dishwashing concentrate; these products are corrosive. There is no other accepted safe alternative to syrup of ipecac. Manual digital stimulation, copper sulfate, salt water, mustard water, apomorphine, and other emetics are unsafe and should not be used.

   e. It is not yet established whether coadministration of activated charcoal with ipecac will result in adequate emesis, although it has been shown that emesis will occur.

B. **Gastric lavage.** Gastric lavage is more invasive than ipecac-induced emesis, but it is a common procedure in most emergency departments and is safe if carefully performed. It is probably slightly more effective than ipecac, especially for recently ingested liquid substances. However, it does not reliably remove undissolved pills or pill fragments (especially sustained-release or enteric-coated products). In addition, the procedure may delay administration of activated charcoal, and may push poisons into the small intestine, especially if the patient is supine or in the right decubitus position. Gastric lavage is probably not necessary for small to moderate ingestions of most substances if activated charcoal can be given promptly.

1. **Indications**

   a. To remove ingested liquid and solid drugs and poisons when the patient has taken a massive overdose.

   b. To administer activated charcoal and cathartics to patients unwilling or unable to swallow them orally.

   c. To dilute and remove corrosive liquids from the stomach and to empty the stomach in preparation for endoscopy.

2. **Contraindications**

   a. Obtunded, comatose, or convulsing patients. Because it may disturb the normal physiology of the esophagus and airway protective mechanisms, gastric lavage must be used with caution in obtunded patients whose airway reflexes are dulled. In such cases, endotracheal intubation with a cuffed endotracheal tube should be performed first to protect the airway.

   b. Ingestion of sustained-release or enteric-coated tablets. Lavage is unlikely to return intact tablets, even through a 40F orogastric hose. In such cases, emesis followed by lavage, or whole bowel irrigation (see p 48), may be preferable to remove as many intact pills as possible.

   c. Ingestion of a corrosive substance is *not* a contraindiction; in fact, many gastroenterologists recommend that immediate lavage be performed after liquid caustic ingestion to remove corrosive material from the stomach and to prepare for endoscopy.

3. Adverse effects

   a. Perforation of the esophagus or stomach.

   b. Nosebleed from nasal trauma during passage of the tube.

   c. Inadvertent tracheal intubation.

   d. Vomiting resulting in pulmonary aspiration of gastric contents in an obtunded patient without airway protection.

4. Technique (see Fig I–9)

   a. Place the patient in the left lateral decubitus position. This helps prevent ingested material from being pushed into the duodenum during lavage.

   b. If the patient is obtunded, protect the airway by intubating the trachea with a cuffed endotracheal tube.

   c. Insert the largest possible gastric tube through the mouth or nose and into the stomach (36–40F in adults; a smaller tube will suffice for liquid poisons). Check tube position with air insufflation while listening over the stomach.

   d. Immediately withdraw as much of the stomach contents as possible, and save the aspirate for possible toxicology screening. If the ingested poison is a toxic chemical that may contaminate hospital personnel (eg, cy-

FIGURE I–9. Gastric lavage.

TABLE I–36. DRUGS AND TOXINS POORLY ADSORBED BY ACTIVATED CHARCOAL[a]

Alkali	Iron
Cyanide[b]	Lithium
Ethanol and other alcohols	Mineral acids
Ethylene glycol	Potassium
Fluoride	

[a]Few studies have been performed to determine in vivo adsorption of these and other toxins to activated charcoal. Adsorption may also depend on the specific type and concentration of charcoal.
[b]Charcoal should still be given because usual doses of charcoal (60–100 g) will adsorb usual lethal ingested doses of cyanide (200–300 mg).

anide, organophosphate insecticide, etc), take steps to immediately isolate it (eg, use a self-contained wall-suction unit).

    e. Administer activated charcoal, 60–100 g (1 g/kg; see **C**, below), down the tube before starting lavage to begin adsorption of material that may enter the intestine during the lavage procedure.

    f. Instill tepid (lukewarm) water or saline, 200–300 mL aliquots, and remove by gravity or active suction. Use repeated aliquots for a total of 2 L or until return is free of pills or toxic material. ***Caution:*** Use of excessive volumes of lavage fluid or plain tap water can result in hypothermia or electrolyte imbalance in infants and small children.

C. Activated charcoal. Activated charcoal is a highly adsorbent powdered material made from distillation of wood pulp. Owing to its very large surface area, it is highly effective in adsorbing most toxins. Only a few toxins are poorly adsorbed to charcoal (Table I–36). Recent studies suggest that activated charcoal given alone without prior gastric emptying is as effective or even more effective than emesis and lavage procedures (see **A** and **B**, above).

    1. Indications

        a. Used after virtually any toxic ingestion to limit drug absorption from the gastrointestinal tract.

        b. Charcoal is usually given even if the offending substance is not known to be well adsorbed to charcoal, in case other substances have been coingested or, as with cyanide, partial adsorption of the ingested poison may be sufficient to limit its toxic effect.

        c. Repeated oral doses of activated charcoal may enhance elimination of some drugs from the bloodstream (see p 52).

    2. Contraindications. Ileus without distension is not a contraindication for a single dose of charcoal.

    3. Adverse effects

        a. Constipation or intestinal impaction/bezoar (may be prevented by coadministration of a cathartic).

        b. Distension of the stomach with potential risk of pulmonary aspiration.

        c. Many commercial charcoal products now available contain charcoal and the cathartic sorbitol in a premixed suspension. Although this is a convenient formulation, repeated doses may cause excessive diarrhea, dehydration, and hypernatremia, especially in young children and elderly persons.

        d. May bind coadministered ipecac or acetylcysteine (not clinically significant).

    4. Technique

        a. Give activated charcoal, 60–100 g (1 g/kg) orally or by gastric tube. If the quantity of ingested substance is known, give at least 10 times the ingested dose of toxin by weight to prevent desorption of the toxin in the lower gastrointestinal tract.

        b. One or 2 additional doses of activated charcoal may be given at 1- or 2-hour intervals to ensure adequate gut decontamination, particularly after large ingestions.

D. Cathartics. Controversy remains over the use of cathartics to hasten elimination of toxins from the gastrointestinal tract. Most toxicologists use cathartics but also recognize that little data exist to support their efficacy.

   1. Indications

      a. To enhance gastrointestinal transit of the charcoal-toxin complex, decreasing the likelihood of desorption of toxin or development of a charcoal bezoar.

      b. To hasten passage of iron tablets and other ingestions not adsorbed by charcoal.

   2. Contraindications

      a. Ileus or intestinal obstruction.

      b. Sodium- and magnesium-containing cathartics should not be used in patients with fluid overload or renal insufficiency, respectively.

      c. There is no role for oil-based cathartics (previously recommended for hydrocarbon poisoning).

   3. Adverse effects

      a. Severe fluid loss, hypernatremia, and hyperosmolarity may result from overuse or repeated doses of cathartics.

      b. Hypermagnesemia may occur in patients with renal insufficiency who are given magnesium-based cathartics.

      c. Abdominal cramping and vomiting may occur, especially with sorbitol.

   4. Technique

      a. Administer cathartic of choice (magnesium citrate 10%, 3–4 mL/kg; or sorbitol 70%, 1–2 mL/kg) along with activated charcoal or mixed together as a slurry.

      b. Repeat one-half the original dose if there is no charcoal stool after 6–8 hours.

E. Whole bowel irrigation. Whole bowel irrigation has become an accepted method for elimination of some toxins from the gut. The technique uses surgical bowel-cleansing polyethylene glycol electrolyte solutions that are formulated to pass through the intestinal tract without being absorbed. These are given in large quantity to force intestinal contents out by sheer volume. There are still some unanswered questions regarding this procedure, including the apparent interaction between activated charcoal and the irrigation solution.

   1. Indications

      a. Large ingestions of iron, lithium, or other drugs poorly adsorbed to activated charcoal.

      b. Possibly, large ingestions of sustained-release or enteric-coated tablets (eg, Theo-dur, Ecotrin, etc) known to be poorly removed by gastric tube, or ingestion of foreign bodies or drug-filled packets or condoms.

   2. Contraindications

      a. Ileus or intestinal obstruction.

      b. Obtunded, comatose, or convulsing patient unless airway is protected.

   3. Adverse effects

      a. Nausea and bloating.

      b. Regurgitation and pulmonary aspiration.

      c. Activated charcoal may not be as effective when given with whole bowel irrigation.

   4. Technique

      a. Administer bowel preparation solution (eg, CoLyte or GoLYTELY), 2 L/h by gastric tube (children, 500 mL/h), until rectal effluent is clear.

      b. Be prepared for large volume stool within 1–2 hours. Pass a rectal tube or, preferably, have the patient sit on a commode.

F. Other oral binding agents. Other binding agents may be given in certain circumstances to trap toxins in the gut, although activated charcoal is the most widely used effective adsorbent. Table I–37 lists some alternative binding agents and the toxin(s) for which they may be useful.

G. Surgical removal. Occasionally, drug-filled packets or condoms, intact tab-

TABLE I–37. SELECTED ORAL BINDING AGENTS

Drug or Toxin	Binding Agent(s)
Calcium	Cellulose sodium phosphate
Chlorinated hydrocarbons	Cholestyramine resin
Digitoxin[a]	Cholestyramine resin
Heavy metals (As, Hg)	Demulcents (egg white, milk)
Iron	Sodium bicarbonate
Lithium	Sodium polystyrene sulfonate (Kayexalate)
Paraquat[a]	Fuller's earth, Bentonite
Potassium	Sodium polystyrene sulfonate (Kayexalate)

[a]Activated charcoal is also very effective.

lets, or tablet concretions persist despite aggressive gastric lavage or whole gut lavage, and surgical removal may be necessary. Consult a regional poison control center (Table I–41, p 53) or a medical toxicologist for advice.

ENHANCED ELIMINATION

Measures to enhance elimination of drugs and toxins have been overemphasized in the past. Although a desirable goal, rapid elimination of most drugs and toxins is frequently not practical and may be unsafe. A logical understanding of pharmacokinetics as they apply to toxicology (toxicokinetics) is necessary for the appropriate use of enhanced removal procedures.

  I. **Assessment.** Three critical questions must be answered.
   A. **Does the patient need enhanced removal?** Ask the following questions: How is the patient doing? Will supportive care enable the patient to recover fully? Is there an antidote or other specific drug that might be used? Important indications for enhanced drug removal include:
      1. Obvious severe or critical intoxication with deteriorating condition despite maximal supportive care (eg, phenobarbital overdose with intractable hypotension).
      2. The normal or usual route of elimination is impaired (eg, lithium overdose in a patient with renal failure).
      3. The patient has ingested a known lethal dose or has a lethal blood level (eg, theophylline, methanol, paraquat).
      4. The patient has underlying medical problems that could increase the hazards of prolonged coma or other complications (eg, severe chronic obstructive pulmonary disease, congestive heart failure).
   B. **Is the drug or toxin accessible to the removal procedure?** For a drug to be accessible to removal by extracorporeal procedures, it should be located primarily within the bloodstream or in the extracellular fluid. If it is extensively distributed to tissues, it is not likely to be easily removed.
      1. **The volume of distribution (Vd)** is a numerical concept that provides an indication of the accessibility of the drug:

      Vd = apparent volume into which the drug is distributed
      = (amount of drug in the body)/(plasma concentration)
      = (mg/kg)/(mg/L) = L/kg

      A drug with a very large Vd has a very low plasma concentration. In contrast, a drug with a small Vd is potentially quite accessible by extracorporeal removal procedures. Table I–38 lists some common volumes of distribution.
      2. **Protein binding** may affect accessibility; highly protein-bound drugs have low free drug concentrations and are difficult to remove by dialysis.
   C. **Will the method work?** Does the removal procedure efficiently extract the toxin from the blood?

TABLE I–38. VOLUME OF DISTRIBUTION (Vd) OF SOME DRUGS AND TOXINS

Large Vd (> 5–10 L/kg)	Small Vd (< 1 L/kg)
Antidepressants	Alcohols
Digoxin	Carbamazepine
Lindane	Lithium
Opiates	Phenobarbital
Phencyclidine (PCP)	Salicylate
Phenothiazines	Theophylline

1. **The clearance (Cl)** is the rate at which a given volume of fluid can be "cleared" of the substance.

   a. The Cl may be calculated from the extraction ratio across the dialysis machine or hemoperfusion column, multiplied by the blood flow rate through the system:

   $$Cl = \text{extraction ratio} \times \text{blood flow rate}$$

   b. A crude urinary Cl may be useful for estimating the effectiveness of fluid therapy for enhancing renal elimination (eg, lithium):

   $$\text{Renal Cl} = \frac{\text{urine level} \times \text{urine flow rate}}{\text{serum level}}$$

   Note: The units of clearance are milliliters per minute. Clearance is not the same as elimination rate (milligrams per minute). If the blood concentration is small, the actual amount of drug removed is also small.

2. **Total clearance** is the sum of all sources of clearance (eg, renal excretion plus hepatic metabolism plus respiratory and skin excretion plus dialysis). If the contribution of dialysis is small compared with the total clearance rate, then the procedure will contribute little to overall elimination rate (Table I–39).

3. The **half-life** $(t\frac{1}{2})$ depends on the volume of distribution and the clearance:

   $$t\frac{1}{2} = \frac{0.693 Vd}{Cl}$$

   where the unit of measurement of Vd is L and of Cl is L/min.

II. Methods available for enhanced elimination

A. **Urinary manipulation.** These methods require that the renal route be a significant contributor to total clearance.

   1. Forced diuresis may increase glomerular filtration rate, and ion trapping by urinary pH manipulation may enhance elimination of polar drugs.

   2. Alkalinization is commonly used for salicylate overdose, but "forced" diuresis (producing urine volumes of up to 1 L/h) is generally not used because of the risk of fluid overload.

B. **Hemodialysis.** Blood is taken from a large vein (usually femoral vein) using a double-lumen catheter and is pumped through the hemodialysis system. The patient must be anticoagulated to prevent clotting of blood in the dialyzer. Drugs and toxins flow passively across the semipermeable membrane down a concentration gradient into a dialysate (electrolyte and buffer) solution. Fluid and electrolyte abnormalities can be corrected concurrently.

   1. Flow rates of up to 300–500 mL/min can be achieved, and clearance rates may reach 200–300 mL/min.

   2. Characteristics of the drug or toxin that enhance its extractability include small size (molecular weight < 500 daltons), water solubility, and low protein binding.

TABLE I–39. ELIMINATION OF SELECTED DRUGS AND TOXINS[a]

Drug or Toxin	Volume of Distribution (L/kg)	Usual Body Clearance (mL/min)	Reported Clearance by:	
			Dialysis (mL/min)	Hemoperfusion[b] (mL/min)
Acetaminophen	0.8–1	400	150	190–300
Amitriptyline	6–10	500–800	NHD[c]	240[d]
Bromide	0.7	5	100	NA[c]
Carbamazepine	1.2	90	NHD	80–90
Digitoxin	0.6	4	10–26	NA
Digoxin	5–6	150–200	NHD	90–140
Ethanol	0.7	100–300	100–200	NHP[c]
Ethchlorvynol	2–4	120–140	20–80	150–300[d]
Ethylene glycol	0.6	200	100–200	NHP
Glutethimide	2.7	200	70	300[d]
Isopropyl alcohol	0.7	30	100–200	NHP
Lithium	0.6–1	25–30	50–150	NHP
Methanol	0.7	40–60	100–200	NHP
Methaqualone	5.8	130–175	23	150–270
Methotrexate	0.5–1	50–100	NA	54
Nortriptyline	20–40	500–1000	24–34	216[d]
Paraquat	2.8	200	10	50–155
Pentobarbital	0.8–1	27	40–55	200–300
Phenobarbital	0.8	2–15	60–75	100–300
Phenytoin	0.6	15–30	NHD	76–189
Procainamide	1.9	650	70	75
N-acetylprocainamide (NAPA)	1.4	220	48	75
Salicylate	0.15	30	35–80	57–116
Theophylline	0.3–0.6	80–120	30–50	60–225
Trichloroethanol	0.6–1.6	25	68–162	119–200

[a]Adapted in part from Pond SM: Diuresis, dialysis, and hemoperfusion: Indications and benefits. *Emerg Med Clin North Am* 1984;2:29.
[b]Hemoperfusion data are mainly for charcoal hemoperfusion.
[c]Abbreviations: NHD = not hemodialyzable; NA = not available; NHP = not hemoperfusable.
[d]Data are for XAD-4 resin hemoperfusion.

   3. **Note:** Smaller, portable dialysis units that utilize a resin column or filter to recycle a smaller volume dialysate ("mini-dialysis") do not efficiently remove drugs or poisons and should not be used.
C. **Hemoperfusion.** Using equipment and vascular access similar to that for hemodialysis, the blood is pumped directly through a column containing an adsorbent material (either charcoal or Amberlite resin). Systemic anticoagulation is required, often in higher doses than for hemodialysis, and thrombocytopenia is a common complication.
   1. Because the drug or toxin is in direct contact with the adsorbent material, drug size, water solubility, and protein binding are not important limiting factors.
   2. For most drugs, hemoperfusion can achieve greater clearance rates than

TABLE I–40. SOME DRUGS REMOVED BY REPEAT-DOSE ACTIVATED CHARCOAL

Carbamazepine	Phenobarbital
Chlordecone	Phenylbutazone
Dapsone	Phenytoin
Digitoxin	Salicylate
Nadolol	Theophylline

hemodialysis. For example, the hemodialysis clearance for phenobarbital is 60–80 mL/min, whereas the hemoperfusion clearance is 200–300 mL/min.

D. Peritoneal dialysis. Dialysate fluid is poured into the peritoneal cavity through a transcutaneous catheter and drained off, and the procedure is repeated with fresh dialysate. The gut wall and peritoneal lining serve as the semipermeable membrane.

    1. Peritoneal dialysis is easier to perform than hemodialysis or hemoperfusion and does not require anticoagulation, but it is only about 10–15% as effective owing to poor extraction ratios and slower flow rates (clearance rates, 10–15 mL/min).

    2. However, peritoneal dialysis can be performed continuously, 24 hours a day: a 24-hour peritoneal dialysis with dialysate exchange every 1–2 hours is approximately equal to 4 hours of hemodialysis.

E. Repeat-dose activated charcoal. Repeated doses of activated charcoal (20–30 g or 0.5–1 g/kg every 2–3 hours) are given orally or via gastric tube. A constant slurry of activated charcoal in the intestinal lumen extracts drug or toxin from the gut wall in a kind of "gut dialysis" quite distinct from simple adsorption of ingested unabsorbed tablets. This technique is easy and noninvasive and has been shown to shorten the half-life of phenobarbital, theophylline, and several other drugs (Table I–40). *Caution:* Repeat-dose charcoal may cause serious fluid and electrolyte disturbance secondary to large-volume diarrhea, especially if premixed charcoal-sorbitol suspensions are used. Also, it should not be used in patients with ileus or obstruction.

DISPOSITION OF THE PATIENT

I. Emergency department discharge or intensive care unit admission?

    A. All patients with potentially serious overdose should be observed for at least 6 hours before transfer to a nonmedical (eg, psychiatric) facility or discharge. If signs or symptoms of intoxication develop during this time, admission for further observation and treatment is required.

    B. Beware of delayed complications from slow absorption of medications (eg, from a tablet concretion or bezoar, or sustained-release or enteric-coated preparations). If specific drug levels are determined, obtain repeated serum levels to be certain that they are decreasing as expected.

    C. Most patients admitted for poisoning or drug overdose will need observation in an intensive care unit, although this depends on the potential for serious cardiorespiratory complications. Any patient with suicidal intent must be kept under close observation.

II. Regional poison control center consultation. Consult with a regional poison control center to determine the need for further observation or admission, administration of antidotes or therapeutic drugs, selection of appropriate laboratory tests, or decisions about extracorporeal removal. An experienced clinical toxicologist is usually available for immediate consultation. See Table I–41 for a list of regional poison control centers (certified by the American Association of Poison Control Centers).

III. Psychosocial evaluation

    A. Psychiatric consultation for suicide risk. All patients with intentional poisoning or drug overdose should have psychiatric evaluation for suicidal intent.

        1. It is not appropriate to discharge a potentially suicidal patient from the emer-

TABLE I–41. AAPCC-CERTIFIED[a] REGIONAL POISON CONTROL CENTERS IN THE USA[b]

State	Poison Center	Phone Number
Alabama	Children's Hospital of Alabama, Birmingham	(800) 292–6678 (AL only) (205) 939–9201
Arizona	Arizona Poison and Drug Information Center, Tucson	(800) 362–0101 (AZ only) (602) 626–6016
	Samaritan Regional Poison Center, Phoenix	(602) 253–3334
California	Fresno Regional Poison Control Center, Fresno	(800) 346–5922 (CA only) (209) 445–1222
	San Diego Regional Poison Center, University of California, San Diego	(800) 876–4766 (CA only) (619) 543–6000
	San Francisco Bay Area Regional Poison Center, San Francisco	(800) 523–2222 (CA only)
	Santa Clara Valley Regional Poison Center, San Jose	(800) 662–9886 (CA only) (408) 299–5112
	UC Davis Medical Center Regional Poison Center, Sacramento	(800) 342–9293 (CA only) (916) 734–3692
Colorado (also Montana)	Rocky Mountain Poison Center, Denver	(303) 629–1123
Florida	Florida Poison Information Center, Tampa	(800) 282–3171 (FL only) (813) 253–4444
Georgia	Georgia Poison Center, Atlanta	(800) 282–5846 (GA only) (404) 589–4400
Indiana	Indiana Poison Center, Indianapolis	(800) 382–9097 (IN only) (317) 929–2323
Maryland	Maryland Poison Center, Baltimore	(800) 492–2414 (MD only) (410) 528 –7701
Massachusetts	Massachusetts Poison Control System, Boston	(800) 682–9211 (MA only) (617) 232–2120
Michigan	Blodgett Regional Poison Center, Grand Rapids	(800) 632–2727 (MI only)
	Poison Control Center, Children's Hospital, Detroit	(313) 745–5711
Minnesota	Hennepin Regional Poison Center, Minneapolis	(612) 347–3141
	Minnesota Regional Poison Center, St Paul	(612) 221–2113
Missouri	Cardinal Glennon Children's Hospital Regional Poison Center, St Louis	(800) 366–8888 (MO only) (314) 772–5200
Montana	*See* Colorado	
Nebraska (also Wyoming)	Mid-Plains Poison Center, Omaha	(800) 955–9119 (NE only) (402) 390–5555
New Jersey	New Jersey Poison Information and Education System, Newark	(800) 962–1253 (NJ only)
New Mexico	New Mexico Poison and Drug Information Center, Albuquerque	(800) 432–6866 (NM only) (505) 843–2551
New York	Hudson Valley Poison Center, Nyack	(800) 336–6997 (914) 353–1000
	Long Island Regional Poison Control Center, East Meadow	(516) 542–2323
	New York City Poison Center, New York City	(212) 340–4494 (212) 764–7667
Ohio	Central Ohio Poison Center, Columbus	(800) 682–7625 (OH only) (614) 228–1323
	Cincinnati Drug and Poison Information Center, Cincinnati	(800) 872–5111 (513) 558–5111

(*continued*)

TABLE I–41. AAPCC-CERTIFIED[a] REGIONAL POISON CONTROL CENTERS IN THE USA[b] (*Continued*)

State	Poison Center	Phone Number
Oregon	Oregon Poison Center, Portland	(800) 452–7165 (OR only) (503) 494–8968
Pennsylvania	Central Pennsylvania Poison Center, Hershey	(800) 521–6110
	Pittsburgh Poison Center, Pittsburgh	(412) 681–6669
	The Poison Center, Philadelphia	(215) 386–2100
Rhode Island	Rhode Island Poison Center, Providence	(401) 277–5727
Texas	North Texas Poison Center, Dallas	(800) 441–0040 (TX only) (214) 590–5000
	Texas State Poison Center, Galveston Houston	(409) 765–1420 (713) 654–1701
Utah	Intermountain Regional Poison Center, Salt Lake City	(800) 456–7707 (UT only) (801) 581–2151
Virginia	Blue Ridge Poison Center, Charlottesville	(800) 451–1428 (804) 924–5543
Washington, DC	National Capitol Poison Center, Washington, DC	(202) 625–3333
West Virginia	West Virginia Poison Center, Charleston	(800) 642–3625 (WV only) (304) 348–4211
Wyoming	*See* Nebraska	

[a]AAPCC, American Association of Poison Control Centers.
[b]AAPCC Regional Certification Committee, April 1993.

gency department without a careful psychiatric evaluation. Most states have provisions for the physician to place an emergency psychiatric hold, forcing involuntary patients to remain under psychiatric observation for up to 72 hours.

2. Patients calling from home after an intentional ingestion should always be referred to an emergency department for medical and psychiatric evaluation.

B. Child abuse (see also p 56) or sexual abuse

1. Children should be evaluated for the possibility that the ingestion was not accidental. Sometimes parents or other adults intentionally give children sedatives or tranquilizers to control their behavior.

2. Accidental poisonings may also warrant social services referral. Occasionally children get into stimulants or other abused drugs that are left around the home. Repeated ingestions suggest overly casual or negligent parental behavior.

3. Intentional overdose in a child or adolescent should raise the possibility of physical or sexual abuse. Teenage girls may have overdosed because of unwanted pregnancy.

IV. Overdose in the pregnant patient

A. In general, it is prudent to check for pregnancy in any young woman with drug overdose or poisoning. Unwanted pregnancy may be a cause for intentional overdose, or special concerns may be raised about treatment of the pregnant patient.

B. Inducing emesis with syrup of ipecac is probably safe in early pregnancy, but protracted vomiting is unwelcome, especially in the third trimester. Gastric lavage or oral activated charcoal is preferable in all trimesters.

C. Some toxins are known to be teratogenic or mutagenic (Table I–42). However, adverse effects to the fetus are generally associated with chronic, repeated use as opposed to acute, single exposure.

TABLE I–42. HUMAN TERATOGENS[a]

Alcohol (ethanol)
Alkylating agents (busulfan, chlorambucil, cyclophosphamide, mustine/mechlorethamine)
Antimetabolic agents (aminopterin, azauridine, cytarabine, fluorouracil, 6-mercaptopurine, methotrexate)
Carbon monoxide
Coumadins
Diethylstilbestrol (DES)
Disulfiram
Heparin
Lithium carbonate
Mercuric sulfide
Methyl mercury
Phenytoin
Polychlorinated biphenyls (PCBs)
Tetracycline
Thalidomide
Tretinoin (retinoic acid)
Trimethadione
Valproic acid

[a]Reference: Bologa-Campeanu M et al: Prenatal adverse effects of various drugs and chemicals: A review of substances of frequent concern to mothers in the community. *Med Toxicol Adverse Drug Exp* 1988;3:307.

SPECIAL CONSIDERATIONS IN PEDIATRIC PATIENTS

Delia A. Dempsey, MD, MS

The majority of calls to poison control centers involve children under 5 years of age. Fortunately, children account for only a minority of serious poisonings requiring emergency hospital treatment. Most common childhood ingestions involve nontoxic substances or nontoxic doses of potentially toxic drugs or products (see p 235). The leading causes of serious or fatal childhood poisoning include iron supplements (see p 189); cyclic antidepressants (see p 147); cardiovascular medications such as digitalis (see p 124), beta blockers (p 99) or calcium antagonists (p 113); methyl salicylate (p 277); and hydrocarbons (p 178).

I. **High-risk populations.** Two age groups are commonly involved in pediatric poisonings: children between 1 and 5 years old, and adolescents.

   A. **Ingestions in toddlers and young children** usually result from oral exploration. Unintentional ingestion in children under 6 months of age or between the ages of 5 and adolescence is rare. In young infants, consider the possibility of intentional administration by an older child or adult. In older children, suspect a suicidal attempt.

   B. **In adolescents and young adults,** overdoses are usually suicidal but may also result from drug abuse or experimentation. Common underlying reasons for adolescents' suicide attempts include: pregnancy; sexual, physical, or mental abuse; school failure; conflict with peers; conflict with homosexual or lesbian orientation; a sudden or severe loss; and alcoholism or illicit drug use. Any adolescent who makes a suicide attempt or gesture needs psychiatric evaluation and follow-up.

II. **Poisoning prevention.** Young children with an unintentional ingestion are at higher risk for a second ingestion than the general pediatric population. After an ingestion, prevention strategies need to be reviewed. If the family does not understand the instructions or it is the second poisoning, consider a home evaluation for childproofing by a public health nurse or other health care professional.

   A. **Childproof** the home, day-care setting, and households the child commonly visits (eg, grandparents, other relatives). Store medicines, chemicals, and cleaning products out of the reach of children or in locked cabinets. Do not store chemicals in food containers, and do not store chemicals in the same cabinets as food. Common places children find medications include visitors' purses or backpacks and bedside tables.

B. Use child-resistant containers to store prescription and nonprescription medications. However, child-resistant containers are not childproof; they only slow down the time it takes a determined child to get into the container.

C. Dispense syrup of ipecac (see p 345) to the home and day-care setting in case of an ingestion.

III. Child abuse. Consider the possibility that the child was intentionally given the drug or toxin. Most states require that all health care professionals report suspected cases of child abuse or neglect, which means that it is not a discretionary decision but a legal obligation to report *any* suspicious incident. The parents or guardians should be informed in a straightforward, nonjudgmental manner that a report is being made under this legal obligation. In serious cases, the suspected abuse report should be made before the child is released, and the local child protective services should decide if it is safe to release the child to the parents or guardians. In unclear situations, the child can be admitted for "observation" to allow time for social services to make an expeditious evaluation. The following should alert medical personnel to the possibility of abuse or neglect:

A. The story does not make sense or does not ring true, or it changes over time, or different people give different stories.

B. The child is nonambulatory (eg, child under 6 months of age). Carefully review how the child gained access to the drug or toxin.

C. The child is over 4–5 years old. Accidental ingestions are rare in older children; suicide attempt and abuse should not be ruled out.

D. The drug ingested was a tranquilizer (eg, haloperidol, chlorpromazine), a drug of abuse (eg, cocaine, heroin), a sedative (eg, diazepam), or ethanol, or the parents are intoxicated.

E. There is a long interval between the time of ingestion and the time the child is taken for medical evaluation.

F. There are signs of physical or sexual abuse or neglect: multiple or unusual bruises; a broken bone or burns; a very dirty, unkempt child; a child with a flat affect or indifferent or inappropriate behavior. A nonpediatrician who suspects physical or sexual abuse in addition to a poisoning should consider a pediatric evaluation.

G. A history of repeated episodes of possible or documented poisonings, or a history of prior abuse.

H. Munchausen syndrome by proxy: Drugs or toxins are given to the child to simulate illness. Most perpetrators are mothers, often with some medical background. This is a rare diagnosis.

IV. Clinical evaluation. The physical and laboratory evaluation is essentially the same as for adults. However, normal vital signs vary with age (see Table I–43).

A. Heart rate. Newborns may have normal heart rates as high as 190/min, and 2 years olds up to 120/min. Abnormal tachycardia or bradycardia suggests the possibility of hypoxemia, in addition to the numerous drugs and poisons that affect heart rate and rhythm (see Tables I–4 through I–7).

B. Blood pressure is a very important vital sign in a poisoned child. The blood pressure cuff must be of the proper size; cuffs that are too small can falsely elevate the pressure. Blood pressures on infants are difficult to obtain by auscultation but are easily obtained by doppler.

1. Many children normally have a lower blood pressure than adults. However, low blood pressure in the context of a poisoning should be regarded as normal only if the child is alert, active, appropriate, and has normal peripheral perfusion.

2. Idiopathic or essential hypertension is rare in children. Elevated blood pressure should be assumed acute in nature, although the systolic blood pressure can be transiently elevated if the child is vigorously crying or screaming. Unless a child's baseline blood pressure is known, values at the upper limit of normal should be assumed "elevated." The decision to treat an elevated blood pressure must be made on an individual basis, based on the clinical scenario and the toxin involved.

TABLE I-43. PEDIATRIC VITAL SIGNS[a]

Age	Respiratory Rate (/min)	Heart Rate (/min)	Blood Pressure (mm Hg)			
			Lower Limit	Average	Upper Limit	Severe
Newborn	30–80	110–190	52/25	50–55[b]	95/72	110/85
1 month	30–50	100–170	64/30	85/50	105/68	120/85
6 months	30–50	100–170	60/40	90/55	110/72	125/85
1 year	20–40	100–160	66/40	90/55	110/72	125/88
2 years	20–30	100–160	74/40	90/55	110/72	125/88
4 years	20–25	80–130	79/45	95/55	112/75	128/88
8 years	15–25	70–110	85/48	100/60	118/75	135/92
12 years	15–20	60–100	95/50	108/65	125/84	142/95

[a]References: Dieckmann RA, Coulter K: Pediatric emergencies. Page 811 in: *Current Emergency Diagnosis and Treatment, 4th ed.* Saunders CE, Ho MT (editors). Appleton & Lange, 1992; Gundy JH: The pediatric physical exam. Page 68 in: *Primary Pediatric Care.* Hoekelman RA et al (editors). Mosby, 1987; Hoffman JIE: Systemic arterial hypertension. Page 1438 in: *Rudolph's Pediatrics,* 19th ed. Rudolph AM et al (editors). Appleton & Lange 1991; Liebman J, Freed MD: Cardiovascular system. Page 447 in: *Nelson's Essentials of Pediatrics.* Behrman RE, Kleigman R (editors). Saunders, 1990; Lum GM: Kidney and urinary tract. Page 624 in: *Current Pediatric Diagnosis and Treatment,* 10th ed. Hathaway WE et al (editors). Appleton & Lange, 1991.
[b]Mean arterial pressure range on the first day of life.

V. Neonates present specific problems, including unique pharmacokinetics and potentially severe withdrawal from prenatal drug exposure.
    A. Neonatal pharmacokinetics. The newborn (birth to 1 month) and infants (1–12 months) are unique from a toxicologic and pharmacologic perspective. Drug absorption, distribution, and elimination are different from those of older children and adults. Incorrect dosing, transplacental passage proximate to the time of birth, breast-feeding, dermal absorption, and intentional poisoning are potential routes of toxic exposure. Of particular importance are enhanced skin absorption and reduced drug elimination, which may lead to toxicity after relatively mild exposure.
        1. Skin absorption. Neonates have a very high surface area to body weight, which predisposes them to poisoning via percutaneous absorption (eg, hexachlorophene, boric acid, alcohols).
        2. Elimination of many drugs (eg, acetaminophen, many antibiotics, caffeine, lidocaine, morphine, phenytoin, theophylline) is prolonged in neonates. For example, the half-life of caffeine is approximately 3 hours in adults but greater than 100 hours in newborns.
    B. Neonatal drug withdrawal may occur in infants with chronic prenatal exposure to illicit or therapeutic drugs. The onset is usually within 72 hours of birth, but an onset as late as 14 days has been reported. Signs usually commence in the nursery and infants are not discharged until clinically stable. However, with early discharge from nurseries becoming the norm, an infant in withdrawal may first present to an emergency department or acute care clinic. The presentation may be as mild as colic or severe as withdrawal seizures or profound diarrhea.
        1. Opioids (especially methadone and heroin; also pentazocine, propoxyphene) are the most common cause of serious neonatal drug withdrawal symptoms. **Other drugs** for which a withdrawal syndrome has been reported include phencyclidine (PCP), cocaine, amphetamines, cyclic antidepressants, phenothiazines, benzodiazepines, barbiturates, ethanol, clonidine, diphenhydramine, lithium, meprobamate, and theophylline. A careful drug history from the mother should include illicit drugs, alcohol, and pre-

scription and over-the-counter medications, and whether she is breast feeding.

2. **The manifestations of neonatal opioid withdrawal** include inability to sleep, irritability, tremulousness, inconsolability, high-pitched incessant cry, hypertonia, hyperreflexia, sneezing and yawning, lacrimation, disorganized suck, poor feeding, vomiting, diarrhea, tachypnea or respiratory distress, tachycardia, autonomic dysfunction, sweating, fevers, and seizures. Morbidity and mortality from untreated opioid withdrawal can be significant and commonly result from weight loss, metabolic acidosis, respiratory alkalosis, dehydration, electrolyte imbalance, and seizures. Withdrawal is a diagnosis of exclusion; immediately rule out sepsis, hypoglycemia, hypocalcemia, and hypoxia, and consider hyperbilirubinemia, hypomagnesemia, hyperthyroidism, and intracranial hemorrhage. Seizures do not usually occur as the only clinical manifestation of opioid withdrawal.

3. **Treatment of neonatal opioid withdrawal** is mainly supportive and includes swaddling, rocking, a subdued room, frequent small feedings with high caloric formula, and IV fluids if necessary. A variety of drugs have been used, including morphine, paregoric, tincture of opium, diazepam, lorazepam, chlorpromazine, and phenobarbital. Numerous abstinence scoring systems exist to objectively evaluate and treat opioid withdrawal. *The scoring and treatment of a neonate in withdrawal should be supervised by a neonatologist or a pediatrician experienced with neonatal withdrawal.*

GENERAL REFERENCES IN CLINICAL TOXICOLOGY

Doull J, Klaassen C, Amdur M (editors): *Casarett and Doull's Toxicology: The Basic Science of Poisons,* 3rd ed. MacMillan, 1990.

Ellenhorn M, Barceloux D: *Medical Toxicology.* Elsevier, 1988.

Goldfrank LR et al (editors): *Goldfrank's Toxicologic Emergencies,* 4th ed. Appleton & Lange, 1990.

Gosselin RE et al: *Clinical Toxicology of Commercial Products,* 6th ed. Williams & Wilkins, 1988.

Haddad LM, Winchester JF (editors): *Clinical Management of Poisoning and Drug Overdose,* 2nd ed. Saunders, 1990.

Rumack BH (editor): *Poisindex* [computerized poison information system]. Micromedex [updated quarterly].

SECTION II. Specific Poisons and Drugs: Diagnosis and Treatment

ACETAMINOPHEN
Kent R. Olson, MD

ANTIDOTE   IPECAC   LAVAGE   CHARCOAL

Acetaminophen (Anacin-3, Liquiprin, Panadol, Paracetamol, Tempra, Tylenol) is a widely used drug found in many over-the-counter and prescription analgesics and cold remedies. When it is combined with another drug such as codeine or propoxyphene, the more dramatic acute symptoms caused by the other toxin may mask the mild and nonspecific symptoms of early acetaminophen toxicity, resulting in missed diagnosis or delayed antidotal treatment. *Common combination products containing acetamino-*

LEGEND

Not Indicated
or
Not Available   Questionable
Value or
Controversial   ANTIDOTE   IPECAC   LAVAGE   CHARCOAL

phen include Comtrex, Darvocet, Excedrin ES, Nyquil, Percocet, Unisom Dual Relief Formula, Sominex 2, Tylenol with codeine, Tylox, Vicks Formula 44-D, and Vicodin.

I. **Mechanism of toxicity.** One of the products of normal metabolism of acetaminophen by the cytochrome P-450 mixed oxidase system is hepatotoxic; normally, this reactive metabolite is rapidly detoxified by glutathione in the liver. However, in overdose, production of the toxic metabolite exceeds glutathione capacity and the metabolite reacts directly with hepatic macromolecules, causing liver injury. Renal damage may occur by the same mechanism owing to renal metabolism. Overdose during pregnancy has been associated with fetal death and spontaneous abortion.

II. **Toxic dose**
   A. **Acute ingestion** of more than 140 mg/kg in children or 6 g in adults is potentially hepatotoxic.
      1. Children younger than 10–12 years of age appear to be less susceptible to hepatotoxicity because of the smaller contribution of cytochrome P-450 to acetaminophen metabolism.
      2. On the other hand, the margin of safety is lower in chronic alcoholics and other patients with induced cytochrome P-450 microsomal enzymes, because more of the toxic metabolite may be produced in these patients.
   B. **Chronic toxicity** has been reported after daily consumption of high therapeutic doses (4–6 g) by alcoholics.

III. **Clinical presentation.** Clinical manifestations depend upon the time after ingestion.
   A. **Early** after acute acetaminophen overdose, there are no symptoms other than anorexia, nausea, or vomiting.
   B. **After 24–48 hours,** when prothrombin time (PT) and transaminase levels rise, hepatic necrosis becomes evident. If acute hepatic failure occurs, encephalopathy and death may ensue. Encephalopathy, metabolic acidosis, and a continuing rise in the PT indicate a poor prognosis. Acute renal failure occasionally occurs, with or without concomitant liver failure.

IV. **Diagnosis** is possible only if the ingestion is suspected early and a serum acetaminophen level is obtained. However, patients may fail to provide the history of acetaminophen ingestion, because they are unable (eg, comatose from another ingestion), unwilling, or unaware of its importance. Therefore, many clinicians routinely order stat acetaminophen levels in all overdose patients, regardless of the history of substance ingested.
   A. **Specific levels.** Obtain a 4-hour postingestion acetaminophen level and use the nomogram (Fig II–1) to predict the range of severity. Falsely elevated acetaminophen levels may occur in the presence of high levels of salicylate and other interferents by certain methods (see Section I, Table I–32, p 40).
   B. **Other useful laboratory studies.** Electrolytes, glucose, BUN, creatinine, liver transaminases, prothrombin time.

V. **Treatment**
   A. **Emergency and supportive measures**
      1. **Spontaneous vomiting** may delay the administration of antidote and charcoal (see below) and should be treated with metoclopramide (see p 352).
      2. Provide general supportive care for hepatic or renal failure if it occurs. **Liver transplant** may be necessary for massive hepatic failure.
   B. **Specific drugs and antidotes.** If the serum level falls above the lower ("probable toxicity") line on the nomogram or if stat serum levels are not immediately available, start antidotal therapy with **acetylcysteine** (NAC, Mucomyst, p 311), 140 mg/kg orally. The effectiveness of this therapy depends on **early treatment,** before the metabolite accumulates; it is of maximal benefit if started within 8–10 hours, and of diminishing value after 12–16 hours (however, treatment should not be withheld, even if the delay is 24 hours or more). If vomiting interferes with oral acetylcysteine administration, give it by gastric tube and use high-dose metoclopramide (60–70 mg IV in adults, see p 352), if necessary.
   C. **Decontamination** (see p 44)
      1. **Prehospital.** Administer activated charcoal, if available. Ipecac-induced emesis may be useful for initial treatment of children at home if it can be given within 30 minutes of exposure.

Figure II–1. Nomogram for prediction of acetaminophen hepatoxicity following acute overdosage. The upper line defines serum acetaminophen concentrations known to be associated with hepatotoxicity; the lower line defines serum levels 25% below those expected to cause hepatotoxicity. To give a margin for error, the lower line should be used as a guide to treatment. (Modified and reproduced, with permission, from Rumack BM, Matthew M: Acetaminophen poisoning and toxicity. *Pediatrics* 1975;**55**:871.)

2. **Hospital.** Administer activated charcoal and a cathartic. Although activated charcoal adsorbs some of the orally administered antidote *n*-acetylcysteine, this effect is not considered clinically important. Gastric emptying is not necessary if charcoal can be given promptly.

D. **Enhanced elimination.** Hemoperfusion effectively removes acetaminophen from the blood but is not generally indicated because antidotal therapy is so effective.

AMANTADINE
Christopher R. Brown, MD

ANTIDOTE   IPECAC   LAVAGE   CHARCOAL

Amantadine (Symmetrel) is an antiviral agent that is also effective in the treatment of Parkinson's disease and for prophylaxis against the parkinsonian side effects of neuroleptic agents. It has also been advocated for use in therapy of cocaine addiction. Although there is limited information about its effects in acute overdose, it has been associated with seizures, arrhythmias, neuroleptic malignant syndrome, and death.

I. **Mechanism of toxicity.** Amantadine is thought to both enhance the release of dopamine and prevent dopamine reuptake in the peripheral and central nervous systems. In addition, it has anticholinergic properties, especially in overdose.

II. **Toxic dose.** The toxic dose has not been determined. Because the elimination of amantadine depends entirely on kidney function, elderly patients with renal insufficiency may develop intoxication with therapeutic doses.

III. **Clinical presentation**

A. **Amantadine intoxication** causes agitation, visual hallucinations, nightmares, disorientation, delirium, slurred speech, ataxia, myoclonus, tremor, and sometimes seizures. Anticholinergic manifestations include dry mouth, urinary retention, and mydriasis. Rarely, ventricular arrhythmias including torsades de pointes (see p 14) and multifocal premature ventricular contractions may occur. Amantadine has also been reported to cause heart failure.

B. Amantadine withdrawal, either after standard therapeutic use or in the days following an acute overdose, may result in hyperthermia and rigidity (possibly a form of neuroleptic malignant syndrome; see p 20).

IV. Diagnosis is based on a history of acute ingestion or by noting the above-mentioned constellation of symptoms and signs in a patient taking amantadine.

    A. Specific levels are not readily available. Serum levels above 1.5 mg/L have been associated with toxicity.

    B. Other useful laboratory studies. Electrolytes, BUN, creatinine, ECG.

V. Treatment

    A. Emergency and supportive measures

        1. Maintain the airway and assist ventilation if necessary (see p 4).

        2. Treat coma (p 18), seizures (p 22), arrhythmias (p 14), and hyperthermia (p 20) if they occur.

        3. Monitor the asymptomatic patient for at least 8–12 hours after acute ingestion.

    B. Specific drugs and antidotes. There is no known antidote. Although some of the manifestations of toxicity are caused by anticholinergic effects of amantadine, physostigmine should not be used.

        1. Treat **tachyarrhythmias** with beta blockers such as propranolol (see p 373) or esmolol (p 338).

        2. Neuroleptic malignant syndrome (NMS) requires urgent cooling measures (p 20) and may respond to specific pharmacologic therapy with dantrolene (p 325). When NMS occurs in the setting of amantadine withdrawal, some have advocated using amantadine as therapy.

    C. Decontamination (see p 44)

        1. Prehospital. Administer activated charcoal, if available. Ipecac-induced emesis may be useful for initial treatment of children at home if it can be given within 30 minutes of exposure.

        2. Hospital. Administer activated charcoal and a cathartic. Gastric emptying is not necessary if activated charcoal can be given promptly.

    D. Enhanced elimination. Amantadine is not effectively removed by dialysis, because the volume of distribution is very large (5 L/kg). The serum elimination half-life ranges from 12 hours to 34 days, depending on renal function. In a patient with no renal function, dialysis or hemoperfusion may be necessary.

AMMONIA
Kent R. Olson, MD

ANTIDOTE   IPECAC   LAVAGE   CHARCOAL

Ammonia is widely used as a refrigerant, a fertilizer, and a household and commercial cleaning agent. Anhydrous ammonia (NH_3) is a highly irritating gas that is very water-soluble. Aqueous solutions of ammonia may be strongly alkaline, depending on the concentration. Solutions for household use are usually 5–10% ammonia, but commercial solutions may be 25–30% or more. Addition of ammonia to chlorine or hypochlorite solutions will produce chloramine gas, an irritant gas with similar properties.

    I. Mechanism of toxicity. Ammonia gas is highly water-soluble and rapidly produces an alkaline corrosive effect on contact with moist tissues such as the eyes and upper respiratory tract. Exposure to aqueous solutions causes corrosive alkaline injury to the eyes, skin, or gastrointestinal tract (see Caustic and Corrosive Agents, p 126).

II. Toxic dose

A. Ammonia gas. The odor of ammonia is detectable at 50 ppm, and eye irritation is common at 100 ppm. The workplace recommended exposure limit (ACGIH TLV-TWA) for anhydrous ammonia gas is 25 ppm as an 8-hour time-weighted average. The level considered immediately dangerous to life or health (IDLH) is 500 ppm.

B. Aqueous solutions. Dilute aqueous solutions of ammonia (eg, < 5%) rarely cause serious burns but are moderately irritating. More concentrated industrial cleaners (eg, 25–30%) are much more likely to cause serious corrosive injury.

III. Clinical presentation. Clinical manifestations depend on physical state and route of exposure.

A. Inhalation of ammonia gas. Symptoms are rapid in onset owing to the high water-solubility of ammonia and include immediate burning of the eyes, nose, and throat, accompanied by coughing. With serious exposure, upper airway swelling may rapidly cause airway obstruction, preceded by croupy cough, hoarseness, and stridor. Bronchospasm with wheezing may occur. With very large exposure, noncardiogenic pulmonary edema may also occur.

B. Ingestion of aqueous solutions. Immediate burning in the mouth and throat is common. With more concentrated solutions, serious esophageal and gastric burns are common, and victims have dysphagia, drooling, and severe throat, chest, and abdominal pain. Hematemesis and perforation of the esophagus or stomach may occur. The absence of oral burns does not rule out significant esophageal or gastric injury.

C. Skin or eye contact with gas or solution. Serious alkaline corrosive burns may occur.

IV. Diagnosis is based on a history of exposure and description of the typical ammonia smell, accompanied by typical irritative or corrosive effects on the eyes, skin, and upper respiratory or gastrointestinal tract.

A. Specific levels. Blood ammonia levels may be elevated (normal 8–33 μmol/L) but are not predictive of toxicity.

B. Other useful laboratory studies. Electrolytes, arterial blood gases or pulse oximetry, chest x-ray.

V. Treatment

A. Emergency and supportive measures. Treatment depends on the physical state and the route of exposure.

1. Inhalation of ammonia gas

a. Observe carefully for signs of progressive upper airway obstruction, and intubate early if necessary (see p 3).

b. Administer humidified supplemental oxygen and bronchodilators for wheezing (p 9). Treat noncardiogenic pulmonary edema (p 8) if it occurs.

c. Asymptomatic or mildly symptomatic patients may be sent home after brief (1–2 hours) observation.

2. Ingestion of aqueous solution. If a solution of 10% or greater has been ingested or if there are any symptoms of corrosive injury (dysphagia, drooling, pain), perform flexible endoscopy to evaluate for serious esophageal or gastric injury. Obtain a chest x-ray to look for mediastinal air, which suggests esophageal perforation.

3. Eye exposure. After eye irrigation, perform fluorescein examination and refer to an ophthalmologist if there is evidence of corneal injury.

B. Specific drugs and antidotes. There is no specific antidote for these or other common caustic burns. Although administration of corticosteroids was previously recommended in hopes of limiting esophageal scarring, this treatment has been proved ineffective and may be harmful in patients with perforation or serious infection.

C. Decontamination

1. Inhalation. Remove immediately from exposure, and give supplemental oxygen if available.

2. Ingestion (see p 44)

    a. Prehospital. Immediately give water or milk by mouth to dilute the ammonia. Do *not* induce emesis, as this may aggravate corrosive effects.

    b. Hospital. Gastric lavage is recommended in order to remove any liquid caustic in the stomach and to prepare for endoscopy; use a small, flexible tube and pass gently to avoid injury to damaged mucosa.

    c. Do *not* use activated charcoal; it does not adsorb ammonia, and it may obscure the endoscopist's view.

3. Skin and eyes. Remove contaminated clothing and wash exposed skin with water. Irrigate exposed eyes with copious amounts of tepid water or saline (see p 41).

D. Enhanced elimination. There is no role for dialysis or other enhanced elimination procedures.

AMPHETAMINES
Neal L. Benowitz, MD

ANTIDOTE   IPECAC   LAVAGE   CHARCOAL

Dextroamphetamine (Dexedrine) and methylphenidate (Ritalin) are used for the treatment of narcolepsy and for attention-deficit disorders in children. Several amphetaminelike drugs (benzphetamine, diethylpropion, phendimetrazine, phenmetrazine, and phenteramine) are marketed as prescription anorectic medications for use in weight reduction (Table II–1). Methamphetamine (crank, speed), 3,4-methylenedioxymethamphetamine (MDMA, ecstasy), and several other amphetamine derivatives (see Lysergic Acid Diethylamide [LSD] and Other Hallucinogens, p 204), as well as a number of prescription drugs, are used orally and intravenously as illicit stimulants. "Ice" is a smokable form of methamphetamine.

Phenylpropanolamine, ephedrine, and other over-the-counter decongestants are discussed on p 253.

I. Mechanism of toxicity. Amphetaminelike drugs act primarily by activating the sympathetic nervous system via central nervous system stimulation, peripheral release of catecholamines, inhibition of neuronal reuptake of catecholamines, or inhibition of monoamine oxidase. The various drugs have different profiles of action resulting from different levels of central nervous system and peripheral stimulation. All these drugs are well absorbed orally and are generally extensively metabolized by the liver. Excretion of most amphetamines is highly dependent on urine pH, with amphetamines being more rapidly eliminated in acid urine.

II. Toxic dose. These drugs have a low therapeutic index, with toxicity at levels only slightly above usual doses. However, a high degree of tolerance can develop after repeated use. Acute ingestion of more than 1 mg/kg of dextroamphetamine (or an equivalent dose of other drugs; see Table II–1) should be considered potentially life-threatening.

III. Clinical presentation

A. Acute central nervous system effects of intoxication include euphoria, talkativeness, anxiety, restlessness, agitation, seizures, and coma. Intracranial hemorrhage may occur owing to hypertension or cerebral vasculitis.

B. Acute peripheral manifestations include sweating, tremor, muscle fasciculations and rigidity, tachycardia, hypertension, acute myocardial ischemia, and infarction (even with normal coronary arteries). Inadvertent intra-arterial injection may cause vasospasm resulting in gangrene; this has also occurred with oral use of DOB (2,5-dimethoxy-4-bromoamphetamine; see Lysergic Acid Diethylamide [LSD] and Other Hallucinogens, p 204).

C. Death may be caused by ventricular arrhythmia, status epilepticus, intracranial hemorrhage, or hyperthermia. **Hyperthermia** frequently results from seizures

TABLE II–1. COMMON AMPHETAMINELIKE DRUGS

Drugs	Clinical Indications	Typical Adult Dose (mg)
Benzphetamine	Anorectant	25–50
Dextroamphetamine	Narcolepsy, hyperactivity (children)	5–15
Diethylpropion	Anorectant	25, 75 (SR)
Fenfluramine	Anorectant	20–40
Mazindol	Anorectant	1–2
Methamphetamine	Narcolepsy, hyperactivity (children)	5–15
Methylphenidate	Hyperactivity (children)	5–20
Phendimetrazine	Anorectant	35, 105 (SR)
Phenmetrazine	Anorectant	25, 75 (SR)
Phentermine	Anorectant	8, 30 (SR)
Pemoline	Narcolepsy, hyperactivity (children)	18.7–75

SR = Sustained-release.

and muscular hyperactivity and may cause brain damage, rhabdomyolysis, and myoglobinuric renal failure (see p 20).

    D. Chronic effects of amphetamine abuse include weight loss, cardiomyopathy, stereotypic behavior (such as picking at the skin), paranoia, and paranoid psychosis. Psychiatric disturbances may persist for days or weeks. Following cessation of habitual use, patients may suffer fatigue, hypersomnia, hyperphagia, and depression lasting several days.

IV. Diagnosis is usually based on a history of amphetamine use and clinical features of sympathomimetic drug intoxication.

    A. Specific levels. Amphetamine and many related drugs can be detected in urine and gastric samples, providing confirmation of exposure. However, quantitative serum levels do not correlate well with severity of clinical effects and are not generally available. Amphetamine derivatives and adrenergic amines will cross-react in immunoassays (see Table I–32, p 40).

    B. Other useful laboratory studies. Electrolytes, glucose, BUN and creatinine, CPK, urinalysis, urine dipstick test for occult hemoglobin (positive in patients with rhabdomyolysis with myoglobinuria), ECG and ECG monitoring, CT scan of the head (if hemorrhage suspected).

V. Treatment

    A. Emergency and supportive measures

        1. Maintain the airway and assist ventilation if necessary (see p 4).

        2. Treat agitation (p 23), seizures (p 22), coma (p 18), and hyperthermia (p 20) if they occur.

        3. Continuously monitor the temperature, other vital signs, and the ECG for a minimum of 6 hours.

    B. Specific drugs and antidotes. There is no specific antidote.

        1. Hypertension (see p 17) is best treated with a parenteral vasodilator such as phentolamine (p 369) or nitroprusside (p 362).

        2. Treat **tachyarrhythmias** (p 13–14) with propranolol (see p 373) or esmolol (p 338).

        3. Treat **arterial vasospasm** as described for ergots (p 158).

    C. Decontamination (see p 44)

        1. Prehospital. Administer activated charcoal, if available. Do **not** induce emesis because of the risk of abrupt onset of seizures.

        2. Hospital. Administer activated charcoal and a cathartic. Gastric emptying is not necessary if activated charcoal can be given promptly.

D. Enhanced elimination. Dialysis and hemoperfusion are not effective. Repeat-dose charcoal has not been studied. Renal elimination of dextroamphetamine may be enhanced by acidification of the urine, but this is not recommended because of the risk of aggravating the nephrotoxicity of myoglobinuria.

ANESTHETICS, LOCAL
Neal L. Benowitz, MD

ANTIDOTE   IPECAC   LAVAGE   CHARCOAL

Local anesthetics are widely used to provide anesthesia via local subcutaneous injection; topical application to skin and mucous membranes; and epidural, spinal, and regional nerve blocks. In addition, lidocaine (see p 349) is used intravenously as an antiarrhythmic agent and cocaine (see p 138) is a popular drug of abuse. Commonly used agents are divided into 2 chemical groups: ester-linked and amide-linked (Table II–2).

Toxicity from local anesthetics (other than cocaine) is usually caused by therapeutic overdosage (ie, excessive dose for local nerve blocks), inadvertent acceleration of intravenous infusions (lidocaine), or accidental injection of products meant for dilution (eg, 20% lidocaine) instead of those formulated for direct administration (2% solution). Acute injection of lidocaine has also been used as a method of homicide.

TABLE II–2. COMMON LOCAL ANESTHETICS[a]

Anesthetic	Maximum Adult Single Dose[a] (mg)
Ester-linked	
Benzocaine[b]	N/A
Butacaine[b]	N/A
Chlorprocaine	800
Cocaine[b]	N/A
Cyclomethylcaine[b]	N/A
Hexylcaine[b]	N/A
Procaine	600
Proparacaine[b]	N/A
Propoxycaine	75
Tetracaine	15
Amide-linked	
Bupivacaine	400
Dibucaine	10
Etidocaine	400
Lidocaine	300
Lidocaine with epinephrine	500
Mepivacaine	400
Prilocaine	600
Other (neither ester- nor amide-linked)	
Dyclonine[b]	N/A

[a]Maximum single dose for subcutaneous infiltration.
[b]Used only for topical anesthesia.

I. Mechanism of toxicity. Local anesthetics bind to sodium channels in nerve fibers, blocking the sodium current responsible for nerve conduction and thereby increasing the threshold for conduction and reversibly slowing or blocking impulse generation. In therapeutic concentrations, this results in local anesthesia. In high concentrations, such actions may result in central nervous system and cardiovascular toxicity. In addition, some local anesthetics (eg, benzocaine) have been reported to cause methemoglobinemia (see p 217).

II. Toxic dose. Systemic toxicity occurs when brain levels exceed a certain threshold. Toxic levels can be achieved with a single large subcutaneous injection, with rapid intravenous injection of a smaller dose, or by accumulation of drug with repeated doses. The recommended maximum single subcutaneous doses of the common agents are listed in Table II–2.

  A. With local subcutaneous injection, peak blood levels are reached in 10–60 minutes, depending on the vascularity of the tissue and whether a vasoconstrictor such as epinephrine has been added.

  B. **Ester-type** drugs are rapidly hydrolyzed by plasma cholinesterase and have short half-lives. **Amide-type** drugs are metabolized by the liver, have longer duration of effect, and may accumulate after repeated doses in patients with hepatic insufficiency.

III. Clinical presentation

  A. Toxicity owing to **local anesthetic effects** includes prolonged anesthesia and, rarely, permanent sensory or motor deficits. Spinal anesthesia may block nerves to the muscles of respiration, causing respiratory arrest, or may cause sympathetic blockade, resulting in hypotension.

  B. Toxicity resulting from **systemic absorption** of local anesthetics affects primarily the central nervous system, with headache, confusion, perioral paresthesias, slurred speech, muscle twitching, convulsions, coma, and respiratory arrest. Cardiotoxic effects include sinus arrest, atrioventricular block, asystole, and hypotension.

  C. **Methemoglobinemia** (see also p 217) may occur after exposure to benzocaine.

  D. **Allergic reactions** (bronchospasm, hives, and shock) are uncommon and occur almost exclusively with ester-linked local anesthetics. Methylparaben, used as a preservative in some multidose vials, may be the cause of some reported hypersensitivity reactions.

  E. Features of toxicity caused by **cocaine** are discussed on p 138.

IV. Diagnosis is based on a history of local anesthetic use and typical clinical features. Abrupt onset of confusion, slurred speech, or convulsions in a patient receiving lidocaine infusion for arrhythmias should suggest lidocaine toxicity.

  A. **Specific levels.** Serum levels of some local anesthetics may confirm their role in producing suspected toxic effects, but these must be obtained promptly because the levels rapidly fall.

  1. Serum concentrations of lidocaine greater than 6–10 mg/L are considered toxic.

  2. Lidocaine is often detected in urine toxicology screening as a result of use either as a local anesthetic (eg, for minor procedures in the emergency department) or as a cutting agent for drugs of abuse.

  B. **Other useful laboratory studies.** Electrolytes, glucose, BUN and creatinine, ECG monitoring, arterial blood gases or pulse oximetry, methemoglobin level (benzocaine).

V. Treatment

  A. **Emergency and supportive measures**

  1. Maintain the airway and assist ventilation if necessary (see p 4).

  2. Treat coma (p 18), seizures (p 22), hypotension (p 15), arrhythmias (p 10), and anaphylaxis (p 26) if they occur. Extracorporeal circulatory assistance (eg, balloon pump or partial cardiopulmonary bypass) has been used for short-term support for patients with acute massive overdose with 20% lidocaine solution.

  3. Monitor vital signs and ECG for at least 6 hours.

B. Specific drugs and antidotes. There is no specific antidote.

C. Decontamination

1. **Parenteral exposure.** Decontamination is not feasible.
2. **Ingestion** (see p 44)
   a. **Prehospital.** Administer activated charcoal, if available. Do **not** induce emesis because of the risk of abrupt onset of seizures.
   b. **Hospital.** Administer activated charcoal and a cathartic. Consider gastric lavage only for large recent ingestion.

D. Enhanced elimination. Because lidocaine has a moderate volume of distribution, hemoperfusion is potentially beneficial, particularly after a massive overdose or when metabolic elimination is impaired because of circulatory collapse or severe liver disease.

ANTIARRHYTHMIC DRUGS
Neal L. Benowitz, MD

ANTIDOTE · IPECAC · LAVAGE · CHARCOAL

Because of their actions on the heart, antiarrhythmic drugs are extremely toxic and overdoses are often life-threatening. Several classes of antiarrhythmic drugs are discussed elsewhere in Section II: type Ia drugs (quinidine, disopyramide, and procainamide; p 271); type II drugs (beta blockers, p 99); type IV drugs (calcium antagonists, p 113); and the older type Ib drugs (lidocaine, p 68; and phenytoin, p 255). This section describes toxicity caused by newer antiarrhythmic drugs: type Ib (tocainide and mexiletine); type Ic (flecainide, encainide, propafenone, and moricizine); and type III (bretylium and amiodarone). Sotalol, which also has type III antiarrhythmic actions, is discussed in the chapter on beta-adrenergic blockers (see p 99).

I. Mechanism of toxicity

A. Type I drugs in general act by inhibiting the fast sodium channel responsible for initial cardiac cell depolarization and impulse conduction. Type Ia and type Ic drugs (which also block potassium channels) slow depolarization and conduction in normal cardiac tissue, and even at normal therapeutic doses the QT (types Ia and Ic) and QRS intervals (type Ic) are prolonged. Type Ib drugs slow depolarization primarily in ischemic tissue and have little effect on normal tissue or on the ECG. In overdose, all type I drugs have the potential to markedly depress myocardial automaticity, conduction, and contractility.

B. Type II and type IV drugs act by blocking beta-adrenergic receptors (type II) or calcium channels (type IV). Their actions are discussed elsewhere (type II, p 99; type IV, p 143).

C. Type III drugs act primarily by blocking potassium channels to prolong the duration of the action potential and the effective refractory period, resulting in QT interval prolongation at therapeutic doses.

1. Intravenous administration of **bretylium** initially causes release of catecholamines from nerve endings, followed by inhibition of catecholamine release.
2. **Amiodarone** is a noncompetitive beta-adrenergic blocker, which may explain its tendency to cause bradyarrhythmias. Amiodarone may also release iodine, and chronic use has resulted in altered thyroid function.

D. Relevant pharmacokinetics. Normal elimination half-lives are summarized in Table II–3. All drugs discussed in this section are widely distributed to body tissues. Most are extensively metabolized, but significant fractions of tocainide (40%), flecainide (30%), and bretylium (> 90%) are excreted unchanged by the kidneys.

II. Toxic dose. In general, these drugs have a narrow therapeutic index, and severe toxicity may occur slightly above or sometimes even within the therapeutic range, especially if combinations of antiarrhythmic drugs are taken together.

A. Ingestion of **twice the daily therapeutic dose** should be considered potentially life-threatening (usual therapeutic doses are given in Table II–3).

B. An exception to this rule of thumb is amiodarone, which is so extensively distributed to tissues that even massive single overdoses produce little or no toxicity (toxicity usually occurs only after accumulation during chronic amiodarone dosing).

III. Clinical presentation

A. Tocainide and mexiletine

1. **Side effects** with therapeutic use may include dizziness, paresthesias, tremor, ataxia, and gastrointestinal disturbance.
2. **Overdose** may cause sedation, confusion, coma, seizures, respiratory arrest, and cardiac toxicity (sinus arrest, AV block, asystole, and hypotension). As with lidocaine, the QRS and QT intervals are usually normal, although they may be prolonged after massive overdose.

B. Flecainide, encainide, propafenone, and moricizine

1. **Side effects** with therapeutic use include dizziness, blurred vision, headache, and gastrointestinal upset. Ventricular arrhythmias (monomorphic or polymorphic ventricular tachycardia; see p 14) may occur at therapeutic levels, especially in persons receiving high doses and those with reduced ventricular function.
2. **Overdose** causes hypotension, bradycardia, AV block, and asystole. The QRS and QT intervals are prolonged.

C. Bretylium

TABLE II–3. ANTIARRHYTHMIC DRUGS

Class	Drug	Usual Half-Life (hrs)	Therapeutic Daily Dose (mg)	Therapeutic Serum Levels (mg/L)	Major Toxicity[a]
Ia	Quinidine and related (p 271)				
Ib	Tocainide	13	1200–2400	5–12	S, B, H
	Mexiletine	12	300–1200	0.8–2	S, B, H
	Lidocaine (p 68)				
	Phenytoin (p 255)				
Ic	Flecainide	15	200–600	0.2–1	B, V, H
	Encainide[b]	12	75–300	[b]	S, B, V, H
	Propafenone[b]	2–10[c]	450–900	0.5–1	S, B, V, H
	Moricizine	2	600–900		B, V, H
II	Beta Blockers (p 99)				
III	Aminodarone	50 days	200–600	0.5–3	B, V, H
	Bretylium	14	5–10 mg/kg (IV loading dose)	0.7–1.5	H
	Sotalol (p 99)				
IV	Calcium Antagonists (p 113)				

[a]Major toxicity: S = Seizures   H = Hypotension
         B = Bradyarrhythmias   V = Ventricular arrhythmias
[b]Active metabolite may contribute to toxicity; level not established.
[c]Genetically slow metabolizers may have half-lives of 10–32 hours. Also, metabolism is nonlinear, so half-lives may be longer in patients with overdose.

    1. The major toxic **side effect** of bretylium is hypotension caused by inhibition of catecholamine release. Orthostatic hypotension may persist for several hours.

    2. After **rapid intravenous injection,** transient hypertension, nausea, and vomiting may occur.

D. Amiodarone

    1. Acute overdose in a person not already on amiodarone is not expected to cause toxicity.

    2. With **chronic use,** amiodarone may cause ventricular arrhythmias (monomorphic or polymorphic ventricular tachycardia; see p 14) or bradyarrhythmias (sinus arrest, AV block). Amiodarone may aggravate cardiac failure and may cause pneumonitis or pulmonary fibrosis, photosensitivity dermatitis, corneal deposits, hypothyroidism or hyperthyroidism, tremor, and ataxia.

IV. Diagnosis is usually based on a history of antiarrhythmic drug use and typical cardiac and electrocardiographic findings. Syncope in any patient taking these drugs should suggest possible drug-induced arrhythmia.

  A. Specific levels. Serum levels are available for most type Ia and type Ib drugs (Table II–3); however, because toxicity is immediately life-threatening, measurement of drug levels is used primarily for therapeutic drug monitoring or to confirm the diagnosis rather than to determine emergency treatment.

  B. Other useful laboratory studies. Electrolytes, glucose, BUN and creatinine, liver enzymes, thyroid panel (chronic amiodarone), ECG and ECG monitoring.

V. Treatment

  A. Emergency and supportive measures

    1. Maintain the airway and assist ventilation if necessary (see p 4).

    2. Treat coma (p 18), seizures (p 22), hypotension (p 15), and arrhythmias (p 10–14) if they occur. ***Note:*** Type Ia antiarrhythmic agents should not be used to treat cardiotoxicity caused by type Ia, type Ic, or type III drugs.

    3. Continuously monitor vital signs and ECG for a minimum of 6 hours after exposure, and admit the patient for 24 hours of intensive monitoring if there is evidence of toxicity.

  B. Specific drugs and antidotes. In patients with intoxication by type Ia or type Ic drugs, QRS prolongation, bradyarrhythmias, and hypotension may respond to **sodium bicarbonate,** 1–2 meq/kg IV (see p 318). The sodium bicarbonate probably reverses cardiac-depressant effects caused by inhibition of the fast sodium channel.

  C. Decontamination (see p 44)

    1. Prehospital. Administer activated charcoal, if available. Ipecac-induced emesis may be useful for initial treatment at the scene (eg, children at home) if it can be given within a few minutes of exposure.

    2. Hospital. Administer activated charcoal and a cathartic. Consider gastric lavage for large ingestions.

  D. Enhanced elimination. Owing to extensive tissue binding with resulting large volumes of distribution, dialysis and hemoperfusion are not likely to be effective for most of these agents. Hemodialysis may be of possible benefit for tocainide or flecainide overdose in patients with renal failure, but prolonged and repeated dialysis would be necessary. No data are available on the effectiveness of repeat-dose charcoal.

ANTIBIOTICS
Olga F. Woo, PharmD

ANTIDOTE   IPECAC   LAVAGE   CHARCOAL

The antibiotic class of drugs has proliferated immensely since the first clinical use of sulfonamide in 1936 and the mass production of penicillin in 1941. In general, harmful effects have resulted from allergic reactions or inadvertent intravenous overdose. Serious toxicity from single acute ingestion is rare. Table II–4 lists common antibiotics and their toxicities.

 I. **Mechanism of toxicity.** The precise mechanisms underlying toxic effects vary depending on the agent and are not well understood. In some cases, toxicity is caused by an extension of pharmacologic effects, while in other cases allergic or idiosyncratic reactions are responsible.
 II. **Toxic dose.** The toxic dose is highly variable, depending on the agent. Life-threatening allergic reactions may occur after subtherapeutic doses in hypersensitive individuals.
III. **Clinical presentation.** After acute oral overdose, most agents cause only nausea, vomiting, and diarrhea. Specific features of toxicity are described in Table II–4.
IV. **Diagnosis** is usually based on the history of exposure.
  A. **Specific levels.** Serum levels for most commonly used antibiotics are usually

TABLE II–4. COMMON ANTIBIOTICS AND THEIR TOXICITIES

Drug	$t_{1/2}$*	Toxic Dose or Serum Level	Toxicity
Aminoglycosides			
Amikacin	2–3 h	> 35 mg/L	Ototoxicity to vestibular and cochlear cells; nephrotoxicity causing proximal tubular damage and acute tubular necrosis; competitive neuromuscular blockade if given rapidly intravenously with other neuromuscular blocking drugs.
Gentamicin	2 h	> 12 mg/L	
Kanamycin	2–3 h	> 30 mg/L	
Neomycin		0.5–1 g/d	
Streptomycin	2.5 h	> 40–50 mg/L	
Tobramycin	2–2.5 h	> 10 mg/L	
Bacitracin		Unknown	Ototoxicity and nephrotoxicity.
Cephalosporins			
Cefazolin	90–120 min	Unknown	Convulsions reported in patients with renal insufficiency.
Cephalothin	30–50 min		
Cephaloridine		6 g/d	Proximal tubular necrosis.
Cefoperazone	102–156 min	Unknown	Disulfiramlike interaction with ethanol; coagulopathy (inhibition of vitamin K_1 production).
Cefamandole	30–60 min		
Moxalactam	114–150 min		
Cefazolin	90–120 min	Unknown	Coagulopathy (inhibition of vitamin K_1 production).
Cefmetazole	72 min		
Chloramphenicol	4 h	> 50 mg/L	Leukopenia, reticulocytopenia; circulatory collapse (gray baby syndrome).
Dapsone	10–50 h	As little as 100 mg in 18-month-old	Methemoglobinemia, sulfhemoglobinemia, hemolysis; metabolic acidosis; hallucinations, confusion; hepatitis.
Erythromycin	1.4 h	Unknown	Abdominal pain; idiosyncratic hepatotoxicity with estolate salt.
Gramicidin		Unknown	Hemolysis.
Isoniazid	0.5–4 h	1–2 g orally	Convulsions, metabolic acidosis (see p 192); hepatotoxicity with chronic use.
Lincomycin, clindamycin	4.4–6.4 h 2.4–3 h	Unknown	Hypotension and cardiopulmonary arrest after rapid intravenous administration.
Metronidazole	8.5 h	5 g/d	Convulsions; at therapeutic doses may cause disulfiramlike interaction with ethanol (see p 155).

(*continued*)

TABLE II–4. COMMON ANTIBIOTICS AND THEIR TOXICITIES (CONTINUED)

Drug	$t_{1/2}$*	Toxic Dose or Serum Level	Toxicity
Nalidixic acid		50 mg/kg/d	Seizures, hallucinations, confusion; visual disturbances; metabolic acidosis; intracranial hypertension.
Nitrofurantoin	20 min.	Unknown	Hemolysis in G6PD-deficient patients.
Penicillins Penicillin	30 min	10 million units/d IV, or CSF > 5 mg/L	Seizures with single high dose or chronic excessive doses in patients with renal dysfunction.
Methicillin	30 min	Unknown	Interstitial nephritis, leukopenia.
Nafcillin	1.0 h	Unknown	Neutropenia.
Ampicillin, amoxicillin	1.5 h 1.3 h	Unknown	Acute renal failure caused by crystal deposition.
Polymyxins Polymyxin B	4.3–6 h	30,000 units/kg/d	Nephrotoxicity and noncompetitive neuromuscular blockade.
Polymyxin E		250 mg IM in a 10-month-old	
Rifampin	1.7 h	100 mg/kg/d	Facial edema, pruritus; headache, vomiting, diarrhea; red urine and tears.
Spectinomycin	1.2–2.8 h		Acute toxicity not reported.
Tetracyclines	6–12 h	> 1 g/d in infants	Benign intracranial hypertension.
		> 4 g/d in pregnancy	Acute fatty liver.
Demeclocycline	10–17 h	Unknown	Nephrogenic diabetes insipidus.
Minocycline	11–26 h	Unknown	Vestibular symptoms.
Sulfonamides		Unknown	Acute renal failure caused by crystal deposition.
Trimethoprim	8–11 h	Unknown	Bone marrow depression.
Vancomycin	4–6 h	> 80 mg/L	Ototoxic and nephrotoxic. Hypotension, skin rash/flushing ("red-man syndrome") associated with IV administration.
Zidovudine (AZT)		Unknown	Seizures (36 g overdose), bone marrow suppression (20 g overdose).

*Normal renal function

available. Serum levels are particularly useful for predicting toxic effects of **aminoglycosides, chloramphenicol,** and **vancomycin.**

  B. **Other useful laboratory studies.** CBC, electrolytes, glucose, BUN and creatinine, liver function tests, urinalysis, methemoglobin level (for patients with dapsone overdose).

V. **Treatment**

  A. **Emergency and supportive measures**

   1. Maintain the airway and assist ventilation if necessary (see p 4).

   2. Treat coma (p 18), seizures (p 22), hypotension (p 15), anaphylaxis (p 26), and hemolysis (See Rhabdomyolysis, p 25) if they occur.

   3. Replace fluid losses resulting from gastroenteritis with intravenous crystalloids.

  B. **Specific drugs and antidotes**

    1. Trimethoprim poisoning. Administer **leucovorin** (folinic acid; see p 348). Folic acid is not effective.

    2. Dapsone overdose. Administer **methylene blue** (see p 351) for symptomatic methemoglobinemia.

C. Decontamination (see p 44)

    1. Prehospital. Administer activated charcoal, if available. Ipecac-induced emesis may be useful for initial treatment at the scene (eg, children at home) if it can be given within a few minutes of exposure.

    2. Hospital. Administer activated charcoal and a cathartic. Gastric emptying is not necessary if activated charcoal can be given promptly.

D. Enhanced elimination. Most antibiotics are excreted unchanged in the urine, so maintenance of adequate urine flow is important. The role of forced diuresis is unclear. Hemodialysis is not usually indicated, except perhaps in patients with renal dysfunction and a high level of a toxic agent.

    1. Charcoal hemoperfusion effectively removes **chloramphenicol** and is indicated after a severe overdose with a high serum level and metabolic acidosis.

    2. Dapsone undergoes enterohepatic recirculation and is more rapidly eliminated with repeat-dose activated charcoal.

ANTICHOLINERGICS
S. Alan Tani, PharmD

ANTIDOTE   IPECAC   LAVAGE   CHARCOAL

Anticholinergic intoxication can occur with a wide variety of prescription and over-the-counter medications and numerous plants and mushrooms. Common drugs that possess anticholinergic activity include antihistamines, antipsychotics, antispasmodics, skeletal muscle relaxants, and cyclic antidepressants (Table II–5). *Common combination products containing anticholinergic drugs* include Atrohist, Donnagel, Donnatal, Hyland's Teething Tablets, Lomotil, Motofen, Ru-Tuss, Urised, and Urispas. Plants and mushrooms containing anticholinergic alkaloids include jimsonweed *(Datura stramonium),* deadly nightshade *(Atropa belladonna),* and the fly agaric *(Amanita muscaria).*

  I. Mechanism of toxicity. Anticholinergic agents competitively antagonize the effects of acetylcholine at peripheral muscarinic and central receptors. Exocrine glands, such as those responsible for sweating and salivation, and smooth and cardiac muscle are mostly affected. Tertiary amines such as atropine are well absorbed centrally, whereas quaternary amines such as glycopyrrolate have less central effect.

  II. Toxic dose. The range of toxicity is highly variable and unpredictable. Fatal atropine poisoning has occurred after as little as 1–2 mg was instilled in the eye of a young child. Intramuscular injection of 32 mg of atropine was fatal in an adult.

 III. Clinical presentation. The anticholinergic syndrome is characterized by warm, dry, flushed skin; dry mouth; mydriasis; delirium; tachycardia; ileus; and urinary retention. Jerky myoclonic movements and choreoathetosis are common. Hyperthermia, coma, and respiratory arrest may occur. Seizures are rare.

 IV. Diagnosis is based on a history of exposure and the presence of typical features such as dilated pupils and flushed skin. A trial dose of physostigmine (see below) can be used to confirm the presence of anticholinergic toxicity: rapid reversal of signs and symptoms is consistent with the diagnosis.

  A. Specific levels. Not generally available. Common over-the-counter agents are usually detectable on general urine toxicology screening.

  B. Other useful laboratory studies. Electrolytes, glucose, arterial blood gases or pulse oximetry, ECG monitoring.

TABLE II–5. COMMON ANTIMUSCARINIC ANTICHOLINERGIC DRUGS[a]

Tertiary Amines	Usual Adult Single Dose (mg)	Quarternary Amines	Usual Adult Single Dose (mg)
Atropine	0.4–1	Anisotropine	50
Dicyclomine	10–20	Glycopyrrolate	1
Hyoscyamine	0.15–0.3	Methantheline	50
Oxyphencyclimine	10	Methscopolamine	2.5
Scopolamine	0.4–1	Propantheline	15
Trihexyphenidyl	6–10		
Benztropine	1–6		

[a]Adapted and reproduced, with permission, from Katzung BG: Cholinoceptor-blocking drugs. Table 8–2 in: *Basic & Clinical Pharmacology*, 4th ed. Katzung BG (editor). Appleton & Lange, 1989.

V. Treatment
A. Emergency and supportive measures
1. Maintain the airway and assist ventilation if needed (see p 4).
2. Treat hyperthermia (p 20), coma (p 18), and seizures (p 22) if they occur.
B. Specific drugs and antidotes.
If a pure anticholinergic poisoning is suspected, a small dose of **physostigmine** (see p 370), 0.5–1 mg IV in an adult, can be given to patients with severe toxicity (eg, hyperthermia, severe delirium, or tachycardia). *Caution:* Physostigmine is capable of causing atrioventricular block, asystole, and seizures, especially in patients with cyclic antidepressant overdose.
C. Decontamination (see p 44)
1. **Prehospital.** Administer activated charcoal, if available. Ipecac-induced emesis may be useful for initial treatment at the scene (eg, children at home) if it can be given within 30 minutes of exposure.
2. **Hospital.** Administer activated charcoal and a cathartic. Gastric emptying is not necessary if activated charcoal can be given promptly.
D. Enhanced elimination.
Hemodialysis, hemoperfusion, peritoneal dialysis, and repeat-dose charcoal are not effective in removing anticholinergic agents.

ANTIDEPRESSANTS (NEWER)
Neal L. Benowitz, MD

ANTIDOTE   IPECAC   LAVAGE   CHARCOAL

Several newer noncyclic antidepressants have been introduced in the past decade, including trazodone (Desyrel), fluoxetine (Prozac), sertraline (Zoloft), paroxetine (Paxil), and bupropion (Wellbutrin). In general, these drugs are much less toxic than the cyclic antidepressants (see p 147), although serious effects such as seizures and hypotension occasionally occur. Drugs in this category are described in Table II–6.
I. Mechanism of toxicity
A. Most agents cause central nervous system depression. Bupropion can also cause seizures, presumably related to inhibition of reuptake of dopamine and norepinephrine.
B. Trazodone produces peripheral alpha-adrenergic blockade, which can result in hypotension and priapism.
C. Serotonin uptake inhibitors (fluoxetine, sertraline, paroxetine, and trazodone)

TABLE II–6. NEWER ANTIDEPRESSANTS

Drug	Action[a]	Usual Adult Daily Dose (mg)	Usual Elimination Half-life (h)[b]
Bupropion	D	200–450	16
Fluoxetine	S	20–80	70
Paroxetine	S	20–50	21
Sertraline	S	50–200	28
Trazodone	S, A	50–400	8

[a]A = alpha-adrenergic blocker; D = dopamine uptake blocker; S = serotonin uptake blocker.
[b]All have active metabolites, many with longer half-lives than the parent drug.

may interact with oral ingestion of tryptophan or with chronic use of a monoamine oxidase (MAO) inhibitor to produce the "serotonin syndrome" (see below and p 21).

   D. None of the drugs in this group has significant anticholinergic effects.
II. Toxic dose. The newer antidepressants generally have a wide therapeutic index, with doses in excess of 10 times the usual therapeutic dose tolerated without serious toxicity. Bupropion can cause seizures in some patients with moderate overdose or even in therapeutic doses.
III. Clinical presentation
   A. Central nervous system. The usual presentation after overdose includes ataxia, sedation, and coma. Respiratory depression may occur, especially with coingestion of alcohol or other drugs. These agents, particularly bupropion, can cause restlessness, anxiety, and agitation. Tremor and seizures are common with bupropion but occur rarely after fluoxetine overdose.
   B. Cardiovascular effects are usually minimal, although trazodone can cause hypotension and orthostatic hypotension, bupropion can cause sinus tachycardia, and fluoxetine may cause minor ST-T wave changes.
   C. Serotonin syndrome (see p 21) is characterized by confusion, hypomania, restlessness, myoclonus, hyperreflexia, diaphoresis, shivering, tremor, incoordination, and hyperthermia. This reaction may be seen when patients taking MAO inhibitors or tryptophan ingest fluoxetine or one of the other serotonin uptake blockers (sertraline, paroxetine, or trazodone), or when MAO inhibitors or tryptophan are given to patients chronically receiving one of these drugs. Because of the long duration of effects of MAO inhibitors and most of the serotonin uptake blockers, this type of adverse interaction can occur up to several weeks after either treatment regimen has been discontinued.
IV. Diagnosis should be suspected in patients with a history of depression who develop lethargy, coma, or seizures. These agents do not generally affect cardiac conduction, and QRS interval prolongation should suggest cyclic antidepressant overdose (see p 147).
   A. Specific levels. Blood and urine assays are not routinely available and are not useful for emergency management. These drugs may or may not appear on routine toxicology screening.
   B. Other useful laboratory studies. Electrolytes, glucose, arterial blood gases or pulse oximetry, ECG monitoring.
V. Treatment
   A. Emergency and supportive measures
      1. Maintain the airway and assist ventilation if needed (see p 4). Administer supplemental oxygen.
      2. Treat coma (p 18), hypotension (p 15), and seizures (p 22) if they occur.
   B. Specific drugs and antidotes. For suspected serotonin syndrome, anecdotal

reports claim benefit from methysergide (Sansert), 2 mg orally every 6 hours for 3 doses (1 case report), and cyproheptadine (Periactin), 4 mg orally every hour for 3 doses (1 case report), presumably because of the serotonin antagonist effects of these drugs.

C. Decontamination (see p 44)

    1. Prehospital. Administer activated charcoal, if available. Ipecac-induced emesis may be useful for initial treatment at the scene (eg, children at home) if it can be given within a few minutes of exposure.

    2. Hospital. Administer activated charcoal and a cathartic. Gastric emptying is not necessary if activated charcoal can be given promptly.

D. Enhanced elimination. Owing to extensive protein binding and large volumes of distribution, dialysis, hemoperfusion, peritoneal dialysis, and repeat-dose charcoal are not effective.

ANTIHISTAMINES
S. Alan Tani, PharmD

ANTIDOTE   IPECAC   LAVAGE   CHARCOAL

Antihistamines (H_1 receptor antagonists) are commonly found in over-the-counter and prescription medications used for motion sickness, control of allergy-related itching, and cough and cold palliation and as sleep aids (Table II–7). Acute intoxication with

TABLE II–7. COMMON H_1 RECEPTOR ANTAGONIST ANTIHISTAMINES[a]

Drug	Usual Duration of Action (hr)	Usual Single Adult Dose (mg)	Sedation
Ethanolamines			
Carbinoxamine	3–4	4–8	++
Dimenhydrinate	4–6	50	+++
Diphenhydramine	4–6	25–50	+++
Doxylamine	4–6	25	+++
Ethylenediamines			
Pyrilamine	4–6	25–50	++
Tripelennamine	4–6	25–50	++
Alkylamines			
Brompheniramine	4–6	4–8	+
Chlorpheniramine	4–6	4–8	+
Piperazines			
Cyclizine	4–6	25–50	+
Meclizine	12–24	25–50	+
Hydroxyzine	6–24	25–50	+
Others			
Astemizole	[b]	10	—
Terfenadine	8–12	60	—

[a]Adapted in part, with permission, from Douglas WW: Histamine and 5-hydroxytryptamine (serotonin) and their antagonists. Table 26–3 in: *Goodman and Gilman's The Pharmacological Basis of Therapeutics*, 7th ed. Gilman AG et al (editors), Macmillan, 1985; and Burkhalter A, Frick OL: Histamine, serotonin, and the ergot alkaloids. Table 16–1 in *Basic & Clinical Pharmacology*, 4th ed. Katzung BG (editor), Appleton & Lange, 1989.
[b]Elimination half-life 7–10 days.

antihistamines results in symptoms very similar to those of anticholinergic poisoning. H_2 receptor blockers (cimetidine, ranitidine, and famotidine) inhibit gastric acid secretion but otherwise share no effects with H_1 agents, do not produce significant intoxication, and are not discussed here. *Common combination products containing antihistamines* include Actifed, Allerest, Caladryl, Contac, Coricidin, Dimetapp, Dristan, Drixoral, Excedrin PM, Nyquil, Nytol, Pamprin, Pediacare, Tavist, Triaminic, Triaminicol, Unisom Dual Relief Formula, and Vicks Pediatric Formula 44.

I. **Mechanism of toxicity.** H_1 blocker antihistamines are structurally related to histamine and antagonize the effects of histamine on H_1 receptor sites. They possess anticholinergic effects (except the "nonsedating" agents terfenadine and astemizole). They may also stimulate or depress the central nervous system, and some agents (eg, diphenhydramine) have local anesthetic and membrane-depressant effects in large doses.

II. **Toxic dose.** The estimated fatal oral dose of diphenhydramine is 20–40 mg/kg. In general, toxicity occurs after ingestion of 3–5 times the usual daily dose. Children are more sensitive to the toxic effects of antihistamines than adults.

III. **Clinical presentation**
   A. Overdose results in many symptoms similar to anticholinergic poisoning: drowsiness, dilated pupils, flushed dry skin, fever, tachycardia, hallucinations, choreoathetoid movements, and delirium. Convulsions and hyperthermia may occur with serious overdose.
   B. Massive **diphenhydramine** overdose has been reported to cause QRS widening and myocardial depression similar to cyclic antidepressant overdose (see p 11 & 147).
   C. QT interval prolongation and torsades-type atypical ventricular tachycardia (see p 14) have been associated with elevated serum levels of **terfenadine** or **astemizole**. These have occurred after overdose, excessive daily dosing, or use of an interacting drug (eg, erythromycin, ketoconazole, itraconazole).

IV. **Diagnosis** is generally based on the history of ingestion and can usually be readily confirmed by the presence of typical anticholinergic syndrome. Toxicology screening will detect most common antihistamines.
   A. **Specific levels.** Not generally available or useful. Common over-the-counter antihistamines are usually detectable on general urine toxicology screening.
   B. **Other useful laboratory studies.** Electrolytes, glucose, arterial blood gases or pulse oximetry, ECG and ECG monitoring (diphenhydramine, terfenadine, astemizole).

V. **Treatment**
   A. **Emergency and supportive measures**
      1. Maintain the airway and assist ventilation if necessary (see p 4).
      2. Treat coma (p 18), seizures (p 22), hyperthermia (p 20), and atypical ventricular tachycardia (p 14) if they occur.
      3. Monitor the patient for at least 6–8 hours after ingestion. For terfenadine or astemizole, consider monitoring for at least 18–24 hours.
   B. **Specific drugs and antidotes.** There is no specific antidote for antihistamine overdose. As for anticholinergic poisoning (see p 75), physostigmine has been used for treatment of severe delirium or tachycardia. However, because antihistamine overdose carries a greater risk for seizures, physostigmine is not recommended. **Sodium bicarbonate** (see p 318), 1–2 meq/kg IV, may be useful for myocardial depression and QRS interval prolongation after massive diphenhydramine overdose.
   C. **Decontamination** (see p 44)
      1. **Prehospital.** Administer activated charcoal, if available. Ipecac-induced emesis may be useful for initial treatment at the scene (eg, children at home) if it can be given within a few minutes of exposure.
      2. **Hospital.** Administer activated charcoal and a cathartic. Consider gastric lavage for massive ingestions.
   D. **Enhanced elimination.** Hemodialysis, hemoperfusion, peritoneal dialysis, and repeat-dose activated charcoal are not effective in removing antihistamines.

ANTIMONY AND STIBINE
Kent R. Olson, MD

ANTIDOTE   IPECAC   LAVAGE   CHARCOAL

Antimony is widely used as a hardening agent in soft metal alloys; for compounding rubber; in flameproofing compounds; and as a coloring agent in dyes, varnishes, paints, and glazes. Exposure to antimony dusts and fumes may also occur during mining and refining of ores and from the discharge of firearms. Organic antimony compounds are used as antiparasitic drugs.

Stibine (antimony hydride, SbH_3) is a colorless gas with the odor of rotten eggs that is produced as a by-product when antimony-containing ores or furnace slag is treated with acid.

I. **Mechanism of toxicity.** The mechanism of antimony and stibine toxicity is not known. Because these compounds are chemically related to arsenic and arsine, their modes of action may be similar.

   A. **Antimony** compounds probably act by binding to sulfhydryl groups and inactivating key enzymes.

   B. **Stibine,** like arsine, may cause hemolysis. It is also an irritant gas.

II. **Toxic dose**

   A. The lethal oral dose of **antimony** in mice is 100 mg/kg; at these doses mice developed eosinophilia and cardiac failure. The recommended workplace limit (ACGIH TLV-TWA) for antimony is 0.5 mg/m³ as an 8-hour time-weighted average.

   B. The recommended workplace limit (ACGIH TLV-TWA) for **stibine** is 0.1 ppm as an 8-hour time-weighted average. The air level considered immediately dangerous to life or health (IDLH) is 40 ppm.

III. **Clinical presentation**

   A. **Acute ingestion of antimony** causes nausea, vomiting, and diarrhea (often bloody). Hepatitis and renal insufficiency may occur. Death is rare if the patient survives the initial gastroenteritis.

   B. **Acute stibine inhalation** causes acute hemolysis, resulting in anemia, jaundice, hemoglobinuria, and renal failure.

   C. **Chronic exposure to antimony dusts and fumes** in the workplace is the most common type of exposure and may result in headache, anorexia, pneumoconiosis, peptic ulcers, and dermatitis (antimony spots). Sudden death presumably resulting from a direct cardiotoxic effect has been reported in workers exposed to antimony trisulfide.

IV. **Diagnosis** is based on a history of exposure and typical clinical presentation.

   A. **Specific levels.** Normal serum and urine antimony levels are below 10 μg/L. Serum and urine concentrations correlate poorly with workplace exposure, but exposure to air concentrations greater than the TLV-TWA will increase urinary levels. Urinary antimony is increased after firearm discharge exposure. There is no established toxic antimony level after stibine exposure.

   B. **Other useful laboratory studies.** CBC, plasma free hemoglobin, electrolytes, BUN, creatinine, urinalysis for free hemoglobin, liver transaminases, bilirubin, prothrombin time (PT).

V. **Treatment**

   A. **Emergency and supportive measures**

      1. **Antimony.** Large-volume intravenous fluid resuscitation may be necessary for shock caused by gastroenteritis (see p 15).

      2. **Stibine.** Blood transfusion may be necessary after massive hemolysis. Treat hemoglobinuria with fluids and bicarbonate as for rhabdomyolysis (see p 25).

   B. **Specific drugs and antidotes.** There is no specific antidote. BAL (dimercaprol) and penicillamine are not effective chelators for antimony, nor are they expected to be effective for stibine.

   C. **Decontamination** (see p 41)

     1. Inhalation. Remove from exposure, and give supplemental oxygen if available. Protect rescuer from exposure.

     2. Ingestion of antimony salts

       a. Prehospital. Administer activated charcoal, if available (although there is no evidence for its effectiveness). Ipecac-induced emesis may be useful for initial treatment at the scene (eg, children at home) if it can be given within a few minutes of exposure.

       b. Hospital. Perform gastric lavage, and administer activated charcoal. Do **not** use cathartics.

   D. Enhanced elimination. Hemodialysis, hemoperfusion, and forced diuresis are **not** effective at removing antimony or stibine. Exchange transfusion may be effective in treating massive hemolysis caused by stibine.

ANTINEOPLASTIC AGENTS
Susan Kim, PharmD

ANTIDOTE   IPECAC   LAVAGE   CHARCOAL

Because of the inherently cytotoxic nature of most chemotherapeutic antineoplastic agents, overdoses are likely to be extremely serious. These agents are classified into 6 categories (Table II–8). Relatively few acute overdoses have been reported for these agents.

  I. Mechanism of toxicity. In general, toxic effects are extensions of the pharmacologic properties of these drugs.

    A. Alkylating agents. These drugs provide highly charged carbon atoms that attack nucleophilic sites on DNA, resulting in alkylation and cross-stranding and thus inhibiting replication and transcription. Binding to RNA or protein moieties appears to contribute little to cytotoxic effects.

    B. Antibiotics. These drugs intercalate within base pairs in DNA, inhibiting DNA-directed RNA synthesis. Another potential mechanism may be generation of cytotoxic free radicals.

    C. Antimetabolites. These agents interfere with DNA synthesis at various stages. For example, methotrexate binds reversibly to dihydrofolate reductase, preventing synthesis of purine and pyrimidine nucleotides.

    D. Hormones. Steroid hormones regulate the synthesis of steroid-specific proteins. The exact mechanism of antineoplastic action is unknown.

    E. Mitotic inhibitors. These agents act in various ways to inhibit orderly mitosis, thereby arresting cell division.

    F. Others. The cytotoxic actions of other antineoplastic drugs result from a variety of mechanisms, including DNA alkylation, blockade of protein synthesis, and inhibition of hormone release.

  II. Toxic dose. Because of the highly toxic nature of these agents (except for hormones), exposure to even therapeutic amounts should be considered potentially serious. Most oral antineoplastic agents are readily absorbed, with peak levels reached within 1–2 hours of ingestion.

  III. Clinical presentation. The organ systems affected by the various agents are listed in Table II–8. The most common sites of toxicity are the hematopoietic and gastrointestinal systems.

    A. Leukopenia is the most common manifestation of bone marrow depression. Thrombocytopenia and anemia may also occur. Death may result from overwhelming infections or hemorrhagic diathesis. With alkylating agents, nadirs occur 1–4 weeks after exposure; while with antibiotics, antimetabolites, and mitotic inhibitors, the nadirs occur 1–2 weeks after exposure.

    B. Gastrointestinal toxicity is also very common. Nausea and vomiting often accompany therapeutic administration, and severe ulcerative gastroenteritis may occur.

TABLE II–8. COMMON ANTINEOPLASTIC AGENTS AND THEIR TOXICITIES

Drug	Major Site(s) of Toxicity[a]	Comments
Alkylating agents		
Busulfan	D+, En+, M+, P++	Pulmonary fibrosis with chronic use.
Carboplatin	G++, An+, M++	Peripheral neuropathy in 4% of patients.
Carmustine (BCNU)	D+, G+, H+, M+, Ex+, P+	Flushing, hypotension, and tachycardia with rapid IV injection.
Chlorambucil	D+, G+, H+, M+, N++	Seizures, confusion, coma reported after overdose.
Cisplatin	An+, G++, M+, N+, P+, R++	Ototoxic, nephrotoxic. Good hydration essential. Hemodialysis not effective.
Cyclophosphamide	Al++, C+, D+, En+, G++, M++, R+	Hemodialysis effective. Acetylcysteine and 2 mercaptoethanesulfonate have been used investigationally to reduce hemorrhagic cystitis.
Ifosfamide	M++, N+, Al++, G+	Urotoxic. Hemorrhagic cystitis, somnolence, confusion, hallucinations, coma seen during therapy.
Lomustine (CCNU)	Al+, G+, H+, M+, P+	Thrombocytopenia, leukopenia, liver and lymph node enlargement after overdose.
Mechlorethamine	D+, G++, M++, N+, Ex+	Lymphocytopenia may occur within 24 hours.
Melphalan	G+, M+	Hemodialysis effective although of questionable need (half-life only 90 minutes).
Pipobroman	G+, M+	
Streptozocin	R++, G+, H+, M+	Renal toxicity in two-thirds of patients. Hypoglycemia from insulin shock a risk.
Thiotepa	An+, G++, M++	Bone marrow suppression usually very severe.
Uracil mustard	G+, M++	Bone marrow suppression first noted as thrombocytopenia, leukopenia.
Antibiotics		
Bleomycin	An++, D++, G+, P++	Pulmonary fibrosis with chronic use. Febrile reaction in 20–25% of patients.
Dactinomycin	Al+, D+, G++, M++, Ex++	Severe inflammatory reaction may occur at previously irradiated sites.
Daunorubicin	Al++, An+, C++, G++, M++, Ex++	Congestive cardiomyopathy may occur after total cumulative dose > 600 mg/m².
Doxorubicin	Al+, An+, C++, D+, G++, M++, Ex++	Cardiotoxicity and cardiomyopathy may occur after total cumulative dose > 55 mg/mg². Arrhythmias after acute overdose. Hemoperfusion may be effective.
Idarubicin	C++, G+, M++, Ex++	Congestive heart failure, acute life-threatening arrhythmias may occur.
Mitomycin	Al+, D+, G++, H+, M+, P+, R+, Ex++	Hemolytic anemia reported with therapeutic doses.

Drug	Codes	Comments
Mitoxantrone	An+, C+, G++, M++	Four reported overdosed patients died from severe leukopenia and infection.
Pentostatin	G+, M+, N++, R++	Central nervous system depression, convulsions, coma seen at high doses.
Plicamycin	An+, D+, G++, H++, M++, N+, Ex+	Coagulopathy, electrolyte disturbances may occur. Check calcium frequently.
Antimetabolites		
Cytarabine	An+, E+, G+, H+, M+	"Cytarabine syndrome": fever, myalgia, bone pain, rash, malaise.
Floxuridine	AI+, G++, M++	
Fludarabine	G+, M++, N++, R+	Blindness, coma, death at high doses.
5-Fluorouracil	AI+, D+, G++, M++, N+	Acute cerebellar syndrome seen.
6-Mercaptopurine	G+, H++, M+	Hemodialysis removes drug but of questionable need (half-life 20–60 minutes).
Methotrexate	AI+, D+, G++, H+, M++, N+, P+, R+	Folinic acid (leucovorin; see p 348) is specific antidote. Hemoperfusion effective.
6-Thioguanine	G+, H+, M+, R+	Hemodialysis probably ineffective owing to rapid intracellular incorporation.
Hormones		
Androgens		
Testolactone	En±, G±	Toxicity unlikely after single acute overdose.
Antiandrogens		
Flutamide	G+	Gynecomastia.
Estrogens		
Diethylstilbestrol	En±, G±	Possible carcinogenic effect on fetus if taken during early pregnancy.
Estramustine	En±, G±, H±, M±	Has both weak estrogenic and alkylating activity.
Polyestradiol	En±, G±	Toxicity unlikely after single acute overdose.
Antiestrogens		
Tamoxifen	AI±, D±, En±, G±	Acute toxic effects unlikely. Hot flashes, vaginal bleeding with chronic use.
Progestins		
Medroxyprogesterone	An±, En±, G±	Acute toxic effects unlikely. May induce porphyria in susceptible patients.
Megestrol	En±, G±	Acute toxic effects unlikely. May induce porphyria in susceptible patients.

(continued)

83

TABLE II–8. COMMON ANTINEOPLASTIC AGENTS AND THEIR TOXICITIES (CONTINUED)

Drug	Major Site(s) of Toxicity[a]	Comments
Other hormones		
Leuprolide	En+	Acute toxic effects unlikely. Initial increase in luteinizing hormone, follicle-stimulating hormone levels.
Mitotic inhibitors		
Etoposide	An+, G+, M++	Myelosuppression major toxicity. Dystonic reaction reported.
Teniposide	An+, G+, M++, Ex+	One report of sudden death from hypotension, cardiac arrhythmias.
Vinblastine	G+, M++, N+, Ex++	Myelosuppression, ileus, syndrome of inappropriate antidiuretic hormone reported after overdose.
Vincristine sulfate	G+, M±, N++, Ex++	Delayed (up to 9 days) seizures, delirium, coma reported after overdoses.
Miscellaneous		
Altretamine	G+, N+, M+	Reversible peripheral neuropathy.
Asparaginase	An++, En+, G+, H++, N++, R+	Bleeding diathesis. Hyperglycemia.
BCG (Intravesical)	G+	Attenuated mycobacterium bovis. Bladder irritation common. Risk of sepsis in immunocompromised patients.
Dacarbazine	Al+, An+, En+, G++, H+, M+, N+, Ex±	May produce flulike syndrome. Photosensitivity reported.
Hydroxyurea	D+, G+, M++	Leukopenia, anemia more common than thrombocytopenia.
Levamisole	G+, N+	May have nicotinic and muscarinic effects at cholinergic receptors. Gastroenteritis, dizziness, headache after 2–5 mg/kg dose reported. Generalized seizures, coma reported during treatment.
Mitotane	Al+, D+, En++, G++, N++	Adrenal suppression; glucocorticoid replacement essential during stress.
Paclitaxel	An++, C+, M+, N+	Severe hypersensitivity reactions, including death, reported. Hypotension, bradycardia, ECG abnormalities, conduction abnormalities may occur.
Procarbazine hydrochloride	An+, D+, En+, G++, M++, N++	Monoamine oxidase inhibitor activity. Disulfiramlike ethanol interaction.
Streptozocin	En+, G+, H+, M+, R++	Destroys pancreatic beta islet cells, may produce acute diabetes mellitus. Niacinamide (see p 359) may be effective in preventing islet cell destruction.

[a] Al = alopecia; An = anaphalaxis allergy or drug fever; C = cardiac; D = dermatologic; En = endocrine; Ex = extravasation risk; G = gastrointestinal; H = hepatic; M = myelosuppressive; N = neurologic; P = pulmonary; R = renal. + = mild to moderate seeverity; ++ = severe toxicity; ± = minimal.

C. **Extravasation** of some antineoplastic drugs at the intravenous injection site may cause severe local injury, with skin necrosis and sloughing.

IV. **Diagnosis** is usually based on the history. Because some of the most serious toxic effects may be delayed until several days after exposure, early clinical symptoms and signs may not be dramatic.

    A. **Specific levels.** Not generally available. For methotrexate, see Table III–6, p 349.

    B. **Other useful laboratory studies.** CBC with differential, platelet count, electrolytes, glucose, BUN and creatinine, liver enzymes, and prothrombin time (PT). ECG may be indicated for cardiotoxic agents, and pulmonary function tests are indicated for agents with known pulmonary toxicity.

V. **Treatment**

    A. **Emergency and supportive measures**

        1. Maintain the airway and assist ventilation if necessary (see p 4).

        2. Treat coma (p 18), seizures (p 22), hypotension (p 15), and arrhythmias (p 10–14) if they occur.

        3. Treat nausea and vomiting with metoclopramide (p 352) and fluid loss caused by gastroenteritis with intravenous crystalloid fluids.

        4. **Bone marrow depression** should be treated with the assistance of an experienced hematologist or oncologist.

        5. **Extravasation.** Immediately stop the infusion and withdraw as much fluid as possible by negative pressure on the syringe. Then give the following specific treatment:

            a. **Dactinomycin, daunorubicin, idarubicin, mitomycin-C, plicamycin, mitoxantrone.** Apply ice compresses to extravasation site for 15 minutes 4 times daily for 3 days. Topical application of dimethyl sulfoxide (DMSO) may be beneficial (commercially available 50% solution is less concentrated than those used in experimental studies, but may be tried). There is no justification for injection of hydrocortisone or sodium bicarbonate.

            b. **Mechlorethamine.** Infiltrate site of extravasation with 10–15 mL of sterile 0.15 molar sodium thiosulfate (dilute 4 mL of 10% thiosulfate with sterile water to a volume of 15 mL); apply ice compresses for 6–12 hours.

            c. **Vincristine** or **vinblastine.** Place heating pad over the area on and off for 24 hours; elevate limb. Local injection of hyaluronidase (150–900 units) may be beneficial.

    B. **Specific drugs and antidotes.** Very few specific treatments or antidotes are available (Table II–8).

    C. **Decontamination** (see p 44)

        1. **Prehospital.** Administer activated charcoal, if available. Ipecac-induced emesis may be useful for initial treatment at the scene (eg, children at home) if it can be given within a few minutes of exposure.

        2. **Hospital.** Administer activated charcoal and a cathartic. Gastric emptying is not necessary following small ingestions if activated charcoal can be given promptly.

    D. **Enhanced elimination.** Because of the rapid intracellular incorporation of most agents, dialysis and other extracorporeal removal procedures are generally not effective (see Table II–8 for exceptions).

ANTISEPTICS AND DISINFECTANTS
Olga F. Woo, PharmD

ANTIDOTE   IPECAC   LAVAGE   CHARCOAL

Antiseptics are applied to living tissue to kill or prevent the growth of microorganisms. **Disinfectants** are applied to inanimate objects to destroy pathogenic microorganisms.

Despite their unproved worth, they are widely used in the household, food industry, and hospitals. This chapter describes toxicity caused by **hydrogen peroxide, potassium permanganate, hexylresorcinol,** and **ichthammol.** All these agents are generally used as dilute solutions and cause little or no toxicity. Hexylresorcinol is commonly found in throat lozenges. For toxicity of other antiseptics and disinfectants, see Iodine (p 187); Mercurochrome (p 210); Isopropyl alcohol (p 193); Pine oil (p 178); and Hypochlorite (p 130).

I. Mechanism of toxicity

A. Hydrogen peroxide is an oxidizing agent, but it is very unstable and readily breaks down to oxygen and water. Generation of oxygen gas in closed body cavities can potentially cause mechanical distention resulting in gastric or intestinal perforation.

B. Potassium permanganate is an oxidant, and the crystalline form or concentrated solutions are corrosive.

C. Hexylresorcinol is related to phenol but is much less toxic, although alcohol-based solutions possess vesicant properties.

D. Ichthammol contains about 10% sulfur in the form of organic sulfonates, and it is keratolytic to tissues.

II. Toxic dose

A. Hydrogen peroxide for household use is available in 3–5% solutions and is mildly irritating; concentrations above 10% are found in some hair-bleaching solutions and are potentially corrosive. A 3-year-old child died after ingesting 40% hydrogen peroxide.

B. Potassium permanganate solutions of greater than 1:5000 strength may cause corrosive burns.

III. Clinical presentation. Most antiseptic ingestions are benign, and mild irritation is self-limited. Spontaneous emesis and diarrhea may occur, especially after a large-volume ingestion.

A. Exposure to **concentrated** solutions may cause corrosive burns on the skin and mucous membranes, and oropharyngeal, esophageal, or gastric injury may occur. Glottic edema has been reported after ingestion of concentrated potassium permanganate.

B. Permanganate may also cause **methemoglobinemia** (see p 217).

C. Hydrogen peroxide ingestion may cause gastric distention and, rarely, perforation. Corrosive injury and air embolus have also been reported with the concentrated (> 10%) form.

IV. Diagnosis is based on a history of exposure and the presence of mild gastrointestinal upset or frank corrosive injury. Solutions of potassium permanganate are dark purple, and skin and mucous membranes are often characteristically stained.

A. Specific levels. Serum drug levels are not useful or available.

B. Other useful laboratory studies. Electrolytes, glucose, methemoglobin level (for potassium permanganate exposure), upright chest x-ray (if suspected gastric perforation).

V. Treatment

A. Emergency and supportive measures

1. After ingestion of concentrated solutions, monitor the airway for swelling and intubate if necessary.

2. Consult a gastroenterologist for possible endoscopy. Most ingestions are benign, and mild irritation is self-limited.

B. Specific drugs and antidotes. No specific antidotes are available for irritant or corrosive effects. If **methemoglobinemia** occurs, administer methylene blue (see p 351).

C. Decontamination

1. Ingestion (see p 44)

    a. Dilute immediately with water or milk.

    b. Perform gastric lavage cautiously. Do **not** induce emesis because of the risk of corrosive injury.

    c. Activated charcoal and cathartics are not effective.

2. **Eyes and skin.** Irrigate the eyes and skin with copious amounts of tepid water. Remove contaminated clothing.

D. **Enhanced elimination.** Enhanced elimination methods are neither necessary nor effective.

ARSENIC
Michael J. Kosnett, MD, MPH

ANTIDOTE   IPECAC   LAVAGE   CHARCOAL

Many inorganic and organic arsenic compounds are used in a variety of industries and commercial products, including wood preservatives, weed killers, herbicides, glass manufacturing, nonferrous alloys, and semiconductors. Arsenic is recovered as a by-product in copper and lead smelting. Natural soil deposits may contaminate artesian well water, particularly in regions of geothermal activity. Some commercial household ant stakes (eg, Grant's Ant Control Ant Stakes) contain arsenic-impregnated gels. Arsenic compounds are used in some veterinary pharmaceuticals and may also occur in some folk remedies and tonics. Arsine gas, a hydride of arsenic, is discussed on p 89.

I. **Mechanism of toxicity.** Arsenic compounds may be organic or inorganic and may contain arsenic in either a pentavalent (arsenate) or trivalent (arsenite) form. Once absorbed, arsenicals disrupt enzymatic reactions vital to cellular metabolism by interacting with sulfhydryl groups (trivalent arsenic) or substituting for phosphate (pentavalent arsenic).

A. Soluble arsenic compounds, which are well absorbed after ingestion or inhalation, pose the greatest risk for human intoxication.

B. Inorganic arsenic dusts (such as arsenic trioxide) are also irritants of the skin, mucous membranes, and respiratory and gastrointestinal tracts. Systemic poisoning can occur after percutaneous absorption.

C. Arsenic exerts clastogenic effects and is a known human carcinogen. Although arsenic compounds of low solubility (eg, gallium arsenide, calcium arsenate, elemental arsenic) have low acute toxicity, they may be retained in the lung after inhalation, possibly increasing cancer risk.

II. **Toxic dose.** The toxicity of arsenic compounds varies considerably based on the valence state, physical state, solubility, and the animal species exposed.

A. **Inorganic arsenic compounds.** In general, trivalent arsenic (As^{+3}) is 2–10 times more toxic than pentavalent arsenic (As^{+5}).

1. Acute ingestion of as little as 100–300 mg of a trivalent arsenic compound (eg, sodium arsenite) could be fatal.

2. In sensitive populations, chronic ingestion of 20–60 µg/kg/d (roughly 1–4 mg/d in an adult) may be associated with signs of chronic poisoning.

3. The OSHA permissible exposure limit (PEL) for workplace exposure to inorganic arsenic compounds is 10 µg/m³ as an 8-hour time-weighted average.

4. A 2- to 3-fold elevation in lung cancer mortality has been detected after 15–25 years of occupational exposure to airborne arsenic concentrations of 300–600 µg/m³. OSHA regulates arsenic as a workplace carcinogen.

B. **Organic arsenic.** In general, pentavalent organic arsenate compounds are less toxic than trivalent inorganic compounds. Marine organisms may contain large quantities of arsenobetaine, an organic trimethylated compound, which is excreted unchanged in the urine and produces no known toxic effects.

III. **Clinical presentation**

A. **Acute exposure** most commonly occurs following accidental, suicidal, or deliberate poisoning by ingestion.

1. **Gastrointestinal effects.** After a delay of minutes to hours, diffuse capillary damage results in hemorrhagic gastroenteritis. Nausea, vomiting, abdomi-

nal pain, and watery diarrhea are common. In severe cases, extensive tissue third-spacing of fluids combined with fluid loss from gastroenteritis may lead to hypotension, shock, and death.

2. **Cardiopulmonary effects.** Congestive cardiomyopathy, cardiogenic or noncardiogenic pulmonary edema, cardiac conduction abnormalities, and QT interval prolongation with polymorphous ventricular tachycardia (see p 14) may occur promptly or after a delay of several days.

3. **Neurologic effects.** Acute poisoning can cause delirium, encephalopathy, and coma. A delayed sensorimotor peripheral neuropathy may appear 2–6 weeks after acute ingestion. Sensory effects, particularly painful dysesthesias, occur early and more commonly in moderate poisoning, while ascending weakness and paralysis may predominate in severe poisoning. Neuromuscular respiratory failure has occurred.

4. **Other effects.** Transverse white striae in the nails (Aldrich-Mees lines) may become apparent months after an acute intoxication. Hair loss may also occur. Pancytopenia, particularly leukopenia, reaches a nadir at 1–3 weeks. Basophilic stippling of red cells may also be present.

B. **Chronic intoxication** is also associated with multisystemic effects, which may include fatigue and malaise, gastroenteritis, leukopenia and anemia (occasionally megaloblastic), sensorimotor peripheral neuropathy, hepatic transaminase elevation, noncirrhotic portal hypertension, and peripheral vascular insufficiency. In addition, skin disorders and cancer may occur.

1. **Skin lesions** take years to manifest (3–7 years for a characteristic pattern of hypo- and hyperpigmentation and hyperkeratoses; up to 40 years for skin cancer) and may occur after lower doses than those causing neuropathy or anemia.

2. **Cancer.** Chronic inhalation is associated with lung cancer. Chronic ingestion may also increase the risk of lung, liver, kidney, and bladder cancer.

IV. **Diagnosis** is usually based on a history of exposure combined with a typical presentation. Suspect acute arsenic poisoning in a patient with abrupt onset of abdominal pain, vomiting, watery diarrhea, and hypotension, possibly in association with multisystem signs and symptoms described above. A garlicky odor on the breath has been described but often is not present. Some arsenic compounds, particularly those of lower solubility, are radiopaque and may be visible on plain abdominal x-ray.

A. **Specific levels.** In the first 2–3 days after acute symptomatic poisoning, total 24-hour urinary excretion is typically in excess of several thousand micrograms (spot urine > 1000 µg/L) and, depending on severity of poisoning, may not return to background levels (< 50 µg/24-hour specimen) for weeks.

1. Ingestion of **seafood,** which may contain very large amounts of nontoxic arsenobetaine, can markedly elevate total urinary arsenic for 2–3 days.

2. **Blood levels** are highly variable and are rarely of value in management. Although whole blood arsenic, normally less than 3 µg/dL, may be elevated early in acute intoxication, it may decline rapidly to the normal range despite persistent elevated urinary excretion and continuing symptoms.

3. **Elevated concentrations of arsenic in nails or hair** (normally < 1 ppm) may persist for months after urine levels normalize, but should be interpreted cautiously owing to the possibility of external contamination.

B. **Other useful laboratory studies.** CBC and smear for basophilic stippling, electrolytes, glucose, BUN and creatinine, liver enzymes, CPK, urinalysis, ECG and ECG monitoring, abdominal and chest x-rays.

V. **Treatment**

A. **Emergency and supportive measures**

1. Maintain the airway and assist ventilation if necessary (see p 4).

2. Treat coma (p 18), shock (p 15), and arrhythmias (p 14) if they occur. Because of the association of arsenic with prolonged QT intervals, avoid quinidine, procainamide, and other type Ia antiarrhythmic agents.

3. Treat hypotension and fluid loss with aggressive use of intravenous crystalloid solutions.
4. Prolonged inpatient support and observation are indicated in patients with significant acute intoxication because cardiopulmonary complications may be delayed for several days.

B. Specific drugs and antidotes

1. In symptomatic patients, administer **BAL** (dimercaprol; see p 317), 3–5 mg/kg IM every 4–6 hours. The antidotal efficacy of BAL has been demonstrated in animals when it is administered promptly (ie, minutes to hours) after exposure. Treatment should not be delayed during the several days commonly required to obtain specific laboratory confirmation.
2. **Dimercaptosuccinic acid** (2,3-DMSA, succimer, p 332), a water-soluble analog of BAL, is also effective. However, it is available in the US only as an oral formulation, which precludes its use early in acute poisoning, when gastroenteritis and splanchnic edema may limit gut absorption. It may be used for oral treatment after the patient has stabilized or in patients with chronic intoxication.
3. The therapeutic end points of chelation are poorly defined; however, once urinary arsenic levels are less than 500 µg/L, endogenous biomethylation and detoxification may obviate the need for further chelation. The value of chelation for treatment of an established neuropathy (or prevention of an incipient neuropathy) has not been proved.

C. Decontamination (see p 44)

1. **Prehospital.** Administer activated charcoal, if available. Ipecac-induced emesis may be useful for initial treatment at the scene (eg, children at home) if it can be given within a few minutes of exposure.
2. **Hospital.** Administer activated charcoal. However, note that animal and in vitro studies suggest that activated charcoal has a relatively poor affinity for inorganic arsenic salts. Consider gastric lavage for large ingestions.

D. Enhanced elimination. Hemodialysis may be of possible benefit in patients with concomitant renal failure, but otherwise contributes minimally to arsenic clearance. There is no known role for diuresis, hemoperfusion, or repeat-dose charcoal.

ARSINE
Kent R. Olson, MD

ANTIDOTE   IPECAC   LAVAGE   CHARCOAL

Arsine is a colorless gas formed when arsenic comes into contact with hydrogen or with reducing agents in aqueous solution. Typically, exposure occurs in metal smelting and refining industries when metals containing arsenic as an alloy react with an acid. Arsine is also used as a dopant in the microelectronics industry.

I. **Mechanism of toxicity.** Arsine enters red blood cells and forms a complex that results in massive intravascular hemolysis. Several explanations are postulated for the hemolysis, including liberation of elemental arsenic and the formation of complexes with sulfhydryl groups essential to erythrocyte enzymes. **Renal failure** is the most common cause of death after arsine exposure. Renal failure is probably secondary to massive hemolysis and hemoglobinuria, but it may also be caused by direct toxic effects on renal tubular cells or deposition of the arsine-hemoglobin-haptoglobin complex.

II. **Toxic dose.** Arsine is the most toxic form of arsenic. The air level considered immediately dangerous to life or health (IDLH) is 6 ppm. Exposure to 250 ppm may be instantly lethal, and exposure to 25–50 ppm for 30 minutes is usually lethal. The recommended workplace limit (ACGIH TLV-TWA) is 0.05 ppm as an 8-hour time-weighted average. The odor threshold is approximately 0.5 ppm.

III. Clinical presentation

A. Because arsine gas is not acutely irritating, inhalation causes **no immediate symptoms.** Those exposed to high concentrations may describe a garliclike odor in the air but more typically are unaware that significant exposure has occurred.

B. After a **latent period of 2–24 hours** (depending on the intensity of exposure), massive hemolysis occurs, with early symptoms of malaise, headache, weakness, dyspnea, nausea, vomiting, abdominal pain, hemoglobinuria, and jaundice. Oliguria and acute renal failure often occur 1–3 days after exposure.

IV. Diagnosis

is based on a history of exposure; it should be suspected in any worker potentially exposed to arsine who develops acute hemolysis. Laboratory evidence of hemolysis includes acute anemia, anisocytosis, and fragmented red cells. Plasma free hemoglobin levels may exceed 2 g/dL, and haptoglobin levels are lowered. Routine urinalysis reveals hemoglobinuria but few intact red blood cells.

A. Specific levels. The urine arsenic concentration may be elevated, but this does not assist in emergency management. Whole blood arsenic concentrations of greater than 0.4 mg/L are associated with fatal cases.

B. Other useful laboratory studies. CBC, plasma free hemoglobin, haptoglobin, blood type and screen (cross-match if needed), BUN and creatinine, urinalysis.

V. Treatment

A. Emergency and supportive measures

1. Treat hemolysis with blood transfusions as needed.

2. Prevent deposition of hemoglobin and arsine complex in the kidney tubules by intravenously administering bicarbonate, fluids, and mannitol, if needed, to maintain an adequate (2–3 mL/kg/h) alkaline urine flow. (See discussion of treatment of rhabdomyolysis, p 25.)

B. Specific drugs and antidotes. BAL and other chelators are *not* effective for arsine-induced intoxication.

C. Decontamination. Remove victim from area. Rescuers should wear self-contained breathing apparatus to protect themselves from exposure.

D. Enhanced elimination. The arsine-haptoglobin-hemoglobin complex is not significantly removed by hemodialysis. Forced alkaline diuresis may prevent renal tubular necrosis but does not enhance removal of the complex.

ASBESTOS
John Balmes, MD

ANTIDOTE   IPECAC   LAVAGE   CHARCOAL

Asbestos is the name given to a group of naturally occurring silicates: chrysotile, amosite, and crocidolite and the asbestiform types of tremolite, actinolite, and anthophylite. Exposure to asbestos is a well-documented cause of pulmonary and pleural fibrosis, lung cancer, and mesothelioma, illnesses that may appear many years after exposure.

I. Mechanism of toxicity. Inhalation of thin fibers longer than 5 μ produces lung fibrosis and cancer in animals (shorter fibers are generally phagocytosed by macrophages and removed from the lungs). The exact mechanism of toxicity is unknown. Smoking cigarettes appears to enhance the likelihood of developing lung disease and malignancy.

II. Toxic dose. A safe threshold of exposure to asbestos has not been established. Balancing potential health risks against feasibility of workplace control, the 1986 OSHA federal asbestos standard set a permissible exposure limit (PEL) of 0.2 fibers per cubic centimeters (fibers/cc) as an 8-hour time-weighted average.

III. Clinical presentation. After a latent period of 15–20 years, the patient may develop one or more of the following clinical syndromes:

A. Asbestosis is a slowly progressive fibrosing disease of the lungs. Pulmonary impairment resulting from lung restriction and decreased gas exchange is common.

B. Pleural plaques typically involve only the parietal pleura and are usually asymptomatic but provide a marker of asbestos exposure. Rarely, significant lung restriction occurs as a result of severe pleural fibrosis involving both parietal and visceral surfaces.

C. Pleural effusions may occur as early as 5–10 years after the onset of exposure and are often unrecognized as asbestos-related.

D. Lung cancer is a common cause of death in patients with asbestos exposure, especially in cigarette smokers. **Mesothelioma** is a malignancy that may affect the pleura or the peritoneum. The incidence of **gastrointestinal cancer** may be increased in asbestos-exposed workers.

IV. Diagnosis is based on a history of exposure to asbestos (usually at least 15–20 years before onset of symptoms) and clinical presentation of one or more of the syndromes described above. Chest x-ray typically shows small, irregular, round opacities distributed primarily in the lower lung fields. Pleural plaques, diffuse thickening, or calcification may be present. Pulmonary function tests reveal decreased vital capacity and total lung capacity and impairment of carbon monoxide diffusion.

A. Specific tests. There are no specific blood or urine tests.

B. Other useful laboratory studies. Chest x-ray, arterial blood gases, pulmonary function tests.

V. Treatment

A. Emergency and supportive measures. Emphasis should be placed on **prevention** of exposure. All asbestos workers should be encouraged to stop smoking and to observe workplace control measures stringently.

B. Specific drugs and antidotes. There are none.

C. Decontamination (see p 41)

1. **Inhalation.** Persons exposed to asbestos dust and those assisting victims should wear protective equipment, including appropriate respirators and disposable gowns and caps. Watering down any dried material will help to prevent its dispersion into the air as dust.

2. **Skin exposure.** Asbestos is not absorbed through the skin. However, it may be inhaled from skin and clothes, so removal of clothes and washing the skin are recommended.

3. **Ingestion.** Asbestos is not known to be harmful by ingestion, so no decontamination is necessary.

D. Enhanced elimination. There is no role for these procedures.

AZIDE, SODIUM
Jo Ellen Dyer, PharmD

ANTIDOTE   IPECAC   LAVAGE   CHARCOAL

Sodium azide is a highly toxic, white crystalline solid. It has recently come into widespread use in automobile airbags: its explosive decomposition to nitrogen gas provides rapid inflation of the airbag. In addition, sodium azide is used in the production of metallic azide explosives, and as a preservative in laboratories. It has no current medical uses, but because of its potent vasodilatory effects, it has been evaluated as an antihypertensive agent.

I. Mechanism of toxicity

A. The mechanism of azide toxicity is unclear. Like cyanide and hydrogen sulfide, azide inhibits iron-containing respiratory enzymes such as cytochrome oxidase, resulting in cellular asphyxiation. Azide is also a potent, direct-acting vasodilator.

  B. Although neutral solutions are stable, acidification rapidly converts the azide salt to **hydrazoic acid**. Hydrazoic acid vapors are pungent and (at high concentrations) explosive. The acute toxicity of hydrazoic acid has been compared to hydrogen cyanide and hydrogen sulfide.

II. Toxic dose. Although several grams of azide are found in an automobile airbag, it is completely consumed and converted to nitrogen during the explosive inflation process, and toxicity has not been reported from exposure to spent airbags.

  A. Inhalation. Irritation symptoms or pungent odor do not give adequate warning of toxicity. The recommended workplace ceiling limit (ACGIH TLV-C) is 0.29 mg/m^3 for sodium azide and 0.11 ppm for hydrazoic acid. Air concentrations as low as 0.5 ppm may result in mucous membrane irritation, hypotension, and headache. A chemist who intentionally sniffed the vapor above a 1% hydrazoic acid solution became hypotensive, collapsed, and recovered 15 minutes later with residual headache. Workers in a lead azide plant exposed to air concentrations of 0.3–3.9 ppm experienced symptoms of headache, weakness, palpitations, mild smarting of the eyes and nose, and a fall in blood pressure. Laboratory workers adjacent to a sulfur analyzer emitting vapor concentrations of 0.5 ppm experienced symptoms of nasal stuffiness without detecting a pungent odor.

  B. Dermal. Industrial workers handling bulk sodium azide experienced headache, nausea, faintness, and hypotension, but it is unclear whether the exposure occurred via dermal absorption or inhalation.

  C. Ingestion. Several serious or fatal poisonings have occurred as a result of laboratory saline or distilled water containing 1–2% azide as a preservative being used for drinking or making tea, rather than as a result of exposure to concentrated material.

  1. Ingestion of several grams can cause death within 1–2 hours.

  2. Ingestion of 700 mg resulted in myocardial failure after 72 hours. Ingestion of 150 mg produced shortness of breath, tachycardia, restlessness, nausea, vomiting, and diarrhea within 15 minutes. Later, polydipsia, T wave changes on ECG, leukocytosis, and numbness occurred, lasting 10 days.

  3. Doses of 0.65–3.9 mg/d up to 2.5 years have been used experimentally as an antihypertensive. The hypotensive effect occurred within one minute. Headache was the only complaint noted in these patients.

III. Clinical presentation

  A. Irritation. Exposure to dust or gas may produce reddened conjunctivas and nasal and bronchial irritation that may progress to pulmonary edema.

  B. Systemic toxicity. Both inhalation and ingestion are associated with a variety of dose-dependent systemic symptoms. Early in the course, hypotension and tachycardia occur that can evolve to bradycardia, ventricular fibrillation, and myocardial failure. Neurologic symptoms include headache, restlessness, facial flushing, loss of vision, faintness, weakness, hyporeflexia, seizures, coma, and respiratory failure. Nausea, vomiting, diarrhea, diaphoresis, and lactic acidosis also appear during the course.

IV. Diagnosis is based on the history of exposure and clinical presentation.

  A. Specific levels. Specific blood levels are not routinely available. A simple qualitative test can be used: azide forms a red precipitate in the presence of ferric chloride.

  B. Other useful laboratory studies. Electrolytes, glucose, arterial blood gases or pulse oximetry, ECG.

V. Treatment. *Caution:* Cases involving severe azide ingestion are potentially dangerous to health care providers. In the acidic environment of the stomach, azide salts are converted to hydrazoic acid, which is highly volatile. Quickly isolate all vomitus or gastric washings, and keep the patient in a well-ventilated area. Wear appropriate respiratory protective gear if available and trained to use it. Dispose of azide with care. Contact with heavy metals, including copper or lead found in water pipes, forms metal azides that may explode.

A. Emergency and supportive measures

1. Protect the airway and assist ventilation (see p 4) if necessary. Insert an intravenous line and monitor the ECG and vital signs.

2. Treat coma (p 18), hypotension (p 15), seizures (p 22), and arrhythmias (p 14) if they occur.

B. Specific drugs and antidotes. There is no specific antidote.

C. Decontamination (see p 41–49)

1. **Inhalation.** Remove victim from exposure and give supplemental oxygen, if available. Rescuers should wear self-contained breathing apparatus and appropriate chemical protective clothing.

2. **Skin.** Remove and bag contaminated clothing and wash affected areas copiously with soap and water.

3. **Ingestion.** See caution statement above; isolate all vomitus or gastric washings to avoid exposure to volatile hydrazoic acid.

   a. **Prehospital.** Administer activated charcoal, if available). Do **not** induce emesis because of the risk of abrupt onset of hypotension or seizures.

   b. **Hospital.** Perform gastric lavage, and administer activated charcoal. The affinity of charcoal for azide is not known.

D. Enhanced elimination. There is no role for dialysis or hemoperfusion in acute azide poisoning.

BARBITURATES
Kent R. Olson, MD

ANTIDOTE   IPECAC   LAVAGE   CHARCOAL

Barbiturates are used as hypnotic and sedative agents, for the induction of anesthesia, and for the treatment of epilepsy and status epilepticus. They are often divided into 4 major groups by their pharmacologic activity and clinical use: **ultrashort-acting, short-acting, intermediate-acting,** and **long-acting** (Table II–9). *Common combination products* containing small amounts of barbiturates include Fiorinal and Donnatal.

I. Mechanism of toxicity

A. All barbiturates cause generalized **depression of neuronal activity** in the brain. These effects are primarily achieved through enhanced GABA-mediated synaptic inhibition. Hypotension that occurs with large doses is caused by depression of central sympathetic tone as well as by direct depression of cardiac contractility.

B. The various agents have different pharmacokinetic properties:

1. **Ultrashort-acting** barbiturates are highly lipid-soluble and rapidly penetrate the brain to induce anesthesia, then are quickly redistributed to other tissues. For this reason, the duration of effect is much shorter than the elimination half-life for these compounds.

2. **Long-acting barbiturates** are distributed more evenly and have long elimination half-lives, making them useful for once-daily treatment of epilepsy. Primidone (Mysoline) is metabolized to phenobarbital and phenylethylmalonamide (PEMA); although phenobarbital accounts for only about 25% of the metabolites, it has the greatest anticonvulsant activity.

II. Toxic dose. The toxic dose of barbiturates varies widely and depends on the drug, the route and rate of administration, and individual patient tolerance. In general, toxicity is likely when the dose exceeds 5–10 times the hypnotic dose. Chronic users or abusers may have striking tolerance to depressant effects.

TABLE II-9. COMMON BARBITURATES[a]

Drug	Normal Elimination Half-Life (h)	Usual Duration of Effect (h)	Usual Hypnotic Dose (Adult) (mg)	Minimum Toxic Level (mg/L)
Ultrashort-acting				
Methohexital	1–2	< 0.5	50–120	> 5
Thiopental	6–46	< 0.5	50–75	> 5
Short-acting				
Pentobarbital	15–48	> 3–4	100–200	> 10
Secobarbital	15–40	> 3–4	100–200	> 10
Intermediate-acting				
Amobarbital	8–42	> 4–6	65–200	> 10
Aprobarbital	14–34	> 4–6	40–160	> 10
Butabarbital	34–42	> 4–6	50–100	> 10
Long-acting				
Mephobarbital	11–67	> 6–12	50–100	> 30
Phenobarbital	80–120	> 6–12	100–320	> 30

[a]References: Harvey SC: Hypnotics and sedatives. Chap 17, pp 339–371, in: *Goodman & Gilman's The Pharmacological Basis of Therapeutics,* 7th ed. Gilman AG et al (editors), Macmillan, 1985; and Ellenhorn MJ, Barceloux DG: *Medical Toxicology.* Pages 576–577. Elsevier, 1988.

    A. The potentially fatal **oral dose** of the shorter-acting agents is 2–3 g, compared with 6–10 g for phenobarbital.

    B. Several deaths were reported in young women undergoing therapeutic abortion after they received rapid **intravenous injections** of 1–3 mg/kg of methohexital.

III. Clinical presentation. The onset of symptoms depends on the drug and the route of administration.

    A. Lethargy, slurred speech, nystagmus, and ataxia are common with mild to moderate intoxication. With higher doses, hypotension, coma, and respiratory arrest commonly occur. With deep coma, the pupils are usually small; the patient may lose all reflex activity and may appear to be dead.

    B. Hypothermia is common in patients with deep coma, especially if the victim has suffered exposure to a cool environment. Hypotension and bradycardia commonly accompany hypothermia.

IV. Diagnosis is usually based on a history of ingestion and should be suspected in any epileptic patient with stupor or coma. Although skin bullae are sometimes seen with barbiturate overdose, these are not specific for barbiturates. Other causes of coma should also be considered (see p 18).

    A. Specific levels. Serum levels of phenobarbital are usually readily available from hospital clinical laboratories; concentrations greater than 60–80 mg/L are usually associated with coma and those greater than 150–200 mg/L with severe hypotension. For short-acting barbiturates, coma is likely when the serum concentration exceeds 20–30 mg/L. Barbiturates are easily detected in routine toxicologic screening.

    B. Other useful laboratory studies. Electrolytes, glucose, BUN, creatinine, arterial blood gases or pulse oximetry, chest x-ray.

V. Treatment

    A. Emergency and supportive measures

        1. Protect the airway and assist ventilation (see p 4) if necessary.

2. Treat coma (p 18), hypothermia (p 19), and hypotension (p 15) if they occur.

B. Specific drugs and antidotes. There is no specific antidote.

C. Decontamination (see p 44)

    1. Prehospital. Administer activated charcoal, if available. Ipecac-induced emesis may be useful for initial treatment at the scene (eg, children at home) if it can be given within a few minutes of exposure.

    2. Hospital. Administer activated charcoal and a cathartic. Consider gastric lavage for massive ingestion.

D. Enhanced elimination

    1. Alkalinization of the urine (p 49) increases the elimination of phenobarbital but not other barbiturates. Its value in acute overdose is unproved, and it may potentially contribute to fluid overload and pulmonary edema.

    2. Repeat-dose activated charcoal has been shown to decrease the half-life of phenobarbital, but there is no evidence that it actually shortens duration of coma.

    3. Hemoperfusion may be indicated for severely intoxicated patients not responding to supportive care (ie, with intractable hypotension).

BARIUM
Olga F. Woo, PharmD

ANTIDOTE   IPECAC   LAVAGE   CHARCOAL

Barium poisonings are uncommon and usually result from accidental contamination of food sources, suicidal ingestion, or occupational inhalation exposure. The water-soluble barium salts (acetate, carbonate, chloride, hydroxide, nitrate, sulfide) are highly toxic, whereas the insoluble salt barium sulfate is nontoxic because it is not absorbed. Soluble barium salts are found in depilatories, fireworks, and rodenticides and are used in the manufacture of glass and in dyeing textiles. Barium sulfide and polysulfide may also produce hydrogen sulfide toxicity (see p 182).

I. Mechanism of toxicity

    A. Systemic barium poisoning is characterized by profound hypokalemia, leading to respiratory and cardiac arrest. The mechanism for the rapid onset of severe hypokalemia is not known; studies have excluded intracellular sequestration of potassium, enhanced renal elimination, and adrenergic stimulation. It is proposed that barium ions have a direct action on muscle cell potassium permeability, which stimulates smooth, striated, and cardiac muscles, resulting in peristalsis, arterial hypertension, muscle twitching, and cardiac arrhythmias.

    B. Inhalation of insoluble inorganic barium salts can cause baritosis, a benign pneumoconiosis.

    C. Pharmacokinetics. Barium is stored in bone and slowly excreted via the feces. Tissue distribution follows a 3-compartment model with half-lives of 3.6, 34, and 1033 days.

II. Toxic dose. The minimum oral toxic dose of soluble barium salts is undetermined but may be as low as 200 mg. Lethal doses range between 1–30 g for various barium salts because absorption is influenced by gastric pH and foods high in sulfate.

III. Clinical presentation. Within minutes to a few hours after ingestion, victims develop profound hypokalemia and skeletal muscle weakness progressing to flaccid paralysis of the limbs and respiratory muscles. Ventricular arrhythmias also occur. Gastroenteritis with severe watery diarrhea, mydriasis with impaired visual accommodation, and central nervous system depression are sometimes present. More often, patients remain conscious even when severely intoxicated.

IV. Diagnosis is based on a history of exposure, accompanied by rapidly progressive hypokalemia and muscle weakness.

    A. Specific levels. Blood barium levels are not routinely available.

    B. Other useful laboratory studies. Electrolytes (potassium), BUN, creatinine, arterial blood gases or pulse oximetry, ECG.

V. Treatment

    A. Emergency and supportive measures

        1. Maintain the airway and assist ventilation if necessary (see p 4).

        2. Treat fluid losses from gastroenteritis with intravenous crystalloids.

        3. Attach a cardiac monitor and observe patient closely for several hours after ingestion.

    B. Specific drugs and antidotes. Administer **potassium chloride** (KCl) at 10–15 meq/h IV to treat symptomatic or severe hypokalemia (see p 35). Large doses of potassium may be necessary (doses as high as 420 meq over 24 hours have been given).

    C. Decontamination (see p 44)

        1. Induce emesis or perform gastric lavage. *Caution:* Rapidly progressive weakness may increase the risk of pulmonary aspiration.

        2. Magnesium sulfate or sodium sulfate (60–100 mL) may be administered orally to precipitate ingested barium as the insoluble sulfate salt.

        3. The efficacy of activated charcoal is not known.

    D. Enhanced elimination

        1. Diuresis with saline and furosemide to obtain a urine flow of 4–6 mL/kg/h may enhance barium elimination.

        2. Hemodialysis and hemoperfusion have not been evaluated in the treatment of serious barium poisoning.

BENZENE
Charles E. Becker, MD

ANTIDOTE   IPECAC   LAVAGE   CHARCOAL

Benzene, a clear volatile liquid with a characteristic pleasant odor, is one of the most widely used industrial chemicals, with more than 2 million workers potentially exposed. It is used as a constituent in gasoline; as a solvent for fats, inks, paints, and plastics; and as a chemical intermediate in the synthesis of a variety of materials. It is generally not present in household products.

   I. Mechanism of toxicity. Like other hydrocarbons, benzene can cause a chemical pneumonia if it is aspirated. See p 178 for a general discussion of hydrocarbon toxicity.

    A. Once absorbed, benzene causes central nervous system depression and may sensitize the myocardium to the arrhythmogenic effects of catecholamines.

    B. Benzene is also known for its chronic effects on the hematopoietic system, which are thought to be caused by the phenolic metabolite.

    C. Benzene is a suspected human carcinogen.

  II. Toxic dose. Benzene is rapidly absorbed by inhalation and ingestion and, to a limited extent, percutaneously.

    A. The estimated lethal **oral** dose is 100 mL, but as little as 15 mL has caused death.

    B. The recommended workplace limit (ACGIH TLV-TWA) for benzene **vapor** is 10 ppm as an 8-hour time-weighted average. A single exposure to 10,000 ppm can be fatal. Chronic exposure to air concentrations well below the threshold for smell (2 ppm) are associated with hematopoietic toxicity.

 III. Clinical presentation

    A. Acute exposure may cause immediate central nervous system effects, including headache, nausea, dizziness, convulsions, and coma. Symptoms of CNS toxicity should be apparent immediately after inhalation or within 30–60 minutes after ingestion. Ventricular arrhythmias may result from sensitization of the myocardium.

B. After **chronic exposure,** hematologic disorders such as aplastic anemia, thrombocytopenia, multiple myeloma, myelofibrosis, preleukemia, and acute leukemia may occur. Chromosomal abnormalities have been reported, although no effects on fertility have been described in women following occupational exposure.

IV. Diagnosis of benzene poisoning is based on a history of exposure and typical clinical findings. With chronic hematologic toxicity, erythrocyte, leukocyte, and thrombocyte counts may first increase before the onset of aplastic anemia.

A. Specific levels

1. Increased urine phenol levels may be useful for following workers' exposure (if diet is carefully controlled for phenol products). Spot urine phenol higher than 20 mg/L suggests excessive occupational exposure. Urinary muconic acid is more specific for benzene exposure.

2. Benzene can also be measured in expired air for up to 5 days after exposure.

3. Blood levels of benzene or metabolites are not clinically useful.

B. Other useful laboratory studies. CBC, electrolytes, BUN, creatinine, liver function tests, ECG monitoring, chest x-ray (if aspiration suspected).

V. Treatment

A. Emergency and supportive measures

1. Maintain the airway and assist ventilation if necessary (see p 4).

2. Treat coma (p 18), seizures (p 22), arrhythmias (p 14), and other complications if they occur.

3. Be cautious with use of any adrenergic agents (eg, epinephrine, metaproterenol, albuterol) because of the possibility of myocardial sensitization.

4. Monitor vital signs and ECG for 12–24 hours after significant exposure.

B. Specific drugs and antidotes. There is no specific antidote.

C. Decontamination (see p 41)

1. **Inhalation.** Immediately move the victim to fresh air and administer oxygen, if available.

2. **Skin and eyes.** Remove clothing and wash the skin; irrigate exposed eyes with copious amounts of water or saline.

3. **Ingestion** (see p 44)

   a. Prehospital. Administer activated charcoal, if available. Do not induce emesis because of the risk of abrupt onset of coma or convulsions.

   b. Hospital. Administer activated charcoal and a cathartic. Consider gastric lavage for a recent (less than 30 minutes) large ingestion.

D. Enhanced elimination. Dialysis and hemoperfusion are not effective.

BENZODIAZEPINES
Karl A. Sporer, MD

ANTIDOTE   IPECAC   LAVAGE   CHARCOAL

The drug class of benzodiazepines contains many compounds that vary widely in potency, duration of effect, presence or absence of active metabolites, and clinical use (Table II–10). In general, death from benzodiazepine overdose is rare, unless the drugs are combined with other central nervous system depressant agents such as ethanol or barbiturates. Newer potent short-acting agents have been considered the sole cause of death in recent forensic cases.

TABLE II–10. BENZODIAZEPINES FOR ORAL USE[a]

Drug	Half-Life (h)	Active Metabolite	Oral Adult Dose (mg)
Alprazolam	10–20	Yes	0.25–0.5
Chlordiazepoxide	5–15	Yes	5–50
Clonazepam	20–30	Yes	0.5–2
Clorazepate	50–80[b]	Yes	3.75–30
Diazepam	30–60	Yes	5–20
Estazolam	10–25	Slight	1–2
Flurazepam	50–100[b]	Yes	15–30
Lorazepam	10–20	No	2–4
Midazolam	2–5	Yes	1–5[c]
Oxazepam	5–10	No	15–30
Prazepam	0.5–2	Yes	20–60
Temazepam	10–17	Slight	15–30
Triazolam	1.5–3	?	0.125–0.5

[a]Adapted in part, with permission, from Harvey SC: Hypnotics and sedatives. Table 17–4 in *Goodman and Gilman's The Pharmacological Basis of Therapeutics.* 7th ed. Gilman AG et al (editors). Macmillan, 1985.
[b]Half-life of active metabolite, to which effects can be attributed.
[c]IM or IV.

I. **Mechanism of toxicity.** Benzodiazepines enhance the action of the inhibitory neurotransmitter gamma-aminobutyric acid (GABA). They also inhibit other neuronal systems by poorly defined mechanisms. The result is generalized depression of spinal reflexes and the reticular activating system. This may cause coma and respiratory arrest.
   A. Respiratory arrest is more likely with newer short-acting triazolobenzodiazepines such as triazolam (Halcion), alprazolam (Xanax), and midazolam (Versed).
   B. Cardiopulmonary arrest has occurred after rapid injection of diazepam, possibly because of CNS-depressant effects or because of the toxic effects of the diluent propylene glycol.
II. **Toxic dose.** In general, the toxic-therapeutic ratio for benzodiazepines is very high. For example, oral overdoses of diazepam have been reported in excess of 15–20 times the therapeutic dose without serious depression of consciousness. In contrast, respiratory arrest has been reported after ingestion of 5 mg of triazolam and after rapid intravenous injection of diazepam, midazolam, and many other benzodiazepines.
III. **Clinical presentation.** Onset of CNS depression may be observed within 30–120 minutes of ingestion, depending on the compound. Lethargy, slurred speech, ataxia, coma, and respiratory arrest may occur. Generally, patients with benzodiazepine-induced coma have hyporeflexia and midposition or small pupils. Hypothermia may occur. Serious complications are more likely when newer short-acting agents are involved or when other depressant drugs have been ingested.
IV. **Diagnosis** is usually based on the history of ingestion or recent injection. The differential diagnosis should include other sedative-hypnotic agents, antidepressants, antipsychotics, and narcotics. Coma and small pupils do not respond to naloxone but will reverse with administration of flumazenil
   A. **Specific levels.** Serum drug levels are often available from regional commercial toxicology laboratories but are rarely of value in emergency management. Urine and blood qualitative screening may provide rapid confirmation of expo-

sure. Certain immunoassays may not detect newer benzodiazepines or those in low concentrations.
  B. **Other useful laboratory studies.** Glucose, arterial blood gases or pulse oximetry.

V. Treatment
A. Emergency and supportive measures
1. Protect the airway and assist ventilation if necessary (see p 4).
2. Treat coma (p 18), hypotension (p 15), and hypothermia (p 19) if they occur. Hypotension usually responds promptly to supine position and intravenous fluids.

B. Specific drugs and antidotes. Flumazenil (see p 340) is a specific benzodiazepine receptor antagonist that can rapidly reverse coma. However, because benzodiazepine overdose by itself is rarely fatal, the role of flumazenil in routine management has yet to be established. It is administered intravenously with a starting dose of 0.1–0.2 mg, repeated as needed up to a total of no more than 3 mg. It has some important potential drawbacks:
1. It may induce seizures in patients with cyclic antidepressant overdose.
2. It may induce acute withdrawal, including seizures and autonomic instability, in patients who are addicted to benzodiazepines.
3. Resedation is common when the drug wears off after 1–2 hours, and repeated dosing is usually required.

C. Decontamination (see p 44)
1. **Prehospital.** Administer activated charcoal, if available. Ipecac-induced emesis may be useful for initial treatment at the scene (eg, children at home) if it can be given within a few minutes of exposure. However, do **not** induce emesis in patients who have ingested newer ultra short-acting agents such as triazolam, because onset of coma may be rapid and abrupt.
2. **Hospital.** Administer activated charcoal and a cathartic. Gastric emptying is not necessary if activated charcoal can be given promptly.

D. Enhanced elimination. There is no role for diuresis, dialysis, or hemoperfusion. Repeat-dose charcoal has not been studied.

BETA-ADRENERGIC BLOCKERS
Neal L. Benowitz, MD

ANTIDOTE   IPECAC   LAVAGE   CHARCOAL

Beta-adrenergic blocking agents are widely used for the treatment of hypertension, arrhythmias, angina pectoris, migraine headaches, and glaucoma. Many patients with beta-blocker overdose will have underlying cardiovascular diseases or will be taking other cardioactive medications, both of which may aggravate beta-blocker overdose. A variety of beta blockers are available, with varying pharmacologic effects and clinical uses (Table II–11).

  I. **Mechanism of toxicity.** Excessive beta-adrenergic blockade is common to overdose with all drugs in this category. Although beta-receptor specificity is seen at low doses, it is lost in overdose.
  A. **Propranolol** and other agents with membrane-depressant (quinidinelike) effects further depress myocardial contractility and conduction. Propranolol is also lipid soluble, which enhances brain penetration and can cause seizures and coma.
  B. **Pindolol** and other agents with partial beta-agonist activity may cause hypertension.
  C. **Sotalol,** which also has type III antiarrhythmic activity, prolongs the QT interval in a dose-dependent manner and may cause torsades des pointes (see p 14) and ventricular fibrillation.

TABLE II–11. COMPARISON OF BETA-ADRENERGIC BLOCKING AGENTS

Drug	Usual Daily Adult Dose (mg/24 h)	Cardio-selective	Membrane Depression	Partial Agonist	Normal Half-life (h)
Acebutolol	400–800	+	+	+	7
Alprenolol	200–800	0	+	++	2–3
Atenolol	50–100	+	0	0	6–9
Betaxolol[a]	10–20	+	0	0	14–22
Carteolol	2.5–10	–	–	+	6
Esmolol[b]		+	0	0	9 min
Labetalol[c]	200–800	0	+	0	3–5
Levobunolol[a]		0	0	0	5–6
Metoprolol	100–450	+	+/–	0	3–4
Nadolol	80–240	0	0	0	14–24
Oxyprenolol	40–480	0	+	++	2
Penbutolol	20–40	–	–	+	5
Pindolol	5–60	0	+	+++	3–4
Propranolol	40–360	0	++	0	2–6
Sotalol[d]	160–480	–	–	–	17
Timolol[a]	20–80	0	0	+/–	4–5

[a]Also available as ophthalmic preparation.
[b]Intravenous infusion 50–200 µg/kg/min.
[c]Alpha-adrenergic blocking activity.
[d]Class III antiarrhythmic activity.

II. **Toxic dose.** The response to beta-blocker overdose is highly variable depending on underlying medical disease or other medications. Susceptible patients may have severe or even fatal reactions to therapeutic doses. There are no clear guidelines, but ingestion of only 2–3 times the therapeutic dose (Table II–11) should be considered potentially life-threatening in all patients. Atenolol and pindolol appear to be less toxic than other agents.

III. **Clinical presentation.** The pharmacokinetics of beta blockers vary considerably, and duration of poisoning may range from minutes to days.
   A. **Cardiac disturbances,** including hypotension and bradycardia, are the most common manifestations of poisoning. Atrioventricular block, intraventricular conduction disturbances, cardiogenic shock, and asystole may occur with severe overdose, especially with membrane-depressant drugs such as propranolol. The ECG usually shows a normal QRS duration with increased PR interval; QRS widening occurs with massive intoxication.
   B. **Central nervous system toxicity** including convulsions, coma, and respiratory arrest is commonly seen with propranolol and other membrane-depressant and lipid-soluble drugs.
   C. **Bronchospasm** is most common in patients with preexisting asthma or chronic bronchospastic disease.
   D. **Hypoglycemia** and **hyperkalemia** may occur.

IV. **Diagnosis** is based on the history of ingestion, accompanied by bradycardia and hypotension. Other drugs that may cause a similar presentation after overdose include sympatholytic and antihypertensive drugs, digitalis, cyclic antidepressants, and calcium channel blockers.

A. **Specific levels.** Measurement of beta-blocker serum levels may confirm the diagnosis but does not contribute to emergency management.

B. **Other useful laboratory studies.** Electrolytes, glucose, BUN, creatinine, arterial blood gases, ECG and ECG monitoring.

V. Treatment

A. Emergency and supportive measures

1. Maintain the airway and assist ventilation if necessary (see p 4).
2. Treat coma (p 18), seizures (p 22), hypotension (p 15), hyperkalemia (p 35), and hypoglycemia (p 32) if they occur.
3. Treat bradycardia (p 10) with atropine, 0.01–0.03 mg/kg IV; isoproterenol (start with 4 µg/min and increase infusion as needed); or cardiac pacing.
4. Treat bronchospasm with nebulized bronchodilators (p 9).
5. Continuously monitor the vital signs and ECG for at least 6 hours after ingestion.

B. Specific drugs and antidotes

1. Bradycardia and hypotension resistant to the above measures should be treated with **glucagon,** 0.1–0.3 mg/kg IV bolus, repeated as needed (see p 342).
2. Wide complex conduction defects caused by membrane-depressant poisoning may respond to **hypertonic sodium bicarbonate** 1–2 meq/kg, as given for cyclic antidepressant overdose (see p 318).
3. Torsades des pointes polymorphous ventricular tachycardia associated with QT prolongation resulting from sotalol poisoning can be treated with **isoproterenol** infusion, **magnesium,** or **overdrive pacing** (see p 14). Correction of hypokalemia may also be useful.

C. Decontamination (see p 44)

1. **Prehospital.** Administer activated charcoal, if available. Ipecac-induced emesis may be useful for initial treatment at the scene if it can be given within a few minutes of exposure.
2. **Hospital.** Administer activated charcoal and a cathartic. Consider gastric lavage for large ingestions, especially involving propranolol. Gastric emptying is not necessary for small ingestions if activated charcoal can be given promptly.

D. Enhanced elimination.
Most beta blockers, especially the more toxic drugs such as propranolol, are highly lipophilic and have a large volume of distribution. For those with a relatively small volume of distribution coupled with a long half-life or low intrinsic clearance (eg, acebutolol, atenolol, nadolol, sotalol), hemoperfusion, hemodialysis, or repeat-dose charcoal may be effective.

BETA-2–ADRENERGIC STIMULANTS
Susan Kim, PharmD

ANTIDOTE   IPECAC   LAVAGE   CHARCOAL

Beta-adrenergic agonists can be broadly categorized as having β_1 and β_2 receptor activity. This section describes the toxicity of several β_2 selective agonists that are commonly available for oral use: albuterol, metaproterenol, ritodrine, and terbutaline (see Table II–12). Nylidrin, a peripheral vasodilator with mixed β_1 and β_2 activity, would be expected to have a similar toxicity profile.

I. **Mechanism of toxicity.** Stimulation of β_2 receptors results in relaxation of smooth muscles in the bronchi, uterus, and skeletal muscle vessels. At high toxic doses, selectivity for β_2 receptors may be lost and β_1 effects may be seen.

II. **Toxic dose.** Generally, single ingestion of more than the total daily dose (see Table II–12) is expected to produce signs and symptoms of toxicity. Dangerously

TABLE II–12. COMMONLY AVAILABLE β_2 SELECTIVE AGONISTS

Drug	Adult Dose (mg/d)	Pediatric Dose (mg/kg/d)	Onset (min)	Duration (h)
Albuterol (Proventil, Ventolin)	8–16	0.3–0.8	30	4–8
Metaproterenol (Alupent)	60–80	0.9–2.0	30	4
Ritodrine (Yutopar)	40–120	N/A	30	4–6
Terbutaline (Brethine)	7.5–20	0.15–0.6	30	4–8

exaggerated responses to therapeutic doses of terbutaline have been reported in pregnant women, presumably as a result of pregnancy-induced hemodynamic changes.

III. **Clinical presentation.** Overdose of these drugs affects primarily the cardiovascular system. Most overdoses, especially in children, result in only mild toxicity.

   A. **Vasodilation** results in reduced peripheral vascular resistance and can lead to significant hypotension. The diastolic pressure is usually reduced to a greater extent than the systolic pressure, resulting in a wide pulse pressure and bounding pulse.

   B. **Tachycardia** is a common reflex response to vasodilation, and may also be caused by direct stimulation of β_1 receptors as β_2 selectivity is lost in high doses. Supraventricular tachycardia or ventricular extrasystoles are occasionally reported.

   C. **Agitation and skeletal muscle tremors** are common. Seizures are rare.

   D. **Metabolic effects** include hypokalemia, hyperglycemia, and lactic acidosis. Hypokalemia is caused by an intracellular shift of potassium rather than true depletion.

IV. **Diagnosis** is based on the history of ingestion. The findings of tachycardia, hypotension with a wide pulse pressure, tremor, and hypokalemia are strongly suggestive. Theophylline overdose (see p 295) may present with similar manifestations.

   A. **Specific levels.** Serum drug levels are not generally available and do not contribute to emergency management.

   B. **Other useful laboratory studies.** Electrolytes, glucose, BUN, creatinine, CPK (if excessive muscle activity suggests rhabdomyolysis), ECG monitoring.

V. Treatment. Most overdoses are mild and do not require aggressive treatment.

   A. **Emergency and supportive measures**

      1. Maintain the airway and assist ventilation if necessary (see p 4).

      2. Monitor the vital signs and ECG for about 4–6 hours after ingestion.

      3. If seizures or altered mental status occur, they are most likely caused by cerebral hypoperfusion, and should respond to treatment of hypotension (see below).

      4. Treat hypotension initially with boluses of intravenous crystalloid, 10–30 mL/kg. If this fails to improve the blood pressure, use a beta-adrenergic blocker (see **B,** below).

      5. Sinus tachycardia rarely requires treatment, especially in children, unless accompanied by hypotension or ventricular dysrhythmias. If treatment is necessary, use beta-adrenergic blockers (see **B,** below).

      6. Hypokalemia does not usually require treatment, since it is transient and does not reflect a total body potassium deficit.

   B. **Specific drugs and antidotes.** Hypotension, tachycardia, and ventricular arrhythmias are caused by excessive beta-adrenergic stimulation, and beta blockers are specific antagonists. Give **propranolol** (see p 373), 0.01–0.03 mg/kg IV, or **esmolol** (see p 338), 25–50 µg/kg/min IV. Use beta blockers cautiously in patients with a prior history of asthma or wheezing.

   C. **Decontamination** (see p 44)

      1. **Prehospital.** Administer activated charcoal, if available. Ipecac-induced

emesis may be useful for initial treatment at the scene (eg, children at home) if it can be given within a few minutes of exposure.

2. **Hospital.** Administer activated charcoal and a cathartic. Gastric emptying is not necessary if activated charcoal can be given promptly.

D. **Enhanced elimination.** There is no role for these procedures.

BODY-BUILDING PRODUCTS
Jo Ellen Dyer, PharmD

ANTIDOTE   IPECAC   LAVAGE   CHARCOAL

There is a lucrative and growing market for any product claimed to improve body image or athletic performance. The incidence of use of anabolic steroids among high school males is estimated to be 6.6%, and use among women is expanding. Various drugs (eg, gamma hydroxybutyrate [GHB]) and other substances sold as nutritional supplements are also promoted for bodybuilding. These so-called bodybuilding agents are commonly available at gymnasiums, through mail order, and in health food stores.

Androgenic steroids have been placed in schedule III of the federal controlled substances act because of the potential for abuse as well as evidence of chronic adverse effects, dependence, and withdrawal syndromes. In an effort to increase or prolong anabolic effects and to evade detection in drug screens, numerous modifications have been made to the basic steroid ring structure. Recognized *parenteral* anabolic steroids are boldenone (a veterinary product), nandrolone, and testosterone and its esters. *Oral* products include danazol, ethylestrenol, fluoxymesterone, methandrostenolone, methyltestosterone (also buccal tablets), oxandrolone, oxymetholone, stanozolol, and testolactone. There are other illicit derivatives for which there is no reliable human information.

Gamma hydroxybutyrate (GHB, Gamma Hydrate, Gamma-OH, Oxybate, Somatomax) was originally investigated as an anesthetic agent until its severe side effects and lack of analgesia were recognized. It is now legally available in the US only under investigational use for treatment of narcolepsy. GHB is promoted as a growth hormone releaser, diet aid, and soporific.

Bodybuilding aids sold as **nutritional supplements** include **chromium picolinate, vanadyl sulfate,** and **spirulina.** The law does not require nutritional supplements to be proved safe and effective prior to sale if there are no labeling drug claims (ie, claims to diagnose, cure, treat, mitigate, prevent disease, or affect structure or function of the human body). The purity of available products has not been evaluated.

I. **Mechanism of toxicity**

A. **Androgenic hormones** act by established molecular mechanisms to induce pleiotropic responses. Virilizing side effects are mediated by androgen receptors, and feminizing effects are mediated by estrogenic metabolites. Anabolic effects refer to the increased protein synthesis and decreased catabolism. Retention of nitrogen, sodium, potassium, phosphate, sulfur, and associated water produces an edema that contributes to short-term weight gain. The exogenous androgens interfere with normal feedback regulation of hormone levels, inhibit pituitary production of luteinizing hormone and follicle-stimulating hormone, and cause testicular atrophy and infertility. The mechanisms causing cholestatic hepatitis, peliosis hepatitis, hepatic carcinoma, and psychologic effects are uncertain. In addition, nonsterile products and needle sharing may lead to infection.

B. **Gamma hydroxybutyrate** is a structural analogue of the neurotransmitters gamma-aminobutyric acid (GABA) and glutamine. It crosses the blood-brain barrier and increases dopamine levels in some areas of the brain. Even though its specific receptor is not defined, GHB has been proposed to act as a neurotransmitter.

C. Chromium. Trivalent chromium III is commonly found in nature and is considered an essential trace element in biologic systems. Trivalent compounds are generally poorly soluble and of low toxicity compared with hexavalent chromium VI compounds (see Chromium, p 135). In **chromium picolinate,** chromium III is chelated by picolinate, an isomer of niacin claimed to enhance the absorption of chromium and to lower cholesterol. Although deficiency is unlikely and supplementation has not been demonstrated to have any consequence in normal individuals, chromium is proported by its boosters to enhance glucose utilization and increase lean muscle mass.

D. Vanadium is a ubiquitous, nonessential trace element found in biologic systems. It occurs in six oxidation states, including pentavalent vanadium, which is used industrially and forms an irritant dust, and tetravalent vanadium, which is currently investigated in diabetic rats for proposed insulinlike effects. Tetravalent vanadium is poorly absorbed from the gastrointestinal tract, binds reversibly to transferrin, and is eliminated through the kidneys. The consequences of dietary supplementation are unknown. As a bodybuilding agent, tetravalent **vanadyl sulfate** is promoted as an insulin enhancer to increase lean muscle mass.

E. Spirulina, a blue-green alga promoted for its amino acid content, often contains **niacin**. It can produce a typical niacin flushing reaction owing to histamine release, which is often alarming to the unexpecting user (see Vitamins, p 306).

II. Toxic dose

A. Androgenic steroids have low acute toxicity. Chronic therapeutic use and chronic overuse in patterns of stacking (using oral and parenteral agents together), pyramiding (progressively increasing the dose), or cycling (interrupting steroid use with periods of abstinence) produce marked psychologic and physiologic effects and dependence.

B. Gamma hydroxybutyrate. Response to low oral doses of GHB is unpredictable, with variability between patients and in the same patient. Narcolepsy studies with 30 mg/kg reported effects including abrupt onset of sleep, hallucinations, and myoclonic movements. Anesthetic studies reported unconsciousness with 50 mg/kg and unarousable coma with 60 mg/kg. Fasting, ethanol, and other depressants may enhance effects of GHB. There have been no fatalities attributed to the use of GHB alone.

C. Chromium III toxicity is unlikely with a single acute dose. Gastrointestinal absorption of trivalent chromium is estimated to be less than 1%; increased bioavailability with chelation to picolinate is not established. The minimum daily requirement for chromium has not been established, but 50–200 μg is estimated to be a safe and adequate daily dose.

D. Vanadium. The estimated average daily dietary intake is 20 μg. Oral ingestion data are not sufficient to establish minimum risk levels of vanadyl sulfate. Ammonium vanadyl tartrate, another tetravalent vanadium compound, produced gastrointestinal symptoms with daily doses of 50–125 mg.

III. Clinical presentation

A. Androgenic steroids. Symptoms other than gastrointestinal upset are unlikely following **acute** oral ingestion.

   1. Classic signs of **chronic** androgenic steroid abuse are pituitary hypogonadism, feminization of males, and virilization of females. Sudden cardiac death may occur owing to alteration of the lipid profile, hypertension, cardiomyopathy, increased aggregation of platelets, and coronary artery spasm. Psychotropic effects include paranoia, psychosis, aggressive behavior, and hypomania. Other effects include acne, immune system suppression, and polycythemia. Cholestatic or peliosis hepatitis and hepatoma are possible hepatic effects.

   2. Children may have accelerated skeletal growth with early fusion of the epiphysis and precocious sexual development.

3. Discontinuing chronic use may produce a withdrawal syndrome consisting of depression and suicidal ideation.

B. Gamma hydroxybutyrate. Patients with acute overdose of GHB commonly present with coma, bradycardia, and myoclonic movements. GHB produces soporific effects and euphoria within 15 minutes of an oral dose. Unconsciousness and profound coma may follow in 30–40 minutes. Delirium and tonic clonic seizures are possible. Bradycardia is more common, but stimulation may cause tachycardia and mild hypertension. Bradypnea with increase in tidal volume is common, and Cheyne-Stokes respiration occurs. Emesis is a common side effect. When GHB is ingested alone, duration of coma is usually short, with responsiveness returning within 2–4 hours and complete resolution of effects within 8 hours.

C. Chromium. Although chromium deficiency has been described, the consequences of chronic overuse are unknown.

D. Vanadium. Excess supplementation of vanadyl sulfate in humans has not been evaluated. Volunteers given doses of 50–125 mg/d of ammonium vanadyl tartrate reported green tongue, intestinal cramps, diarrhea, and black stools.

E. Spirulina ingestion may cause a niacin-related flushing reaction (see p 306).

IV. Diagnosis is usually based on history of use of bodybuilding aids and characteristic clinical manifestations. Keep in mind that since some of these agents are illegal, the user may not admit to their use.

A. Specific levels

1. Urine screens are an effective way to determine recent use of anabolic steroids, but may not be sensitive to all available androgens.

2. Assays are not generally available for GHB.

3. Serum chromium levels are not routinely available, and would not be effective in determining small changes caused by chronic supplementation. Normal serum chromium is 0.04–0.35 µg/L. Normal urine excretion averages less than 10 µg/d.

4. Serum vanadium levels in normal persons are 2–4 µg/L, but are not routinely available. Normal urine excretion averages less than 8 µg/d.

B. Other useful laboratory studies. Electrolytes, glucose, BUN, creatinine, liver function tests. **In steroid users,** also obtain cholesterol, and x-rays should be evaluated in young patients to determine bone maturation and effect on epiphyseal centers.

V. Treatment

A. Emergency and supportive measures

1. Maintain the airway and assist ventilation if necessary (p 4).

2. Treat coma (p 18), seizures (p 22), and bradycardia or other arrhythmias (p 10–14) if they occur.

3. Patients with niacin-related flush from spirulina may benefit from diphenhydramine (p 331).

B. Specific drugs and antidotes. There are no specific antidotes available. Flumazenil has not been evaluated in GHB toxicity.

C. Decontamination (see p 44). Androgenic steroids and nutritional supplements are generally used chronically, so patients are unlikely to benefit from decontamination.

1. Prehospital. Give activated charcoal if available. Do **not** induce emesis because of the risk of rapidly developing coma.

2. Hospital. Administer activated charcoal and cathartic. For recent acute ingestion of GHB, perform gastric lavage. Because GHB is rapidly absorbed after ingestion, gastric emptying may not be useful if the ingestion is small (eg, < 1 tsp) or more than 1 hour has passed.

D. Enhanced elimination. There is no evidence for efficacy of enhanced removal procedures such as dialysis or hemoperfusion. There is no evidence that chelation is beneficial for chromium III removal. Chelation of vanadium with penicillamine, BAL, and calcium sodium EDTA has been suggested; however, there is no human evidence to support its use.

BORIC ACID AND BORATES
Olga F. Woo, PharmD

ANTIDOTE   IPECAC   LAVAGE   CHARCOAL

Boric acid has been used for many years in a variety of products as an antiseptic and as a fungistatic agent in baby talcum powder. Boric acid powder (99%) is still used as a pesticide against ants and cockroaches. In the past, widespread and indiscriminate use resulted in many cases of severe poisoning owing to chronic absorption of boric acid through broken or abraded skin. Epidemics have also occurred in which boric acid was added to infant formula. Although such cases of chronic toxicity seldom occur now, acute ingestion by children at home is common.

I. **Mechanism of toxicity.** The mechanism of borate poisoning is unknown. Boric acid is not highly corrosive. It probably acts as a generalized cellular poison. Organ systems most commonly affected are the gastrointestinal tract, brain, liver, and kidney.

Pharmacokinetics: The volume of distribution (Vd) is 0.17–0.50 L/kg. Elimination is mainly through the kidneys, and 85–100% of a dose may be found in the urine over 5–7 days. The elimination half-life is 12–27 hours.

II. **Toxic dose**

A. The **acute** single oral toxic dose is highly variable, but serious poisoning is reported to occur with 1–3 g in newborns, 5 g in infants, and 20 g in adults. A teaspoon of 99% boric acid contains 3–4 g. Most accidental ingestions in children result in minimal or no toxicity.

B. **Chronic** ingestion or application to abraded skin is much more serious than acute single ingestion. Serious toxicity and death occurred in infants ingesting 5–15 g in formula over several days; serum borate levels were 400–1600 mg/L.

III. **Clinical presentation**

A. Following oral or dermal absorption, the earliest symptoms are gastrointestinal with vomiting and diarrhea. Emesis and diarrhea may have a blue-green color. Significant dehydration and renal failure can occur, with death caused by profound shock.

B. Neurologic symptoms of hyperactivity, agitation, and seizures may occur early.

C. An erythrodermic rash (boiled lobster appearance) is followed by exfoliation after 2–5 days. Alopecia totalis has been reported.

IV. **Diagnosis** is based on a history of exposure, the presence of gastroenteritis (possibly with blue-green emesis), exfoliative rash, and elevated serum borate levels.

A. **Specific levels.** Serum borate levels are not generally available, and may not correlate accurately with the level of intoxication. Analysis of blood for borates can be obtained from National Medical Services, Inc., telephone (215) 657-4900, or consult a local laboratory. Normal blood levels are less than 5 mg/L.

B. **Other useful laboratory studies.** Electrolytes, glucose, BUN, creatinine, urinalysis.

V. **Treatment**

A. **Emergency and supportive measures**

1. Maintain the airway and assist ventilation if necessary (see p 4).

2. Treat coma (p 18), seizures (p 22), hypotension (p 15), and renal failure (p 36) if they occur.

B. **Specific drugs and antidotes.** There is no specific antidote.

C. **Decontamination** (see p 44)

1. **Prehospital.** Administer activated charcoal, if available. Ipecac-induced emesis may be useful for initial treatment at the scene (eg, children at home) if it can be given within a few minutes of exposure.

  2. Hospital. Administer activated charcoal (although boric acid is not well-adsorbed). Consider gastric lavage for large ingestions.
 D. Enhanced elimination. Hemodialysis is effective and is indicated after massive ingestions and for supportive care of renal failure. Peritoneal dialysis has not proved effective in enhancing elimination in infants.

BOTULISM
Olga F. Woo, PharmD

ANTIDOTE   IPECAC   LAVAGE   CHARCOAL

Botulism dates back to the 1700s as a recognized cause of fatal food poisoning. Rare outbreaks still occur in the USA, usually associated with improper home canning of foods. Recently, new sources of botulism have been discovered, such as improperly prepared or stored pot pies, fried onions, and baked potatoes; **wound botulism** in parenteral drug abusers; and **infant botulism.**

 I. Mechanism of toxicity
  A. Botulism is caused by a heat-labile neurotoxin (botulin) produced by the bacteria *Clostridium botulinum.* Different strains of the bacterium produce 7 distinct exotoxins: A, B, C, D, E, F, and G; types A, B, and E are most frequently involved in human disease. Botulin toxin irreversibly binds to cholinergic nerve terminals and prevents acetylcholine release from the axon. Severe muscle weakness results, and death is caused by respiratory failure.
  B. Botulinum spores are ubiquitous in nature but are not dangerous unless they are allowed to germinate in an anaerobic environment with a pH greater than 4.6. Incompletely cooked foods left out at ambient temperatures for several hours may produce lethal amounts of botulin toxin. The spores can be destroyed by pressure cooking at a temperature of at least 120 °C (250 °F) for 30 minutes. The toxin can be destroyed by boiling at 100 °C (212 °F) for one minute or heating at 80 °C (176 °F) for 20 minutes.
 II. Toxic dose. Botulin toxin is extremely potent; as little as one taste of botulin-contaminated food (approximately 0.05 µg of toxin) may be fatal.
 III. Clinical presentation
  A. Classic botulism occurs after ingestion of preformed toxin in contaminated food. The incubation period is usually 18–36 hours after ingestion but can vary from a few hours to 8 days. The earlier the onset of symptoms, the more severe the illness. Initial symptoms may suggest a flulike syndrome: sore throat, dry mouth, and gastrointestinal upset. Later, diplopia, ptosis, dysarthria, and other cranial nerve weaknesses occur, followed by progressive descending paralysis and finally respiratory arrest. The patient's mentation is clear, and there is no sensory loss. Pupils may be dilated and unreactive or normal. Constipation may occur.
  B. Infant botulism is not caused by ingestion of preformed toxin but by in vivo production of toxin in the immature infant gut. Infants 1 week to 6 months old (most are 2–6 months) who are breast-fed and those given honey may have a higher risk of developing the disease, which is characterized by hypotonia, constipation, tachycardia, difficulty in feeding, head lag, and diminished gag reflex. It is rarely fatal, and infants usually recover strength within 4–6 weeks.
  C. Wound botulism occurs mostly in young adult intravenous drug abusers, and occasionally results from infected surgical wounds. The organism germinates in an infected injection site and produces toxin in vivo. Typical manifestations of botulism occur after an incubation period of 4–14 days.
 IV. Diagnosis is based on a high index of suspicion in any patient with a dry sore throat, clinical findings of descending cranial nerve palsies or gastroenteritis, and a history of ingestion of home-canned food. Symptoms may be slow in onset but are sometimes rapidly progressive. Electromyography may reveal normal conduc-

tion velocity but decreased motor action potential and no incremental response to repetitive stimulation.

The differential diagnosis includes myasthenia gravis, Eaton-Lambert syndrome, and the Fisher variant of Guillain-Barré syndrome.

A. Specific levels. Diagnosis is confirmed by determination of the toxin in serum, stool, or wound; although these tests are useful for public health investigation, they cannot be used to determine initial treatment because the analysis takes more than 24 hours to perform. Obtain serum, stool, wound pus, vomitus, gastric contents, and suspect food for toxin analysis by the local or state health department. The results may be negative if the samples were collected late or the quantity of toxin is small.

B. Other useful laboratory studies. Electrolytes, blood sugar, arterial blood gases, electromyogram, CSF if CNS infection is suspected.

V. Treatment

A. Emergency and supportive measures
   1. Maintain the airway and assist ventilation if necessary (see p 4).
   2. Obtain arterial blood gases and observe closely for respiratory weakness; respiratory arrest can occur abruptly.

B. Specific drugs and antidotes
   1. Classic and wound botulism
   a. Botulin **antitoxin** (see p 320) binds the circulating free toxin and prevents the progression of illness; however, it does not reverse established neurologic manifestations. Available antitoxins are bivalent (AB) and trivalent (ABE); trivalent antitoxin is preferred unless the exact toxin is known.
      (1) Consult the local health department or Centers for Disease Control, Atlanta, Ga; telephone (404) 329-2888 (24-hour number).
      (2) Determine sensitivity to horse serum prior to treatment.
      (3) Administer 1 vial every 4 hours for at least 4–5 doses or until no toxin is present in serum.
   b. Guanidine may be useful as adjunctive therapy in enhancing release of acetylcholine at the nerve terminal and improving ocular and limb paralysis but not respiratory paralysis. The dose is 15–50 mg/kg/d divided into 4–5 doses.
   2. Infant botulism. Trivalent antitoxin is not recommended for infant botulism, but clinical trials are underway in California with human tissue-derived botulism immune globulin (BIG). In California, contact the state Department of Health Services, telephone (510) 540-2646. The use of oral antibiotics and cathartics is controversial.

C. Decontamination (see p 44)
   1. Prehospital. Induce emesis if recent ingestion of known or suspected contaminated material has occurred.
   2. Hospital. If recent ingestion is suspected, perform gastric lavage and administer activated charcoal and a cathartic.

D. Enhanced elimination. There is no role for enhanced elimination; the toxin binds rapidly to nerve endings, and any free toxin can be readily detoxified with antitoxin.

BROMATES

Kathryn H. Keller, PharmD

ANTIDOTE   IPECAC   LAVAGE   CHARCOAL

Bromate poisoning was most common during the 1940s and 1950s when it was a popular ingredient in home permanent neutralizers. Less toxic substances have been substituted for bromates in kits for home use, but poisonings still occur occasionally from professional products (bromate-containing permanent wave neutralizers have been ingested in suicide attempts by professional hairdressers). Commercial bakeries often use bromate salts to improve bread texture, and bromates are components of fusing material for some explosives. Bromates were previously used in matchstick heads. Bromate-contaminated sugar was the cause of one reported epidemic of bromate poisoning.

I. Mechanism of toxicity. The mechanism is not known. The bromate ion is toxic to the cochlea, causing irreversible hearing loss, and nephrotoxic, causing acute tubular necrosis. Bromates may be converted to hydrobromic acid in the stomach, causing gastritis. Bromates are also strong oxidizing agents, capable of oxidizing hemoglobin to methemoglobin.

II. Toxic dose. The acute ingestion of 200–500 mg/kg of potassium bromate is likely to cause serious poisoning. Ingestion of 2–4 oz of 2% potassium bromate solution caused serious toxicity in children. The sodium salt is believed to be less toxic.

III. Clinical presentation
- **A.** Within 2 hours of ingestion, victims develop gastrointestinal symptoms, including vomiting (occasionally with hematemesis), diarrhea, and epigastric pain. This may be accompanied by restlessness, lethargy, coma, and convulsions.
- **B.** An asymptomatic phase of a few hours may follow before overt renal failure develops. Anuria is usually apparent within 1–2 days of ingestion; renal failure may be irreversible.
- **C.** Tinnitus and irreversible sensorineural deafness occurs between 4–16 hours after ingestion in adults, but deafness may be delayed for several days in children.
- **D.** Hemolysis and thrombocytopenia have been reported in some pediatric cases.
- **E.** Methemoglobinemia (see p 217) has been reported, but is rare.

IV. Diagnosis is based on a history of ingestion, especially if accompanied by gastroenteritis, hearing loss, or renal failure.
- **A. Specific levels.** Bromates may be reduced to bromide in the serum, but bromide levels do not correlate with the severity of poisoning. There are qualitative tests for bromates, but serum concentrations are not available.
- **B. Other useful laboratory studies.** CBC, electrolytes, glucose, BUN, creatinine, urinalysis, audiometry, methemoglobin.

V. Treatment
- **A. Emergency and supportive measures**
  1. Maintain the airway and assist ventilation if necessary (see p 4).
  2. Treat coma (p 18) and seizures (p 22) if they occur.
  3. Replace fluid losses, treat electrolyte disturbances caused by vomiting and diarrhea, and monitor renal function. Perform hemodialysis as needed for support of renal failure.
- **B. Specific drugs and antidotes**
  1. **Sodium thiosulfate** (see p 376) may theoretically reduce bromate to the less toxic bromide ion. There are few data to support the use of thiosulfate, but in the recommended dose it is benign. Administer 10% thiosulfate solution, 10–50 mL (0.2–1 mL/kg) IV.
  2. Treat methemoglobinemia with **methylene blue** (see p 351).
- **C. Decontamination** (see p 44)
  1. **Prehospital**
     a. Sodium bicarbonate (baking soda), 1 tsp in 8 oz of water, given orally may prevent formation of hydrobromic acid in the stomach.
     b. Administer activated charcoal, if available. Ipecac-induced emesis may be useful for initial treatment at the scene (eg, children at home) if it can be given within a few minutes of exposure.
  2. **Hospital**
     a. For large recent ingestions, consider gastric lavage with a **2% sodium bicarbonate** solution to prevent formation of hydrobromic acid in the stomach.

b. Administer activated charcoal and a cathartic.

D. Enhanced elimination. The bromate ion may be removed by hemodialysis, but this treatment has not been carefully evaluated. Since bromates are primarily excreted renally, initiating hemodialysis early in the course of a documented large ingestion may be prudent therapy to prevent irreversible hearing loss and renal failure.

BROMIDES
Delia A. Dempsey, MD

ANTIDOTE   IPECAC   LAVAGE   CHARCOAL

Bromide was once used as a sedative and an effective anticonvulsant, and until 1975 it was the major ingredient in a variety of over-the-counter products such as Bromo-Seltzer and Dr. Miles' Nervine. Currently, bromide is still found in photographic chemicals and as the bromide salt or other constituent of numerous medications. Bromism (chronic bromide intoxication) has been reported with some bromide-containing drugs (halothane and pyridostigmine), but not others (eg, dextromethorphan hydrobromide, brompheniramine, ipratropium bromide). Bromide is also found in some sources of well water, and it may be released from some bromide-containing hydrocarbons (eg, methyl bromide, ethylene dibromide, and halothane). Foodstuff fumigated with methyl bromide may contain residual bromide, but the amounts are too small to cause toxicity.

I. **Mechanism of toxicity.** Bromide ion substitutes for chloride in various membrane transport systems, particularly within the nervous system. It is preferentially reabsorbed over chloride by the kidney. Up to 30% of chloride may be replaced in the body. With high bromide levels, the membrane-depressant effect progressively impairs neuronal transmission. The half-life of bromide is about 12 days, and bioaccumulation occurs with chronic exposure. Bromide is excreted in breast milk. It crosses the placenta, and neonatal bromism has been described.

II. **Toxic dose.** The adult therapeutic dose of bromide is 3–5 g. One death has been reported after ingestion of 100 g of sodium bromide. Chronic consumption of 0.5–1 g per day may cause bromism.

III. **Clinical presentation.** Death is rare. Acute oral overdose usually causes nausea and vomiting from gastric irritation. Chronic intoxication can result in a variety of neurologic, psychiatric, gastrointestinal, and dermatologic effects.

   A. Neurologic and **psychiatric** manifestations are protean and include restlessness, irritability, ataxia, confusion, hallucinations, psychosis, weakness, stupor, and coma. At one time bromism was responsible for 5–10% of admissions to psychiatric facilities.

   B. Gastrointestinal effects include nausea and vomiting (acute ingestion) and anorexia and constipation (chronic use).

   C. Dermatologic effects include acneiform, pustular, or erythematous rashes. Up to 25% of patients are affected.

IV. **Diagnosis.** Consider bromism in any confused or psychotic patient with a high serum chloride level and a low or negative anion gap. The serum chloride level is often falsely elevated owing to interference by bromide in the analytic test: the serum chloride is elevated by 0.8 meq/L for each 1 meq/L (or 8 mg/dL) of bromide present.

   A. Specific levels. A specific serum bromide level may be obtained. *Check units carefully:* 80 mg/L = 1 meq/L = 8 mg/dL = 8 mg% = 0.08 mg/mL). The threshold for detection by usual methods is 50 mg/L. Therapeutic levels are 50–100 mg/L (0.6–1.2 meq/L); sedation may occur with levels of 100–500 mg/L (1.2–6 meq/L); bromide levels above 500 mg/dL (6 meq/L) are common in patients with florid bromism; and levels above 3000 mg/L (40 meq/L) may be fatal.

B. Other useful laboratory studies. Electrolytes, glucose, BUN, creatinine, abdominal x-ray (bromide is radiopaque).

V. Treatment

A. Emergency and supportive measures

1. Protect the airway and assist ventilation if needed (see p 4).

2. Treat coma if it occurs (see p 18).

B. Specific drugs and antidotes. There is no specific antidote. However, administering chloride will promote bromide excretion (see below).

C. Decontamination (see p 44)

1. Prehospital. Ipecac-induced emesis may be useful for initial treatment at the scene (eg, children at home) if it can be given within a few minutes of exposure.

2. Hospital. After recent ingestion, induce emesis or perform gastric lavage, and administer a cathartic. Activated charcoal does not adsorb inorganic bromide ion, but it may adsorb organic bromides, and should also be used if other drug ingestion is suspected.

D. Enhanced elimination. Bromide is eliminated entirely by the kidney. The serum half-life can be dramatically reduced with fluids and chloride loading. Administer **sodium chloride** intravenously as half-normal saline (D50.5NS) at a rate sufficient to obtain a urine output of 4–6 mL/kg/h. **Furosemide,** 1 mg/kg, may assist urinary excretion. Hemodialysis may rarely be indicated in patients with renal insufficiency or severe toxicity. Hemoperfusion is not effective.

CADMIUM
Kent R. Olson, MD

ANTIDOTE   IPECAC   LAVAGE   CHARCOAL

Cadmium (Cd) is found in sulfide ores, along with zinc and lead. The metallic form is used in electroplating because of its anticorrosive properties; the metallic salts are used as pigments and stabilizers in plastics; and cadmium alloys are used in soldering and welding and in nickel-cadmium batteries. Cadmium solder in water pipes and cadmium pigments in pottery can be sources of contamination of water and acidic foods.

I. Mechanism of toxicity. Inhaled cadmium is at least 60 times more toxic than the ingested form. Fumes and dust may cause delayed chemical pneumonitis and resultant pulmonary edema and hemorrhage. Ingested cadmium is a gastrointestinal tract irritant. Once absorbed, cadmium is bound to metallothionein and filtered by the kidney, where renal tubule damage may occur.

II. Toxic dose

A. Inhalation. The ACGIH-recommended threshold limit value (TLV-TWA) for air exposure to cadmium dusts and salts fumes is 0.05 mg/m^3 as an 8-hour time-weighted average. The ceiling value (TLV-C) for fumes is 0.05 mg/m^3. Exposure to 5 mg/m^3 inhaled for 8 hours may be lethal.

B. Ingestion. Cadmium salts in solutions of greater than 15 mg/L may induce vomiting. The lethal oral dose ranges from 350 to 8900 mg.

III. Clinical presentation

A. Acute inhalation may cause cough, wheezing, headache, fever, and, if severe, chemical pneumonitis and noncardiogenic pulmonary edema within 12–24 hours after exposure.

B. Acute oral ingestion of cadmium salts causes nausea, vomiting, abdominal cramps, and diarrhea, sometimes bloody, within minutes after exposure. Deaths after oral ingestion result from shock or acute renal failure.

IV. Diagnosis is based on a history of exposure and the presence of respiratory complaints (after inhalation) or gastroenteritis (after ingestion).

A. Specific levels. Whole blood cadmium levels may confirm the exposure. Very little cadmium is excreted in the urine, and urine determinations are of no value. Measures of tubular microproteinuria (beta-microglobulin, retinol-binding protein, albumin, metallothionein) are used to monitor the toxic effect of cadmium on the kidney.

B. Other useful laboratory studies. CBC, electrolytes, glucose, BUN, creatinine, arterial blood gases or oximetry, chest x-ray.

V. Treatment

A. Emergency and supportive measures

1. **Inhalation.** Monitor arterial blood gases and obtain chest x-ray. Observe for at least 6–8 hours and treat wheezing and pulmonary edema (see p 7–9) if they occur. After significant exposure, it may be necessary to observe for 1–2 days for delayed-onset noncardiogenic pulmonary edema.

2. **Ingestion.** Treat fluid loss caused by gastroenteritis with intravenous crystalloid fluids (see p 15).

B. Specific drugs and antidotes. There is no evidence that chelation therapy (eg, with BAL, EDTA, or penicillamine) is effective.

C. Decontamination

1. **Inhalation.** Remove the victim from exposure and give supplemental oxygen, if available.

2. **Ingestion** (see p 44)

   a. **Prehospital.** Administer activated charcoal, if available (uncertain benefit). Do *not* induce emesis because of the irritant nature of cadmium salts.

   b. **Hospital.** Perform gastric lavage. Administer activated charcoal, although the efficacy of charcoal is unknown. Do not give cathartics if the patient has diarrhea.

D. Enhanced elimination. There is no role for dialysis, hemoperfusion, or repeat-dose charcoal.

CAFFEINE
Christopher R. Brown, MD

ANTIDOTE   IPECAC   LAVAGE   CHARCOAL

Caffeine is the most widely used psychoactive substance. Besides its well-known presence in coffee, it is available in many over-the-counter and prescription oral medications and as injectable caffeine sodium benzoate (occasionally used for neonatal apnea). Caffeine is widely used as an anorexiant, a coanalgesic, a diuretic, and a sleep suppressant. Although caffeine has a wide therapeutic index and rarely causes serious toxicity, there are many documented cases of accidental, suicidal, and iatrogenic intoxication, some resulting in death.

I. **Mechanism of toxicity.** Caffeine is a trimethylxanthine closely related to theophylline. It acts primarily through inhibition of the adenosine receptor. In addition, with overdose there is considerable β_1- and β_2-adrenergic stimulation secondary to release of endogenous catecholamines.

Caffeine is 100% absorbed orally with a volume of distribution of 0.7–0.8 L/kg. Its elimination half-life ranges from 3 hours in healthy smokers to 10 hours in nonsmokers. In infants less than 2–3 months old, metabolism is extremely slow and the half-life may exceed 24 hours.

II. **Toxic dose.** The reported lethal oral dose is 10 g (150–200 mg/kg), although one case report documents survival after a 24-g ingestion. In children, ingestion of 35 mg/kg may lead to moderate toxicity. Coffee contains 50–200 mg of caffeine per cup depending on how it is brewed. Infants younger than 2–3 months of age metabolize caffeine very slowly and may become toxic after repeated doses. As with theophylline, chronic administration of excessive doses may cause serious toxicity with relatively low serum concentrations compared with acute single ingestion.

III. Clinical presentation

A. The earliest symptoms with **acute** caffeine poisoning are usually anorexia, tremor, and restlessness. These are followed by nausea, vomiting, tachycardia, and confusion. With serious intoxication, delirium, seizures, supraventricular and ventricular tachyarrhythmias, hypokalemia, and hyperglycemia may occur. Hypotension is caused by excessive β_2-mediated vasodilation and is characterized by a low diastolic pressure and a wide pulse pressure.

B. Chronic high-dose caffeine intake can lead to "caffeinism" (nervousness, irritability, anxiety, tremulousness, muscle twitching, insomnia, palpitations, and hyperreflexia).

IV. Diagnosis is suggested by the history of caffeine exposure or the constellation of nausea, vomiting, tremor, tachycardia, seizures, and hypokalemia (also consider theophylline; see p 295).

A. Specific levels. Serum caffeine levels are not routinely available in hospital laboratories but can be determined at regional commercial toxicology laboratories. Toxic concentrations may be detected by cross-reaction with theophylline assays (see Table I–32, p 40). Coffee drinkers have caffeine levels of 1–10 mg/L, while levels of 80 mg/L have been associated with death. The level associated with a high likelihood of seizures is unknown.

B. Other useful laboratory studies. Electrolytes, glucose, ECG monitoring.

V. Treatment

A. Emergency and supportive measures

1. Maintain the airway and assist ventilation if necessary (see p 4).
2. Treat seizures (p 22) and hypotension (p 15) if they occur.
3. Hypokalemia usually resolves without aggressive treatment.
4. Monitor ECG and vital signs for at least 6 hours after ingestion or until serum level is documented to be decreasing.

B. Specific drugs and antidotes. Beta blockers effectively reverse cardiotoxic effects mediated by excessive beta-adrenergic stimulation. Treat tachyarrhythmias or hypotension with intravenous **propranolol,** 0.01–0.02 mg/kg (see p 373), or **esmolol,** 25–100 µg/kg/min (see p 338), beginning with low doses and titrating to effect. Because of its short half-life and cardioselectivity, esmolol is preferred.

C. Decontamination (see p 44)

1. **Prehospital.** Administer activated charcoal, if available. Ipecac-induced emesis may be useful for initial treatment at the scene (eg, children at home) if it can be given within a few minutes of exposure.
2. **Hospital.** Administer activated charcoal and a cathartic. Gastric emptying is not necessary if activated charcoal can be given promptly, although gastric lavage should be considered for massive ingestion.

D. Enhanced elimination. Repeat-dose activated charcoal (see p 52) may enhance caffeine elimination. Seriously intoxicated patients (with multiple seizures, significant tachyarrhythmias, or intractable hypotension) may require charcoal hemoperfusion (see p 51).

CALCIUM ANTAGONISTS
Neal L. Benowitz, MD

ANTIDOTE   IPECAC   LAVAGE   CHARCOAL

Calcium antagonists (also known as calcium channel blockers) are widely used to treat angina pectoris, coronary spasm, hypertension, hypertrophic cardiomyopathy, supraventricular cardiac arrhythmias, and migraine headache. Toxicity from calcium antagonists may occur with therapeutic use (often owing to drug interactions) or as a result of accidental or intentional overdose. Overdoses of calcium antagonists are fre-

quently life-threatening and represent an increasingly important source of drug-induced mortality.

  I. Mechanism of toxicity. Calcium antagonists slow the influx of calcium through
     cellular calcium channels. Currently marketed agents act primarily on vascular smooth
     muscle and the heart. They result in coronary and peripheral vasodilation, reduced
     cardiac contractility, slowed (AV) nodal conduction, and depressed sinus node ac-
     tivity. Lowering of blood pressure through a fall in peripheral vascular resistance
     may be offset by reflex tachycardia, although this reflex response may be blunted
     by depressant effects on contractility and sinus node activity. Table II–13 summa-
     rizes usual doses, sites of activity, and half-lives of common calcium antagonists.
     A. In usual therapeutic doses, amlodipine, felodipine, isradipine, nicardipine,
         nifedipine, and nitrendipine act primarily on blood vessels, whereas verapamil
         and diltiazem act on both the heart and blood vessels. In overdose, however,
         this selectivity may be lost.
     B. Bepridil, used primarily for refractory angina pectoris, has verapamil-like effects
         on the heart, inhibits the fast sodium channel, and has type III antiarrhythmic
         activity. Bepridil also has proarrhythmic effects, especially in the presence of
         hypokalemia.
     C. Important **drug interactions** may result in toxicity. Hypotension is more likely
         to occur in patients taking beta blockers, nitrates, or both, especially if they are
         hypovolemic after diuretic therapy. Patients taking disopyramide or other de-
         pressant cardioactive drugs and those with severe underlying myocardial dis-
         ease are also at risk for hypotension. Life-threatening bradyarrhythmias, in-
         cluding asystole, may occur when beta blockers and verapamil are given
         together parenterally. Propranolol also inhibits the metabolism of verapamil.
 II. Toxic dose. Usual therapeutic daily doses for each agent are listed in Table II–13.
     The toxic/therapeutic ratio is relatively small, and serious toxicity may occur with
     therapeutic doses. Any dose greater than the usual therapeutic range should be
     considered potentially life-threatening. Note that many of the common agents are
     available in sustained-release formulations, which can result in delayed onset or
     sustained toxicity.
III. Clinical presentation
     A. The primary features of calcium antagonist intoxication are **hypotension** and
         bradycardia. Hypotension may be caused by peripheral vasodilation, reduced
         cardiac contractility, slowed heart rate, or a combination of all of these. Brady-
         cardia may result from sinus bradycardia, second- or third-degree atrioventric-
         ular block, or sinus arrest with junctional rhythm. Most calcium antagonists do

TABLE II–13. COMMON CALCIUM ANTAGONISTS[a]

Drug	Usual Adult Daily Dose (mg)	Elimination Half-Life (h)	Primary Site(s) of Activity
Amlodipine	2.5–10	30–50	V
Bepridil	200–400	42	M, V
Diltiazem	90–360 (PO) 0.25 mg/kg (IV)	4	M, V
Felodipine	5–30	10	V
Isradipine	5–25	8	V
Nicardipine	60–120	3	V
Nifedipine	30–120	4	V
Nitrendipine	40–80	12	V
Verapamil	120–480 (PO) 0.075–0.15 mg/kg (IV)	3–7	M, V

[a]Major toxicity: M = myocardial (decreased contractility, AV block); V = vascular (vasodilation).

not affect intraventricular conduction, so the QRS duration is usually unaffected. The PR interval is prolonged even with therapeutic doses of verapamil. Bepridil prolongs the QT interval and may cause ventricular arrhythmias, including torsades des pointes (see p 14).

B. Noncardiac manifestations of intoxication include nausea and vomiting, abnormal mental status (stupor, confusion), metabolic acidosis (probably resulting from hypotension), and hyperglycemia (owing to blockade of insulin release).

IV. Diagnosis.
The findings of hypotension and bradycardia, particularly with sinus arrest or AV block, in the absence of QRS interval prolongation should suggest calcium antagonist intoxication. The differential diagnosis should include beta blockers and other sympatholytic drugs (see p 27–28).

A. Specific levels. Serum drug levels are not widely available.

B. Other useful laboratory studies. Electrolytes, glucose, BUN, creatinine, arterial blood gases or oximetry, ECG and ECG monitoring.

V. Treatment
A. Emergency and supportive measures
1. Maintain the airway and assist ventilation if necessary (see p 4).
2. Treat coma p 18), hypotension (p 15), and bradyarrhythmias (p 10) if they occur. The use of cardiopulmonary bypass to allow time for liver metabolism has been reported in a patient with massive verapamil poisoning.
3. Monitor the vital signs and ECG for at least 6 hours after alleged ingestion. Admit symptomatic patients for at least 24 hours.

B. Specific drugs and antidotes
1. **Calcium** (see p 323) usually promptly reverses the depression of cardiac contractility, but it does **not** affect sinus node depression or peripheral vasodilation and has variable effects on AV nodal conduction. Administer **calcium chloride** 10%, 10 mL (0.1–0.2 mL/kg) IV, or **calcium gluconate** 10%, 20 mL (0.3–0.4 mL/kg) IV. Repeat doses as needed; aim to increase the serum calcium by 3–4 mg/dL to a maximum of 13 mg/dL.
2. **Glucagon** (see p 342), **epinephrine** (see p 337), and amrinone (Inocor, 0.75 mg/kg IV followed by infusion of 5–10 μg/kg/min) have been reported to increase blood pressure in patients with refractory hypotension. Glucagon and epinephrine can also increase the heart rate.
3. Outside the USA, **4-aminopyridine** may be available as an antidote for calcium antagonist intoxication.

C. Decontamination (see p 44)
1. **Prehospital.** Administer activated charcoal, if available. Ipecac-induced emesis may be useful for initial treatment at the scene (eg, children at home) if it can be given within a few minutes of exposure.
2. **Hospital.** Administer activated charcoal and a cathartic; also, consider gastric lavage for all but the most trivial ingestions.
3. For large ingestions of a sustained-release preparation, consider whole bowel irrigation (see p 48) in addition to repeated doses of charcoal (see p 47). Continue charcoal administration for up to 48–72 hours.

D. Enhanced elimination.
Owing to extensive protein binding, dialysis and hemoperfusion are not effective. Repeat-dose activated charcoal has not been evaluated, but may serve as an adjunct to gastrointestinal decontamination after overdose with sustained-release preparations.

CAMPHOR AND OTHER ESSENTIAL OILS
Ilene B. Anderson, PharmD

ANTIDOTE   IPECAC   LAVAGE   CHARCOAL

Camphor is one of several essential oils (volatile oils) derived from natural plant products that have been used for centuries as topical rubefacients and counterirritant agents for analgesic and antipruritic purposes (Table II–14). Camphor and other essential oils are found in many over-the-counter remedies such as Campho-Phenique (10.8% camphor, 4.66% phenol), Vicks Vaporub (4.73% camphor, 2.6% menthol, 1.2% eucalyptus oil, 4.5% turpentine spirits), camphorated oil (20% camphor), and Mentholatum (9% camphor, 1.35% menthol, 1.96% eucalyptus oil, 1.4% turpentine spirits). Toxic effects have occurred primarily when camphorated oil was mistakenly administered instead of castor oil, and in accidental pediatric ingestions.

I. **Mechanism of toxicity.** After topical application, essential oils produce inflammation followed by a feeling of comfort, but if ingested they can cause systemic toxicity. Most essential oils cause central nervous system stimulation or depression. **Camphor** is a central nervous system stimulant that causes seizures shortly after ingestion. The underlying mechanism is unknown. Camphor is rapidly absorbed from the gastrointestinal tract and is metabolized by the liver. It is not known whether metabolites contribute to toxicity.

II. **Toxic dose.** Serious poisonings and death have occurred in children after ingestion of as little as 1 g of camphor. This is equivalent to just 10 mL of Campho-Phenique or 5 mL of camphorated oil. Recovery after ingestion of 42 g in an adult has been reported. The concentrations of other essential oils range from 1 to 20%; doses of 5–15 mL are considered potentially toxic.

III. **Clinical presentation**

A. **Oral.** Manifestations of **acute** oral overdose usually occur within 5–30 minutes after ingestion. Burning in the mouth and throat occurs immediately, followed by nausea and vomiting. Ataxia, drowsiness, confusion, restlessness, delirium, muscle twitching, and coma may occur. Camphor typically causes abrupt onset of seizures about 20–30 minutes after ingestion. Death may result from central nervous system depression and respiratory arrest or may be secondary to sta-

TABLE II–14. SOME ESSENTIAL OILS

Name	Comments
Birch oil	Contains 98% methyl salicylate (equivalent to 1.4 g aspirin per mL; see Salicylates, p 277).
Camphor	Pediatric toxic dose 1 g (see text).
Cinnamon oil	Stomatitis and skin burns can result from prolonged contact. Potent antigen. Smoked as a hallucinogen.
Clove oil	Contains 80–90% eugenol. Clove cigarettes may cause irritant tracheobronchitis, hemoptysis.
Ecalyptus oil	Contains 70% eucalyptol. Toxic dose is 5 mL; may cause rapid CNS depression.
Eugenol	A phenol derived from clove oil; used in dentistry for its disinfectant property.
Guaiacol	Nontoxic.
Lavender oil	Used in doses of 0.1 mL as a carminative. Contains trace amounts of coumarin (see p 143). May cause photosensitization.
Menthol	An alcohol derived from various mint oils. Toxic dose is 2 g.
Myristica oil	Nutmeg oil. A carminative in a dose of 0.03 mL. Used as a hallucinogen (2–4 tbsp of ground nutmeg can cause psychogenic effects).
Pennyroyal oil	Fatal coma and hepatic necrosis occurred after ingestion of 30 mL by an 18-year-old woman. N-acetylcysteine may be effective in preventing hepatic necrosis.
Peppermint oil	Contains 50% menthol. Toxic dose is 5–10 g.
Thymol	Used as an antiseptic (see phenol, p 249).
Turpentine oils	Toxic dose 15 mL in children; 140 mL in adults may be fatal. Can cause pneumonitis if aspirated.
Wintergreen oil	Contains methyl salicylate 98% (equivalent to 1.4 g aspirin per mL; see Salicytes, p 277).

tus epilepticus. **Chronic** camphor intoxication may produce symptoms similar to Reye's syndrome.
- **B.** Prolonged **skin contact** may result in a burn.
- **C.** **Smoking** (eg, clove cigarettes) or inhaling essential oils may cause tracheo-bronchitis.

IV. Diagnosis is usually based on a history of exposure. The pungent odor of camphor and other volatile oils is usually apparent.
- **A. Specific levels.** Serum drug levels are not available.
- **B. Other useful laboratory studies.** Electrolytes, glucose, liver transaminases, arterial blood gases (if patient is comatose or in status epilepticus).

V. Treatment
- **A. Emergency and supportive measures**
  1. Maintain the airway and assist ventilation if necessary (see p 4).
  2. Treat seizures (p 22) and coma (p 18) if they occur.
- **B. Specific drugs and antidotes.** There are no specific antidotes for camphor. **N-acetylcysteine** (see p 311) may be effective for preventing hepatic injury after pennyroyal oil ingestion.
- **C. Decontamination** (see p 44)
  1. **Prehospital.** Administer activated charcoal, if available. Do **not** induce emesis because of the risk of abrupt onset of seizures.
  2. **Hospital.** Administer activated charcoal and a cathartic. Gastric emptying is not necessary for small ingestions if activated charcoal can be given promptly.
- **D. Enhanced elimination.** The volumes of distribution of camphor and other essential oils are extremely large, and it is unlikely that any enhanced removal procedure will remove significant amounts of camphor. Poorly substantiated case reports have recommended hemoperfusion.

CAPTOPRIL AND RELATED DRUGS
Olga F. Woo, PharmD

ANTIDOTE   IPECAC   LAVAGE   CHARCOAL

Benazepril, captopril, enalapril, fosinopril, lisinopril, quinapril, and ramipril are angiotensin-converting enzyme (ACE) inhibitors introduced in the last decade for the treatment of renovascular and resistant idiopathic hypertension. The few reports of acute overdose with these drugs suggest that toxicity is mild.

- **I. Mechanism of toxicity.** These agents inhibit vasoconstriction by inhibiting the enzyme peptidyldipeptide carboxyhydrolase, which converts angiotensin I to angiotensin II. All of the agents except captopril and lisinopril must be metabolized to their active moieties (eg, enalapril is converted to enalaprilat).

  Pharmacokinetics: The volume of distribution (Vd) of these drugs is fairly small (0.7 L/kg for captopril). The parent drugs are rapidly converted to their active metabolites, with half-lives of 0.75–1.5 hours. The active metabolites have elimination half-lives of 5.9–35 hours.

- **II. Toxic dose.** Only mild toxicity has resulted from large overdoses of up to 5 g of captopril and 300 mg of enalapril. Bradycardia has been reported with therapeutic doses of enalapril. No fatalities have been reported from acute poisonings.

- **III. Clinical presentation.** Mild hypotension, usually responsive to fluid therapy, has been the only toxic effect seen with acute overdose. Bradycardia may also occur. Hyperkalemia has been reported with therapeutic use, especially in patients with renal insufficiency and those taking nonsteroidal anti-inflammatory drugs.

- **IV. Diagnosis** is based on a history of exposure.
  - **A. Specific levels.** A radioimmunoassay is available to measure serum levels of

ACE inhibitors, but blood levels are not readily available and do not correlate with clinical effects.

B. **Other useful laboratory studies.** Electrolytes, glucose, BUN, creatinine.

V. **Treatment**

A. **Emergency and supportive measures.** Treat hypotension with supine positioning and intravenous fluids (see p 15) if it occurs. Vasopressors are rarely necessary.

B. **Specific drugs and antidotes.** No specific antidote is available.

C. **Decontamination** (see p 44)

1. **Prehospital.** Administer activated charcoal, if available. Ipecac-induced emesis may be useful for initial treatment at the scene (eg, children at home) if it can be given within a few minutes of exposure.

2. **Hospital.** Administer activated charcoal and a cathartic. Gastric emptying is not necessary if activated charcoal can be given promptly.

D. **Enhanced elimination.** Hemodialysis may effectively remove these drugs but is not likely to be indicated clinically.

CARBAMATE INSECTICIDES
Olga F. Woo, PharmD

| ANTIDOTE | IPECAC | LAVAGE | CHARCOAL |

Carbamate insecticides are less toxic than organophosphates, although their clinical effects are similar. They are found in a variety of commercial veterinary and pesticide products widely used in agriculture. Most household insect sprays contain carbamates. An acute outbreak of aldicarb poisoning occurred in California in 1985 after ingestion of contaminated watermelons.

I. **Mechanism of toxicity.** Like organophosphates, carbamates inhibit acetylcholinesterase enzyme, which allows excessive accumulation of acetylcholine at muscarinic, nicotinic, and central nervous system receptors. Unlike the case with organophosphates, this inhibition is short-lived and reversible.

Carbamates are absorbed by inhalation, ingestion, and through the skin (with the exception of aldicarb, most carbamates are relatively poorly absorbed dermally compared with organophosphates).

II. **Toxic dose.** There is wide variability in the potency of carbamates (Table II–15).

TABLE II–15. CARBAMATE INSECTICIDES[a]

Highly Toxic (LD_{50} < 50 mg/kg)	Moderately Toxic (LD_{50} < 200 mg/kg)	Low Toxicity (LD_{50} > 200 mg/kg)
Aldicarb	Thiodicarb	MTMC (Metacrate)
MIPC (Isoprocarb)	Dioxacarb	Ethiofencarb
Oxamyl	Promecarb	BPMC (Fenocarb)
Carbofuran	Bufencarb	MPMC (Meobal)
Mexacarbate	Carbosulfan	Isoprocarb
Isolan	Benfuracarb	Carbaryl
Methomyl	Propoxur	XMC (Cosban)
Methiocarb	Pirimicarb	
Aldoxycarb	Trimethacarb	
Formetanate		
Aminocarb		
Mecarbam		
Bendiocarb		
Dimetilan		

[a]Listed in decreasing order of potency.

Aldicarb is an important carbamate because it is relatively more potent, undergoes extensive enterohepatic recirculation, and is translocated systemically by certain plants (eg, melons) and concentrated in their fruit.

III. Clinical presentation. Signs and symptoms of cholinergic excess usually occur within 30 minutes but may not develop until 1–2 hours after exposure. Clinical manifestations are the same as those seen with organophosphates (see p 240), but the duration of toxicity is usually shorter (< 6 hours) and symptoms are self–limited.

IV. Diagnosis is based on a history of exposure and the characteristic presentation of muscarinic, nicotinic, and central nervous system acetylcholine excess.

    A. Specific levels. Red blood cell cholinesterase and plasma pseudocholinesterase are not reliable indicators of carbamate poisoning because enzyme activity rapidly and spontaneously recovers within several minutes or hours. Thus, normal levels do not rule out intoxication. Also, because the range of normal enzyme activity is broad and interindividual variability is high, intoxication may be present despite normal enzyme activity. However, a depression of 25% or more from an individual's baseline value is indicative of exposure. Samples should be analyzed immediately, because in vitro hydrolysis of the carbamate can occur.

    B. Other useful laboratory studies. Electrolytes, glucose, BUN, creatinine, arterial blood gases or oximetry.

V. Treatment

    A. Emergency and supportive measures

        1. Maintain the airway and assist ventilation if necessary (see p 4). Administer supplemental oxygen.

        2. Treat coma (p 18) and seizures (p 22) if they occur.

        3. Observe for 4–6 hours. Few patients require prolonged observation.

    B. Specific treatment

        1. Administer **atropine,** 0.5–2 mg (0.01–0.04 mg/kg) IV or IM every 15 minutes until manifestations of muscarinic toxicity (eg, symptomatic bradycardia, bronchorrhea, or wheezing) are reversed (see p 315).

        2. Pralidoxime (see p 371) is not generally recommended, because cholinesterase enzyme inhibition is reversible. However, if a combination of carbamate and organophosphate poisoning has occurred, pralidoxime should be given.

    C. Decontamination (see p 41–49)

        1. Skin and eyes. Remove all contaminated clothing and wash affected skin copiously with soap and water, including the hair and under the nails. Irrigate exposed eyes with copious tepid water or saline.

        2. Ingestion. Administer activated charcoal. Do *not* induce emesis because of the risk of sudden seizures, coma, or respiratory depression. Gastric lavage is probably not necessary following small ingestions if activated charcoal is given promptly.

    D. Enhanced elimination. Dialysis and hemoperfusion are not indicated because the duration of toxicity is brief and effective antidotal therapy is available. Repeat-dose activated charcoal is theoretically applicable to aldicarb poisoning, because aldicarb undergoes enterohepatic recirculation.

CARBAMAZEPINE
Olga F. Woo, PharmD

ANTIDOTE   IPECAC   LAVAGE   CHARCOAL

Carbamazepine was introduced in the US in 1974 for the treatment of trigeminal neuralgia. Since then it has become a first-line drug for the treatment of temporal lobe epilepsies and a variety of other seizure disorders.

I. **Mechanism of toxicity.** Most toxic manifestations appear to be related to its anti-cholinergic effects. In addition, presumably because its chemical structure is similar to that of the tricyclic antidepressant imipramine, acute carbamazepine overdose can potentially cause seizures (mainly in patients with preexisting seizure disorders) and cardiac conduction disturbances (rare).

Pharmacokinetics: Carbamazepine is slowly and erratically absorbed from the gastrointestinal tract, and peak levels may be delayed for 6–24 hours, particularly after an overdose (continued absorption for up to 72 hours has been reported). The volume of distribution (Vd) is 1.4 L/kg, up to 3 L/kg after overdose. Up to 28% of a dose is eliminated in the feces, and there is enterohepatic recycling. The parent drug is metabolized to its 10,11-epoxide, which is as active as the parent compound. The normal elimination half-life is approximately 15–24 hours for carbamazepine and 5–10 hours for the epoxide.

II. **Toxic dose.** Acute ingestion of over 10 mg/kg may result in a blood level above the therapeutic range of 4–8 mg/L. The recommended maximum dose is 1600 mg/d in adults (30 mg/kg/d in children, to a maximum of 1 g). Death has occurred after adult ingestion of 6–60 g, but survival has been reported after an 80-g ingestion. Life-threatening toxicity occurred after ingestion of 5.8–10 g in adults and 2 g (148 mg/kg) in a 23-month-old child.

III. **Clinical presentation**
  A. Ataxia, nystagmus, ophthalmoplegia, mydriasis, and sinus tachycardia are common with mild to moderate overdose. With more serious intoxication, myoclonus, seizures, hyperthermia, coma, and respiratory arrest may occur. Atrioventricular block and bradycardia have been reported in some elderly patients. Based upon its structural similarity to cyclic antidepressants, carbamazepine might potentially cause QRS and QT interval prolongation.
  B. After an acute overdose, manifestations of intoxication may be delayed for several hours because of erratic absorption. Cyclic coma and rebound relapse of symptoms may be caused by continued absorption from a tablet mass as well as enterohepatic circulation of the drug.
  C. Chronic use has been associated with mild leukopenia and thrombocytopenia. Aplastic anemia is extremely rare.

IV. **Diagnosis** is based on a history of exposure and clinical signs such as ataxia, stupor, and tachycardia, along with elevated serum levels.
  A. **Specific levels.** Obtain a stat serum carbamazepine level and repeat levels every 4–6 hours to rule out delayed or prolonged absorption. Serum levels greater than 10 mg/L are associated with ataxia and nystagmus. Serious intoxication may occur with serum levels greater than 20 mg/L, although there is poor correlation between levels and severity of clinical effects. Death occurred in a patient who had a peak concentration of 120 µg/mL. The epoxide metabolite is nearly equipotent, and specific epoxide levels may be useful (the metabolite may cross-react with EMIT assays).
  B. **Other useful laboratory studies.** CBC, electrolytes, glucose, arterial blood gases or oximetry, ECG monitoring.

V. **Treatment**
  A. **Emergency and supportive measures**
    1. Maintain the airway and assist ventilation if necessary (see p 4). Administer supplemental oxygen.
    2. Treat seizures (p 22), coma (p 18), and arrhythmias (p 10–14) if they occur.
    3. Asymptomatic patients should be observed for a minimum of 6 hours after ingestion.
  B. **Specific drugs and antidotes.** There is no specific antidote. Physostigmine is *not* recommended for anticholinergic toxicity.
  C. **Decontamination** (see p 44)
    1. **Prehospital.** Administer activated charcoal, if available. Ipecac-induced emesis may be useful for initial treatment at the scene (eg, children at home) if it can be given within a few minutes of exposure.

2. **Hospital.** Administer activated charcoal and a cathartic. Gastric lavage is not necessary after small to moderate ingestions if activated charcoal can be given promptly.

3. For massive ingestions, consider repeated doses of activated charcoal and possibly whole bowel irrigation (see p 48).

D. **Enhanced elimination.** In contrast to tricyclic antidepressants, the volume of distribution of carbamazepine is small, making it accessible to enhanced removal procedures.

1. **Repeat-dose activated charcoal** is effective and may increase clearance by up to 50%. However, it may be difficult to perform safely in a patient with obtundation and ileus, and there is no demonstrated benefit on morbidity or mortality.

2. **Charcoal hemoperfusion** is highly effective and may be indicated for severe intoxication (eg, status epilepticus, cardiotoxicity) unresponsive to standard treatment.

3. Peritoneal dialysis and hemodialysis do not effectively remove carbamazepine because it is 80% protein-bound.

CARBON MONOXIDE
Kent R. Olson, MD

ANTIDOTE   IPECAC   LAVAGE   CHARCOAL

Carbon monoxide (CO) is a colorless, odorless, tasteless, and nonirritating gas produced by the incomplete combustion of any carbon-containing material. Common sources of human exposure include smoke inhalation in fires; automobile exhaust fumes; faulty or poorly ventilated charcoal, kerosene, or gas stoves; and, to a lesser extent, cigarette smoke and methylene chloride (see p 220).

I. **Mechanism of toxicity.** Toxicity is a consequence of cellular hypoxia and ischemia.

A. Carbon monoxide binds to hemoglobin with an affinity 250 times that of oxygen, resulting in reduced oxyhemoglobin saturation and decreased blood oxygen-carrying capacity. In addition, the oxyhemoglobin dissociation curve is displaced to the left, impairing oxygen delivery at the tissues.

B. Carbon monoxide may also directly inhibit cytochrome oxidase, further disrupting cellular function, and it is known to bind to myoglobin, possibly contributing to impaired myocardial contractility.

C. In animal models of intoxication, damage is most severe in areas of the brain that are highly sensitive to ischemia, and often correlates with the severity of systemic hypotension.

D. **Fetal hemoglobin** is more sensitive to binding by carbon monoxide, and fetal or neonatal levels may be twice as high as maternal levels.

II. **Toxic dose.** The recommended workplace limit (ACGIH TLV-TWA) for carbon monoxide is 25 ppm as an 8-hour time-weighted average. The level considered immediately dangerous to life or health (IDLH) is 1500 ppm (0.15%). Several minutes of exposure to 1000 ppm (0.1%) may result in 50% saturation of carboxyhemoglobin.

III. **Clinical presentation.** Symptoms of intoxication are predominantly in organs with high oxygen consumption such as the brain and heart.

A. The majority of patients complain of headache, dizziness, and nausea. Patients with coronary disease may experience angina or myocardial infarction. With more severe exposures, impaired thinking, syncope, coma, convulsions, cardiac arrhythmias, hypotension, and death may occur. Although blood carboxyhemoglobin levels may not correlate reliably with the severity of intoxication, levels greater than 40 are usually associated with obvious intoxication (Table II–16).

TABLE II–16. CARBON MONOXIDE POISONING[a]

Estimated Carbon Monoxide Concentration	Carboxy-hemoglobin (%)	Symptoms[b]
Less than 35 ppm (cigarette smoking)	5	None, or mild headache.
0.005% (50 ppm)	10	Slight headache, dyspnea on vigorous exertion.
0.01% (100 ppm)	20	Throbbing headache, dyspnea with moderate exertion.
0.02% (200 ppm)	30	Severe headache, irritability, fatigue, dimness of vision.
0.03–0.05% (300–500 ppm)	40–50	Headache, tachycardia, confusion, lethargy, collapse.
0.08–0.12% (800–1200 ppm)	60–70	Coma, convulsions.
0.19% (1900 ppm)	80	Rapidly fatal.

[a]Reproduced, with permission, from *Current Emergency Diagnosis & Treatment*, 3rd ed. Ho MT, Saunders CE (editors). Appleton & Lange, 1990.
[b]Symptoms and signs of toxicity do not always correlate with measured carboxyhemoglobin level.

B. Survivors of serious poisoning may suffer numerous overt neurologic sequelae consistent with an hypoxic-ischemic insult, ranging from gross deficits such as parkinsonism and persistent vegetative state to subtler personality and memory disorders.

C. Exposure during pregnancy may result in fetal demise.

IV. Diagnosis is not difficult if there is a history of exposure (eg, the patient was found in a car in a locked garage) but may be elusive if not suspected in less obvious cases. There are no specific reliable clinical findings; cherry red skin coloration or bright red venous blood is highly suggestive but not frequently noted. The routine arterial blood gas measures oxygen dissolved in plasma but does not directly measure oxygen saturation or oxygen content and therefore is usually misleadingly normal. Pulse oximetry also gives falsely normal readings.

   A. Specific levels. Obtain a specific carboxyhemoglobin concentration (see Table II–16).

   B. Other useful laboratory studies. Electrolytes, glucose, BUN, creatinine, ECG, pregnancy test.

V. Treatment

   A. Emergency and supportive measures

   1. Maintain the airway and assist ventilation if necessary (see p 4). If smoke inhalation has also occurred, consider early intubation for airway protection (p 3).

   2. Treat coma (p 18) and seizures (p 22) if they occur.

   3. Continuously monitor the ECG for several hours after exposure.

   4. Because smoke often contains other toxic gases, consider the possibility of cyanide poisoning (p 145), methemoglobinemia (p 217), and irritant gas injury (p 176).

   B. Specific drugs and antidotes. Administer **oxygen** in the highest possible concentration (100%). Breathing 100% oxygen reduces the half-time of the carboxyhemoglobin complex from 6 hours (in room air) to approximately 1 hour. Use a tight-fitting mask and high-flow oxygen with a reservoir (non-rebreather) or administer the oxygen by endotracheal tube. Treat until the carboxyhemoglobin level is less than 5%.

   C. Decontamination (see p 41). Remove the patient immediately from exposure and give supplemental oxygen. Rescuers exposed to potentially high concentrations of carbon monoxide should wear self-contained breathing apparatus.

D. Enhanced elimination. Hyperbaric oxygen provides 100% oxygen under 2–3 atm of pressure and can enhance elimination of carbon monoxide (half-time reduced to 20–30 minutes). It may be useful in patients with severe intoxication who do not respond rapidly to oxygen at atmospheric pressure, or for pregnant women or newborns, when there is ready access to a chamber. However, long-distance transport of an unstable patient for hyperbaric treatment may be risky, and it remains controversial whether hyperbaric oxygen is clinically more effective than 100% oxygen administered at atmospheric pressure. Consult a regional poison control center (see p 153) for advice and for the location of nearby hyperbaric chambers.

CARBON TETRACHLORIDE
Diane Liu, MD, MPH

ANTIDOTE   IPECAC   LAVAGE   CHARCOAL

Carbon tetrachloride (CCl_4, tetrachloromethane) was once widely used as a dry cleaning solvent, degreaser, spot remover, fire extinguisher agent, and anthelmintic. Because of its liver toxicity and known carcinogenicity in animals, its role has become limited; it is now used mainly as a fumigant and as an intermediate in chemical manufacturing.

I. **Mechanism of toxicity.** Carbon tetrachloride is a central nervous system depressant and a potent hepatic and renal toxin. It may also sensitize the myocardium to arrhythmogenic effects of catecholamines. The mechanism of hepatic and renal toxicity is thought to be a result of a toxic free radical intermediate of metabolism. Chronic use of metabolic enzyme inducers such as phenobarbital and ethanol increase the toxicity of carbon tetrachloride. Carbon tetrachloride is a known animal and suspected human carcinogen.

II. **Toxic dose**
   A. Toxicity from **inhalation** is dependent on the concentration in air and the duration of exposure. Symptoms have occurred after exposure to 160 ppm for 30 minutes. The recommended workplace limit (ACGIH TLV-TWA) is 5 ppm as an 8-hour time-weighted average, and the air level considered immediately dangerous to life or health (IDLH) is 300 ppm.
   B. **Ingestion** of as little as 5 mL has been reported to be fatal.

III. **Clinical presentation**
   A. Persons exposed to carbon tetrachloride from acute inhalation, skin absorption, or ingestion may present with nausea, vomiting, dizziness, and confusion. With serious intoxication, coma and cardiac arrhythmias may occur.
   B. Severe and sometimes fatal renal and hepatic damage may become apparent after 1–3 days.

IV. **Diagnosis** is based on a history of exposure and the clinical presentation of central nervous system depression, arrhythmias, and hepatic necrosis. The liquid is radiopaque and may be visible on abdominal x-ray after acute ingestion.
   A. **Specific levels.** Serum levels are not available in most commercial laboratories. Qualitative screening for chlorinated hydrocarbons (Fujiwara test) may be positive after massive overdose.
   B. **Other useful laboratory studies.** Electrolytes, glucose, BUN, creatinine, liver transaminases, prothrombin time (PT), ECG monitoring.

V. **Treatment**
   A. **Emergency and supportive measures**
      1. Maintain the airway and assist ventilation if necessary (see p 4).
      2. Treat coma (p 18) and arrhythmias (p 14) if they occur. ***Caution:*** Avoid use of epinephrine because it may induce or aggravate arrhythmias. Tachyarrhythmias caused by myocardial sensitization may be treated with

propranolol, 1–2 mg IV (see p 373), or **esmolol,** 25–100 µg/kg/min IV (see p 338).

B. Specific treatment. Acetylcysteine (NAC; see p 311) may minimize hepatic and renal toxicity by providing a scavenger for the toxic intermediate. Although its use for carbon tetrachloride poisoning has not been studied in humans, acetylcysteine is widely used without serious side effects for treatment of acetaminophen overdose. If possible, it should be given within the first 12 hours after exposure.

C. Decontamination (see p 41–49)
1. **Inhalation.** Remove from exposure and give supplemental oxygen, if available.
2. **Skin and eyes.** Remove contaminated clothing and wash affected skin with copious soap and water. Irrigate exposed eyes with copious saline or water.
3. **Ingestion** (see p 44)
a. **Prehospital.** Administer activated charcoal, if available. Ipecac-induced emesis may be useful for initial treatment if it can be given immediately after the ingestion, but is generally avoided because of the risk of abrupt onset of coma.
b. **Hospital.** Perform gastric lavage, and administer activated charcoal and a cathartic.

D. Enhanced elimination. There is no role for dialysis, hemoperfusion, or other enhanced removal procedures.

CARDIAC GLYCOSIDES
Neal L. Benowitz, MD

ANTIDOTE   IPECAC   LAVAGE   CHARCOAL

Cardiac glycosides are found in several plants, including oleander, foxglove, lily of the valley, red squill, and rhododendron, and in toad venom (*Bufo spp,* which may be found in some Chinese herbal medications). Cardiac glycosides are used therapeutically in tablet form as digoxin and digitoxin. Digoxin is also available in liquid-filled capsules with greater bioavailability.

I. Mechanism of toxicity. Cardiac glycosides inhibit the function of the sodium-potassium-ATPase pump. After acute overdose, this results in hyperkalemia (with chronic intoxication, the serum potassium level is usually normal or low owing to concurrent diuretic therapy). Vagal tone is potentiated, and sinus and atrioventricular node conduction velocity is decreased. Automaticity in Purkinje fibers is increased.

Pharmacokinetics: The bioavailability of digoxin ranges from 60–80%; for digitoxin more than 90% is absorbed. The volume of distribution (Vd) of digoxin is very large (5–10 L/kg), whereas for digitoxin the Vd is small (about 0.5 L/kg). Peak effects occur after a delay of 6–12 hours. The elimination half-life of digoxin is 30–50 hours, and for digitoxin is 5–8 days (owing to enterohepatic recirculation).

II. Toxic dose. Acute ingestion of as little as 1 mg of digoxin in a child or 3 mg of digoxin in an adult can result in serum concentrations well above the therapeutic range. More than these amounts of digoxin and other cardiac glycosides may be found in just a few leaves of oleander or foxglove. Generally, children appear to be more resistant than adults to the cardiotoxic effects of cardiac glycosides.

III. Clinical presentation. Intoxication may occur after acute accidental or suicidal ingestion or with chronic therapy. Signs and symptoms depend on the chronicity of the intoxication.
A. With **acute overdose,** vomiting, hyperkalemia, sinus bradycardia, sinoatrial arrest, and second- or third-degree atrioventricular block are common. Ventricular tachycardia or fibrillation may occur.

B. With **chronic intoxication,** visual disturbances, weakness, sinus bradycardia, atrial fibrillation with slowed ventricular response rate or junctional escape rhythm, and ventricular arrhythmias (ventricular bigeminy or trigeminy, ventricular tachycardia, bidirectional tachycardia, and ventricular fibrillation) are common. Accelerated junctional tachycardia and paroxysmal atrial tachycardia with block are frequently seen. Hypokalemia and hypomagnesemia from chronic diuretic use may be evident and appear to worsen the tachyarrhythmias.

IV. **Diagnosis** is based on a history of recent overdose or characteristic arrhythmias (eg, bidirectional tachycardia, accelerated junctional rhythm) in a patient receiving chronic therapy. Hyperkalemia suggests acute ingestion but may also be seen with very severe chronic poisoning. Serum potassium levels higher than 5.5 meq/L are associated with severe poisoning.

A. **Specific levels.** Stat digoxin or digitoxin levels are recommended, although they may not correlate accurately with severity of intoxication. This is especially true after acute ingestion, when the serum level is high for 6–12 hours before tissue distribution is complete. After use of digitalis-specific antibodies, the radioimmunoassay digoxin level is falsely markedly elevated. Therapeutic levels of digoxin are 0.5–2 ng/mL; of digitoxin, 10–30 ng/mL.

B. **Other useful laboratory studies.** Electrolytes, BUN, creatinine, serum magnesium, ECG and ECG monitoring.

V. **Treatment**

A. **Emergency and supportive measures**
   1. Maintain the airway and assist ventilation if necessary (see p 4).
   2. Monitor the patient closely for at least 12–24 hours after significant ingestion because of delayed tissue distribution.
   3. Treat **hyperkalemia** (p 35), if greater than 5.5 meq/L, with sodium bicarbonate (1 meq/kg), glucose (0.5 g/kg IV) with insulin (0.1 unit/kg IV), or sodium polystyrene sulfonate (Kayexalate, 0.5 g/kg orally). Do **not** use calcium; it may worsen ventricular arrhythmias. Mild hyperkalemia may actually protect against tachyarrhythmias.
   4. Treat **bradycardia** or **heart block** with atropine, 0.5–2 mg IV (p 315); a temporary pacemaker may be needed for persistent symptomatic bradycardia.
   5. **Ventricular tachyarrhythmias** may respond to lidocaine (p 349) or phenytoin (p 370), or to correction of low potassium or magnesium. Avoid quinidine, procainamide, and bretylium.

B. **Specific drugs and antidotes. Fab fragments of digoxin-specific antibodies (Digibind)** are indicated for significant poisoning (eg, severe hyperkalemia, symptomatic arrhythmias not responsive to drugs described above), and possibly for prophylactic treatment in a massive oral overdose with high serum levels. Digibind rapidly binds to digoxin and, to a lesser extent, digitoxin and other cardiac glycosides. The inactive complex that is formed is rapidly excreted in the urine. Details of Digibind dose calculation and infusion rate are given on p 329.

C. **Decontamination** (see p 44)
   1. **Prehospital.** Administer activated charcoal, if available. Ipecac-induced emesis may be useful for initial treatment at the scene (eg, children at home) if it can be given within a few minutes of exposure.
   2. **Hospital.** Administer activated charcoal and a cathartic. Gastric emptying is not necessary if activated charcoal can be given promptly.

D. **Enhanced elimination** (see p 49)
   1. Because of its large volume of distribution, **digoxin** is not effectively removed by dialysis or hemoperfusion. Repeat-dose activated charcoal may be useful in patients with severe renal insufficiency, in whom clearance of digoxin is markedly diminished.
   2. **Digitoxin** has a small volume of distribution and also undergoes extensive enterohepatic recirculation, and its elimination can be markedly enhanced by repeat-dose charcoal.

CAUSTIC AND CORROSIVE AGENTS
Kent R. Olson, MD

ANTIDOTE   IPECAC   LAVAGE   CHARCOAL

A wide variety of chemical and physical agents may cause corrosive injury. These include mineral and organic acids, alkalies, oxidizing agents, denaturants, some hydrocarbons, and agents causing exothermic reactions. Although the mechanism and the severity of injury may vary, the consequences of mucosal damage and permanent scarring are shared by all agents. **Button batteries** are small disk-shaped batteries used in watches, calculators, and cameras. They contain caustic metal salts such as mercuric chloride that may cause corrosive injury.

I. **Mechanism of toxicity**
  A. **Acids** cause an immediate coagulation-type necrosis that creates an eschar, which tends to self-limit further damage.
  B. In contrast, **alkalies** cause a liquefactive necrosis with saponification and continued penetration into deeper tissues, resulting in extensive damage.
  C. **Other agents** may act by alkylating or denaturing cellular proteins or by defatting surface tissues.
  D. **Button batteries** cause injury by corrosive effects resulting from leakage of the corrosive metal salts, by direct impaction of the disk-shaped foreign body, and possibly by local discharge of electrical current at the site of impaction.

II. **Toxic dose.** There is no specific toxic dose or level, because the concentration of corrosive solutions and the potency of caustic effect vary widely. The concentration or the pH of the solution may indicate the potential for serious injury. For alkalies, the titratable alkalinity is a better predictor of corrosive effect than the pH.

III. **Clinical presentation**
  A. **Inhalation** of corrosive gases (eg, chlorine, ammonia) may cause upper respiratory tract injury, with stridor, hoarseness, wheezing, and noncardiogenic pulmonary edema. Pulmonary symptoms may be delayed after exposure to gases with low water solubility (eg, nitrogen dioxide, phosgene; see p 176).
  B. **Eye or skin** exposure to corrosive agents usually results in immediate pain and redness, followed by blistering. Conjunctivitis and lacrimation are common. Serious full-thickness burns and blindness can occur.
  C. **Ingestion** of corrosives can cause oral pain, dysphagia, drooling, and pain in the throat, chest, or abdomen. Esophageal or gastric perforation may occur, manifested by severe chest or abdominal pain, signs of peritoneal irritation, or pancreatitis. Free air may be visible in the mediastinum or abdomen on x-ray. Hematemesis and shock may occur. Systemic acidosis has been reported following acid ingestion and may be partly caused by absorption of hydrogen ions. Scarring of the esophagus or stomach may result in permanent stricture formation and chronic dysphagia.
  D. **Systemic toxicity** can occur after inhalation, skin exposure, or ingestion of a variety of agents (Table II–17).
  E. **Button batteries** usually cause serious injury only if they become impacted in the esophagus, leading to perforation into the aorta or mediastinum. Most cases involve large (25 mm in diameter) batteries. If button batteries reach the stomach without impaction in the esophagus, they nearly always pass uneventfully via the stools within several days.

IV. **Diagnosis** is based on a history of exposure to a corrosive agent and characteristic findings of skin, eye, or mucosal irritation or redness and the presence of injury to the gastrointestinal tract. Victims with oral or esophageal injury nearly always have drooling or pain on swallowing.
  A. **Endoscopy.** Esophageal or gastric injury is unlikely after ingestion if the patient is completely asymptomatic, but studies have repeatedly shown that a small number of patients will have injury in the absence of oral burns or obvious

TABLE II–17. EXAMPLES OF SYSTEMIC SYMPTOMS FROM CORROSIVE AGENTS[a]

Corrosive Agent	Systemic Symptoms
Formaldehyde	Metabolic acidosis; formate poisoning
Hydrofluoric acid	Hypocalcemia; hyperkalemia
Methylene chloride	CNS depression; cardiac arrhythmias; converted to carbon monoxide
Oxalic acid	Hypocalcemia; renal failure
Paraquat	Pulmonary fibrosis
Permanganate	Methemoglobinemia
Phenol	Seizures, coma; hepatic and renal damage
Phosphorus	Hepatic and renal injury
Picric acid	Renal injury
Silver nitrate	Methemoglobinemia
Tannic acid	Hepatic injury

[a]Reference: Edelman PA: Chemical and electrical burns. Pages 183–202 in: *Management of the Burned Patient.* Achauer BM (editor). Appleton & Lange, 1987.

dysphagia. For this reason, many authorities recommend endoscopy for all patients regardless of symptoms.

 B. X-rays of the chest and abdomen will usually reveal impacted button batteries. X-rays may also demonstrate air in the mediastinum from esophageal perforation or free abdominal air from gastric perforation.

 C. Specific levels. See specific chemical. Urine mercury levels have been reported elevated after button battery ingestion.

 D. Other useful laboratory studies. CBC, electrolytes, glucose, arterial blood gases, chest x-ray, upright abdominal x-ray.

V. Treatment

 A. Emergency and supportive measures

  1. Inhalation. Give supplemental oxygen, and observe closely for signs of progressive airway obstruction or noncardiogenic pulmonary edema (see p 4).

  2. Ingestion

   a. Immediately give water or milk to drink.

   b. If esophageal or gastric perforation is suspected, obtain immediate surgical or endoscopic consultation.

 B. Specific drugs and antidotes. For most agents, there is no specific antidote. (See p 180 for hydrofluoric acid burns and p 249 for phenol burns.) In the past, corticosteroids were used by many clinicians in the hope of reducing scarring, but this treatment has been proved ineffective. Moreover, steroids may be harmful in the patient with perforation by masking early signs of inflammation and inhibiting resistance to infection.

 C. Decontamination (see p 41–49). *Caution:* Rescuers should use appropriate respiratory and skin protective equipment.

  1. Inhalation. Remove from exposure; give supplemental oxygen if available.

  2. Skin and eyes. Remove all clothing; wash skin and irrigate eyes with copious water or saline.

  3. Ingestion (see p 44)

   a. Immediately give water or milk to drink. Do *not* induce emesis or give pH-neutralizing solutions (eg, dilute vinegar or bicarbonate).

   b. Gastric lavage to remove the corrosive material is controversial but is probably beneficial in acute liquid corrosive ingestion, and it will be required before endoscopy anyway. Use a soft flexible tube and lavage with repeated aliquots of water or saline, frequently checking the pH of the washings.

c. In general, do **not** give activated charcoal, as it may interfere with visibility at endoscopy. Charcoal may be appropriate if the ingested agent can cause significant systemic toxicity.

d. Button batteries lodged in the esophagus must be removed immediately by endoscopy to prevent rapid perforation. Batteries in the stomach or intestine should not be removed unless signs of perforation or obstruction develop.

D. Enhanced elimination. In general, there is no role for any of these procedures (see specific chemical).

CHLORATES
Kathryn H. Keller, PharmD

ANTIDOTE   IPECAC   LAVAGE   CHARCOAL

Potassium chlorate is a component of some matchheads; barium chlorate (see also p 95) is used in the manufacture of fireworks and explosives; sodium chlorate is still a major ingredient of some weed killers used in commercial agriculture; and other chlorate salts are used in dye production. Safer and more effective compounds have replaced chlorate in toothpaste and antiseptic mouthwashes. Chlorate poisoning is similar to bromate intoxication (see p 108), but chlorates are more likely to cause intravascular hemolysis and methemoglobinemia.

I. Mechanism of toxicity. Chlorates are potent oxidizing agents and also attack sulfhydryl groups, particularly in red blood cells and the kidneys. Chlorates cause methemoglobin formation as well as increased red blood cell membrane fragility, which may result in intravascular hemolysis. Renal failure is probably caused by a combination of direct cellular toxicity and hemolysis.

II. Toxic dose. The minimum toxic dose in children is not established, but is estimated to range from 1 g in infants to 5 g in older children. Children may ingest up to 1–2 matchbooks without toxic effect (each matchhead may contain 10–12 mg of chlorate). The adult lethal dose was estimated to be 7.5 g in one case but is probably closer to 20–35 g. A 26-year-old woman survived a 150- to 200-g ingestion.

III. Clinical presentation. Within a few minutes to hours after ingestion, abdominal pain, vomiting, and diarrhea may occur. Methemoglobinemia is common (see p 217). Massive hemolysis, hemoglobinuria, and acute tubular necrosis may occur over 1–2 days after ingestion. Coagulopathy and hepatic injury have been described.

IV. Diagnosis is usually based on a history of exposure and the presence of methemoglobinemia and hemolysis.

A. Specific levels. Serum levels are not available, nor are they useful.

B. Other useful laboratory studies. CBC, plasma free hemoglobin, electrolytes, glucose, BUN, creatinine, methemoglobin level, prothrombin time (PT), liver transaminases, urinalysis. Coagulation studies if coagulopathy suspected.

V. Treatment

A. Emergency and supportive measures

1. Maintain the airway and assist ventilation if necessary (see p 4).

2. Treat coma (p 18), hemolysis, hyperkalemia (p 35), and renal (p 36) or hepatic failure (p 37) if they occur.

3. Massive hemolysis may require blood transfusions. To prevent renal failure resulting from deposition of free hemoglobin in the kidney tubules, administer intravenous fluids and sodium bicarbonate.

B. Specific drugs and antidotes

1. Treat methemoglobinemia with **methylene blue** (see p 351), 1–2 mg/kg

(0.1–0.2 mL/kg) of 1% solution. Methylene blue is reportedly most effective when used early in mild cases, but has poor effectiveness in severe cases where hemolysis has already occurred.

2. Intravenous **sodium thiosulfate** (see p 376) may inactivate the chlorate ion and has been reported successful in anecdotal reports. However, this treatment has not been clinically tested. Administration as a lavage fluid may potentially produce some hydrogen sulfide, and so is contraindicated.

C. Decontamination (see p 44)

1. **Prehospital.** Administer activated charcoal, if available. Ipecac-induced emesis may be useful for initial treatment at the scene (eg, children at home) if it can be given within a few minutes of exposure. *Note:* Spontaneous emesis is common after significant ingestion.

2. **Hospital.** Administer activated charcoal and a cathartic. Gastric emptying is not necessary after small ingestions if activated charcoal can be given promptly.

D. Enhanced elimination. Chlorates are eliminated mainly through the kidney; elimination may be hastened by hemodialysis, especially in patients with renal insufficiency. Exchange transfusion and peritoneal dialysis have been used in a few cases.

CHLORINATED HYDROCARBON PESTICIDES
Olga F. Woo, PharmD

ANTIDOTE   IPECAC   LAVAGE   CHARCOAL

Chlorinated hydrocarbon pesticides are widely used in agriculture, structural insect control, and malaria control programs around the world. Lindane is used medicinally for the treatment of lice and scabies. Chlorinated hydrocarbons are of major toxicologic concern, and many (eg, DDT, chlordane) are now banned from commercial use because they persist in the environment and accumulate in biologic systems.

I. **Mechanism of toxicity.** Chlorinated hydrocarbons are "axon poisons" that interfere with transmission of nerve impulses, especially in the brain, resulting in behavioral changes, involuntary muscle activity, and depression of the respiratory center. They may also sensitize the myocardium to arrhythmogenic effects of catecholamines, and many can cause liver or renal injury, possibly owing to generation of toxic metabolites. In addition, some chlorinated hydrocarbons may be carcinogenic.

Pharmacokinetics: Chlorinated hydrocarbons are well absorbed from the gastrointestinal tract, across the skin, and by inhalation. They are highly lipid-soluble and accumulate with repeated exposure. Elimination does not follow first-order kinetics; compounds are slowly released from body stores over days to several months or years.

II. **Toxic dose.** The acute toxic doses of these compounds are highly variable, and reports of acute human poisonings are limited. Table II–18 ranks the relative toxicity of several common compounds.

A. **Ingestion** of as little as 1 g of lindane can produce seizures in a child, and 10–30 g is considered lethal in an adult. The estimated adult lethal oral dose of aldrin and chlordane is 3–7 g; of dieldrin, 2–5 g. A 49-year-old man died after ingesting 12 g of endrin. A 20-year-old man survived a 60-g endosulfan ingestion but was left with a chronic seizure disorder.

B. **Skin absorption** is a significant route of exposure, especially with aldrin, dieldrin, and endrin. Extensive or repeated (as little as 2 applications on 2 successive days) whole-body application of lindane to infants has resulted in seizures and death.

III. **Clinical presentation.** Shortly after acute ingestion, nausea and vomiting occur, followed by confusion, tremor, obtundation, coma, seizures, and respira-

TABLE II–18. COMMON CHLORINATED HYDROCARBONS

Highly Toxic (animal oral LD_{50} < 50 mg/kg)	Moderately Toxic (animal oral LD_{50} > 50 mg/kg)	Low Toxicity (animal oral LD_{50} > 1 g/kg)
Aldrin	Chlordane	Ethylan (Perthane)
Dieldrin	DDT	Hexachlorobenzene
Endrin	Heptachlor	Methoxychlor
Endosulfan	Kepone	
	Lindane	
	Mirex	
	Toxaphene	

tory depression. Because chlorinated hydrocarbons are highly lipid-soluble, the duration of toxicity may be prolonged.

    A. Recurrent or delayed-onset seizures have been reported.

    B. Arrhythmias may occur owing to myocardial sensitivity to catecholamines.

    C. Signs of hepatitis or renal injury may develop.

IV. Diagnosis is based on the history of exposure and clinical presentation.

    A. Specific levels. Chlorinated hydrocarbons can be measured in the serum, but levels are not routinely available.

    B. Other useful laboratory studies. Electrolytes, glucose, BUN, creatinine, hepatic transaminases, prothrombin time (PT), ECG monitoring.

V. Treatment

    A. Emergency and supportive measures

        1. Maintain the airway and assist ventilation if necessary (see p 4). Administer supplemental oxygen.

        2. Treat seizures (p 22), coma (p 18), and respiratory depression (p 7) if they occur. Ventricular arrhythmias may respond to beta-adrenergic blockers such as propranolol (p 373) or esmolol (see p 338).

        3. Attach electrocardiographic monitor, and observe the patient for at least 6–8 hours.

    B. Specific drugs and antidotes. There is no specific antidote.

    C. Decontamination (see p 41–49)

        1. Skin and eyes. Remove contaminated clothing and wash affected skin with copious soap and water, including hair and nails. Irrigate exposed eyes with copious tepid water or saline. Rescuers must take precautions to avoid personal exposure.

        2. Ingestion

            a. Prehospital. Administer activated charcoal, if available. Do **not** induce emesis because of the risk of abrupt onset of seizures.

            b. Hospital. Administer activated charcoal and a cathartic. Consider gastric lavage for large ingestions.

    D. Enhanced elimination (see p 49)

        1. Repeat-dose activated charcoal or cholestyramine resin may be administered to enhance elimination by interrupting enterohepatic circulation.

        2. Exchange transfusion, peritoneal dialysis, hemodialysis, and hemoperfusion are not likely to be beneficial because of the large volume of distribution of these chemicals.

CHLORINE
Kent R. Olson, MD

ANTIDOTE   IPECAC   LAVAGE   CHARCOAL

Chlorine is a yellowish-green gas with an irritating odor, used widely in chemical manufacturing, bleaching, and (as hypochlorite) in swimming pool disinfectant and cleaning agents. **Hypochlorite** is an aqueous solution produced by the reaction of chlorine gas with water; most household bleach solutions contain 3–5% hypochlorite; swimming pool disinfectants and industrial strength cleaners may contain up to 20% hypochlorite. Addition of acid to hypochlorite solution may release chlorine gas. Addition of ammonia to hypochlorite solution may release chloramine, a gas with similar properties.

I. **Mechanism of toxicity.** Chlorine gas produces a corrosive effect on contact with moist tissues such as the eyes and upper respiratory tract. Exposure to aqueous solutions causes corrosive injury to the eyes, skin, or gastrointestinal tract (see p 126). Chloramine is less water-soluble and may produce more indolent or delayed irritation.

II. **Toxic dose**

A. **Chlorine gas.** The recommended workplace limit (ACGIH TLV-TWA) for chlorine gas is 0.5 ppm (1.5 mg/m^3) as an 8-hour time-weighted average. The level considered immediately dangerous to life or health (IDLH) is 25 ppm.

B. **Aqueous solutions.** Dilute aqueous hypochlorite solutions (3–5%) commonly found in homes rarely cause serious burns but are moderately irritating. However, more concentrated industrial cleaners (20% hypochlorite) are much more likely to cause serious corrosive injury.

III. **Clinical presentation**

A. **Inhalation of chlorine gas.** Symptoms are rapid in onset owing to the relatively high water solubility of chlorine. Immediate burning of the eyes, nose, and throat occurs, accompanied by coughing. Wheezing may also occur, especially in patients with preexisting bronchospastic disease. With serious exposure, upper airway swelling may rapidly cause airway obstruction, preceded by croupy cough, hoarseness, and stridor. With massive exposure, noncardiogenic pulmonary edema (chemical pneumonitis) may also occur.

B. **Skin or eye contact with gas or concentrated solution.** Serious corrosive burns may occur. Manifestations are similar to those of other corrosive exposures (see p 126).

C. **Ingestion of aqueous solutions.** Immediate burning in the mouth and throat is common, but no further injury is expected after ingestion of 3–5% hypochlorite. With more concentrated solutions, serious esophageal and gastric burns may occur, and victims often have dysphagia, drooling, and severe throat, chest, and abdominal pain. Hematemesis and perforation of the esophagus or stomach may occur.

IV. **Diagnosis** is based on a history of exposure and description of the typical irritating odor, accompanied by irritative or corrosive effects on the eyes, skin, or upper respiratory or gastrointestinal tract.

A. **Specific levels.** There are no specific serum levels.

B. **Other useful laboratory studies.** With **ingestion,** CBC, electrolytes, chest and abdominal x-rays; with **inhalation,** arterial blood gases or oximetry, chest x-ray.

V. **Treatment**

A. **Emergency and supportive measures**

1. **Inhalation of chlorine gas**

a. Immediately give humidified supplemental oxygen. Observe carefully for signs of progressive upper airway obstruction, and intubate the trachea if necessary (see p 3).

b. Use bronchodilators for wheezing (p 9–10), and treat noncardiogenic pulmonary edema (p 8) if it occurs.

2. **Ingestion of hypochlorite solution.** If solution of 10% or greater has been ingested, or if there are any symptoms of corrosive injury (dysphagia, drooling, pain), flexible endoscopy is recommended to evaluate for serious esophageal or gastric injury. Obtain chest and abdominal x-rays to look for mediastinal or intra-abdominal air, which suggest perforation.

B. **Specific drugs and antidotes.** There is no proved specific treatment for this or other common caustic burns or inhalations. Administration of corticosteroids is unproved and may be harmful in patients with perforation or serious infection.

C. Decontamination (see p 41–49)
   1. **Inhalation.** Remove immediately from exposure, and give supplemental oxygen if available.
   2. **Skin and eyes.** Remove contaminated clothing, and flush exposed skin immediately with copious water. Irrigate exposed eyes with water or saline.
   3. **Ingestion of hypochlorite solution**
      a. **Prehospital.** Immediately give water or milk by mouth. Do **not** induce emesis.
      b. **Hospital.** Gastric lavage is recommended after concentrated liquid ingestion, in order to remove any corrosive material in the stomach and to prepare for endoscopy; use a small flexible tube to avoid injury to damaged mucosa.
      c. Do **not** use activated charcoal; it may obscure the endoscopist's view.
   D. Enhanced elimination. There is no role for enhanced elimination.

CHLOROFORM
Diane Liu, MD, MPH

ANTIDOTE   IPECAC   LAVAGE   CHARCOAL

Chloroform (trichloromethane) is a chlorinated hydrocarbon solvent used as a raw material in the production of Freon and as an extractant and solvent in the chemical and pharmaceutical industry. Because of its hepatic toxicity, it is no longer used as a general anesthetic or anthelmintic agent. Chronic low-level exposure may occur in some municipal water supplies owing to chlorination of biologic methanes.

I. **Mechanism of toxicity.** Chloroform is a direct central nervous system depressant. In addition, as with other chlorinated hydrocarbons, it may potentiate cardiac arrhythmias by sensitizing the myocardium to catecholamines. Hepatic and renal toxicity is probably caused by metabolism to a highly reactive intermediate, possibly a free radical or phosgene. Chloroform is embryotoxic and is a suspected human carcinogen.

II. **Toxic dose**
   A. The fatal **oral** dose of chloroform may be as little as 10 mL, although survival after ingestion of more than 100 mL has been reported. The oral LD_{50} in rats is 2000 mg/kg.
   B. The **air level** considered immediately dangerous to life or health (IDLH) is 1000 ppm. The recommended workplace limit (ACGIH TLV-TWA) is 10 ppm as an 8-hour time-weighted average.

III. **Clinical presentation**
   A. **Skin or eye contact** results in irritation and defatting. Mucous membrane irritation is seen with ingestion or inhalation.
   B. **Inhalation or ingestion.** Mild to moderate systemic toxicity includes headache, nausea, vomiting, confusion, and drunkenness. More severe exposures may cause coma, respiratory arrest, and ventricular arrhythmias. Hepatic and renal injury may be apparent 1–3 days after exposure.

IV. **Diagnosis** is based on history and clinical presentation. Be aware that hepatic and renal toxicity may be delayed.
   A. **Specific levels.** Blood, urine, or breath concentrations may document exposure but are rarely available and are not useful for acute management.
   B. **Other useful laboratory studies.** Electrolytes, BUN, creatinine, liver transaminases, prothrombin time (PT), ECG monitoring.

V. **Treatment**
   A. **Emergency and supportive measures**
      1. Maintain the airway and assist ventilation if necessary (see p 4).
      2. Treat coma (p 18) and arrhythmias (p 14) if they occur. Avoid use of epi-

nephrine or other sympathomimetic amines, which may precipitate arrhythmias. Tachyarrhythmias caused by myocardial sensitization may be treated with **propranolol,** 1–2 mg IV (see p 373), or **esmolol,** 25–100 μg/kg/min IV (see p 338).

   3. Monitor ECG for at least 4–6 hours after exposure.

B. Specific drugs and antidotes. Acetylcysteine (NAC; see p 311) may be helpful in preventing hepatic and renal damage by scavenging toxic metabolic intermediates, but no controlled study has been performed.

C. Decontamination (see p 41–49)

   1. Inhalation. Remove victim from exposure and give supplemental oxygen if available.

   2. Skin and eyes. Remove contaminated clothing and wash exposed skin with soap and water. Irrigate exposed eyes with copious tepid water or saline.

   3. Ingestion

      a. Prehospital. Administer activated charcoal, if available. Do *not* induce emesis with ipecac because of the risk of abrupt onset of coma.

      b. Hospital. Perform gastric lavage, and administer activated charcoal and a cathartic.

D. Enhanced elimination. There is no documented efficacy for forced diuresis, hemodialysis, hemoperfusion, or repeat-dose charcoal.

CHLOROPHENOXY HERBICIDES
Kent R. Olson, MD

ANTIDOTE   IPECAC   LAVAGE   CHARCOAL

Chlorophenoxy compounds have been widely used as herbicides. Agent Orange was a mixture of the chlorophenoxy herbicides 2,4-D (dichlorophenoxyacetic acid) and 2,4,5-T (trichlorophenoxyacetic acid) that also contained small amounts of the highly toxic contaminant TCDD (2,3,7,8-tetrachlorodibenzo-*p*-dioxin; see p 154). Commercially available 2,4-D no longer contains TCDD.

  I. Mechanism of toxicity. In plants, the compounds act as growth hormone stimulators. Their mechanism of toxicity in animals is not known. In animal studies, widespread muscle damage occurs and the cause of death is usually ventricular fibrillation. Massive rhabdomyolysis has been described in human cases.

  II. Toxic dose. The minimum toxic dose of 2,4-D in humans is 3–4 g or 40–50 mg/kg, and death has occurred after adult ingestion of 6.5 g.

 III. Clinical presentation. Tachycardia, muscle weakness, and muscle spasms occur shortly after ingestion and may progress to profound muscle weakness and coma. Massive rhabdomyolysis and severe and intractable hypotension have been reported, resulting in death within 24 hours. Hepatitis and renal injury may occur.

 IV. Diagnosis depends on a history of exposure and the presence of muscle weakness and elevated serum creatine phosphokinase (CPK).

   A. Specific levels are not routinely available.

   B. Other useful laboratory studies. Electrolytes, glucose, BUN, creatinine, creatine phosphokinase (CPK), urinalysis (occult heme test positive in the presence of myoglobin), liver enzymes, ECG and ECG monitoring.

  V. Treatment

   A. Emergency and supportive measures

      1. Maintain the airway and assist ventilation if necessary (see p 4).

      2. Treat coma (p 18), hypotension (p 15), and rhabdomyolysis (p 25) if they occur.

      3. Monitor the patient closely for at least 6–12 hours after ingestion because of the potential for delayed onset of symptoms.

   B. Specific drugs and antidotes. There is no specific antidote.

C. Decontamination (see p 44)

   1. Prehospital. Administer activated charcoal, if available. Ipecac-induced emesis may be useful for initial treatment at the scene (eg, children at home) if it can be given within a few minutes of exposure.

   2. Hospital. Administer activated charcoal, then perform gastric lavage. Following lavage, give an additional dose of charcoal and a cathartic.

D. Enhanced elimination. There is no proved role for these procedures, although alkalinization of the urine may promote excretion of 2,4-D.

CHLOROQUINE AND OTHER AMINOQUINOLINES
Neal L. Benowitz, MD

ANTIDOTE   IPECAC   LAVAGE   CHARCOAL

Chloroquine and other aminoquinolines are used in the prophylaxis or therapy of malaria and other parasitic diseases. Chloroquine and hydroxychloroquine are also used in the treatment of rheumatoid arthritis. Drugs in this class include chloroquine phosphate (Aralen), amodiaquine hydrochloride (Camoquin), hydroxychloroquine sulfate (Plaquenil), mefloquine (Lariam), primaquine phosphate, and quinacrine hydrochloride (Atabrine). Chloroquine overdose is common, especially in countries where malaria is prevalent, and the mortality rate is 10–30%.

I. Mechanism of toxicity. Chloroquine and related drugs are highly tissue-bound (volume of distribution is 200 L/kg) and are eliminated very slowly from the body (half-life of 280 hours).

   A. Chloroquine blocks the synthesis of DNA and RNA and also has some quinidinelike cardiotoxicity.

   B. Primaquine and **quinacrine** are oxidizing agents and can cause methemoglobinemia or hemolytic anemia (especially in patients with G6PD deficiency).

II. Toxic dose. The therapeutic dose of chloroquine phosphate is 500 mg once a week for malaria prophylaxis, or 2.5 g over 2 days for treatment of malaria. Deaths have been reported in children after doses as low as 300 mg; the lethal dose of chloroquine for an adult is estimated at 30–50 mg/kg.

III. Clinical presentation

   A. Mild to moderate chloroquine overdose results in dizziness, nausea and vomiting, abdominal pain, headache and visual disturbances (sometimes including irreversible blindness), auditory disturbances (sometimes leading to deafness), agitation, and neuromuscular excitability.

   B. Severe chloroquine overdose may cause convulsions, coma, shock, and respiratory or cardiac arrest. Quinidinelike cardiotoxicity may be seen, including sinoatrial arrest, depressed myocardial contractility, QRS or QT interval prolongation, heart block, and ventricular arrhythmias. Severe hypokalemia sometimes occurs and may contribute to arrhythmias.

   C. Primaquine and **quinacrine** intoxication commonly cause gastrointestinal upset and may also cause severe methemoglobinemia (see p 217) or hemolysis; chronic treatment can cause ototoxicity and retinopathy.

   D. Amodiaquine in therapeutic doses has caused severe and even fatal neutropenia.

   E. Mefloquine in therapeutic use or overdose may cause dizziness, vertigo, hallucinations, psychosis, and seizures.

IV. Diagnosis. The findings of gastritis, visual disturbances, and neuromuscular excitability, especially if accompanied by hypotension, QRS or QT interval widening, or ventricular arrhythmias, should suggest chloroquine overdose. Hemolysis or methemoglobinemia should suggest primaquine or quinacrine overdose.

   A. Specific levels. Chloroquine levels can be measured in blood but are not generally available. Because chloroquine is concentrated intracellularly, whole blood measurements are 5-fold higher than serum or plasma levels.

1. Plasma (trough) concentrations of 10–20 ng/mL (0.01–0.02 mg/L) are effective in the treatment of various types of malaria.
2. Cardiotoxicity may be seen with serum levels of 1 mg/L (1000 ng/mL); serum levels reported in fatal cases have ranged from 1–210 mg/L (average, 55 mg/L).

B. **Other useful laboratory studies.** Electrolytes, glucose, BUN, creatinine, ECG and ECG monitoring. With **primaquine** or **quinacrine,** also include CBC, free plasma hemoglobin, methemoglobin.

V. Treatment

A. Emergency and supportive measures

1. Maintain the airway and assist ventilation if necessary (see p 4).
2. Treat seizures (p 22), coma (p 18), hypotension (p 15), and methemoglobinemia (p 217) if they occur.
3. Treat massive hemolysis with blood transfusions if needed, and prevent hemoglobin deposition in the kidney tubules by alkaline diuresis (as for rhabdomyolysis; see p 25).
4. Continuously monitor the ECG for at least 6–8 hours.

B. Specific drugs and antidotes

1. Treat cardiotoxicity as for quinidine poisoning (see p 000) with **sodium bicarbonate** (see p 318), 1–2 meq/kg IV.
2. **Epinephrine** infusion (see p 337) may be useful in treating hypotension via combined vasoconstrictor and inotropic actions.
3. High-dose **diazepam** (2 mg/kg IV, given over 30 minutes) has been reported to reduce mortality in animals and to ameliorate cardiotoxicity in human cases. However, the mechanism of protection is unknown and its routine use is not recommended.

C. Decontamination (see p 44)

1. **Prehospital.** Administer activated charcoal, if available. Ipecac-induced emesis may be useful for initial treatment at the scene (eg, children at home) if it can be given within a few minutes of exposure.
2. **Hospital.** Administer activated charcoal and a cathartic. Perform gastric lavage for significant ingestions (eg, > 30–50 mg/kg). Gastric emptying is probably not necessary after small ingestions if activated charcoal can be given promptly.

D. Enhanced elimination. Because of extensive tissue distribution, enhanced removal procedures are ineffective.

CHROMIUM
Charles E. Becker, MD

ANTIDOTE   IPECAC   LAVAGE   CHARCOAL

Chromium is a hard silver-colored metal used in chrome plating, pigments, and oxidizing agents. Electroplaters, welders, lithographers, and metal and textile workers are among those potentially exposed. Most chromium salts with human health effects occur in 1 of 2 valence states: trivalent (chromic oxide, chromic sulfate) or hexavalent (chromium trioxide, chromic anhydride, chromic acid, dichromate salts).

I. Mechanism of toxicity

A. **Trivalent chromium** compounds and chromate salts of lead, zinc, barium, bismuth, and silver are relatively less toxic than hexavalent compounds, owing to lower solubility and a smaller redox potential.

B. **Hexavalent compounds** are soluble and are more readily absorbed from the gastrointestinal tract, skin, and lungs. Hexavalent chromium salts are strong oxidizing agents that may oxidize hemoglobin to produce methemoglobinemia. They also produce corrosive burns by denaturation of tissue protein.

C. Chromic acid is a strong acid, while some chromate salts are strong bases.

II. Toxic dose

A. Inhalation. The recommended workplace limit (ACGIH TLV-TWA) for chromium metal and divalent or trivalent compounds is 0.5 mg/m^3 as an 8-hour time-weighted average; for insoluble chromates, chromite dust, and soluble hexavalent compounds, the TLV-TWA is 0.05 mg/m^3.

B. Skin. Skin burns may enhance systemic absorption, and death has occurred after a 10% surface area burn.

C. Ingestion. Serious toxicity has occurred from ingestion of as little as 500 mg of hexavalent chromium. The estimated lethal dose of chromic acid is 1–2 g; of potassium dichromate, 6–8 g. Drinking water standards are set at 50 μg/L (1 micromol/L) total chromium.

III. Clinical presentation

A. Inhalation. Inhalation can cause upper respiratory tract irritation, wheezing, and pulmonary edema (which may be delayed for several hours after exposure).

B. Skin and eyes. Acute contact may cause severe corneal injury, deep skin burns, and oral or esophageal burns. Hypersensitivity dermatitis may result.

C. Ingestion. Ingestion may cause immediate hemorrhagic gastroenteritis; resulting massive fluid and blood loss may cause shock and oliguric renal failure. Hemolysis, hepatitis, and cerebral edema have been reported. Chromates are capable of oxidizing hemoglobin, but clinically significant methemoglobinemia is relatively uncommon after acute overdose.

IV. Diagnosis is based on a history of exposure and clinical manifestations of skin and mucous membrane burns, gastroenteritis, and shock.

A. Specific levels. Blood levels are not useful in emergency management, nor are they widely available. Detection in the urine may confirm exposure; normal urine levels are less than 20 μg/L.

B. Other useful laboratory studies. CBC, plasma free hemoglobin and haptoglobin (if hemolysis suspected), electrolytes, glucose, BUN, creatinine, liver transaminases, urinalysis (for hemoglobin), arterial blood gas or pulse oximetry, methemoglobin, chest x-ray.

V. Treatment

A. Emergency and supportive measures

1. Inhalation. Give supplemental oxygen. Treat wheezing (see p 9–10), and monitor closely for several hours for development of noncardiogenic pulmonary edema (p 8).

2. Ingestion

a. Treat hemorrhagic gastroenteritis with aggressive fluid and blood replacement (p 15). Consider endoscopy to rule out esophageal or gastric burns.

b. Treat hemoglobinuria resulting from hemolysis with alkaline diuresis as for rhabdomyolysis (p 25).

B. Specific drugs and antidotes

1. Chelation therapy (eg, with BAL) is not effective.

2. After oral ingestion of hexavalent compounds, **ascorbic acid** has been suggested to assist the conversion of hexavalent to less toxic trivalent compounds. For each 0.135 g of chromium compound ingested, give 1 g of ascorbic acid orally.

3. Acetylcysteine (see p 311) has been used in several animal studies and one human case of dichromate poisoning.

C. Decontamination (see p 41–49)

1. Inhalation. Remove victim from exposure and give supplemental oxygen, if available.

2. Skin. Remove contaminated clothing and wash exposed areas immediately with copious soap and water. EDTA (see p 335) 10% ointment may facilitate removal of chromate scabs.

 3. Eyes. Irrigate copiously with tepid water or saline and perform fluorescein examination to rule out corneal injury if pain or irritation persists.

 4. Ingestion (see p 44)

  a. Prehospital. Give milk or water to dilute corrosive effects. Do *not* induce emesis owing to the potential for corrosive injury.

  b. Hospital. Perform gastric lavage. Administer activated charcoal, although there is no evidence for its efficacy. Do *not* give charcoal if immediate endoscopy is planned.

 D. Enhanced elimination. There is no evidence for efficacy of enhanced removal procedures such as dialysis or hemoperfusion.

CLONIDINE AND RELATED DRUGS
Olga F. Woo, PharmD

ANTIDOTE IPECAC LAVAGE CHARCOAL

Clonidine and the related centrally acting adrenergic inhibitors **guanabenz** and **methyldopa** are commonly used for the treatment of hypertension. Clonidine has also been used to alleviate opioid and nicotine withdrawal symptoms. Clonidine overdose is a common pediatric problem that may occur after ingestion of pills or the newer long-acting skin patches. **Oxymetazoline** and **tetrahydrozoline** are nasal decongestants that may cause toxicity identical to that of clonidine.

 I. Mechanism of toxicity. All agents decrease central sympathetic outflow by stimulating α_2-adrenergic (inhibitory) receptors in the brain.

  A. Clonidine, oxymetazoline, and **tetrahydrozoline** may also stimulate peripheral α_1-receptors, resulting in vasoconstriction and transient hypertension.

  B. Guanabenz is structurally similar to guanethidine, a ganglionic blocker, and has some neuron-blocking action.

  C. Methyldopa may further decrease sympathetic outflow by metabolism to a false neurotransmitter (alpha-methylnorepinephrine) or by decreasing plasma renin activity.

  D. Pharmacokinetics. See Table II–19.

 II. Toxic dose

  A. Clonidine. As little as one tablet of 0.1 mg clonidine has produced toxic effects in children; however, 10 mg shared by twin 34-month-old girls was not lethal. Adults have survived acute ingestions with as much as 18.8 mg. No fatalities from acute overdoses have been reported.

  B. Guanabenz. Mild toxicity developed in adults who ingested 160–320 mg and in a 3-year-old who ingested 12 mg. Severe toxicity developed in a 19-month-old who ingested 28 mg. A 3-year-old child had moderate symptoms after ingesting 480 mg. All these children had recovered by 24 hours.

  C. Methyldopa. More than 2 g in adults is considered a toxic dose, and death was reported in an adult after an ingestion of 25 g. The therapeutic dose of methyldopa for children is 10–65 mg/kg/d, and the higher dose is expected to cause mild symptoms.

 III. Clinical presentation. Manifestations of intoxication result from generalized sympathetic depression and include pupillary constriction, lethargy, coma, apnea, bradycardia, hypotension, and hypothermia. Paradoxic hypertension, caused by stimulation of peripheral α_1-receptors, may occur with clonidine, oxymetazoline, and tetrahydrozoline (and possibly guanabenz) and is usually transient. The onset of symptoms is usually within 30–60 minutes, although peak effects may occur

TABLE II–19. PHARMACOKINETIC PROPERTIES OF CLONIDINE AND RELATED DRUGS

Drug	Volume of Distribution (L/kg)	Peak Absorption (h)	Elimination Half-life (h)
Clonidine	3–5.5	2–3	5–13[a]
Guanabenz	7.4–17	2–5	7–14
Methyldopa	0.24	3–4	4–14

[a] 17–41 h in renal failure.

6–12 hours after ingestion, with full recovery within 24 hours.

IV. Diagnosis should be suspected in patients with pinpoint pupils, respiratory depression, hypotension, and bradycardia. Clonidine overdose may mimic opioid overdose but does not usually respond to administration of naloxone.

   A. Specific levels. Serum drug levels are not routinely available or clinically useful.

   B. Other useful laboratory studies. Electrolytes, glucose, arterial blood gases or oximetry.

V. Treatment. Patients usually recover within 24 hours with supportive care.

   A. Emergency and supportive measures

   1. Protect the airway and assist ventilation if necessary (see p 4).

   2. Treat coma (p 18), hypotension (p 15), bradycardia (p 10), and hypothermia (p 19) if they occur. These signs usually resolve with supportive measures such as fluids, atropine, dopamine, and warming.

   B. Specific drugs and antidotes

   1. **Naloxone** (see p 355) has been reported to reverse signs and symptoms of clonidine overdose, but this has not been confirmed. However, because the overdose mimics opioid intoxication, naloxone is indicated because narcotics may also have been ingested.

   2. **Tolazoline,** a central α_2-receptor antagonist, has been recommended by some, but the response is highly variable and it should not be used.

   C. Decontamination (see p 44)

   1. **Prehospital.** Administer activated charcoal, if available. Ipecac-induced emesis may be useful for initial treatment at the scene (eg, children at home) if it can be given immediately after exposure.

   2. **Hospital.** Administer activated charcoal and a cathartic. Gastric emptying is not necessary if activated charcoal can be given promptly.

   D. Enhanced elimination. There is no evidence that enhanced removal procedures are effective.

COCAINE
Neal L. Benowitz, MD

ANTIDOTE   IPECAC   LAVAGE   CHARCOAL

Cocaine is one of the most popular drugs of abuse. It may be sniffed into the nose (snorted), smoked, or injected intravenously. Occasionally it is combined with heroin and injected (speedball). Cocaine purchased on the street is usually of high purity, but it may occasionally contain substitute stimulants such as caffeine (see p 112), phenylpropanolamine (p 253), ephedrine (p 253), or phencyclidine (p 248).

The "free base" form of cocaine is preferred for smoking because it volatilizes at a lower temperature and is not as easily destroyed by heat as the crystalline hydrochloride salt. Free base is made by dissolving cocaine salt in an aqueous alkaline solution and then extracting the free base form with a solvent such as ether. Heat is sometimes applied to hasten solvent evaporation, creating a fire hazard. "Crack" cocaine is produced by using sodium bicarbonate to create the alkaline aqueous solution, which is then dried.

I. **Mechanism of toxicity.** The primary actions of cocaine are local anesthetic effects (see p 68), central nervous system stimulation, and inhibition of neuronal uptake of catecholamines.

A. Central nervous system stimulation and inhibition of catecholamine uptake result in a state of generalized sympathetic stimulation very similar to that of amphetamine intoxication (see p 66).

B. Cardiovascular effects of high doses of cocaine, presumably related to blockade of cardiac cell sodium channels, include depression of conduction and contractility.

C. Cocaine is well absorbed from all routes, and toxicity has been described after mucosal application as a local anesthetic. Smoking and intravenous injection produce maximum effects within 1–2 minutes, while oral or mucosal absorption may take up to 20–30 minutes. Once absorbed, cocaine is eliminated by metabolism and hydrolysis with a half-life of about 60 minutes.

D. In the presence of ethanol, cocaine is transesterified to **cocaethylene**, which has similar pharmacologic effects and a longer half-life than cocaine.

II. **Toxic dose.** The toxic dose is highly variable and depends on individual tolerance, the route of administration, and the presence of other drugs, as well as other factors. Rapid intravenous injection or smoking may produce transient high brain and heart levels resulting in convulsions or cardiac arrhythmias, whereas the same dose swallowed or snorted may produce only euphoria.

A. The usual maximum recommended dose for intranasal local anesthesia is 100–200 mg (1–2 mL of 10% solution).

B. A typical "line" of cocaine to be snorted contains 20–30 mg or more. Crack is usually sold in pellets or "rocks" containing 100–150 mg.

C. Ingestion of 1 g or more of cocaine is very likely to be fatal.

III. **Clinical presentation**

A. **Central nervous system manifestations** of toxicity may occur within minutes after smoking or intravenous injection or may be delayed for 30–60 minutes after snorting, mucosal application, or oral ingestion.

1. Initial euphoria may be followed by anxiety, agitation, delirium, psychosis, tremulousness, muscle rigidity or hyperactivity, and seizures. High doses may cause respiratory arrest.

2. Seizures are usually brief and self-limited; status epilepticus should suggest continued drug absorption (as from ruptured cocaine-filled condoms in the gastrointestinal tract) or hyperthermia.

3. Coma may be caused by a postictal state, hyperthermia, or intracranial hemorrhage resulting from cocaine-induced hypertension.

4. With chronic cocaine use, insomnia, weight loss, and paranoid psychosis may occur. A "washed-out" syndrome has been observed in cocaine abusers after a prolonged binge, consisting of profound lethargy and deep sleep that may last for several hours, followed by spontaneous recovery.

B. **Cardiovascular toxicity** may also occur rapidly after smoking or intravenous injection and is mediated by sympathetic overactivity.

1. Fatal ventricular tachycardia or fibrillation may occur.

2. Severe hypertension may cause hemorrhagic stroke or aortic dissection.

3. Coronary artery spasm and/or thrombosis may result in myocardial infarction, even in patients with no coronary disease. Diffuse myocardial necrosis similar to catecholamine myocarditis, and chronic cardiomyopathy have been described.

4. Shock may be caused by myocardial, intestinal, or brain infarction, hyperthermia, tachyarrhythmias, or hypovolemia produced by extravascular fluid sequestration owing to vasoconstriction.

5. Renal failure may result from shock, renal arterial spasm, or rhabdomyolysis with myoglobinuria.

C. Death is usually caused by a sudden fatal arrhythmia, status epilepticus, intracranial hemorrhage, or hyperthermia. Hyperthermia is usually caused by seizures, muscular hyperactivity, or rigidity and is typically associated with rhabdomyolysis, myoglobinuric renal failure, coagulopathy, and multiple organ failure.

D. A variety of **other effects** have occurred after smoking or snorting cocaine.

    1. Chest pain without ECG evidence of myocardial ischemia is common. The presumed basis is musculoskeletal, and may be associated with chest wall muscle rhabdomyolysis.

    2. Pneumothorax and pneumomediastinum cause pleuritic chest pain, and the latter is often recognized by a "crunching" sound ("Hammond's crunch") heard over the anterior chest.

    3. Nasal septal perforation may occur after chronic snorting.

    4. Accidental subcutaneous injection of cocaine may cause localized necrotic ulcers ("coke burns"), and wound botulism (see p 107) has been reported.

E. Body "packers" or **"stuffers."** Persons attempting to smuggle cocaine may swallow large numbers of tightly packed cocaine-filled condoms ("body packers"). Street vendors suddenly surprised by a police raid may quickly swallow their wares, often without carefully wrapping or closing the packets or vials ("body stuffers"). The swallowed condoms, packets, or vials may break open, releasing massive quantities of cocaine. The packages are sometimes, but not always, visible on plain abdominal x-ray.

IV. Diagnosis is based on a history of cocaine use or typical features of sympathomimetic intoxication. Skin marks of chronic intravenous drug abuse, especially with scarring from coke burns, and nasal septal perforation after chronic snorting suggest cocaine use. Chest pain with electrocardiographic evidence of ischemia or infarction in a young, otherwise healthy person also suggests cocaine use.

A. Specific levels. Serum cocaine levels are not routinely available and do not assist in emergency management. Cocaine and its metabolite benzoylecgonine are easily detected in the urine and provide qualitative confirmation of cocaine use.

B. Other useful laboratory studies. Electrolytes, glucose, BUN, creatinine, creatine phosphokinase (CPK), urinalysis, urine myoglobin, ECG and ECG monitoring, CT head scan (if hemorrhage is suspected), abdominal x-ray (if cocaine-filled condom or packet ingestion is suspected).

V. Treatment

  A. Emergency and supportive measures

    1. Maintain the airway and assist ventilation if necessary (see p 4).

    2. Treat coma (p 18), agitation (p 23), seizures (p 22), hyperthermia (p 20), arrhythmias (p 10–14), and hypotension (p 15) if they occur.

    3. Angina pectoris may be treated with nitrates or calcium channel blockers such as nifedipine (p 360). For acute myocardial infarction, consider thrombolytic therapy if there are no contraindications (eg, intracranial hemorrhage, aortic dissection).

    4. Monitor vital signs and ECG for several hours. Patients with suspected coronary artery spasm should be admitted to a coronary care unit, and because of reports of persistent or recurrent coronary spasm up to several days after initial exposure, consider use of an oral calcium antagonist such as nifedipine or diltiazem and/or cardiac nitrates for 2–4 weeks after discharge.

  B. Specific drugs and antidotes. There is no specific antidote. Although propranolol was previously recommended as the drug of choice for treatment of cocaine-induced hypertension, it may in fact produce paradoxic worsening of hypertension because of blockade of β_2-mediated vasodilation; **propranolol** (p 373) or **esmolol** (p 338) may be used **in combination** with a vasodilator such as **phentolamine** (p 369). Beta blockers may be used alone for treatment of tachyarrhythmias.

C. Decontamination (see p 44). Decontamination is not necessary after smoking, snorting, or intravenous injection. After **ingestion:**

1. **Prehospital.** Administer activated charcoal, if available. Do *not* induce emesis because of the risk of abrupt onset of seizures.

2. **Hospital.** Administer activated charcoal and a cathartic. Gastric emptying is not necessary if activated charcoal can be given promptly.

3. For ingestion of cocaine-filled condoms or packets, give repeated doses of activated charcoal and consider whole bowel irrigation (see p 48). If large ingested packets (ie, Ziploc bags) are not removed by these procedures, laparotomy and surgical removal may be necessary.

D. Enhanced elimination. Because cocaine is extensively distributed to tissues and rapidly metabolized, dialysis and hemoperfusion procedures are not effective. Acidification of the urine does not significantly enhance cocaine elimination and may aggravate myoglobinuric renal failure.

COLCHICINE
Neal L. Benowitz, MD

ANTIDOTE   IPECAC   LAVAGE   CHARCOAL

Colchicine is marketed in tablets used for treatment of gout and familial Mediterranean fever and is found in certain plants: autumn crocus or meadow saffron *(Colchicum autumnale)* and glory lily *(Gloriosa superba)*. Colchicine overdose is extremely serious, with considerable mortality that is often delayed.

I. **Mechanism of toxicity.** Colchicine inhibits mitosis of dividing cells and, in high concentration, is a general cellular poison. Colchicine is rapidly absorbed and extensively distributed to body tissues.

II. **Toxic dose.** The maximum therapeutic dose of colchicine is 8–10 mg in one day. Tablets contain 0.5–0.6 mg. Fatalities have been reported with single ingestions of as little as 7 mg. In a series of 150 cases, doses of 0.5 mg/kg were associated with diarrhea and vomiting but not death; 0.5–0.8 mg/kg with marrow aplasia and 10% mortality. Ingestions of parts of colchicine-containing plants have resulted in severe toxicity and death.

III. **Clinical presentation.** Colchicine poisoning affects many organ systems, with toxic effects occurring over days to weeks.

A. Following **acute overdose,** symptoms are typically delayed for 2–12 hours and include nausea, vomiting, abdominal pain, and severe bloody diarrhea. Shock results from depressed cardiac contractility and fluid loss into the gastrointestinal tract and other tissues. **Death** usually occurs after 8–36 hours and is caused by respiratory failure, intractable shock, or sudden cardiac arrest. Other manifestations of acute colchicine poisoning include acute myocardial injury, rhabdomyolysis with myoglobinuria, disseminated intravascular coagulation, and acute renal failure.

B. **Late complications** include bone marrow suppression, particularly leukopenia and thrombocytopenia (4–5 days) and alopecia (2–3 weeks). Chronic colchicine therapy may produce myopathy (proximal muscle weakness and elevated creatinine kinase levels) and polyneuropathy.

IV. **Diagnosis.** A syndrome beginning with severe gastroenteritis, shock, rhabdomyolysis, and acute renal failure and, several days later, leukopenia and thrombocytopenia should suggest colchicine poisoning. A history of gout or familial Mediterranean fever in the patient or family member is also suggestive.

A. **Specific levels.** Measurement of levels in blood and urine is neither available nor clinically useful.

B. **Other useful laboratory studies.** CBC, electrolytes, glucose, BUN, creatinine, creatine phosphokinase (CPK), urinalysis, ECG monitoring.

V. Treatment

A. Emergency and supportive measures.
Provide aggressive supportive care, with careful monitoring and treatment of fluid and electrolyte disturbances.

1. Anticipate sudden respiratory or cardiac arrest, and maintain the airway and assist ventilation if necessary (see p 4).

2. Treatment of shock (p 15) may require large amounts of crystalloid fluids, possibly blood (to replace loss from hemorrhagic gastroenteritis), and pressor agents such as dopamine (p 334).

3. Infusion of sodium bicarbonate and mannitol is recommended if there is evidence of rhabdomyolysis (p 25).

4. Bone marrow depression requires specialized intensive care. Severe neutropenia requires patient isolation and management of febrile episodes as for other neutropenic conditions. Platelet transfusions may be required to control bleeding.

B. Specific drugs and antidotes.
No specific antidotes are available.

C. Decontamination (see p 44).

1. **Prehospital.** Administer activated charcoal, if available. Ipecac-induced emesis may be useful for initial treatment at the scene (eg, children at home) if it can be given within a few minutes of exposure.

2. **Hospital.** Administer activated charcoal and a cathartic. Consider gastric lavage for large ingestions.

D. Enhanced elimination.
Because colchicine is highly bound to tissues, with a large volume of distribution, hemodialysis and hemoperfusion are ineffective. Colchicine undergoes enterohepatic recirculation, so **repeat-dose charcoal** might be expected to accelerate elimination, although this has not been documented.

COPPER
Kent R. Olson, MD

ANTIDOTE   IPECAC   LAVAGE   CHARCOAL

Copper is widely used in its elemental metal form, in metal alloys, and in the form of copper salts. Elemental metallic copper is used in electrical wiring and plumbing materials, and copper salts are used as pesticides and algicides. Because of its toxicity, copper sulfate is no longer used as an emetic. The copper alloy brass is an important source of exposure because of leaching of copper ions into acidic beverages stored in brass containers.

I. Mechanism of toxicity

A. **Elemental metallic copper** is poorly absorbed orally and has little toxicity. However, inhalation of copper dust or fumes may cause chemical pneumonitis or a syndrome similar to metal fumes fever (see p 214).

B. **Copper sulfate** salt is highly irritating, depending on the concentration, and may produce mucous membrane irritation and gastroenteritis.

C. **Systemic absorption** can produce hepatic and renal tubular injury. Hemolysis has been associated with copper exposure from hemodialysis equipment or absorption through burned skin.

II. Toxic dose

A. **Inhalation.** The recommended workplace limit (ACGIH TLV-TWA) for copper fumes is 0.2 mg/m^3; for dusts and mists, it is 1 mg/m^3.

B. **Ingestion** of more than 250 mg of copper sulfate can produce vomiting, and larger ingestions can potentially cause hepatic and renal injury.

III. Clinical presentation

A. **Inhalation of copper fumes** or **dusts** may cause cough, dyspnea, fever, and pulmonary infiltrates (see also Metal fumes fever, p 214).

B. **Ingestion of copper salts** rapidly causes metallic taste, epigastric burning, vomiting, and diarrhea. The vomitus may be blue-green. Hypotension may occur, presumably owing to fluid loss from gastroenteritis, and oliguric renal failure may follow. Hepatitis has been reported. Deaths within the first 24 hours after ingestion have resulted from shock.

IV. **Diagnosis** is based on a history of ingestion of copper salts accompanied by gastroenteritis, of inhalation of copper fumes, or of welding accompanied by fever and respiratory complaints.

   A. **Specific levels.** If copper salt ingestion is suspected, a serum copper level should be obtained. Normal serum copper concentrations average 1 mg/L, and this doubles during pregnancy. Serum copper levels above 5 mg/L are considered very toxic. Whole blood copper levels may correlate better with acute intoxication because acute excess copper is carried in the red blood cell; however, blood copper levels are not as widely available.

   B. **Other useful laboratory studies.** BUN, creatinine, hepatic transaminases, arterial blood gases or oximetry, chest x-ray.

V. **Treatment**

   A. **Emergency and supportive measures**

      1. **Inhalation of copper fumes** or **dusts.** Give supplemental oxygen if indicated by arterial blood gases, and treat bronchospasm (see p 9–10) and chemical pneumonitis (p 8) if they occur. Symptoms are usually short-lived and resolve without specific treatment.

      2. **Ingestion of copper salts**

         a. Treat shock caused by gastroenteritis with aggressive intravenous fluid replacement and, if necessary, pressor drugs (p 15).

         b. Consider endoscopy to rule out corrosive esophageal or stomach injury, depending on the concentration of the solution and the patient's symptoms.

   B. **Specific drugs and antidotes. BAL** (dimercaprol; see p 317) and **penicillamine** (see p 366) are effective chelating agents and should be used in seriously ill patients with large ingestion.

   C. **Decontamination**

      1. **Inhalation.** Remove victim from exposure and give supplemental oxygen if available.

      2. **Ingestion** (see p 44)

         a. Perform gastric lavage. Do **not** induce emesis because it may worsen gastroenteritis.

         b. Administer activated charcoal, although there is no documentation of its effectiveness.

   D. **Enhanced elimination.** Dialysis, hemoperfusion, and repeat-dose charcoal are not effective in enhancing elimination. Hemodialysis may be required for supportive care of patients with acute renal failure, and it can marginally increase the elimination of the copper-chelator complex.

COUMARIN AND RELATED RODENTICIDES
Ilene B. Anderson, PharmD

ANTIDOTE   IPECAC   LAVAGE   CHARCOAL

Dicumarol and other natural anticoagulants are found in sweet clover. Coumarin derivatives are used both therapeutically and as rodenticides. Warfarin (Coumadin) is widely used as a therapeutic anticoagulant, but is no longer popular as a rodenticide because rats and mice have become resistant. The most common rodenticides available today contain long-acting **"superwarfarin"** anticoagulants such as brodifacoum, diphacinone, bromadiolone, chlorophacinone, difenacoum, pindone, and valone, which have profound and prolonged anticoagulant effects. Common commercial products include D-con Mouse Prufe (warfarin 0.054%), D-con Mouse Prufe II (brodifacoum 0.005%), Ramik (diphacinone 0.005%), and Talon-G (brodifacoum 0.005%).

I. **Mechanism of toxicity.** All these compounds inhibit hepatic synthesis of the vitamin K–dependent coagulation factors II, VII, IX, and X. Only the synthesis of new factors is affected, and the anticoagulant effect is delayed until currently circulating factors have been degraded. Peak effects are usually not observed for 2–3 days because of the long half-lives of the factors VII, IX, and X (24–60 hours).

   A. The duration of anticoagulant effect after a single dose of **warfarin** is usually 5–7 days.

   B. **Superwarfarin** products may continue to produce significant anticoagulation for weeks to months after a single ingestion.

II. **Toxic dose.** The toxic dose is highly variable.

   A. Generally, a single small ingestion of **warfarin** (eg, 10–20 mg) will not cause serious intoxication (most warfarin-based rodenticides contain 0.05% warfarin). In contrast, chronic or repeated ingestion of even small amounts (eg, 2 mg/d) can produce significant anticoagulation. Patients with hepatic dysfunction, malnutrition, or a bleeding diathesis are at greater risk.

   B. **Superwarfarins** are extremely potent and have prolonged effects even after a single small ingestion (ie, as little as 1 mg in an adult).

   C. Multiple **drug interactions** are known to alter the anticoagulant effect of warfarin (Table II–20).

III. **Clinical presentation.** Excessive anticoagulation may cause ecchymoses, subconjunctival hemorrhage, bleeding gums, or evidence of internal hemorrhage (eg, hematemesis, melena, or hematuria). The most immediately life-threatening complications are massive gastrointestinal bleeding and intracranial hemorrhage.

   A. Anticoagulant effects may be apparent within 8–12 hours, but most commonly they are delayed for at least 1–2 days after ingestion.

   B. Evidence of continuing anticoagulant effect may persist for days, weeks, or even months with superwarfarin products.

IV. **Diagnosis** is based on the history and evidence of anticoagulant effect. It is important to identify the exact product ingested to ascertain whether a superwarfarin is involved.

   A. **Specific levels.** Blood levels of anticoagulants are not available, nor are they helpful.

      1. Anticoagulant effect is best quantified by baseline and daily repeated measurement of the **prothrombin time** (PT), which may not be elevated until 1–2 days after ingestion. A normal PT 48–72 hours after exposure rules out significant ingestion.

      2. Blood levels of clotting factors II, VII, IX, and X will be decreased, but these measurements are not routinely available.

TABLE II–20. EXAMPLES OF DRUG INTERACTIONS WITH COUMARIN[a]

Increased anticoagulant effect	Decreased anticoagulant effect
Allopurinol	Barbiturates
Chloral hydrate	Carbamazepine
Cimetidine	Cholestyramine
Disulfiram	Glutethimide
Indomethacin and other nonsteroidal anti-inflammatory agents	Oral contraceptives
Quinidine	Rifampin
Salicylates	
Sulfonamides	

[a]Adapted and reproduced, with permission, from Olson KR, Becker CE: Poisoning. In: *Current Emergency Diagnosis & Treatment*, 3rd ed. Ho MT, Saunders CE (editors). Appleton & Lange, 1990.

B. Other useful laboratory studies. CBC, blood type and cross-match.

V. Treatment

A. Emergency and supportive measures. If significant bleeding occurs, be prepared to treat shock with transfusions and fresh-frozen plasma, and obtain immediate neurosurgical consultation if intracranial bleeding is suspected.

1. Take care not to precipitate hemorrhage in severely anticoagulated patients; prevent falls and other trauma. If possible, avoid use of nasogastric or endotracheal tubes or central intravenous lines.

2. Avoid drugs that may enhance bleeding or decrease metabolism of the anticoagulant (Table II–20).

B. Specific drugs and antidotes. Vitamin K$_1$ (phytonadione), but *not* vitamin K$_3$ (menadione), effectively restores the production of clotting factors. It should be given if there is evidence of significant anticoagulation. *Note,* however, that if it is given prophylactically after an acute ingestion, the 48 hour prothrombin time cannot be used to determine severity of the overdose, and the patient will have to be monitored for a minimum of 5 days after the last vitamin K$_1$ dose.

1. Give 5–10 mg of **vitamin K$_1$** very slowly IV or SC (see p 377). *Caution:* Vitamin K-mediated reversal of anticoagulation may be dangerous for patients who require constant anticoagulation (eg, for prosthetic heart valves). Very minute doses should be given to titrate for partial effect. **Repeated doses** of vitamin K may be required, especially in patients who have ingested a long-acting superwarfarin product. Doses as high as 200 mg/d have been used.

2. Because vitamin K will not restore clotting factors for several hours, patients with active hemorrhage may require **fresh-frozen plasma** or **fresh whole blood.**

C. Decontamination (see p 44)

1. **Prehospital.** Administer activated charcoal, if available. Ipecac-induced emesis may be useful for initial treatment at the scene (eg, children at home) if it can be given within 30 minutes of exposure.

2. **Hospital.** Administer activated charcoal and a cathartic. Gastric emptying is not necessary if activated charcoal can be given promptly, and should be avoided in the person who is already anticoagulated.

D. Enhanced elimination. There is no role for enhanced elimination procedures.

CYANIDE
Paul D. Blanc, MD, MSPH

ANTIDOTE   IPECAC   LAVAGE   CHARCOAL

Cyanide is a highly reactive chemical with a variety of uses, including chemical synthesis, laboratory analysis, and metal plating. Aliphatic nitriles (acrylonitrile, propionitrile) used in plastics manufacturing are metabolized to cyanide. The vasodilator drug nitroprusside releases cyanide on exposure to light or through metabolism. Natural sources of cyanide (amygdalin and many other cyanogenic glycosides) are found in apricot pits, cassava, and many other plants and seeds, some of which may be important depending on ethnobotanical practices. Acetonitrile, a component of some artificial nail glue removers, has caused several pediatric deaths.

Hydrogen cyanide is a gas easily generated by mixing acid with cyanide salts and is a common combustion by-product of burning plastics, wool, and many other natural and synthetic products. Hydrogen cyanide poisoning is an important cause of death in fires, and deliberate cyanide exposure remains an important instrument of homicide and suicide.

I. Mechanism of toxicity. Cyanide is a chemical asphyxiant; binding to cellular cytochrome oxidase, it blocks the aerobic utilization of oxygen. Unbound cyanide is detoxified by metabolism to thiocyanate, a much less toxic compound that is slowly excreted in the urine.

II. **Toxic dose**
   A. Exposure to **hydrogen cyanide gas** (HCN) at low levels (150–200 ppm) can be fatal. The air level considered immediately dangerous to life or health (IDLH) is 50 ppm. The recommended workplace ceiling limit (ACGIH TLV-C) for HCN is 10 ppm (11 mg/m^3). HCN is well-absorbed across the skin.
   B. Adult **ingestion** of as little as 200 mg of the sodium or potassium salt may be fatal. Solutions of cyanide salts can be absorbed through intact skin.
   C. Acute cyanide poisoning is relatively rare with nitroprusside infusion (at normal infusion rates) or after ingestion of amygdalin-containing seeds (unless they have been pulverized).

III. **Clinical presentation.** Abrupt onset of profound toxic effects shortly after exposure is the hallmark of cyanide poisoning. Symptoms include headache, nausea, dyspnea, and confusion. Syncope, seizures, coma, agonal respirations, and cardiovascular collapse ensue rapidly after heavy exposure.
   A. Brief delay may occur if the cyanide is ingested as a salt, especially if it is in a capsule or if there is food in the stomach.
   B. Delayed onset (minutes to hours) may also occur after ingestion of nitriles and plant cyanogenic glycosides, because of metabolism to cyanide.
   C. Chronic neurologic sequelae may follow severe cyanide poisoning.

IV. **Diagnosis** is based on a history of exposure or the presence of rapidly progressive symptoms and signs. Severe lactic acidosis is usually present with significant exposure. The **measured venous oxygen saturation** may be elevated owing to blocked cellular oxygen consumption. The classic "bitter almond" aroma of hydrogen cyanide may or may not be noted, because of genetic variability in the ability to appreciate the smell.
   A. **Specific levels.** Cyanide determinations are rarely of use in emergency management because they cannot be performed rapidly enough to influence initial treatment. In addition, they must be interpreted with caution because of a variety of complicating technical factors.
      1. Whole blood levels higher than 0.5–1 mg/L are considered toxic.
      2. Smokers may have levels up to 0.1 mg/L.
      3. Rapid nitroprusside infusion may produce levels as high as 1 mg/L.
   B. **Other useful laboratory studies.** Electrolytes, glucose, serum lactate, arterial blood gas, mixed venous oxygen saturation, carboxyhemoglobin (if smoke inhalation exposure).

V. **Treatment**
   A. **Emergency and supportive measures.** Treat all cyanide exposures as potentially lethal.
      1. Maintain the airway and assist ventilation if necessary (see p 4). Administer supplemental oxygen.
      2. Treat coma (p 18), hypotension (p 15), and seizures (p 22) if they occur.
      3. Start an intravenous line and monitor the patient's vital signs and ECG closely.
   B. **Other useful laboratory studies**
      1. The **Lilly cyanide antidote kit** consists of amyl and sodium nitrites (see p 361), which produce cyanide-scavenging methemoglobinemia, and sodium thiosulfate (see p 376), which accelerates the conversion of cyanide to thiocyanate.
         a. Break a pearl of **amyl nitrite** under the nose of the victim; and administer **sodium nitrite,** 300 mg IV (6 mg/kg for children). *Caution:* Nitrite-induced methemoglobinemia can be extremely dangerous and even lethal. Nitrite should *not* be given if the symptoms are mild or if the diagnosis is uncertain, especially if concomitant carbon monoxide poisoning is suspected.

b. Administer **sodium thiosulfate,** 12.5 g IV. Thiosulfate is relatively benign and may be given empirically if the diagnosis is uncertain.

2. The most promising alternative antidote is **hydroxocobalamin** (see p 344). It is currently undergoing investigational trials in the USA.

3. Hyperbaric oxygen has no proven role in cyanide poisoning treatment.

C. Decontamination (see p 41–49). *Caution:* Avoid contact with cyanide-containing salts or solutions, and avoid inhaling vapors from vomitus (may give off hydrogen cyanide gas).

1. Inhalation. Remove victim from hydrogen cyanide exposure and give supplemental oxygen, if available. Each rescuer should wear a positive-pressure, self-contained breathing apparatus and, if possible, chemical protective clothing.

2. Skin. Remove and isolate all contaminated clothing and wash affected areas with copious soap and water.

3. Ingestion (see p 44). Even though charcoal has a relatively low affinity for cyanide, it will effectively bind the doses often ingested (eg, 100–500 mg).

a. Prehospital. Immediately administer activated charcoal, if available. Do *not* induce emesis unless victim is more than 20 minutes from a medical facility and charcoal is not available.

b. Hospital. Immediately place a gastric tube and administer activated charcoal, then perform gastric lavage. Give additional activated charcoal and a cathartic after the lavage.

D. Enhanced elimination. There is no role for hemodialysis or hemoperfusion in cyanide poisoning treatment. Hemodialysis may be indicated in patients with renal insufficiency who develop high thiocyanate levels while on extended nitroprusside therapy.

CYCLIC ANTIDEPRESSANTS
Neal L. Benowitz, MD

ANTIDOTE   IPECAC   LAVAGE   CHARCOAL

Cyclic antidepressants, also called tricyclic antidepressants, are commonly taken in overdose by suicidal patients and represent a major cause of poisoning hospitalizations and deaths. Currently available cyclic antidepressants are described in Table II–21. Amitriptyline is also marketed in combination with chlordiazepoxide (Limbitrol) or perphenazine (Etrafon, Triavil).

Cyclobenzaprine (Flexeril), a centrally acting muscle relaxant, is structurally related to the cyclic antidepressants but exhibits minimal cardiotoxic and variable CNS effects. **Newer antidepressants** such as trazodone, fluoxetine, and paroxetine are discussed on p 76. **Monoamine oxidase inhibitors** are discussed on page 222.

I. Mechanism of toxicity. Cyclic antidepressant toxicity affects primarily the cardiovascular and central nervous systems.

A. Cardiovascular effects. Several mechanisms contribute to cardiovascular toxicity:

1. Anticholinergic effects and inhibition of neuronal reuptake of catecholamines result in tachycardia and mild hypertension.

2. Peripheral alpha-adrenergic blockade induces vasodilation.

3. Membrane-depressant (quinidinelike) effects cause myocardial depression and cardiac conduction disturbances by inhibition of the fast sodium channel that initiates the cardiac cell action potential. Metabolic acidosis may contribute to cardiotoxicity by further depressing the fast sodium channel.

B. Central nervous system effects. These result in part from anticholinergic tox-

TABLE II–21. CYCLIC ANTIDEPRESSANTS

Drug	Usual Adult Daily Dose (mg)	Usual Half-Life (h)	Toxicity[a]
Amitriptyline	75–200	19	A, C, S
Amoxapine	150–300	8	S
Clomipramine	100–250	32	A, C, S
Cyclobenzaprine	20–40	24	A
Desipramine	75–200	22	A, C, S
Doxepin	75–300	17	A, C, S
Imipramine	75–200	18	A, C, S
Maprotiline	75–300	40	C, S
Nortriptyline	75–150	28	A, C, S
Protriptyline	20–40	78	A, C, S
Trimipramine	75–200	23	A, C, S

[a]A = anticholinergic; C = cardiovascular; S = seizures.

icity (eg, sedation and coma), but seizures are probably a result of inhibition of reuptake of norepinephrine or serotonin in the central nervous system or other central effects.

C. Relevant pharmacokinetics
  1. Anticholinergic effects of the drugs may retard gastric emptying, resulting in slow or erratic absorption.
  2. Cyclic antidepressants are primarily metabolized by the liver, with only a small fraction excreted unchanged in the urine. Active metabolites may contribute to toxicity; several drugs are metabolized to other well-known cyclic antidepressants (eg, amitriptyline to nortriptyline, imipramine to desipramine).
  3. Most of these drugs are extensively bound to body tissues and plasma proteins, resulting in very large volumes of distribution and long elimination half-lives (Table II–21).

II. Toxic dose. Most of the cyclic antidepressants have a narrow therapeutic index so that doses of less than 10 times the therapeutic daily dose may produce severe intoxication. In general, ingestion of 10–20 mg/kg is potentially life-threatening.

III. Clinical presentation. Cyclic antidepressant poisoning may produce 3 major toxic syndromes: anticholinergic, cardiovascular, and seizures. Depending on the dose and the drug, patients may experience some or all of these toxic effects. Symptoms usually begin within 30–40 minutes of ingestion but may be delayed owing to erratic gut absorption. Patients who are initially awake may abruptly lose consciousness or develop seizures without warning.

A. Anticholinergic effects include sedation, delirium, coma, dilated pupils, dry skin and mucous membranes, diminished sweating, tachycardia, diminished or absent bowel sounds, and urinary retention. Myoclonic or myokymic jerking is common with anticholinergic intoxication and may be mistaken for seizure activity.

B. Cardiovascular toxicity manifests as abnormal cardiac conduction, arrhythmias, and hypotension.
  1. Typical electrocardiographic findings include sinus tachycardia with prolongation of the PR, QRS, and QT intervals. Varying degrees of atrioventricular block may be seen. Prolongation of the QRS complex to 0.12 s or longer is a fairly reliable predictor of serious cardiovascular and neurologic toxicity

(except in the case of amoxapine, which causes seizures and coma with no change in the QRS interval).

2. Sinus tachycardia accompanied by QRS interval prolongation may resemble ventricular tachycardia (see Fig I–4, p 12). True ventricular tachycardia and fibrillation may also occur. Atypical or polymorphous ventricular tachycardia (torsades des pointes; see Fig I–5, p 15) associated with QT interval prolongation may occur with therapeutic dosing, but is actually uncommon in overdose. Development of bradyarrhythmias usually indicates a severely poisoned heart and carries a poor prognosis.

3. Hypotension caused by venodilation is common and usually mild. In severe cases, hypotension results from myocardial depression and may be refractory to treatment; some patients die with progressive intractable cardiogenic shock. Pulmonary edema is also common in severe poisonings.

C. Seizures are common with cyclic antidepressant toxicity and may be recurrent or persistent. The muscular hyperactivity from seizures and myoclonic jerking, combined with diminished sweating, can lead to severe hyperthermia (see p 20), resulting in rhabdomyolysis, brain damage, multisystem failure, and death.

D. Death from cyclic antidepressant overdose usually occurs within a few hours of admission and may result from ventricular fibrillation, intractable cardiogenic shock, or status epilepticus with hyperthermia. Sudden death several days after apparent recovery has occasionally been reported, but in all such cases there was evidence of continuing cardiac toxicity within 24 hours of death.

IV. Diagnosis. Cyclic antidepressant poisoning should be suspected in any patient with lethargy, coma, or seizures accompanied by QRS interval prolongation. QRS interval prolongation greater than 0.12 s in the limb leads suggests severe poisoning. However, with amoxapine, seizures and coma may occur with no widening of the QRS interval.

A. Specific levels. Plasma levels of some of the cyclic antidepressants can be measured by clinical laboratories. Therapeutic concentrations are usually less than 0.3 µg/mL (300 ng/mL). Total concentrations of parent drug plus metabolite of 1 µg/mL (1000 ng/mL) or greater are usually associated with serious poisoning. Generally, plasma levels are not used in emergency management because the QRS interval and clinical manifestations of overdose are reliable and more readily available indicators of toxicity.

B. Other useful laboratory studies. Electrolytes, glucose, BUN, creatinine, creatine phosphokinase (CPK), urinalysis for myoglobin, arterial blood gases or oximetry, 12-lead ECG and continuous ECG monitoring, chest x-ray.

V. Treatment

A. Emergency and supportive measures

1. Maintain the airway and assist ventilation if necessary (see p 4). **Caution:** Respiratory arrest can occur abruptly and without warning.

2. Treat coma (p 18), seizures (p 22), hyperthermia (p 20), hypotension (p 15), and arrhythmias (p 10–14) if they occur.

3. If seizures are not immediately controlled with usual anticonvulsants, paralyze the patient with a neuromuscular blocker such as pancuronium (p 357) to prevent hyperthermia, which may induce further seizures, and lactic acidosis, which aggravates cardiotoxicity. **Note:** Paralysis abolishes the muscular manifestations of seizures, but has no effect on brain seizure activity. After paralysis, EEG monitoring is necessary to determine the efficacy of anticonvulsant therapy.

4. Continuously monitor the temperature, other vital signs, and ECG in asymptomatic patients for a minimum of 6 hours, and admit patients to an intensive care setting for at least 24 hours if there are any signs of toxicity.

B. Specific drugs and antidotes

1. In patients with QRS interval prolongation or hypotension, administer **sodium bicarbonate** (see p 318), 1–2 meq/kg IV, and repeat as needed to maintain the arterial pH between 7.45–7.55. Sodium bicarbonate may re-

verse membrane-depressant effects by increasing extracellular sodium concentrations and by a direct effect of pH on the fast sodium channel.
  2. Although **physostigmine** has been widely advocated in the past, it should ***not*** be routinely administered to patients with cyclic antidepressant poisoning; it may aggravate conduction disturbances, causing asystole, further impair myocardial contractility, worsening hypotension, and contribute to seizures.
  C. Decontamination (see p 44)
    1. **Prehospital.** Administer activated charcoal, if available. Do ***not*** induce emesis because of the risk of abrupt onset of seizures.
    2. **Hospital.** Administer activated charcoal and a cathartic. Perform gastric lavage for large ingestions (eg, > 20–30 mg/kg). Gastric emptying is probably not necessary for smaller ingestions if activated charcoal can be given promptly.
  D. Enhanced elimination. Owing to extensive tissue and protein binding with resulting large volume of distribution, dialysis and hemoperfusion are not effective. Although repeat-dose charcoal has been reported to accelerate cyclic antidepressant elimination, the data are not convincing.

DAPSONE
Kathryn Meier, PharmD

ANTIDOTE   IPECAC   LAVAGE   CHARCOAL

Dapsone is an antibiotic used for many years to treat leprosy and rare dermatologic conditions. Recently, its major use is for prophylaxis against *Pneumocystis carinii* infections in patients with AIDS and other immunodeficiency disorders. Absorption of dapsone is delayed: peak plasma levels occur between 4 and 8 hours after ingestion. Dapsone is metabolized by two primary routes, acetylation and p-450 oxidation. Acetylated dapsone can be metabolized back to dapsone or oxidized by the p-450 system. Both dapsone and its acetylated metabolite undergo enterohepatic recirculation. The average elimination half-life is 30 hours after a therapeutic dose, and as long as 77 hours after an overdose.
  I. Mechanism of toxicity. Toxic effects are caused by the p-450 metabolites and include methemoglobinemia, sulfhemoglobinemia, and Heinz body hemolytic anemia—all of which decrease the oxygen-carrying capacity of the blood.
    A. Dapsone metabolites oxidize the ferrous iron hemoglobin complex to the ferric state, resulting in methemoglobinemia.
    B. Sulfhemoglobinemia occurs when dapsone metabolites sulfate the pyrrole hemoglobin ring; this is an irreversible reaction, and there is no antidote.
    C. Hemolysis may occur owing to depletion of intracellular glutathione by oxidative metabolites. There is no antidote.
  II. Toxic dose. The therapeutic dose ranges from 50 to 300 mg/d. Chronic daily dosing of 100 mg has resulted in methemoglobin levels of 5–8%. Hemolysis has not been reported at doses less than 300 mg/d. Persons with glucose-6-phosphate dehydrogenase (G6PD) deficiency, congenital hemoglobin abnormalities, and underlying hypoxemia may experience greater toxicity at lower doses. Death has occurred with overdose of 1.4 g and greater.
  III. Clinical presentation includes methemoglobinemia, sulfhemoglobinemia, and intravascular hemolysis. Clinical manifestations are more severe in patients with underlying medical conditions that may contribute to hypoxemia.
    A. Methemoglobinemia (see p 217) causes cyanosis and dyspnea. Drawn blood may appear dark, "chocolate" brown when the methemoglobin level is greater than 15–20%. Because of the long half-life of dapsone and its metabolites,

methemoglobinemia may persist for several days, requiring repeated antidotal treatment.

B. **Sulfhemoglobinemia** also decreases oxyhemoglobin saturation and is unresponsive to methylene blue, so patients may continue to appear cyanotic even after receiving antidotal treatment.

C. **Hemolysis.** Heinz bodies may be seen, but hemolysis may be delayed in onset 2–3 days after the ingestion.

IV. **Diagnosis** is based on a history of dapsone use, and should be suspected in any immunocompromised patient with a suspected drug overdose, particularly since manifestations of toxicity may be delayed. Although there are many agents that can cause methemoglobinemia, there are very few that produce both detectable sulfhemoglobin and a prolonged, recurrent methemoglobinemia.

A. **Specific levels.** Dapsone levels are not routinely available.

1. Methemoglobinemia (see p 217) is suspected when a cyanotic patient fails to respond to high-flow oxygen or cyanosis persists despite a normal arterial PO_2 (note that pulse oximetry is not a reliable indicator of oxygen saturation in patients with methemoglobinemia). Specific methemoglobin concentrations can be measured using a multiwave cooximeter. Qualitatively, a drop of blood on white filter paper will appear brown when the level is greater than 15–20%.

2. Sulfhemoglobin is difficult to detect, in part because its spectrophotometric absorbance is similar to methemoglobin. If a crystal of potassium cyanide is added to a blood sample, methemoglobin will become red, but not if significant sulfhemoglobin is present.

B. **Other useful laboratory studies.** CBC (with differential smear to look for reticulocytes and Heinz bodies), glucose, electrolytes, liver transaminases, bilirubin, arterial blood gases.

V. **Treatment**

A. **Emergency and supportive measures**

1. Maintain the airway and assist ventilation if needed (p 4). Administer supplemental oxygen.

2. If hemolysis occurs, administer intravenous fluids and alkalinize the urine, as for rhabdomyolysis (see p 25), in order to prevent acute renal tubular necrosis. For severe hemolysis, blood transfusions may be required.

3. Mild symptoms may resolve without intervention, although it may take 2–3 days.

B. **Specific drugs and antidotes**

1. **Methylene blue** (see p 351) is indicated in the symptomatic patient with a methemoglobin level greater then 15% or with lower levels if even minimal compromise of oxygen-carrying capacity is potentially harmful (eg, severe pneumonia, anemia, myocardial ischemia).

a. Give 1–2 mg/kg (0.1–0.2 mL/kg of 1% solution) over several minutes. Therapeutic response may be delayed up to 30 minutes.

b. Serious overdoses usually require repeated dosing every 6–8 hours for 2–3 days because of the prolonged half-life of dapsone and its metabolites.

c. Methylene blue is ineffective for sulfhemoglobin, and can cause hemolysis in patients with G6PD deficiency. Excessive doses may worsen methemoglobinemia.

2. Other therapies such as ascorbic acid, cimetidine, and vitamin E have been proposed, but their efficacy is unproved.

C. **Decontamination** (see p 44)

1. **Prehospital.** Administer activated charcoal, if available. Ipecac-induced emesis may be useful for initial treatment at the scene (eg, children at home) if it can be given within a few minutes of exposure.

2. **Hospital.** Administer activated charcoal and a cathartic. Gastric emptying is not necessary after a small ingestion if activated charcoal can be given

promptly, but it should be considered for large overdose, even if it has been more than 60 minutes since the ingestion (one report documented tablet fragment return 5 hours after ingestion).

D. Enhanced elimination (see p 49)

1. **Repeat-dose activated charcoal** interrupts enterohepatic recirculation and is very effective, reducing the half-life from 77 to 13.5 hours in one report. Continue charcoal for at least 48–72 hours.

2. **Charcoal hemoperfusion** can reduce the half-life to 1.5 hours, and might be considered in a severe intoxication unresponsive to conventional treatment. Hemodialysis is ineffective because dapsone and its metabolites are highly protein-bound.

DETERGENTS
Olga F. Woo, PharmD

ANTIDOTE   IPECAC   LAVAGE   CHARCOAL

Detergents, familiar and indispensable products in the home, are synthetic surface-active agents chemically classified as **anionic, nonionic,** or **cationic** (Table II–22). Most products also contain bleaching (chlorine-releasing), bacteriostatic (low concentration of quaternary ammonium compound), or enzymatic agents. Accidental ingestion of detergents by children is very common, but severe toxicity rarely occurs.

I. Mechanism of toxicity. Detergents may precipitate and denature protein, are irritating to tissues, and possess keratolytic and corrosive actions.

A. Anionic and **nonionic** detergents are only mildly irritating, but **cationic** detergents are more hazardous because quaternary ammonium compounds may be caustic (benzalkonium chloride solutions of 10% have been reported to cause corrosive burns).

B. Low-phosphate detergents and **electric dishwasher** soaps often contain alkaline corrosive agents such as sodium metasilicate, sodium carbonate, and sodium tripolyphosphate.

C. The **enzyme-containing** detergents may cause skin irritation and have sensitizing properties; they may release bradykinin and histamine, causing bronchospasm.

II. Toxic dose. No minimum or lethal toxic doses have been established. Mortality and serious morbidity are rare. Cationic and dishwasher detergents are more dangerous than anionic and nonionic products.

III. Clinical presentation. Immediate spontaneous emesis often occurs after oral ingestion. Large ingestions may produce intractable vomiting, diarrhea, and hematemesis. Exposures to the eye may cause mild to serious corrosive injury depending on the specific product. Dermal contact generally causes a mild erythema or rash.

A. Phosphate-containing products may produce hypocalcemia and tetany.

B. Methemoglobinemia was reported in a 45-year-old woman after copious irrigation of a hydatid cyst with a 0.1% solution of cetrimide, a cationic detergent.

TABLE II–22. COMMON CATIONIC DETERGENTS

Pyridinium compounds	Quaternary ammonium compounds	Quinolinium compounds
Cetalkonium chloride	Benzalkonium chloride	Dequalinium chloride
Cetrimide	Benzethonium chloride	
Cetrimonium bromide		
Cetylpyridinium chloride		
Stearalkonium chloride		

IV. Diagnosis is based on a history of exposure and prompt onset of vomiting. A sudsy or foaming mouth may also suggest exposure.

    A. Specific levels. There are no specific blood or urine levels.

    B. Other useful laboratory studies. Electrolytes, glucose, calcium and phosphate (after ingestion of phosphate-containing products), methemoglobin (cationic detergents).

V. Treatment

    A. Emergency and supportive measures

        1. In patients with protracted vomiting or diarrhea, administer intravenous fluids to correct dehydration and electrolyte imbalance (see p 15).

        2. If corrosive injury is suspected, consult a gastroenterologist for possible endoscopy.

    B. Specific drugs and antidotes. If symptomatic hypocalcemia occurs after ingestion of a phosphate-containing product, administer intravenous **calcium** (see p 323). If methemoglobinemia occurs, administer **methylene blue** (see p 351).

    C. Decontamination (see p 44)

        1. Ingestion. Dilute orally with small amounts of water or milk. A significant ingestion is unlikely if spontaneous emesis has not already occurred.

            a. Do **not** induce emesis because of the risk for corrosive injury.

            b. Consider gastric lavage after large ingestions of cationic, corrosive, or phosphate-containing detergents.

            c. Activated charcoal is not effective.

        2. Eyes and skin. Irrigate with copious amounts of tepid water or saline. Consult an ophthalmologist if eye pain persists or if there is significant corneal injury on fluorescein examination.

    D. Enhanced elimination. There is no role for these procedures.

DEXTROMETHORPHAN
Kent R. Olson, MD

| ANTIDOTE | IPECAC | LAVAGE | CHARCOAL |

Dextromethorphan is a common antitussive agent found in many over-the-counter cough and cold preparations. Many ingestions occur in children, but severe intoxication is rare. Dextromethorphan is often found in combination products containing antihistamines (see p 78), decongestants (p 253), ethanol (p 160), or acetaminophen (p 61). *Common combination products containing dextromethorphan include Nyquil Nighttime Cold Medicine, Triaminic Nite Lite, Pediacare 1, Pediacare 3, Robitussin DM, Robitussin CF, Triaminic DM, and Vicks Pediatric Formula 44.*

    I. Mechanism of toxicity. Dextromethorphan is the *d*-isomer of the opioid analgesic levorphanol. Although it has approximately equal antitussive efficacy as codeine, dextromethorphan has no apparent analgesic or addictive properties and produces relatively mild opioid effects in overdose. It also is reported to have anticholinergic properties.

    Dextromethorphan is well absorbed orally, and effects are apparent within 15–30 minutes. The duration of effect is normally 3–6 hours.

    II. Toxic dose. The toxic dose is highly variable and depends largely on other ingredients in the ingested product. Symptoms usually occur when the amount of dextromethorphan ingested exceeds 10 mg/kg. The usual recommended adult daily dose of dextromethorphan is 60–120 mg/d; in children age 2–5 years, up to 30 mg/d.

III. Clinical presentation

    A. Mild intoxication produces clumsiness, ataxia, nystagmus, and restlessness. Visual and auditory hallucinations have been reported.

    B. With **severe poisoning,** stupor, coma, and respiratory depression may occur, especially if alcohol has been coingested. The pupils may be constricted or dilated. A few cases of seizures have been reported after ingestions of more than 20–30 mg/kg.

    C. Severe hyperthermia, muscle rigidity, and hypertension may occur with **therapeutic doses** in patients taking **monoamine oxidase inhibitors** (see p 222). The mechanism is not known, but may be related to serotonin syndrome (see p 21).

IV. Diagnosis should be considered with ingestion of any over-the-counter cough suppressant, especially when there is nystagmus, ataxia, and lethargy. Because dextromethorphan is often combined with other ingredients (eg, antihistamines, phenylpropanolamine, acetaminophen), suspect mixed ingestion.

    A. Specific levels. Serum levels are not generally available, nor are they clinically useful. Blood ethanol and acetaminophen levels should be obtained if those drugs are contained in the ingested product.

    B. Other useful laboratory studies. Electrolytes, glucose, ethanol, acetaminophen, arterial blood gases (if respiratory depression suspected).

V. Treatment

    A. Emergency and supportive measures. Most patients with mild symptoms (ie, restlessness, ataxia, mild drowsiness) can be observed for 4–6 hours and discharged if they are improving.

        1. Maintain the airway and assist ventilation if needed (see p 4).

        2. Treat seizures (p 22) and coma (p 18) if they occur.

    B. Specific drugs and antidotes. Although **naloxone** (see p 355) has been reported effective in doses of 0.06–0.4 mg, other cases have failed to respond to as much as 2.4 mg. If the patient exhibits signs of opioid intoxication (eg, coma, pinpoint pupils), administer 0.4–2 mg naloxone IV, with repeat doses as needed.

    C. Decontamination (see p 44)

        1. Prehospital. Administer activated charcoal, if available. Ipecac-induced emesis may be useful for initial treatment at the scene (eg, children at home) if it can be given within a few minutes of exposure.

        2. Hospital. Administer activated charcoal and a cathartic. Gastric emptying is not necessary if activated charcoal can be given promptly.

    D. Enhanced elimination. The volume of distribution of dextromethorphan is very large, and there is no role for enhanced removal procedures.

DIOXINS
Paul D. Blanc, MD, MSPH

      ANTIDOTE   IPECAC   LAVAGE   CHARCOAL

Polychlorinated dibenzodioxins (PCDDs) and dibenzofurans (PCDFs) are a group of highly toxic substances commonly known as dioxins. PCDDs are formed during the production of certain organochlorines (trichlorophenoxyacetic acid [2,4,5-T], silvex, hexachlorophene, pentachlorophenol, etc), and PCDFs are formed by the combustion of these and other compounds such as polychlorinated biphenyls (PCBs; see p 268). Agent Orange, a herbicide used in Vietnam, contained small quantities of a dioxin (2,3,7,8-tetrachlorodibenzo-*p*-dioxin, TCDD) as a contaminant.

    I. Mechanism of toxicity. Dioxins are highly lipid-soluble and are concentrated in the fat and the thymus. Dioxins are known to induce porphyrinogen synthesis and oxidative cytochrome P-450 metabolism and have a variety of effects on various organ systems. The actual mechanism of toxicity is unknown. They are mutagenic and are suspected human carcinogens.

II. Toxic dose. Dioxins are extremely potent animal toxins. The FDA-suggested "no effect" level for inhalation is 70 ng/d per person. The oral 50% lethal dose (LD_{50}) in animals varies from 0.0006 to 0.045 mg/kg. Daily dermal exposure to 10–30 ppm in oil or 100–3000 ppm in soil produces toxicity in animals. Chloracne is likely with daily dermal exposure exceeding 100 ppm.

III. Clinical presentation

    A. Acute symptoms after exposure include irritation of the skin, eyes, and mucous membranes and nausea, vomiting, and myalgias.

    B. After a latency period of up to several weeks, chloracne, porphyria cutanea tarda, hirsutism, or hyperpigmentation may occur. Elevated levels of hepatic transaminases and blood lipids may be found. Polyneuropathies with sensory impairment and lower extremity motor weakness have been reported.

    C. Death in laboratory animals occurs a few weeks after a lethal dose and is caused by a "wasting syndrome" characterized by reduced food intake and loss of body weight.

IV. Diagnosis is difficult and rests mainly on history of exposure; the presence of chloracne provides strong supporting evidence. Although 2,4,5-T no longer contains TCDD as a contaminant, possible exposures to PCDDs and PCDFs occur during many types of chemical fires (eg, PCBs), and the possibility of exposure results in considerable public and individual anxiety.

    A. Specific levels. It is difficult and expensive to detect dioxins in human blood or tissue, and there is no established correlation with symptoms. Unexposed persons have a mean of 7 pg of 2,3,7,8-TCDD per gram of serum lipid, compared to workers producing trichlorophenols who had a mean of 220 pg/g.

    B. Other useful laboratory studies. Glucose, electrolytes, BUN, creatinine, liver transaminases and liver function tests, uroporphyrins (if porphyria suspected).

V. Treatment

    A. Emergency and supportive measures. Treat skin, eye, and respiratory irritation symptomatically.

    B. Specific drugs and antidotes. There is no specific antidote.

    C. Decontamination (see p 41–49)

        1. Inhalation. Remove victim from exposure and give supplemental oxygen, if available.

        2. Eyes and skin. Remove contaminated clothing and wash affected skin with copious soap and water; irrigate exposed eyes with copious tepid water or saline. Personnel involved in decontamination should wear protective gear appropriate to the suspected level of contamination.

        3. Ingestion

            a. Prehospital. Administer activated charcoal, if available. Ipecac-induced emesis may be useful for initial treatment at the scene (eg, children at home) if it can be given within a few minutes of exposure.

            b. Hospital. Administer activated charcoal and a cathartic. Gastric emptying is not necessary if activated charcoal can be given promptly.

    D. Enhanced elimination. There is no known role for these procedures.

DISULFIRAM
Charles E. Becker, MD

ANTIDOTE   IPECAC   LAVAGE   CHARCOAL

Disulfiram (Antabuse) is an antioxidant drug used in the treatment of alcoholism. When a person taking disulfiram ingests alcohol, a well-defined unpleasant reaction occurs, the fear of which provides a negative incentive to drink.

I. **Mechanism of toxicity.** Disulfiram is well absorbed orally and is highly fat-soluble. Its mechanisms of toxicity include:
   A. Inhibition of aldehyde dehydrogenase, resulting in accumulation of acetaldehyde after ethanol ingestion.
   B. Depletion of norepinephrine in terminal presynaptic nerve endings owing to inhibition of dopamine betahydroxylase, causing orthostatic hypotension.

II. **Toxic dose**
   A. **Disulfiram overdose.** Ingestion of 3 g or more may cause toxicity.
   B. **Disulfiram-ethanol interaction.** Ingestion of as little as 7 mL of ethanol can cause a severe reaction in patients taking as little as 200 mg/d of disulfiram. Mild reactions have been reported after use of cough syrup, after-shave lotions, and other alcohol-containing products.

III. **Clinical presentation**
   A. **Acute disulfiram overdose** may cause vomiting, ataxia, confusion, lethargy, seizures, and coma. Hypersensitivity hepatitis has occurred, including several deaths resulting from hepatic failure.
   B. **Disulfiram-ethanol interaction.** Shortly after ingestion of ethanol, the patient receiving chronic disulfiram therapy develops flushing, throbbing headache, dyspnea, anxiety, vertigo, vomiting, and confusion. Orthostatic hypotension with warm extremities is very common.

   The severity of the reaction usually depends on the dose of disulfiram and ethanol. Reactions do not usually occur unless the patient has been on oral disulfiram therapy for at least 1 day; the reaction may occur up to several days after the last dose of disulfiram. Disulfiram has been implanted subcutaneously, leading to reactions after alcohol consumption that are milder but of longer duration.

IV. **Diagnosis** of disulfiram overdose is based on a history of acute ingestion and the presence of central nervous system symptoms. The disulfiram-ethanol interaction is diagnosed in a patient with a history of chronic disulfiram use and possible exposure to ethanol who exhibits a characteristic hypotensive flushing reaction.
   A. **Specific levels.** Blood disulfiram levels are not of value in diagnosis or treatment. Blood acetaldehyde levels may be elevated during the disulfiram-ethanol reaction, but this information is of little value in acute management.
   B. **Other useful laboratory studies.** Electrolytes, glucose, BUN, creatinine, liver transaminases, ethanol level.

V. **Treatment**
   A. **Emergency and supportive measures**
      1. **Acute disulfiram overdose**
         a. Maintain the airway and assist ventilation if necessary (see p 4).
         b. Treat coma (p 18) and seizures (p 22) if they occur.
      2. **Disulfiram-ethanol interaction**
         a. Maintain the airway and assist ventilation if necessary (see p 4).
         b. Treat orthostatic hypotension with supine position and large quantities of intravenous fluids (eg, saline). If a pressor agent is needed, norepinephrine (see p 363) is preferred over dopamine.
   B. **Specific drugs and antidotes.** There is no specific antidote.
   C. **Decontamination** (see p 44)
      1. **Acute disulfiram overdose**
         a. **Prehospital.** Administer activated charcoal, if available. Ipecac-induced emesis may be useful for initial treatment at the scene (eg, children at home) if it can be given within a few minutes of exposure.
         b. **Hospital.** Administer activated charcoal and a cathartic. Gastric emptying is not necessary if activated charcoal can be given promptly.
      2. **Disulfiram-ethanol interaction.** Decontamination procedures are not likely to be of benefit once the reaction begins (unless a very large ethanol ingestion has occurred, in which case gastric lavage should be performed, followed by administration of activated charcoal).

D. Enhanced elimination. Hemodialysis is not indicated for disulfiram overdose, but it may remove ethanol and acetaldehyde and has been reported to be effective in treating the acute disulfiram-ethanol interaction. This is not likely to be necessary in patients receiving adequate fluid and pressor support. There are no data to support the use of repeat-dose activated charcoal for any of the disulfiram syndromes.

DIURETICS
Olga F. Woo, PharmD

ANTIDOTE   IPECAC   LAVAGE   CHARCOAL

Diuretics are commonly prescribed for the management of essential hypertension. Adverse effects from chronic use or misuse are more frequently encountered than those from acute overdose. Overdoses are generally benign, and no serious outcomes have resulted from acute ingestion. Common currently available diuretics are listed in Table II–23.

I. **Mechanism of toxicity.** The toxicity of these drugs is associated with their pharmacologic effects to decrease fluid volume and promote electrolyte loss: dehydration, hypokalemia or hyperkalemia, and hypochloremic alkalosis. Electrolyte imbalance may lead to cardiac arrhythmias and may enhance digitalis toxicity (see p 124). Diuretics are classified according to the pharmacologic mechanisms by which they affect solute and water loss (Table II–23).

II. **Toxic dose.** Minimum toxic doses have not been established. Significant dehydration or electrolyte imbalance is unlikely if the amount ingested is less than the usual recommended daily dose (Table II–23). High doses of intravenous ethacrynic acid and furosemide can cause ototoxicity, especially when administered rapidly and in patients with renal failure.

III. **Clinical presentation.** Lethargy, weakness, hyporeflexia, and dehydration may be present. The onset of symptoms may be delayed for 2–4 hours until diuretic action is obtained. Spironolactone is very slow, with maximal effects after the third day. Spironolactone and other potassium-sparing agents may cause hyperkalemia. Hyperglycemia and hyperuricemia may occur, especially with thiazide diuretics. Carbonic anhydrase inhibitors may induce metabolic acidosis.

IV. **Diagnosis** is based on a history of exposure and evidence of dehydration and acid-base or electrolyte imbalance.
  A. Specific levels are not routinely available nor clinically useful.
  B. Other useful laboratory studies. Electrolytes, glucose, BUN, creatinine, ECG.

V. **Treatment**
  A. Emergency and supportive measures
    1. Replace fluid loss with intravenous crystalloid solutions, and correct electrolyte abnormalities (see Potassium, p 35).
    2. Monitor the ECG until the potassium level is normalized.
  B. Specific drugs and antidotes. There are no specific antidotes.
  C. Decontamination (see p 44)
    1. Prehospital. Administer activated charcoal, if available. Ipecac-induced emesis may be useful for initial treatment at the scene (eg, children at home) if it can be given within a few minutes of exposure.
    2. Hospital. Administer activated charcoal. Do not use a cathartic if the patient appears dehydrated. Gastric emptying is not necessary if activated charcoal can be given promptly.
  D. Enhanced elimination. No experience with extracorporeal removal of diuretics has been reported.

TABLE II–23. COMMON DIURETICS

Drug	Half-Life (h)	Maximum Adult Daily Dose (mg)
Carbonic anhydrase inhibitors		
Acetazolamide	1.5–8	1000
Dichlorphenamide	—	200
Methazolamide	14	300
Loop diuretics		
Bumetanide	1–1.5	2
Ethacrynic acid	2–4	200
Furosemide	1	600
Mercurial		
Mersalyl	—	200
Potassium-sparing		
Amiloride	21–144	20
Spironolactone	1.4	200
Triamterene	1.5–2	300
Thiazides		
Bendroflumethiazide	3–4	20
Benzthiadiozide	—	200
Chlorthalidone	40–65	200
Chlorothiazide	1–2	2000
Cyclothiazide	—	6
Flumethiazide	—	2000
Hydrochlorothiazide	5.6–14.8	200
Hydroflumethiazide	17	200
Indapamide	14–16	5
Methyclothiazide	—	10
Metolazone	5.3	20
Polythiazide	27	4
Quinethazone	—	200
Trichlomethiazide	2.3–7.3	4

ERGOT DERIVATIVES
Neal L. Benowitz, MD

ANTIDOTE   IPECAC   LAVAGE   CHARCOAL

Ergot derivatives are used primarily to treat migraine headache and to a lesser extent to enhance uterine contraction postpartum. Ergots are produced by the fungus *Claviceps purpurea,* which may grow on rye and other grains. Specific ergot-containing drugs include ergotamine (Cafergot, Ergomar, Gynergen, Ergostat), methysergide (Sansert), dihydroergotamine (DHE-45), and ergonovine (Ergotrate). Some ergoloid derivatives (dihydroergocornine, dihydroergocristine, and dihydroergocryptine) have been used in combination (Hydergine, Deapril-ST) for the treatment of dementia.

 I. Mechanism of toxicity. Ergot derivatives directly stimulate vasoconstriction and uterine contraction, antagonize alpha-adrenergic and serotonin receptors, and may also dilate some blood vessels via a central nervous system sympatholytic action. The relative contribution of each of these mechanisms to toxicity depends on the particular ergot alkaloid and its dose.

 Sustained vasoconstriction causes most of the serious toxicity; reduced blood flow causes local tissue hypoxia and ischemic injury, resulting in tissue edema and local thrombosis, worsening ischemia and causing further injury. At a certain point, reversible vasospasm progresses to irreversible vascular insufficiency and limb gangrene.

 II. Toxic dose. Death has been reported in a 14-month-old child after acute ingestion of 12 mg of ergotamine. However, most cases of severe poisoning occur with chronic overmedication for migraine headaches rather than acute single overdose. Daily doses of 10 mg or more of ergotamine are usually associated with toxicity. There are many case reports of vasospastic complications with normal therapeutic dosing.

 III. Clinical presentation. Mild intoxication causes nausea and vomiting. Serious poisoning results in vasoconstriction that may involve many parts of the body. Owing to persistence of ergots in tissues, vasospasm may continue for up to 10–14 days.

 A. Involvement of the extremities causes paresthesias, pain, pallor, coolness, and loss of peripheral pulses in the hands and feet; gangrene may ensue.

 B. Other complications of vasospasm include coronary ischemia and myocardial infarction, abdominal angina and bowel infarction, renal infarction and failure, visual disturbances and blindness, and stroke. Psychosis, seizures, and coma occur rarely.

 C. Chronic use of **methysergide** occasionally causes retroperitoneal fibrosis.

 IV. Diagnosis is based on a history of ergot use and clinical findings of vasospasm.

 A. Specific levels. Ergotamine levels are not widely available, and blood concentrations do not correlate well with toxicity, although ergotamine levels higher than 1.8 ng/mL have been associated with minor toxicity.

 B. Other useful laboratory studies. CBC, electrolytes, BUN, creatinine, ECG. Arteriography of the affected vascular bed is occasionally indicated.

 V. Treatment

 A. Emergency and supportive measures

 1. Maintain the airway and assist ventilation if necessary (see p 4).

 2. Treat coma (p 18) and convulsions (p 22) if they occur.

 3. Immediately discontinue ergot treatment. Hospitalize patients with vasospastic symptoms and treat promptly to prevent complications.

 B. Specific drugs and antidotes

 1. Peripheral ischemia requires prompt vasodilator therapy and anticoagulation to prevent local thrombosis.

 a. Administer intravenous **nitroprusside** (see p 362), starting with 1–2 μg/kg/min, or intravenous **phentolamine** (p 369), starting with 0.5 mg/min, increasing the infusion rate until ischemia is improved or systemic hypotension occurs. Intra-arterial infusion is occasionally required. **Nifedipine** (p 360) or other calcium antagonists may also enhance peripheral blood flow.

 b. Administer **heparin,** 5000 units IV followed by 1000 units/h (in adults), with adjustments in the infusion rate to maintain the activated coagulation time (ACT) or the activated partial thromboplastin time (APTT) approximately 2 times baseline.

 2. Coronary spasm. Administer **nitroglycerin,** 0.15–0.6 mg sublingually or 5–20 μg/min IV; or **nifedipine** (p 360), 10–20 mg orally (adult doses). Intracoronary artery nitroglycerin may be required if there is no response to intravenous infusion.

 C. Decontamination after acute ingestion (see p 44).

 1. Prehospital. Administer activated charcoal, if available. Ipecac-induced emesis may be useful for initial treatment at the scene (eg, children at home) if it can be given within a few minutes of exposure.

2. **Hospital.** Administer activated charcoal and a cathartic. Gastric emptying is not necessary if activated charcoal can be given promptly.

D. **Enhanced elimination.** Dialysis and hemoperfusion are not effective. Repeat-dose charcoal has not been studied, but because of extensive tissue distribution of ergots it is not likely to be useful.

ETHANOL
Kent R. Olson, MD

| ANTIDOTE | IPECAC | LAVAGE | CHARCOAL |

Commercial beer, wine, and liquors contain varying amounts of ethanol. Ethanol is also found in a variety of colognes, perfumes, after-shaves, mouthwashes, some rubbing alcohols, many food flavorings (eg, vanilla, almond, and lemon extracts), pharmaceutical preparations (eg, elixirs), and many other products. Ethanol is frequently ingested recreationally and is also a common coingestant with other drugs in suicide attempts.

I. **Mechanism of toxicity**

A. **Central nervous system depression** is the principal effect of acute ethanol intoxication. Ethanol has additive effects with other central nervous system depressants such as barbiturates, benzodiazepines, antidepressants, and antipsychotics.

B. **Hypoglycemia** may be caused by impaired gluconeogenesis in patients with depleted glycogen stores (particularly small children and poorly nourished persons).

C. Ethanol intoxication and chronic alcoholism also predispose patients to trauma, exposure-induced hypothermia, and a number of metabolic derangements that may easily be overlooked in the "drunk" patient.

II. **Toxic dose.** The volume of distribution of ethanol is 0.7 L/kg, or about 50 liters in the average adult. Generally, 0.7 g/kg pure ethanol (approximately 3–4 drinks) will produce a blood ethanol concentration of 100 mg/dL (0.1 g/dL), considered legally drunk in many states.

A. A level of 100 mg/dL is enough to inhibit gluconeogenesis and cause hypoglycemia but by itself is not enough to cause coma.

B. The level sufficient to cause deep coma or respiratory depression is highly variable, depending on the individual's degree of tolerance to ethanol: Although levels above 300 mg/dL usually cause coma in novice drinkers, chronic alcoholics may be awake with levels of 500–600 mg/dL or higher.

III. **Clinical presentation**

A. **Acute intoxication**

1. With **mild to moderate intoxication,** patients exhibit euphoria, mild incoordination, ataxia, nystagmus, and impaired judgment and reflexes. Social inhibitions are loosened, and boisterous or aggressive behavior is common. Hypoglycemia may occur.

2. With **deep intoxication,** coma, respiratory depression, and pulmonary aspiration may occur. In these patients, the pupils are usually small and the temperature, blood pressure, and pulse rate are often decreased. Rhabdomyolysis may result from prolonged immobilization on a hard floor.

B. **Chronic ethanol abuse** produces gastrointestinal bleeding from gastritis, ulcers, Mallory-Weiss tears, or esophageal varices; pancreatitis; hepatitis, cirrhosis, and hepatic encephalopathy; hypokalemia, hypophosphatemia, and hypomagnesemia; thiamine deficiency (Wernicke's encephalopathy); alcoholic ketoacidosis; and decreased resistance to infections.

    C. Alcohol withdrawal from chronic high-level use usually causes tremulousness, anxiety, sympathetic nervous system overactivity, and convulsions. Occasionally, this may progress to **delirium tremens**, a life-threatening syndrome of severe autonomic hyperactivity, hyperthermia, and delirium, which has significant morbidity and mortality if untreated.

    D. Other problems. Ethanol abusers sometimes intentionally or accidentally ingest ethanol substitutes such as isopropyl alcohol (see p 193), methanol (p 215), or ethylene glycol (p 163). In addition, ethanol may serve as the vehicle for swallowing large numbers of pills in a suicide attempt. Disulfiram (Antabuse, p 155) use can cause a serious acute reaction with ethanol.

IV. Diagnosis of ethanol intoxication is usually simple, based on the history of ingestion, the characteristic smell of fresh alcohol or the fetid odor of acetaldehyde and other metabolic products, and the presence of nystagmus, ataxia, and altered mental status. It is imperative to consider other etiologies that may accompany or mimic intoxication, such as hypoglycemia, head trauma, hypothermia, meningitis, or intoxication with other drugs or poisons.

    A. Specific levels. Ethanol levels are easily and rapidly determined by most hospital laboratories and, depending on the method used, are accurate and specific.

        1. In general, there is only rough correlation between blood levels and clinical presentation; however, an ethanol level below 300 mg/dL in a comatose patient should initiate a search for alternative causes.

        2. If ethanol levels are not readily available, the ethanol concentration may be estimated by calculating the osmolar gap (see p 30).

    B. Suggested laboratory studies. Glucose, electrolytes, BUN, creatinine, liver transaminases, prothrombin time (PT), magnesium, arterial blood gases or oximetry, chest x-ray (if aspiration suspected).

V. Treatment

    A. Emergency and supportive measures

        1. Acute intoxication. Treatment is mainly supportive.

            a. Protect the airway to prevent aspiration (see p 2), and intubate and assist ventilation if needed (p 3).

            b. Give glucose and thiamine (p 19), and treat coma (p 18) and seizures (p 22) if they occur.

            c. Correct hypothermia with gradual rewarming (p 19).

            d. Most patients will recover within 4–6 hours.

        2. Alcohol withdrawal. Treat with benzodiazepines (eg, diazepam, 2–10 mg IV initially, repeated as needed; see p 327) or phenobarbital (see p 368).

    B. Specific drugs and antidotes. There is no commercially available specific ethanol receptor antagonist, but there are anecdotal reports of arousal after administration of naloxone, 2–5 mg IV (see p 355).

    C. Decontamination (see p 44). Because ethanol is rapidly absorbed, emesis or gastric lavage is usually not indicated unless a substantial ingestion has occurred within a few minutes of presentation or other drug ingestion is suspected.

        1. Prehospital. Ipecac-induced emesis may be useful for initial treatment at the scene (eg, children at home) if it can be given within a few minutes of exposure.

        2. Hospital. Perform gastric lavage if the ingestion was large and recent (within 30–45 minutes). Activated charcoal does not efficiently adsorb ethanol but may be given, especially if other toxins were ingested.

    D. Enhanced elimination. Elimination normally occurs at a fixed rate, approximately 20–30 mg/dL/h. Hemodialysis efficiently removes ethanol, but enhanced removal is rarely needed because supportive care is usually sufficient. Hemoperfusion and forced diuresis are not effective.

ETHYLENE DIBROMIDE
Janet Weiss, MD

ANTIDOTE   IPECAC   LAVAGE   CHARCOAL

Ethylene dibromide (EDB, dibromoethane) is a volatile liquid produced by the bromination of ethylene. EDB is used as a lead scavenger in leaded gasoline and as a pesticide and fumigant in soil and on grain, fruits, and vegetables. Because EDB has been classified as a suspected human carcinogen, its use as a pesticide has been restricted since 1984.

I. Mechanism of toxicity
A. Liquid EDB is an irritant capable of causing chemical burns. Inhalation of EDB vapor produces respiratory tract irritation and delayed-onset pulmonary edema.

B. Once absorbed systemically, EDB is converted to active metabolites that become irreversibly bound to macromolecules, including DNA, and inhibit enzymes. Metabolism of EDB involves an oxidative pathway (cytochrome p-450) and a conjugation pathway (glutathione). The liver is a principal target organ for toxicity.

II. Toxic dose
A. Inhalation. Because EDB is a suspected carcinogen (ACGIH category A2), no safe workplace exposure limit has been determined. Exposure to vapor concentrations greater than 200 ppm can produce lung irritation, and 400 ppm may be immediately dangerous to life or health (IDLH).

B. Ingestion of 4.5 mL of liquid EDB has resulted in death.

III. Clinical presentation
A. Inhalation of EDB vapor causes irritation of the eyes and upper respiratory tract. Pulmonary edema usually occurs within 1–6 hours but may be delayed as long as 48 hours after exposure.

B. Skin exposure produces painful local inflammation, swelling, and blistering.

C. Oral ingestion causes prompt vomiting and diarrhea.

D. Systemic manifestations of intoxication include central nervous system depression, seizures, and metabolic acidosis. Skeletal muscle necrosis, acute renal failure, and hepatic necrosis have also been reported in fatal cases.

IV. Diagnosis of EDB poisoning is based on a history of exposure and evidence of upper airway and eye irritation (in case of inhalation) or gastroenteritis (after ingestion). EDB vapor has a strong chemical odor.
A. Specific levels. EDB is detectable in expired air, blood, and tissues, although levels are not useful in emergency management. Serum bromide levels may be elevated (> 0.1 meq/L) in severe cases, because bromide is released from EDB in the body.

B. Other useful laboratory studies. Electrolytes, glucose, BUN, creatinine, liver transaminases, creatine phosphokinase (CPK), arterial blood gases, chest x-ray.

V. Treatment
A. Emergency and supportive measures
1. Maintain the airway and assist ventilation if necessary (see p 4).
2. After inhalation exposure, anticipate and treat wheezing, airway obstruction, and pulmonary edema (p 7–10). Monitor blood gases, provide supplemental oxygen if needed, and avoid fluid overload.
3. Treat coma (p 18), seizures (p 22), rhabdomyolysis (p 25), and metabolic acidosis (p 30) if they occur.

B. Specific drugs and antidotes. There is no specific antidote. There is some experimental evidence in animals that administration of *n*-acetylcysteine (see p 311) may improve outcome.

C. Decontamination (see p 41). *Caution:* Rescuers should use self-contained breathing apparatus and wear protective clothing to avoid personal exposure.

1. **Inhalation.** Remove the victim from exposure and provide supplemental oxygen, if available.
2. **Skin and eyes.** Remove and safely discard all contaminated clothing, and wash exposed skin with copious soap and water. Irrigate exposed eyes with tepid saline or water.
3. **Ingestion** (see p 44)
    a. **Prehospital.** Administer activated charcoal, if available. Do *not* induce emesis because of corrosive effects and the risk of rapid onset of coma or seizures.
    b. **Hospital.** Perform gastric lavage if the patient presents within 30 minutes of ingestion or has ingested a large quantity (more than 1–2 oz). Administer activated charcoal and a cathartic.
D. **Enhanced elimination.** There is no role for dialysis or hemoperfusion, diuresis, or repeat-dose charcoal.

ETHYLENE GLYCOL AND OTHER GLYCOLS
Ilene B. Anderson, PharmD

ANTIDOTE   IPECAC   LAVAGE   CHARCOAL

Ethylene glycol is the primary ingredient (up to 95%) in antifreeze. It is sometimes intentionally consumed as an alcohol substitute by alcoholics and is tempting to children because of its sweet taste. Intoxication by ethylene glycol itself causes inebriation and mild gastritis; in addition, its metabolic products cause metabolic acidosis, renal failure, and death. Other glycols may also produce toxicity (Table II–24).

I. **Mechanism of toxicity**
   A. **Ethylene glycol** is metabolized by alcohol dehydrogenase to glycoaldehyde, which is then metabolized to glycolic, glyoxylic, and oxalic acids. These acids, along with excess lactic acid, are responsible for the anion gap metabolic acidosis. Oxalate readily precipitates with calcium to form insoluble calcium oxalate crystals. Tissue injury is caused by widespread deposition of oxalate crystals and the toxic effects of glycolic and glyoxylic acids.
   B. **Other glycols** (Table II–24). Propylene and dipropylene glycols are of relatively low toxicity. Polypropylene glycol and high molecular weight polyethylene glycols are poorly absorbed and virtually nontoxic. However, diethylene glycol and glycol ethers produce toxic metabolites with toxicity similar to that of ethylene glycol.

II. **Toxic dose.** The approximate lethal oral dose of 95% ethylene glycol (eg, antifreeze) is 1.5 mL/kg; however, survival has been reported following ingestion of 2 L in a patient who received treatment within 1 hour of ingestion.

III. **Clinical presentation**
   A. **Ethylene glycol**
      1. **During the first 3–4 hours** after acute ingestion, the victim may appear intoxicated as if by ethanol. The osmolar gap (see p 30) is increased, but there is no initial acidosis. Gastritis with vomiting may also occur.
      2. **After a delay of 4–12 hours,** evidence of intoxication by metabolic products occurs, with anion gap acidosis, hyperventilation, convulsions, coma, cardiac conduction disturbances, and arrhythmias. Renal failure is common but usually reversible. Pulmonary edema and cerebral edema may also occur. Hypocalcemia with tetany has been reported.
   B. **Other glycols** (Table II–24). Diethylene glycol and glycol ethers are extremely toxic and may produce acute renal failure and metabolic acidosis. Calcium oxalate crystals may or may not be present.

IV. **Diagnosis** of ethylene glycol poisoning is usually based on the history of anti-

TABLE II–24. TOXICITY OF OTHER GLYCOLS

Compound	Toxicity and Comments	Treatment
Propylene glycol	Relatively low toxicity. Lactic acidosis, central nervous system depression, coma, hypoglycemia, seizures, and hemolysis have been reported rarely after massive exposures or chronic exposures in high risk patients. Risk factors include: renal insufficiency, small infants, epilepsy, or burn patients with extensive dermal application of propylene glycol. Osmolar gap, anion gap, and lactate may be elevated. Levels: 70 mg/dL resulted in lactic acidosis and central nervous system depression in a patient with azotemia; 6–42 mg/dL did not result in toxicity after acute infusion; 70 mg/dL resulted in lactic acidosis with a lactate level equal to 24 meq/L without an osmolar gap following chronic infusion; 1059 mg/dL was reported in an 8-month-old with extensive burn injuries after repeated dermal application (the child experienced cardiopulmonary arrest); and 400 mg/dL was measured in an epileptic patient who experienced status epilepticus, respiratory depression, elevated osmolar gap, and metabolic acidosis. Metabolites are lactate and pyruvate. Molecular weight is 76.	Supportive care, sodium bicarbonate. There is no role for ethanol therapy. Hemodialysis is effective but rarely indicated.
Dipropylene glycol	Relatively low toxicity. Central nervous system depression, hepatic injury, and renal damage have occurred in animal studies after massive exposures. There are no reports of acidosis or lactate elevation. Molecular weight is 134.	Supportive care. Therre is no role for ethanol therapy.
Polyethylene glycols	Very low toxicity. A group of compounds with molecular weights ranging from 200 to more than 4000. High molecular weight compounds (> 500) are poorly absorbed and are rapidly excreted by the kidneys. Low molecular weight compounds (200–400) may result in metabolic acidosis, renal failure, hypercalcemia, and elevation in the osmolar gap after massive oral ingestions or repeated dermal applications in patients with extensive burn injuries. Alcohol dehydrogenase metabolizes polyethylene glycols.	Supportive care.
Diethylene glycol	Highly nephrotoxic; similar to ethylene glycol. Renal failure, coma, acidosis, and death have been reported in 5 patients with extensive burn injuries after repeated dermal application. Calcium oxalate crystals have not been reported in human poisonings but have been seen in animal studies. Molecular weight is 106.	Supportive care. The role of ethanol therapy is unknown. In animal studies, bicarbonate therapy was as effective as ethanol therapy.

(continued)

TABLE II–24. TOXICITY OF OTHER GLYCOLS (CONTINUED)

Compound	Toxicity and Comments	Treatment
Ethylene glycol mono butyl ether (EGMBE, 2-butoxyethanol, butyl cellosolve)	May result in hematologic effects; similar to ethylene glycol. ARDS has been reported in one patient. Oxalate crystals, renal dysfunction, and increased osmolar gap may or may not occur. Levels of 432 µg/mL have been associated with coma, hypotension, and acidosis without an osmolar gap, oxalate crystals, or renal dysfunction. Animal studies indicate that EGMBE is metabolized in part to ethylene glycol and that pyrazole (an alcohol dehydrogenase blocker) prevents toxicity, but the affinity of alcohol dehydrogenase for EGMBE is unknown. Molecular weight is 118.	Ethanol may be effective.
Ethylene glycol mono ethyl ether (EGMEE, ethyl cellosolve)	May result in hematologic effects; similar to ethylene glycol. Teratogenic effects have been reported in humans and animals. Calcium oxalate crystals have been reported in animals. Animal studies indicate that EGMEE is metabolized in part to ethylene glycol; however, the affinity of alcohol dehydrogenase is higher for EGMEE than for ethanol. Molecular weight is 90.	Ethanol may be effective.
Ethylene glycol mono methyl ether (EGMME, methyl cellosolve)	May result in hematologic effects; similar to ethylene glycol. Oligospermia has been reported with chronic exposure in humans. Teratogenic effects have been reported in animals. Delayed toxic effects (8 and 18 hours postingestion) similar to ethylene glycol have been reported. Calcium oxalate crystals may or may not occur. Cerebral edema, hemorrhagic gastritis, and degeneration of the liver and kidneys were reported in one autopsy. Animal studies indicate that EGMEE is metabolized in part to ethylene glycol; however, the affinity of alcohol dehydrogenase is about the same for EGMEE as for ethanol. Molecular weight is 76.	Ethanol may be effective.
Dioxane (dimer of ethylene glycol)	May cause coma, liver, and kidney damage. The vapor (> 300 ppm) may result in mucous membrane irritation. Dermal exposure to the liquid may have a defatting action. Metabolites unknown. Molecular weight is 88.	Role of ethanol is unknown, but it may be effective.

165

freeze ingestion, typical symptoms, and elevation of the osmolar and anion gaps. Oxalate or hippurate crystals may be present in the urine. Because many antifreeze products also contain fluorescein, the urine may fluoresce under Wood's lamp, depending on the amount of time since ingestion and on the urine concentration.

A. Specific levels. Tests for ethylene glycol levels are usually available from regional commercial toxicology laboratories but are difficult to obtain quickly.

1. Serum levels higher than 50 mg/dL are usually associated with serious intoxication, although lower levels do not rule out poisoning if the parent compound has already been metabolized (in such a case, the anion gap should be markedly elevated). Calculation of the osmolar gap (see p 30) may be used to estimate the ethylene glycol level.
2. False-positive ethylene glycol levels can be caused by elevated triglycerides (see Table I–32, p 40).
3. In the absence of a serum ethylene glycol level, if the osmolar and anion gaps are both normal and the patient is asymptomatic, then serious ingestion is not likely to have occurred.

B. Other useful laboratory studies. Electrolytes, glucose, BUN, creatinine, calcium, hepatic transaminases, urinalysis (for crystals and Wood's lamp examination), osmolality (freezing point method), arterial blood gases, ECG monitoring.

V. Treatment

A. Emergency and supportive measures

1. Maintain the airway and assist ventilation if necessary (see p 4). Administer supplemental oxygen.
2. Treat coma (p 18), convulsions (p 22), cardiac arrhythmias (p 10–14), and metabolic acidosis (p 30) if they occur. Observe the patient for several hours to monitor for development of metabolic acidosis, especially if symptomatic or known coingestion of ethanol.
3. Treat hypocalcemia with intravenous calcium gluconate or calcium chloride (p 323).

B. Specific drugs and antidotes

1. Administer **ethanol** (see p 339) to saturate the enzyme alcohol dehydrogenase and prevent metabolism of ethylene glycol to its toxic metabolites. Indications for ethanol therapy include:
   a. Ethylene glycol level higher than 20 mg/dL.
   b. History of ethylene glycol ingestion accompanied by an osmolar gap greater than 5 mosm/L not accounted for by ethanol or other alcohols.
   c. Anion gap acidosis accompanied by history of glycol ingestion or presence of oxalate crystalluria or positive Wood's lamp examination of urine.
2. Administer **pyridoxine** (see p 375), **folate** (p 341), and **thiamine** (p 375), cofactors required for the metabolism of ethylene glycol that may alleviate toxicity by enhancing metabolism of glyoxylic acid to nontoxic metabolites.

C. Decontamination (see p 44)

1. **Prehospital.** Ipecac-induced emesis may be useful for initial treatment at the scene (eg, children at home) if it can be given within a few minutes of exposure.
2. **Hospital.** Perform gastric lavage as quickly as possible. Activated charcoal does not efficiently adsorb glycols.

D. Enhanced elimination. The volume of distribution of ethylene glycol is 0.7–0.8 L/kg, making it accessible to enhanced elimination procedures. **Hemodialysis** efficiently removes ethylene glycol and its toxic metabolites, and rapidly corrects acidosis and electrolyte and fluid abnormalities.

1. Indications for hemodialysis:
   a. Suspected ethylene glycol poisoning with osmolar gap greater than 10 mosm/L not accounted for by ethanol or other alcohols.
   b. Any ethylene glycol intoxication accompanied by renal failure.

c. Ethylene glycol serum concentration greater than 20–50 mg/dL.
2. The minimum serum concentration of ethylene glycol associated with serious toxicity is not known; dialysis should be continued until the osmolar and anion gaps are normalized. Ethanol infusion must be increased during dialysis (see p 339) and should be continued for at least 24 hours after the last dialysis because of possible rebound elevation of ethylene glycol levels.

ETHYLENE OXIDE
Charles E. Becker, MD

ANTIDOTE   IPECAC   LAVAGE   CHARCOAL

Ethylene oxide is a highly penetrating gas, widely used in hospitals as a sterilizer of medical equipment and supplies. It is also an important industrial chemical, used as a solvent, plasticizer, and chemical intermediate.

I. Mechanism of toxicity. Ethylene oxide is an alkylating agent and reacts directly with proteins and DNA to cause cell death. Direct contact with the gas causes irritation of the eyes, mucous membranes, and lungs. Ethylene oxide is probably mutagenic, teratogenic, and carcinogenic in humans.

II. Toxic dose. The recommended workplace limit (ACGIH TLV-TWA) in air is 1 ppm as an 8-hour time-weighted average. The air level considered immediately dangerous to life or health (IDLH) is 800 ppm. The odor threshold is approximately 700 ppm, giving the gas poor warning properties. High levels of ethylene oxide can occur when sterilizers malfunction or with the opening or replacing of ethylene oxide tanks.

III. Clinical presentation
   A. Ethylene oxide is a potent mucous membrane irritant, and can cause eye and oropharyngeal irritation, bronchospasm, and pulmonary edema. Cataract formation has been described after significant eye exposure. Exposure to the liquid can cause vesicant injury to the skin.
   B. Neurotoxicity, including convulsions and delayed peripheral neuropathy, may occur after exposure.
   C. Other systemic effects include cardiac arrhythmias when ethylene oxide is used with the carrier gas Freon.
   D. Leukemia has been described in workers chronically exposed to relatively low levels of ethylene oxide.

IV. Diagnosis is based on a history of exposure and typical upper airway irritant effects. Detection of ethylene oxide odor indicates significant exposure. Industrial hygiene sampling is necessary to document air levels of exposure.
   A. Specific levels. Serum levels are not available. Ethylene oxide DNA adducts may indicate exposure but are not available for clinical use.
   B. Other useful laboratory studies. Arterial blood gases or pulse oximetry, chest x-ray.

V. Treatment
   A. Emergency and supportive measures. Monitor closely for several hours after exposure.
      1. Maintain the airway and assist ventilation if necessary (see p 4). Treat bronchospasm (p 9–10) and pulmonary edema (p 8) if they occur.
      2. Treat coma (p 18), convulsions (p 22), and arrhythmias (p 10–14) if they occur.
   B. Specific drugs and antidotes. There is no specific antidote.
   C. Decontamination (see p 41)
      1. Remove the victim from the contaminated environment immediately and administer oxygen. Rescuers should wear self-contained breathing apparatus and chemical protective clothing.

    2. Remove all contaminated clothing and wash exposed skin. For eye exposures, irrigate copiously with tepid water or saline.

   D. Enhanced elimination. There is no role for these procedures.

FLUORIDE
Kathryn H. Meier, PharmD

ANTIDOTE   IPECAC   LAVAGE   CHARCOAL

Fluoride-liberating chemicals are used in some insecticides, rodenticides, aluminum production, vitamins or dietary supplements, and various products to prevent dental caries (eg, Luride drops). It is commonly added to community drinking water. It is also found in hydrofluoric acid (see p 180). Soluble fluoride salts are rapidly absorbed within 30 minutes, and are more toxic (see Table II–25). Fluoride is slowly eliminated in urine and sweat.

   I. Mechanism of toxicity. Toxicity results from direct cytotoxic and metabolic effects as well as binding to calcium and magnesium causing hypocalcemia and hypomagnesemia. Specific effects include: impaired oxidative phosphorylation and glycolysis, enhanced proteolytic processes, impaired blood coagulation, myocardial irritability, impaired neurotransmission, and tetany.

  II. Toxic dose. Vomiting and abdominal pain are common with ingestions of 3–5 mg/kg elemental fluoride (see Table II–25); hypocalcemia and muscular symptoms appear with ingestions of 5–10 mg/kg. Death has been reported in a 3-year-old child following ingestion of 16 mg/kg and in adults with doses in excess of 32 mg/kg.

 III. Clinical presentation. Nausea and vomiting frequently occur within 30–60 minutes of ingestion. Symptoms of more serious intoxication include skeletal muscle weakness, tetanic contractions, respiratory muscle weakness, and respiratory arrest. Cardiac dysrhythmias may be associated with hypocalcemia, hypomagnesemia, and hyperkalemia.

 IV. Diagnosis is usually based on a history of ingestion. Symptoms of abdominal distress, muscle weakness, hypocalcemia, and hyperkalemia suggest fluoride intoxication.

    A. Specific levels. The normal serum fluoride concentration is less than 20 µg/L (ng/mL) but varies considerably with diet and water source. Serum fluoride concentrations are generally difficult to obtain and thus are of limited utility for acute overdose management.

    B. Other useful laboratory studies. Electrolytes, glucose, BUN, creatinine, calcium, albumin (to assess free calcium), magnesium, ECG. If severe tetany: creatine phosphokinase (CPK).

   V. Treatment

    A. Emergency and supportive measures

TABLE II–25. FLUORIDE-CONTAINING COMPOUNDS

Compound	Elemental Fluoride (%)
Soluble salts	
Hydrogen fluoride	95
Sodium fluoride	45
Sodium fluosilicate	61
Less soluble salts	
Cryolite	54
Sodium monofluorophosphate	13
Stannous fluoride	24

1. Maintain the airway and assist ventilation if necessary (see p 4).
2. Monitor ECG and serum calcium for at least 4–6 hours, and admit symptomatic patients to an intensive care setting.

B. Specific drugs and antidotes. When clinically significant hypocalcemia is present, administer **intravenous calcium** (p 323), 10–20 mL (0.1–0.2 mL/kg). Treat hypomagnesemia with intravenous **magnesium sulfate**, 1–2 g.

C. Decontamination (see p 44)

    1. Prehospital. Administer **calcium** salts (eg, calcium carbonate [Tums], calcium lactate, or milk) to form insoluble complexes with fluoride, minimizing absorption. Magnesium-containing antacids may also bind fluoride, although there are no reports of their use. Ipecac-induced emesis may be useful for initial treatment of children at home who have ingested more than 5–10 mg/kg elemental fluoride, if the ipecac can be given within a few minutes of exposure.

    2. Hospital. Following recent ingestion, induce emesis or perform gastric lavage. Administer **calcium** salts as discussed above. Activated charcoal does not adsorb fluoride and is not likely to be beneficial.

D. Enhanced elimination. Although fluoride is a small ion with minimal protein binding, it rapidly binds to free calcium and bone; therefore, hemodialysis and hemoperfusion are unlikely to be beneficial.

FLUOROACETATE
Gerald Joe, PharmD

ANTIDOTE   IPECAC   LAVAGE   CHARCOAL

Fluoroacetate, also known as compound 1080, sodium monofluoroacetate (SMFA), and sodium fluoroacetate, is one of the most toxic substances known. In the past, it was used primarily as a rodenticide by licensed pest control companies, but it has been removed from the US market because of its hazard. It is a tasteless, odorless, water soluble white crystalline powder. Fluoroacetamide (compound 1081) is a similar compound with similar toxicity.

I. Mechanism of toxicity. Fluoroacetate is metabolized to the toxic compound fluorocitrate, which blocks cellular metabolism by inhibiting the Krebs cycle. Clinical effects of poisoning are delayed (from 30 minutes to several hours) until fluoroacetate is metabolized to fluorocitrate.

II. Toxic dose. Inhalation or ingestion of as little as 1 mg of fluoroacetate is sufficient to cause serious toxicity. Death is likely after ingestion of more than 5 mg/kg.

III. Clinical presentation. After a delay of minutes to several hours, manifestations of diffuse cellular poisoning become apparent: nausea, vomiting, diarrhea, metabolic acidosis, renal failure, agitation, confusion, seizures, coma, respiratory arrest, pulmonary edema, and ventricular arrhythmias may occur.

IV. Diagnosis is based on a history of ingestion and clinical findings, which may be delayed for several hours. Poisoning with fluoroacetate may mimic poisoning with other cellular toxins such as hydrogen cyanide and hydrogen sulfide, although with these poisons the onset of symptoms is usually more rapid.

    A. Specific levels. There is no assay available.

    B. Other useful laboratory studies. Electrolytes, glucose, BUN, creatinine, arterial blood gases, chest x-ray.

V. Treatment

    A. Emergency and supportive measures

        1. Maintain the airway and assist ventilation if necessary (see p 4). Administer supplemental oxygen.

        2. Replace fluid losses from gastroenteritis with intravenous saline or other crystalloids.

3. Treat shock (p 15), seizures (p 22), and coma (p 18) if they occur. Monitor the ECG for at least 4–6 hours.

B. Specific drugs and antidotes. There is no available antidote. Monoacetin (glyceryl monoacetate) has been used experimentally in monkeys, but is not available or recommended for human use.

C. Decontamination (see p 44)

   1. Prehospital. If it is available, immediately administer activated charcoal. Do *not* induce emesis unless the victim is more than 20 minutes from a medical facility.

   2. Hospital. Immediately place a gastric tube and administer activated charcoal, then perform gastric lavage. Following lavage, give an additional dose of activated charcoal and a cathartic.

   3. Skin exposure. Remove contaminated clothing and wash exposed skin thoroughly.

D. Enhanced elimination. There is no role for any enhanced removal procedure.

FOOD POISONING: BACTERIAL
Susan Kim, PharmD

ANTIDOTE   IPECAC   LAVAGE   CHARCOAL

Foodborne illness is one of the most common causes of epidemic gastroenteritis. In general, common bacterial food poisoning is relatively mild and self-limited, with recovery within 24 hours. However, severe and even fatal poisoning may occur with listeriosis, salmonellosis, or botulism (see p 107). Poisoning following consumption of fish and shellfish is discussed on p 172. Mushroom poisoning is discussed on p 223.

I. Mechanism of toxicity. Gastroenteritis may be caused by invasive bacterial infection of the intestinal mucosa or by a toxin elaborated by bacteria. Bacterial toxins may be preformed in food that is improperly prepared and improperly stored before use, or may be produced in the gut by the bacteria after they are ingested (Table II–26).

II. Toxic dose. The toxic dose depends on the type of bacteria or toxin and its concentration in the ingested food, as well as individual susceptibility or resistance. Some of the preformed toxins (eg, staphylococcal toxin) are heat-resistant and once in the food are not removed by cooking or boiling.

III. Clinical presentation. Commonly, a delay or "incubation period" of from 2 hours to 3 days precedes the onset of symptoms (Table II–26).

   A. Gastroenteritis is the most common finding, with nausea, vomiting, abdominal cramps, and diarrhea. Significant fluid and electrolyte abnormalities may occur, especially in young children or elderly patients.

   B. Fever, bloody stools, and **fecal leukocytosis** are common with invasive bacterial infections.

   C. Systemic infection can result from salmonella, shigella, or listeria. **Listeriosis** can cause sepsis and meningitis, particularly in the elderly and immunocompromised persons. Infection during pregnancy produce a mild, flulike illness in the mother but serious intrauterine infection resulting in fetal death, neonatal sepsis, or meningitis.

IV. Diagnosis. Bacterial food poisoning is often difficult to distinguish from common viral gastroenteritis, unless the incubation period is short and there are multiple victims who ate similar foods at one large gathering. The presence of many white blood cells in a stool smear suggests invasive bacterial infection. With any epidemic gastroenteritis, consider other foodborne illnesses, such as seafood (see next section), botulism (p 107), and mushrooms (p 223).

TABLE II-26. SUMMARY OF BACTERIAL FOOD POISONING

Organism	Incubation Period	Mechanism	Common Foods
Bacillus cereus	1–6 h and 8–16 h	Toxins produced in food and patient	Reheated fried rice.
Campylobacter	1–2 days	Invasive	Water; direct contact.
Clostridium perfringens	6–16 h	Toxin produced in food and patient	Meats, gravy.
Escherichia coli (toxigenic)	12–72 h	Toxin produced in patient	Water, meats
Listeria monocytogenes	Unknown	Invasive	Milk, soft cheeses.
Salmonella	12–36 h	Invasive	Meat, dairy, bakery foods; water; direct contact.
Shigella	1–7 days	Invasive	Water; fruits, vegetables.
Staphylococcus aureus	1–6 h	Toxin preformed in food; heat-resistant	Very common; meats, dairy, bakery foods.
Vibrio parahemolyticus	8–30 h	Invasive *and* toxin produced in patient	Shellfish; water.

A. Specific levels. There are no specific assays that will assist clinical management.

    1. Stool culture may differentiate *Salmonella, Shigella,* and *Campylobacter* infections.

    2. Blood and **cerebrospinal fluid** may grow invasive organisms, especially *Listeria* (and rarely, *Salmonella* or *Shigella*).

    3. Food samples should be saved for bacterial culture and toxin analysis, primarily for use by public health investigators.

B. Other useful laboratory studies. CBC, electrolytes, glucose, BUN, creatinine.

V. Treatment

  A. Emergency and supportive measures

    1. Replace fluid and electrolyte losses with intravenous saline or other crystalloid solutions (patients with mild illness may tolerate oral rehydration). Patients with hypotension may require large-volume intravenous fluid resuscitation.

    2. Antiemetic agents are acceptable for symptomatic treatment, but strong antidiarrheal agents such as Lomotil (diphenoxylate plus atropine; should *not* be used because they may prolong the course of the infection.

  B. Specific drugs and antidotes. There are no specific antidotes.

    1. In patients with invasive bacterial infection, antibiotics may be used once the stool culture reveals the specific bacteria responsible. Empiric treatment with ciprofloxacin or trimethoprim-sulfamethoxazole is commonly given while awaiting culture results.

    2. Pregnant women who have eaten *Listeria*-contaminated foods should be treated empirically, even if only mildly symptomatic, to prevent serious intrauterine infection. The antibiotic of choice is ampicillin, with gentamicin added for severe infection.

  C. Decontamination. There is no role for gut decontamination.

  D. Enhanced elimination. There is no role for enhanced removal procedures.

FOOD POISONING: FISH AND SHELLFISH
Susan Kim, PharmD

ANTIDOTE   IPECAC   LAVAGE   CHARCOAL

A variety of toxins may produce illness after ingestion of fish or shellfish. The most common types of seafood-related toxins include **ciguatera, scombroid, neurotoxic shellfish poisoning, paralytic shellfish poisoning, tetrodotoxin,** and **domoic acid**. Shellfish-induced *bacterial* diarrhea is described in the previous section (see p 170).

I. **Mechanism of toxicity.** The mechanism varies with each toxin. The toxins are all heat-stable; therefore, cooking the seafood does not prevent illness.

   A. **Ciguatera.** The toxin is produced by dinoflagellates, which are then consumed by reef fish. The mechanism of intoxication is uncertain, but may involve increased sodium permeability in sodium channels and stimulation of central or ganglionic cholinergic receptors.

   B. **Scombroid.** Scombrotoxin is a mixture of histamine and other histaminelike compounds produced when histidine in fish tissue decomposes.

   C. **Neurotoxic shellfish.** The mechanism appears to involve stimulation of sodium channels, resulting in depolarization of nerve fibers.

   D. **Paralytic shellfish.** Dinoflagellates ("red tide") produce saxitoxin, which is concentrated by filter-feeding clams and mussels. Saxitoxin blocks sodium conductance and neuronal transmission in skeletal muscles.

   E. **Tetrodotoxin,** produced in the skin of puffer fish, California newts, and some South American frogs, is similar to saxitoxin and blocks sodium conductance and neuronal transmission in skeletal muscles.

   F. **Domoic acid** is produced by phytoplanktons, which are concentrated by filter-feeding fish and shellfish. The toxin is thought to bind to glutamate receptors, causing neuroexcitatory responses.

II. **Toxic dose.** The concentration of toxin varies widely depending on geographic and seasonal factors. The amount of toxin necessary to produce symptoms is unknown. Saxitoxin is extremely potent; the estimated lethal dose in humans is 0.3–1 mg, and contaminated mussels may contain 15–20 mg.

III. **Clinical presentation.** The onset of symptoms and clinical manifestations vary with each toxin (Table II–27). In the majority of cases, the seafood appears normal with no adverse smell or taste (scombroid may have a peppery taste).

   A. **Ciguatera.** Intoxication produces vomiting and watery diarrhea 1–6 hours after ingestion, followed by headache, malaise, myalgias, paresthesias of the mouth and extremities, ataxia, blurred vision, photophobia, reversal of hot and cold sensation, extreme pruritus, hypotension, bradycardia, and rarely, seizures and respiratory arrest.

   B. **Scombroid.** Symptoms begin rapidly (minutes to 3 hours) after ingestion. Gastroenteritis, headache, and skin flushing are sometimes accompanied by urticaria and bronchospasm.

   C. **Neurotoxic shellfish.** Onset is within a few minutes to 3 hours. Gastroenteritis is accompanied by paresthesias of the mouth, face, and extremities; muscular weakness; and respiratory arrest.

   D. **Paralytic shellfish.** Vomiting, diarrhea, and facial paresthesias usually begin within 30 minutes of ingestion. Headache, myalgias, dysphagia, weakness, and ataxia have been reported. In serious cases respiratory arrest may occur after 1–12 hours.

   E. **Tetrodotoxin.** Symptoms occur within 30–40 minutes after ingestion and include vomiting, paresthesias, salivation, twitching, diaphoresis, weakness, and dysphagia. Hypotension, bradycardia, and respiratory arrest may occur up to 6–24 hours after ingestion.

   F. **Domoic acid.** Symptoms begin from 15 minutes to 38 hours after ingestion

TABLE II–27. SUMMARY OF FISH AND SHELLFISH INTOXICATIONS

Type	Onset	Common Sources	Syndrome
Ciguatera	1–6 h	Barracuda, red snapper, grouper	Gastroenteritis, hot and cold reversal, paresthesias, myalgias, weakness.
Domoic acid	Minutes to hours	Mussels, clams, anchovies	Gastroenteritis, headache, myoclonus, seizures, coma. Persistent neuropathy and memory impairment.
Scombroid	Minutes to hours	Tuna, mahi mahi, bonita, mackerel	Gastroenteritis, flushed skin, urticaria, wheezing.
Neurotoxic shellfish	Minutes to 3 h	Mussels	Gastroenteritis, ataxia, paresthesias.
Paralytic shellfish	Within 30 minutes	Mussels and clams, "red tide"	Gastroenteritis, paresthesias, ataxia, respiratory paralysis.
Tetrodotoxin	Within 30–40 minutes	Puffer fish, sun fish, porcupine fish, California newt	Vomiting, paresthesias, muscle twitching, diaphoresis, weakness, respiratory paralysis.

and consist of gastroenteritis accompanied by unusual neurologic toxicity including fasciculations, mutism, severe headache, hemiparesis, and myoclonus. Coma, seizures, hypotension, and profuse bronchial secretions have been reported with severe intoxication. Long-term sequelae include persistent severe anterograde memory loss, motor neuropathy, and axonopathy.

IV. **Diagnosis** depends on a history of ingestion and is more likely to be recognized when multiple victims present after consumption of a common meal. Scombroid may be confused with an allergic reaction because of the histamine-induced urticaria.

  A. **Specific levels** are not generally available. However, when epidemic poisoning is suspected, state public health departments or the Centers for Disease Control may be able to analyze suspect food for toxins.

  B. **Other useful laboratory studies.** Electrolytes, glucose, BUN, creatinine, arterial blood gases, ECG monitoring, stool for bacterial culture.

V. **Treatment**

  A. **Emergency and supportive measures.** Most cases are mild and self-limited and require no specific treatment. However, because of the risk of respiratory arrest, all patients should be observed for several hours.

    1. Maintain the airway and assist ventilation if necessary (see p 4).

    2. Replace fluid and electrolyte losses from gastroenteritis with intravenous crystalloid fluids.

  B. **Specific drugs and antidotes**

    1. **Scombroid** intoxication can be treated symptomatically with antihistamines, including diphenhydramine (see p 331) and cimetidine, 300 mg IV. Rarely, bronchodilators may also be required.

    2. **Ciguatera.** There are anecdotal reports of successful treatment with intravenous mannitol, 0.5–1 g/kg.

  C. **Decontamination** (see p 44)

    1. **Prehospital.** Administer activated charcoal, if available. Ipecac-induced emesis may be useful for initial treatment at the scene if it can be given within a few minutes of exposure.

    2. **Hospital.** Administer activated charcoal and a cathartic. Consider gastric lavage if ingestion occurred within the preceding hour.

  D. **Enhanced elimination.** There is no role for these procedures.

FORMALDEHYDE
John Balmes, MD

Formaldehyde is a gas with a pungent odor commonly used in the processing of paper, fabrics, and wood products and for the production of urea foam insulation. Low-level formaldehyde exposure has been found in clothing stores selling clothing treated with formaldehyde-containing crease-resistant resins, in mobile homes, and in tightly enclosed rooms built with large quantities of formaldehyde-containing products used in construction materials. Formaldehyde aqueous solution (formalin) is used in varying concentrations (usually 37%) as a disinfectant and tissue fixative. Stabilized formalin may also contain 6–15% methanol.

I. Mechanism of toxicity
  A. Formaldehyde causes precipitation of proteins and will cause coagulation necrosis of exposed tissue. The gas is highly water-soluble and when inhaled produces immediate local irritation of the upper respiratory tract and has been reported to cause spasm and edema of the larynx.
  B. Metabolism of formaldehyde produces formic acid, which may accumulate and produce metabolic acidosis.
  C. Formaldehyde is a known animal and suspected human carcinogen.

II. Toxic dose
  A. Inhalation. The recommended workplace ceiling limit (ACGIH TLV-C) is 0.3 ppm which should not be exceeded at any time. The air level considered immediately dangerous to life or health (IDLH) is 100 ppm.
  B. Ingestion of as little as 30 mL of 37% formaldehyde solution has been reported to cause death in an adult.

III. Clinical presentation
  A. Formaldehyde gas exposure produces irritation of the eyes, and inhalation can produce cough, wheezing, and noncardiogenic pulmonary edema.
  B. Ingestion of formaldehyde solutions may cause severe corrosive esophageal and gastric injury, depending on the concentration. Lethargy and coma have been reported. Metabolic (anion gap) acidosis may be caused by formic acid accumulation from metabolism of formaldehyde or methanol.
  C. Hemolysis has occurred when formalin was accidentally introduced into the blood through contaminated hemodialysis equipment.

IV. Diagnosis is based on a history of exposure and evidence of mucous membrane, respiratory, or gastrointestinal tract irritation.
  A. Specific levels
    1. Plasma formaldehyde levels are not useful, but formate levels may indicate severity of intoxication.
    2. Methanol (see p 215) and formate levels may be helpful in cases of intoxication by formalin solutions containing methanol.
  B. Other useful laboratory studies. Electrolytes, glucose, BUN, creatinine, osmolar gap.

V. Treatment
  A. Emergency and supportive measures
    1. Maintain the airway and assist ventilation if necessary (see p 14).
    2. **Inhalation.** Treat bronchospasm (p 9–10) and pulmonary edema (p 8) if they occur. Administer supplemental oxygen, and observe for at least 4–6 hours.
    3. **Ingestion**
      a. Treat coma (p 18) and shock (p 15) if they occur.
      b. Administer intravenous saline or other crystalloids to replace fluid losses caused by gastroenteritis. Avoid fluid overload in patients with inhalation exposure because of the risk of pulmonary edema.
      c. Treat metabolic acidosis with sodium bicarbonate (p 30).

B. Specific drugs and antidotes

1. If a **methanol-containing** solution has been ingested, then evaluate and treat with **ethanol** and **folic acid** as for methanol poisoning (see p 215).

2. **Formate** intoxication caused by formaldehyde alone should be treated with **folic acid** (see p 341), but ethanol infusion is not effective.

C. Decontamination (see p 41). Rescuers should wear self-contained breathing apparatus and appropriate chemical protective clothing if handling a heavily contaminated patient.

1. **Inhalation.** Remove from exposure and give supplemental oxygen, if available.

2. **Skin and eyes.** Remove contaminated clothing and wash exposed skin with soap and water. Irrigate exposed eyes with copious tepid water or saline; perform fluorescein examination to rule out corneal injury if pain and lacrimation persist.

3. **Ingestion** (see p 44). Depending on concentration of solution and patient symptoms, consider endoscopy to rule out esophageal or gastric injury.

   a. **Prehospital.** Administer activated charcoal, if available. Do *not* induce emesis because of the risk of corrosive injury.

   b. **Hospital.** Perform gastric lavage. Administer activated charcoal (although note that charcoal may obscure view during endoscopy).

D. Enhanced elimination

1. **Hemodialysis** is effective in removing methanol and formate and in correcting severe metabolic acidosis. Indications for hemodialysis include severe acidosis or osmolar gap (see p 30) greater than 10 mosm/L.

2. **Alkalinization** of the urine helps promote excretion of formate.

FREONS (FLUORINATED HYDROCARBONS)
Kent R. Olson, MD

| ANTIDOTE | IPECAC | LAVAGE | CHARCOAL |

Freons (fluorinated hydrocarbons) are widely used as aerosol propellants, in refrigeration units, and as degreasing agents. Some fire extinguishers contain Freons. Most of these compounds are gases at room temperature, but some are liquids (Freons 11, 21, 113, 114) and may be ingested. Many Freons contain chlorine in addition to fluorine (eg, dichlorofluoromethane, dichlorodifluoromethane, chlorodifluoromethane).

I. Mechanism of toxicity

A. Freons are mild central nervous system depressants. They may also displace oxygen from the air, causing hypoxemia. Freons are well-absorbed by inhalation or ingestion and are usually rapidly excreted in the breath within 15–60 minutes.

B. As with chlorinated hydrocarbons, Freons may potentiate cardiac arrhythmias by sensitizing the myocardium to catecholamines.

C. Direct freezing of the skin, with frostbite, may occur if the skin is exposed to rapidly expanding gas as it escapes from a pressurized tank.

D. Freons containing chlorine may decompose to the irritant gases phosgene and hydrochloric acid (see p 176) if they are burned at high temperature, as may happen in a fire or if a refrigeration line is cut by a welding torch or electric arc.

II. Toxic dose

A. Inhalation. The toxic air level is quite variable, depending on the specific agent (see Table IV–13, p 402).

B. Ingestion. The toxic dose by ingestion is not known.

III. Clinical presentation

A. Skin or mucous membrane exposure may result in skin defatting and erythema. Frostbite may occur after exposure to rapidly expanding compressed gas.

B. Systemic effects of moderate exposure include headache, nausea and vomiting, confusion, and drunkenness. More severe intoxication may result in coma or respiratory arrest. Ventricular arrhythmias may occur even with moderate exposures. A number of deaths, presumably caused by ventricular fibrillation, have been reported after Freon abuse by "sniffing" or "huffing" Freon products from plastic bags.

IV. Diagnosis is based on a history of exposure and clinical presentation. Many chlorinated and aromatic hydrocarbon solvents may cause identical symptoms.

   A. Specific levels. Expired-breath monitoring is possible, and blood levels may be obtained to document exposure, but these are not useful in emergency clinical management.

   B. Other useful laboratory studies. Arterial blood gases or oximetry, ECG monitoring.

V. Treatment

   A. Emergency and supportive measures

     1. Maintain the airway and assist ventilation if necessary (see p 4).

     2. Treat coma (p 18) and arrhythmias (p 10–14) if they occur. Avoid epinephrine or other sympathomimetic amines that may precipitate ventricular arrhythmias. Tachyarrhythmias caused by myocardial sensitization may be treated with **propranolol** (see p 373), 1–2 mg IV, or **esmolol** (see p 338), 25–100 µg/kg/min IV.

     3. Monitor the ECG for 4–6 hours.

   B. Specific drugs and antidotes. There is no specific antidote.

   C. Decontamination (see p 41)

     1. Inhalation. Remove victim from exposure, and give supplemental oxygen if available.

     2. Ingestion (see p 44)

       a. Prehospital. Administer activated charcoal, if available. Do *not* induce emesis because of rapid absorption and the risk of abrupt onset of central nervous system depression.

       b. Hospital. Administer activated charcoal and cathartic, although the efficacy of charcoal is unknown. Perform gastric lavage only if the ingestion was recent (less than 30 minutes) and large.

   D. Enhanced elimination. There is no documented efficacy for diuresis, hemodialysis, hemoperfusion, or repeat-dose charcoal.

GASES, IRRITANT
John Balmes, MD

ANTIDOTE   IPECAC   LAVAGE   CHARCOAL

A vast number of compounds produce irritant effects when inhaled in their gaseous form. The most common source of exposure to irritant gases is in industry, but significant exposures may occur in a variety of circumstances, such as after mixing cleaning agents at home, with smoke inhalation in structural fires, or after highway tanker spills.

I. Mechanism of toxicity. Irritant gases are often divided into 2 major groups based on their water solubility (Table II–28).

   A. Highly soluble gases (eg, ammonia, chlorine) are readily adsorbed by the upper respiratory tract and rapidly produce their primary effects on moist mucous membranes in the eyes, nose, and throat.

   B. Less soluble gases (eg, phosgene, nitrogen dioxide) are not rapidly adsorbed by the upper respiratory tract and can be inhaled deeply into the lower respiratory tract to produce delayed-onset pulmonary toxicity.

TABLE II–28. CHARACTERISTICS OF SOME COMMON IRRITANT TOXIC GASES

Gas	TLV^a(ppm)	IDLH^b (ppm)
High water solubility		
Ammonia	25	500
Formaldehyde	0.3 (C)	100
Hydrogen chloride	5 (C)	100
Hydrogen fluoride	3(C)	20
Nitric acid	2	100
Sulfur dioxide	2	100
Moderate water solubility		
Acrolein	0.1	5
Chlorine	0.5	25
Fluorine	1	25
Low water solubility		
Nitric oxide	25	100
Nitrogen dioxide	3	50
Ozone	0.1 (C)	10
Phosgene	0.1	2

^{a}TLV = ACGIH recommended exposure limit as an 8-hour time-weighted average for a 40-hour workweek (TLV-TWA). "(C)" indicates ceiling limit, which should not be exceeded at any time (TLV-C).
^{b}IDLH = Air level considered immediately dangerous to life or health, defined as the maximum air concentration from which one could reasonably escape within 30 minutes without any escape-impairing symptoms or any irreversible health effects.

II. **Toxic dose.** The toxic dose varies depending on the properties of the gas. Table II–28 illustrates the workplace exposure limits (TLV-TWA) and the levels immediately dangerous to life or health (IDLH) for several common irritant gases.

III. **Clinical presentation.** All these gases may produce irritant effects to the upper and lower respiratory tract, but warning properties and the onset and location of primary symptoms depend largely on the water solubility of the gas and the concentration of exposure.

A. **Highly soluble gases.** Because of the good warning properties (upper respiratory tract irritation) of highly soluble gases, voluntary prolonged exposure to even low concentrations is unlikely.

1. Low-level exposure causes rapid onset of mucous membrane and upper respiratory tract irritation; conjunctivitis, rhinitis, skin erythema and burns, sore throat, cough, wheezing, and hoarseness are common.

2. With high-level exposure, laryngeal edema, tracheobronchitis, and abrupt airway obstruction may occur. Irritation of the lower respiratory tract and lung parenchyma causes tracheobronchial mucosal sloughing, chemical pneumonitis, and noncardiogenic pulmonary edema.

B. **Less soluble gases.** Because of poor warning properties owing to minimal upper respiratory tract effects, prolonged exposure to moderate levels of these gases often occurs; therefore, chemical pneumonitis and pulmonary edema are more common. The onset of pulmonary edema may be delayed up to 12–24 hours or even longer.

C. **Sequelae.** Although most patients who suffer toxic inhalation injury will recover without any permanent impairment, bronchiectasis, bronchiolitis obliterans, persistent asthma, and pulmonary fibrosis can occur.

IV. **Diagnosis** is based on a history of exposure and the presence of typical irritant upper or lower respiratory effects. Arterial blood gases and chest x-ray may reveal early evidence of chemical pneumonitis or pulmonary edema. Whereas highly soluble gases have good warning properties and the diagnosis is not difficult, less soluble gases may produce minimal symptoms shortly after exposure; therefore, a high index of suspicion and repeated examinations are required.

A. Specific levels. There are no specific blood levels.

B. Other useful laboratory studies. Arterial blood gases or oximetry, chest x-ray.

V. Treatment

A. Emergency and supportive measures

1. Immediately assess the airway: hoarseness or stridor suggests laryngeal edema, which necessitates direct laryngoscopy and endotracheal intubation if swelling is present (see p 2). Assist ventilation if necessary (p 7).

2. Give supplemental oxygen, and treat bronchospasm with aerosolized bronchodilators (p 9–10).

3. Monitor arterial blood gases or oximetry, chest x-ray, and pulmonary function. Treat pulmonary edema if it occurs (p 18).

4. For victims of smoke inhalation, consider the possibility of concurrent intoxication by carbon monoxide (p 121) or cyanide (p 145).

B. Specific drugs and antidotes. There is no specific antidote for any of these gases.

C. Decontamination (see p 41). Remove victim from exposure and give supplemental oxygen if available. Rescuers should take care to avoid personal exposure; in most cases, self-contained breathing apparatus should be worn.

D. Enhanced elimination. There is no role for enhanced elimination.

HYDROCARBONS
Kent R. Olson, MD

ANTIDOTE   IPECAC   LAVAGE   CHARCOAL

Hydrocarbons, or petroleum distillates, are widely used in the petroleum, plastic, agricultural, and chemical industries as solvents, degreasers, fuels, and pesticides. In its broadest definition, a hydrocarbon is any chemical containing hydrogen and carbon (essentially, any organic compound). There are many subcategories of hydrocarbons, including: aliphatic (saturated carbon structure); alicyclic (ring compounds); aromatic (containing one or more benzene ring structures); halogenated (containing chlorine, bromine, or fluoride atoms); alcohols and glycols; ethers; ketones; carboxylic acids, and many others. The present chapter emphasizes toxicity caused by common household hydrocarbons. See also specific chemicals elsewhere in Section II and in Section IV, Table IV–13 (p 402).

I. Mechanism of toxicity. Toxicity from hydrocarbons may be caused by direct injury from pulmonary aspiration, or systemic intoxication after ingestion, inhalation, or skin absorption (Table II–29). Many hydrocarbons are also irritating to the eyes and skin.

A. Pulmonary aspiration. Most hydrocarbons are capable of inducing chemical pneumonia if aspirated. The risk of aspiration is greatest for those agents that have a low viscosity (eg, petroleum naphtha, furniture polish).

B. Ingestion

1. **Aliphatic hydrocarbons** and **simple petroleum distillates** such as lighter fluid, kerosene, furniture polish, and gasoline are poorly absorbed from the gastrointestinal tract and do not pose a significant risk of systemic toxicity after ingestion, as long as they are not aspirated.

2. In contrast, many **aromatic** and **halogenated hydrocarbons, alcohols, ethers, ketones,** and other **substituted or complex hydrocarbons** are capable of causing serious systemic toxicity, such as coma, seizures, and cardiac arrhythmias.

TABLE II–29. RISK OF TOXICITY FROM HYDROCARBON INGESTION

Common Compounds	Risk of Systemic Toxicity After Ingestion	Risk of Chemical Aspiration Pneumonia	Treatment
No systemic toxicity, high viscosity Petrolatum jelly, motor oil	Low	Low	None.
No systemic toxicity, low viscosity Gasoline, kerosene, petroleum naphtha, mineral seal oil, petroleum ether	Low	High	Observe for pneumonia; do **not** empty stomach.
Unknown or uncertain systemic toxicity Turpentine, pine oil	Uncertain	High	Observe for pneumonia; do **not** empty stomach if ingestion is < 2 mL/kg.
Systemic toxins Camphor, phenol, halogenated, or aromatic compounds	High	High	Observe for pneumonia; perform gastric lavage or give activated charcoal or do both.

C. **Inhalation** of any hydrocarbon vapors in an enclosed space may cause intoxication as a result of systemic absorption or by displacing oxygen from the atmosphere.
II. **Toxic dose.** The toxic dose is highly variable depending on the agent involved and whether it is aspirated, ingested, or inhaled.
  A. **Pulmonary aspiration** of as little as a few milliliters may produce chemical pneumonia.
  B. **Ingestion** of as little as 10–20 mL of some systemic toxins, such as camphor or carbon tetrachloride, may cause serious or fatal poisoning.
  C. For recommended **inhalation** exposure limits for common hydrocarbons, see Table IV–13, p 402.
III. **Clinical presentation**
  A. If **pulmonary aspiration** has occurred, there is usually immediate onset of coughing, gagging, or choking. This may progress within a few hours to tachypnea, wheezing, and severe chemical pneumonitis. Death may ensue from secondary bacterial infection and other respiratory complications.
  B. **Ingestion** often causes abrupt nausea and vomiting, occasionally with hemorrhagic gastroenteritis. Some compounds may be absorbed and produce systemic toxicity.
  C. **Systemic toxicity** caused by ingestion of a toxic hydrocarbon, or inhalation of any hydrocarbon gas or vapor, is highly variable depending on the compound but usually includes confusion, ataxia, lethargy, and headache. With significant exposure, syncope, coma, and respiratory arrest may occur. Cardiac arrhythmias may occur owing to myocardial sensitization. This is most commonly reported with chlorinated and fluorinated compounds and aromatic derivatives. With many agents, hepatic and renal injury may occur.
  D. **Skin or eye contact** may cause local irritation, burns, or corneal injury. Chronic exposure often causes a defatting dermatitis resulting from removal of oils from the skin. Some agents are absorbed through the skin.
IV. **Diagnosis**
  A. **Aspiration pneumonitis.** Diagnosis is based on a history of exposure and the presence of respiratory symptoms such as coughing, choking, and wheezing. If these symptoms are not present within 4–6 hours of exposure, it is very unlikely that chemical pneumonitis will occur. Chest x-ray and arterial blood gases or oximetry may assist in the diagnosis of chemical pneumonitis.
  B. **Systemic intoxication.** Diagnosis is based on a history of ingestion or inhalation, accompanied by the appropriate systemic clinical manifestations.

   C. Specific levels. Specific levels are generally not available or useful.

   D. Other useful laboratory studies. Suspected aspiration pneumonitis: arterial blood gases or oximetry, chest x-ray. Suspected significant inhalation or ingestion of a toxic compound: electrolytes, glucose, BUN, creatinine, liver transaminases, ECG monitoring.

V. Treatment

A. Emergency and supportive measures

   1. General. Provide basic supportive care for all symptomatic patients, whether from aspiration, ingestion, or inhalation:

     a. Maintain the airway and assist ventilation if necessary (see p 4). Administer supplemental oxygen.

     b. Monitor arterial blood gases or oximetry, chest x-ray, and ECG and admit symptomatic patients to an intensive care setting.

     c. Use epinephrine and other sympathomimetic amines with caution in patients with significant hydrocarbon intoxication, because arrhythmias may be induced.

   2. Pulmonary aspiration. Patients who remain asymptomatic after 4–6 hours of observation may be discharged. In contrast, if the patient is coughing on arrival, aspiration has probably occurred.

     a. Administer supplemental oxygen, and treat bronchospasm (see p 9–10), hypoxia (p 8), and pneumonia (p 8) if they occur.

     b. Do *not* use steroids or prophylactic antibiotics.

   3. Ingestion. In the vast majority of accidental childhood ingestions, less than 5–10 mL is actually swallowed and systemic toxicity is rare. Treatment is primarily supportive.

B. Specific drugs and antidotes

   1. There is no specific antidote for general hydrocarbon aspiration pneumonia; corticosteroids are of no proved value.

   2. Specific drugs or antidotes may be available for systemic toxicity of some hydrocarbons (eg, acetylcysteine for carbon tetrachloride, methylene blue for methemoglobin formers; etc).

C. Decontamination

   1. Inhalation. Move the victim to fresh air and administer oxygen, if available.

   2. Skin and eyes. Remove contaminated clothing and wash exposed skin with water and soap. Irrigate exposed eyes with copious tepid water or saline, and perform fluorescein examination for corneal injury.

   3. Ingestion (see p 44). For agents with no known systemic toxicity, gut decontamination is neither necessary nor desirable because any gut-emptying procedure may increase the risk of aspiration. For systemic toxins:

     a. Prehospital. Administer activated charcoal, if available. Do *not* induce emesis, because systemic complications such as seizures and coma may occur rapidly or abruptly.

     b. Hospital. Administer activated charcoal and a cathartic. Consider gastric lavage for large recent ingestions.

D. Enhanced elimination. There is no known role for any of these procedures.

HYDROGEN FLUORIDE AND HYDROFLUORIC ACID
Kent R. Olson, MD

ANTIDOTE   IPECAC   LAVAGE   CHARCOAL

Hydrogen fluoride (HF) is an irritant gas that liquifies at 19.5 °C; in aqueous solution it produces hydrofluoric acid. HF gas is used in chemical manufacturing. In addition, it may be released from fluorosilicates, fluorocarbons, or Teflon when heated over

350 °C. Hydrofluoric acid (aqueous HF solution) is widely used as a rust remover, in glass etching, and in the manufacture of silicon semiconductor chips. Hydrofluoric acid poisoning usually occurs after skin contact, although ingestions occasionally occur.

I. **Mechanism of toxicity.** Hydrogen fluoride is a skin and respiratory irritant. Hydrofluoric acid is actually a relatively weak acid (the dissociation constant is about 1000 times less than that of hydrochloric acid), and toxic effects result primarily from the highly reactive fluoride ion.

   A. HF is able to penetrate tissues deeply, where the highly cytotoxic fluoride ion is released and cellular destruction occurs.

   B. In addition, fluoride readily precipitates with calcium; this may cause local bone demineralization and systemic hypocalcemia.

II. **Toxic dose.** Toxicity depends on the air levels of hydrogen fluoride or concentration of aqueous HF solutions.

   A. **Hydrogen fluoride gas.** The recommended workplace ceiling limit (ACGIH TLV-C) for HF gas is 3 ppm; 20 ppm is considered immediately dangerous to life or health (IDLH). A 5-minute exposure to air concentrations of 50–250 ppm is likely to be lethal.

   B. **Aqueous solutions.** Solutions of 50–70% are highly toxic and produce immediate pain; intermediate concentrations (20–40%) may cause little pain initially but result in deep injury after 1–8 hours; weak solutions (5–15%) cause almost no pain on contact but may cause delayed serious injury after 12–24 hours. Most household products containing aqueous HF contain 5–8% or less.

III. **Clinical presentation.** Symptoms and signs depend on the type of exposure (gas or liquid) and the concentration.

   A. **Inhalation of HF gas.** Inhalation of HF produces eye and nose irritation, sore throat, coughing, and bronchospasm. After a delay of up to several hours, chemical pneumonia and pulmonary edema may occur.

   B. **Skin exposure.** After acute exposure to weak (5–15%) or intermediate (20–40%) solutions, there may be no symptoms because the pH effect is relatively weak. Strong (50–70%) solutions have better warning properties because of immediate pain. After a delay of 1–12 hours, progressive redness, swelling, skin blanching, and pain occur owing to deep penetration by the fluoride ion. The exposure is typically through a pinhole-sized defect in a rubber glove, and the fingertip is the most common site of injury. The pain is progressive and unrelenting. Severe deep-tissue destruction may occur, including full-thickness skin loss and destruction of underlying bone.

   C. **Ingestion** of HF may cause corrosive injury to the mouth, esophagus, and stomach.

   D. **Systemic hypocalcemia** and **hyperkalemia** may occur after ingestion or following skin burns involving a large body surface area or highly concentrated solutions.

IV. **Diagnosis** is based on a history of exposure and typical findings. Immediately after exposure to weak or intermediate solutions, there may be few or no symptoms even though potentially severe injury may develop later.

   A. **Specific levels.** Serum fluoride concentrations are not useful after acute exposure but may be used in evaluating chronic occupational exposure. Normal serum fluoride is less than 20 μg/L.

   B. **Other useful laboratory studies.** Electrolytes, calcium, ECG monitoring.

V. **Treatment**

   A. **Emergency and supportive measures**

      1. Maintain the airway and assist ventilation if necessary (see p 4). Administer supplemental oxygen. Treat pulmonary edema (p 8) if it occurs.

      2. Patients with HF ingestion should be evaluated for corrosive injury, with consultation by a gastroenterologist or surgeon for possible endoscopy (p 126).

      3. Monitor the ECG and serum calcium and potassium levels; give intravenous calcium (p 323 see below) if there is evidence of hypocalcemia or severe hyperkalemia.

B. Specific drugs and antidotes. Calcium (see p 323) rapidly precipitates fluoride ion and is an effective antidote for fluoride skin exposure and for systemic hypocalcemia resulting from absorbed fluoride.

  1. Skin burns. For exposures involving the hands or fingers, immediately consult an experienced hand surgeon, medical toxicologist, or Poison Control Center (see Table I–41, p 53). The nail may need to be removed, and occasionally calcium will need to be given by the intra-arterial route. *Caution:* Do *not* use calcium *chloride* for subcutaneous or intra-arterial injections; this form contains a larger proportion of calcium ion and may cause vasospasm and tissue necrosis.

    a. Topical. Apply a gel containing calcium gluconate or carbonate (see p 323); or soak in a quaternary ammonium solution such as Zephiran (1.3 g per liter of water) or an Epsom salt solution. If pain is not significantly improved within 30–60 minutes, consider SC or intra-arterial injection.

    b. Subcutaneous. Inject calcium gluconate 5–10% subcutaneously in affected areas, using a 27- or 30-gauge needle and no more than 0.5 mL per digit or 1 mL/cm^2 in other regions.

    c. Intra-arterial. Injection of calcium by the intra-arterial route (see p 323) may be necessary for burns involving several digits or subungual areas.

  2. Systemic hypocalcemia or hyperkalemia. Administer calcium gluconate 10%, 2–4 mL/kg IV, or calcium chloride 10%, 1–2 mL/kg IV.

C. Decontamination (see p 41). Rescuers entering a contaminated area should wear self-contained breathing apparatus and appropriate protective clothing to avoid personal exposure.

  1. Inhalation. Immediately remove from exposure and give supplemental oxygen, if available. The use of 2.5% calcium gluconate by nebulization is recommended by some authorities.

  2. Skin. Immediately flood exposed areas with water. Then soak in solution of Epsom salts (magnesium sulfate) or calcium; immediate topical use of calcium or magnesium may prevent deep burns. Some facilities that frequently manage HF cases prepare a 2.5% calcium gluconate gel (in water-based jelly), and this is highly effective if rapidly available. After skin penetration by HF, topical treatment is relatively ineffective and calcium injections (see above) may be required.

  3. Eyes. Flush with copious water or saline. The use of weak (1–2%) calcium gluconate solution is not established.

  4. Ingestion (see p 44)

    a. Prehospital. Immediately give any available magnesium-containing (Epsom salts, magnesium hydroxide, etc) or calcium-containing (calcium carbonate or milk) substance by mouth. Do *not* induce emesis because of the risk of corrosive injury. Activated charcoal is not effective.

    b. Hospital. Perform gastric lavage. Administer magnesium- or calcium-containing substance as in **a.**, above.

D. Enhanced elimination. There is no role for enhanced elimination procedures.

HYDROGEN SULFIDE
Kent R. Olson, MD

ANTIDOTE   IPECAC   LAVAGE   CHARCOAL

Hydrogen sulfide is a highly toxic, flammable, colorless gas that is heavier than air. It is produced naturally by decaying organic matter and is also a by-product of many industrial processes. Hazardous levels may be found in petroleum refineries, tanneries, mines, pulp-making factories, sulfur hot springs, carbon disulfide production, hot asphalt fumes, and pools of sewage sludge or liquid manure.

I. **Mechanism of toxicity.** Hydrogen sulfide causes cellular asphyxia by inhibition of the cytochrome oxidase system, similar to the action of cyanide. Because it is rapidly absorbed by inhalation, symptoms occur nearly immediately after exposure. Hydrogen sulfide is also a mucous membrane irritant.

II. **Toxic dose.** The characteristic rotten egg odor of hydrogen sulfide is detectable at concentrations as low as 0.025 ppm. The recommended workplace limit (ACGIH TLV-TWA) is 10 ppm as an 8-hour time-weighted average, with a short-term exposure limit (STEL) of 15 ppm. Marked respiratory tract irritation occurs with levels of 50–100 ppm. Olfactory nerve paralysis occurs with levels of 100–150 ppm. The level considered immediately dangerous to life or health (IDLH) is 300 ppm. Pulmonary edema occurs at levels of 300–500 ppm. Levels of 600–800 ppm are rapidly fatal.

III. **Clinical presentation**
   A. **Irritant effects.** Upper airway irritation, burning eyes, and blepharospasm may occur at relatively low levels. Skin exposure can cause painful dermatitis. Chemical pneumonitis and noncardiogenic pulmonary edema may occur after a delay of several hours.
   B. **Acute systemic effects** include headache, nausea and vomiting, dizziness, confusion, seizures, and coma. Massive exposure may cause immediate cardiovascular collapse, respiratory arrest, and death.

IV. **Diagnosis** is based on a history of exposure and rapidly progressive manifestations of airway irritation and cellular asphyxia, with sudden collapse. The victim or coworkers may describe the smell of rotten eggs, but because of olfactory nerve paralysis the absence of this smell does not rule out exposure.
   A. **Specific levels.** Serum levels are not available. Sulfhemoglobin is not thought to be produced after hydrogen sulfide exposure.
   B. **Other useful laboratory studies.** Electrolytes, glucose, arterial blood gases, chest x-ray.

V. **Treatment**
   A. **Emergency and supportive measures.** *Note:* Rescuers should use self-contained breathing apparatus to prevent personal exposure.
      1. Maintain the airway and assist ventilation if necessary (see p 4). Administer high-flow humidified supplemental oxygen. Observe for several hours for delayed-onset chemical pneumonia or pulmonary edema (p 8).
      2. Treat coma (p 18), seizures (p 22), and hypotension (p 15) if they occur.
   B. **Specific drugs and antidotes.** Theoretically, administration of nitrites (see p 361) to produce methemoglobinemia may promote conversion of sulfide ion to sulfhemoglobin, which is far less toxic. However, there is limited evidence for the effectiveness of nitrites, and they can cause serious adverse effects.
   C. **Decontamination** (see p 41). Remove the victim from exposure and give supplemental oxygen, if available.
   D. **Enhanced elimination.** There is no role for enhanced elimination procedures. Although hyperbaric oxygen therapy has been promoted for treatment of hydrogen sulfide poisoning, this is based on anecdotal cases and there is no convincing rationale or scientific evidence for its effectiveness.

HYMENOPTERA
Evan T. Wythe, MD

ANTIDOTE   IPECAC   LAVAGE   CHARCOAL

Venomous insects are grouped into 4 families of the order Hymenoptera: Apidae (honeybees), Bombidae (bumblebees), Vespidae (wasps, hornets, and yellow jackets), and Formicidae (ants). With the exception of Vespidae, most bees sting only when disturbed or when the hive is threatened. Yellow jackets may attack without provocation and are the most common cause of insect-induced anaphylactic reactions.

I. **Mechanism of toxicity.** The venoms of the Hymenoptera are complex mixtures of enzymes and are delivered by various methods. The venom apparatus is located in the posterior abdomen of the females.

   A. The terminal end of the stinger of the **Apidae** (honeybee) is barbed, so the stinger remains in the victim and some or all of the venom apparatus will be torn from the body of the bee, resulting in its death as it flies away. The musculature surrounding the venom sac continues to contract for several minutes, causing venom to be persistently ejected. The **Bombidae** and **Vespidae** have nonbarbed stingers that remain functionally intact after a sting, resulting in their ability to inflict multiple stings.

   B. The envenomating **Formicidae** have secretory venom glands in the posterior abdomen and envenomate either by injecting venom through a stinger or by spraying venom from the posterior abdomen into a bite wound produced by their mandibles.

II. **Toxic dose.** The dose of venom delivered per sting may vary from none to the entire contents of the venom gland. The toxic response is highly variable depending on individual sensitivity. Some insects, such as wasps, have the ability to sting several times, increasing the venom load. Disturbing an ant nest may result in as many as 3000–5000 stings within seconds.

III. **Clinical presentation.** The patient may present with signs of envenomation or an allergic reaction.

   A. **Envenomation.** Once venom is injected, there is usually immediate onset of severe pain followed by a local inflammatory reaction, which may include erythema, wheal formation, ecchymosis, edema, vesiculation and blisters, itching, and a sensation of warmth. Multiple stings, and very rarely severe single stings, may also produce vomiting, diarrhea, hypotension, syncope, cyanosis, dyspnea, rhabdomyolysis, coagulopathy, and death.

   B. **Allergic reactions.** About 50 deaths occur annually in the USA from immediate hypersensitivity (anaphylactic) reactions characterized by urticaria, angioedema, bronchospasm, and shock. Most anaphylactic reactions occur within 15 minutes of envenomation. Rarely, delayed-onset reactions may occur, including Arthus reactions (arthralgias, fever), nephritis, transverse myelitis, and Guillain-Barré syndrome.

IV. **Diagnosis** is usually obvious from the history of exposure and typical findings.

   A. **Specific levels** are not available.

   B. **Other useful laboratory studies.** None.

V. **Treatment**

   A. **Emergency and supportive measures**

      1. Monitor the victim closely for at least 30–60 minutes.

      2. Treat anaphylaxis (see p 26), if it occurs, with epinephrine (p 337) and diphenhydramine (p 331). Persistent urticaria may respond to the addition of cimetidine, 300 mg orally or IV. Persons known to be sensitive to Hymenoptera venom should wear medical alert jewelry and carry an epinephrine emergency kit at all times.

      3. In most cases the painful localized tissue response will resolve in a few hours without therapy. Some symptomatic relief may be obtained by topical application of ice, papain (meat tenderizer), or creams containing corticosteroids or antihistamines.

      4. Provide tetanus prophylaxis if appropriate.

   B. **Specific drugs and antidotes.** There is no available antidote.

   C. **Decontamination.** Examine the sting site carefully for any retained stingers; these can be removed by gentle scraping with a knife blade or key (do **not** squeeze the stinger with forceps or fingers; this may release more venom). Wash the area with soap and water.

   D. **Enhanced elimination.** These procedures are not applicable.

HYPOGLYCEMIC AGENTS
Susan Kim, PharmD

ANTIDOTE   IPECAC   LAVAGE   CHARCOAL

Agents used to lower blood glucose are divided into 2 groups: the oral hypoglycemics and insulin products. The **oral hypoglycemic agents** are sulfonylureas, and all produce qualitatively similar blood glucose-lowering effects; they differ primarily by potency and duration of action. All **insulin** products are given by the parenteral route, and all produce effects similar to those of endogenous insulin; they differ by antigenicity and by onset and duration of effect. Table II–30 lists the various available hypoglycemic agents.

I. Mechanism of toxicity
    A. Oral hypoglycemic agents. Hypoglycemia is produced primarily by stimulating endogenous pancreatic insulin secretion and secondarily by enhancing peripheral insulin receptor sensitivity and by reducing glycogenolysis.

    B. Insulin. Blood glucose is lowered directly by stimulation of cellular uptake and metabolism of glucose. Cellular glucose uptake is accompanied by intracellular shift of potassium and magnesium. Insulin also promotes glycogen formation and lipogenesis.

II. Toxic dose
    A. Oral hypoglycemic agents. Toxic dose depends on the agent and the total dose or duration of overdose. Toxicity may also occur owing to drug interactions, resulting in impaired elimination of the oral agent.

        1. Acetohexamide. Two 500-mg tablets has caused hypoglycemic coma in an adult.

        2. Chlorpropamide, 500–750 mg/d for 2 weeks, has caused hypoglycemia in adults.

        3. Glyburide. Acute overdose (10–15 mg) in a child produced profound hypoglycemic coma. In a 79-year-old nondiabetic person, 5 mg caused hypoglycemic coma.

TABLE II–30. PHARMACOLOGIC PROFILES OF HYPOGLYCEMIC AGENTS

Agent	Onset (h)	Peak (h)	Duration[a] (h)
Insulins			
Regular insulin	0.5–1	2–3	5–7
Rapid insulin zinc	0.5–1	4–7	12–16
Insulin zinc	1–2	8–12	18–24
Isophane insulin (NPH)	1–2	8–12	18–24
Prolonged insulin zinc	4–8	16–18	36
Protamine zinc	4–8	14–20	36
Oral hypoglycemic agents			
Glipizide	0.25–0.5	0.5–2	< 24
Glyburide	0.25–1	1–2	24
Chlorpropamide	1	3–6	24–72
Tolazamide	1	4–6	14–20
Tolbutamide	1	5–8	6–12
Acetohexamide	2	4	12–24

[a]Duration of hypoglycemic effects after overdose may be much longer, especially with glyburide (up to 5 days) and chlorpropamide.

4. **Interactions** with the following drugs may increase the risk of hypoglycemia: other hypoglycemics; sulfonamides; propranolol; salicylates; clofibrate; probenecid; dicumarol; cimetidine; monoamine oxidase inhibitors; and alcohol. In addition, coingestion of alcohol may occasionally produce a disulfiramlike interaction (see p 155).

5. **Hepatic** or **renal insufficiency** may impair drug elimination and result in hypoglycemia.

B. **Insulin.** Severe hypoglycemic coma and permanent neurologic sequelae have occurred after injections of 800–3200 units of insulin. Orally administered insulin is not absorbed and is not toxic.

III. **Clinical presentation.** All agents cause hypoglycemia, which may be delayed in onset depending on the agent used and the route of administration (ie, subcutaneous vs intravenous). Manifestations of hypoglycemia include agitation, confusion, coma, seizures, tachycardia, and diaphoresis. The serum potassium and magnesium levels may also be depressed. Note that in patients receiving beta-adrenergic blocking agents (see p 99), many of the manifestations of hypoglycemia (tachycardia, diaphoresis) may be blunted or absent.

IV. **Diagnosis.** Overdose of an hypoglycemic agent should be suspected in any patient with hypoglycemia. Other causes of hypoglycemia that should be considered include alcohol ingestion (especially in children) and hepatic failure.

A. **Specific levels**

1. Tolazamide, tolbutamide, and chlorpropamide serum concentrations can be determined in most regional commercial toxicology laboratories, but have little utility in acute clinical management.

2. Exogenously administered animal insulin can be distinguished from endogenous insulin (ie, in a patient with hypoglycemia caused by insulinoma) by determination of C peptide (present with endogenous insulin secretion).

B. **Other useful laboratory studies.** Glucose, electrolytes, magnesium, ethanol.

V. **Treatment**

A. **Emergency and supportive measures**

1. Maintain the airway and assist ventilation if necessary (see p 4).

2. Treat coma (p 18) and seizures (p 22) if they occur.

B. **Specific drugs and antidotes**

1. Administer concentrated **glucose** (see p 343) as soon as possible after drawing a baseline blood sample for later blood glucose determination. In adults, give 50% dextrose ($D_{50}W$), 1–2 mL/kg; in children, use 25% dextrose ($D_{25}W$), 2–4 mL/kg.

2. Follow serum glucose levels closely for several hours after the last dose of dextrose. Give repeated glucose boluses and administer 5–10% dextrose (D_5–D_{10}) as needed to maintain the serum glucose level at or above 100 mg/dL.

3. For patients with oral hypoglycemic overdose, consider intravenous **diazoxide** (see p 328) if 5% dextrose infusions do not maintain satisfactory glucose concentrations.

C. **Decontamination** (see p 44)

1. **Oral hypoglycemic agents**

a. **Prehospital.** Administer activated charcoal, if available. Ipecac-induced emesis may be useful for initial treatment at the scene (eg, children at home) if it can be given within a few minutes of exposure.

b. **Hospital.** Administer activated charcoal and a cathartic. Gastric emptying is not necessary if activated charcoal can be given promptly.

2. **Insulin**

a. Orally ingested insulin is not absorbed and produces no toxicity, so gut decontamination is not necessary.

b. Local excision of tissue at the site of massive intradermal injection has been performed, but the general utility of this procedure has not been established.

D. **Enhanced elimination.** Alkalinization of the urine (pH 8 or greater) increases the renal elimination of chlorpropamide. Forced diuresis and dialysis procedures are of no known value for other hypoglycemic agents. The high degree of protein binding of the sulfonylureas suggests that dialysis procedures would not generally be effective. However, charcoal hemoperfusion reduced the serum half-life of chlorpropamide in a patient with renal failure.

IODINE
Olga F. Woo, PharmD

ANTIDOTE   IPECAC   LAVAGE   CHARCOAL

The chief use of iodine is for its antiseptic property. It is bactericidal, sporicidal, protozoacidal, cysticidal, and virucidal. Because it is poorly soluble in water, liquid formulations are usually prepared as a tincture in ethanol (50% or higher). Iodoform, iodochlorhydroxyquin, iodophors (povidine-iodine), and sodium and potassium iodides also exert their bactericidal effect by liberating iodine. Lugol's solution (5% iodine and 10% potassium iodide) is used in the treatment of hyperthyroidism and for the prevention of radioactive iodine absorption after nuclear accidents. The antiarrhythmic drug amiodarone releases iodine and may cause thyrotoxicosis after prolonged use.

I. **Mechanism of toxicity.** Iodine is corrosive because of its oxidizing properties. When ingested, iodine is poorly absorbed but may cause severe gastroenteritis. Iodine is readily inactivated by starch to convert it to iodide, which is nontoxic. In the body, iodine is rapidly converted to iodide and stored in the thyroid gland.

II. **Toxic dose** depends on the product and the route of exposure. Iodophors and iodoform liberate only small amounts of iodine and are generally nontoxic and noncaustic.

   A. **Iodine vapor.** The ACGIH recommended workplace ceiling limit (TLV-C) for iodine vapor is 0.1 ppm. The air level considered immediately dangerous to life or health (IDLH) is 10 ppm.

   B. **Skin and mucous membranes.** Strong iodine tincture (7% iodine and 5% potassium iodide in 83% ethanol) may cause burns, but USP iodine tincture (2% iodine and 2% sodium iodide in 50% ethanol) is not likely to produce corrosive damage.

   C. **Ingestion.** Reported fatal doses vary from 200 mg to more than 20 g of iodine; an estimated mean lethal dose is approximately 2–4 g of free iodine. USP iodine tincture contains 100 mg iodine per 5 mL, and strong iodine tincture contains 350 mg of iodine per 5 mL. Iodine ointment contains 4% iodine. Consider ethanol toxicity with large exposures (see p 160).

III. **Clinical presentation.** The manifestations of iodine poisoning are largely related to its corrosive effect on mucous membranes.

   A. **Inhalation** of iodine vapor can cause severe pulmonary irritation leading to pulmonary edema.

   B. **Skin and eye** exposures may result in severe corrosive burns. Exposures on the skin from strong iodine tincture may cause dermal necrosis and systemic absorption of iodine.

   C. **Ingestion** can cause corrosive gastroenteritis with vomiting, hematemesis, and diarrhea, which can result in significant volume loss and circulatory collapse. Pharyngeal swelling and glottic edema have been reported. Mucous membranes are usually stained brown, and the vomitus may be blue if starchy foods are already present in the stomach.

   D. **Chronic** ingestions or absorption may result in hypothyroidism and goiter. Iodides cross the placenta, and neonatal hypothyroidism and death from respiratory distress secondary to goiter have been reported.

IV. **Diagnosis** is based on a history of exposure and evidence of corrosive injury. Mucous membranes are usually stained brown, and vomitus may be blue.

A. Specific levels. Iodide levels are not clinically useful but may confirm exposure.

B. Other useful laboratory studies. For serious corrosive injury: CBC, electrolytes, BUN, creatinine. For serious inhalation: arterial blood gases or oximetry, chest x-ray.

V. Treatment

A. Emergency and supportive measures

1. Maintain the airway and perform endotracheal intubation if airway edema is progressive (see p 2–3). Treat bronchospasm (see p 9–10) and pulmonary edema (p 8) if they occur.
2. Treat fluid loss from gastroenteritis aggressively with intravenous crystalloid solutions.
3. If corrosive injury to the esophagus or stomach is suspected, consult a gastroenterologist to perform endoscopy.

B. Specific drugs and antidotes.
Sodium thiosulfate may convert iodine to iodide and tetrathionate, but is not recommended for intravenous use because iodine is rapidly converted to iodide in the body.

C. Decontamination (see p 41)

1. **Inhalation.** Remove victim from exposure.
2. **Skin and eyes.** Remove contaminated clothing and flush exposed skin with water. Irrigate exposed eyes copiously with tepid water or saline for at least 15 minutes.
3. **Ingestion** (see p 44)
   a. **Prehospital.** Do *not* induce emesis because of the corrosive effects of iodine. Administer a starchy food (potato, flour, cornstarch) or milk to lessen gastrointestinal irritation.
   b. **Hospital.** For large exposures, consider gastric lavage, using milk, cornstarch, or sodium thiosulfate. Activated charcoal is of unknown efficacy.

D. Enhanced elimination.
Once absorbed into the circulation, iodine is rapidly converted to the far less toxic iodide. Therefore, there is no need for enhanced drug removal.

IPECAC SYRUP
Kathryn H. Keller, PharmD

ANTIDOTE   IPECAC   LAVAGE   CHARCOAL

Ipecac syrup is an extract of the ipecacuanha plant. Its principle active ingredients are emetine and cephaeline. Syrup of ipecac is widely available over the counter as an effective, rapidly acting emetic agent. Presently, the major source of poisoning is chronic intoxication resulting from intentional misuse by patients with eating disorders. Cases of "Munchausen's syndrome by proxy," in which a parent repeatedly administers ipecac to a child, have also been reported.

I. Mechanism of toxicity

A. Acute ingestion of ipecac causes vomiting by irritation of the gastric mucosa and by stimulation of the central chemoreceptor trigger zone.

B. Chronic repeated dosing results in interstitial edema, focal connective tissue proliferation, and necrosis of skeletal and myocardial muscle fibers. The normal cellular architecture is disrupted, and clinical myopathy occurs.

II. Toxic dose.
Toxicity depends on the formulation and whether the exposure is acute or chronic.

A. Acute ingestion of 60–120 mL of **syrup of ipecac** is not likely to cause serious poisoning. However, the **fluid extract,** which is approximately 14 times more potent than syrup of ipecac, has caused death after ingestion of as little as 10 mL.

B. Chronic dosing results in cumulative toxicity because of the slow elimination of emetine. Daily ingestion of 90–120 mL of syrup of ipecac for 3 months has caused death from cardiomyopathy.

III. Clinical presentation

A. Acute ingestion of ipecac causes nausea and vomiting. In patients with depressed airway protective reflexes, pulmonary aspiration of gastric contents may occur. Prolonged or forceful emesis may cause gastritis, gastric rupture, pneumomediastinum, retropneumoperitoneum, or Mallory-Weiss tears of the cardioesophageal junction. One fatal case of intracerebral hemorrhage was reported in an elderly patient following a single therapeutic dose of ipecac syrup.

B. Chronic intoxication. In patients with chronic misuse, dehydration and electrolyte abnormalities (eg, hypokalemia) are common secondary to frequent vomiting and diarrhea, and myopathy or cardiomyopathy may develop. Symptoms of myopathy include muscle weakness and tenderness, hyporeflexia, and elevated serum creatine phosphokinase (CPK). Cardiomyopathy, with congestive heart failure and arrhythmias, may be fatal.

IV. Diagnosis is based on a history of ingestion. Chronic ipecac poisoning should be suspected in any patient with a known eating disorder and evidence of dehydration, electrolyte imbalance, or myopathy, or in a young child with repeated unexplained episodes of vomiting, diarrhea, and failure to thrive. The electrocardiogram may show prolonged QRS and QT intervals, flat or inverted T waves, and supraventricular and ventricular arrhythmias.

A. Specific levels. Emetine may be detected in the urine, and its presence may provide qualitative confirmation of ipecac exposure but does not correlate with the degree of effect. It is not part of a routine toxicology screen and must be specifically requested.

B. Other useful laboratory studies. Electrolytes, BUN, creatinine, creatine phosphokinase (CPK), lactate dehydrogenase (LDH), ECG.

V. Treatment

A. Emergency and supportive measures

1. Correct fluid and electrolyte abnormalities with intravenous fluids and potassium as needed.
2. Diuretics and pressor support may be required in patients with congestive cardiomyopathy.
3. Monitor the ECG for 6–8 hours, and admit patients with evidence of myopathy or cardiomyopathy. Treat arrhythmias with standard drugs (see p 14).

B. Specific drugs and antidotes. There is no specific antidote.

C. Decontamination (acute ingestions only; see p 44).

1. **Prehospital.** Administer activated charcoal, if available. Do *not* administer ipecac.
2. **Hospital.** Administer activated charcoal. Consider gastric lavage for very large ingestions.

D. Enhanced elimination. There is no known role for enhanced elimination. The alkaloids are highly bound to muscle tissue.

IRON
Olga F. Woo, PharmD

ANTIDOTE   IPECAC   LAVAGE   CHARCOAL

Iron is widely used for treatment of anemia, for prenatal supplementation, and as a common daily vitamin supplement. Because of its wide availability (often in large, non-childproof containers) and its presumed innocence as a common over-the-counter product, it remains one of the most common childhood ingestions, and is the leading cause of fatal poisonings in children. There are many different iron preparations, containing various amounts of iron salts. Most children's preparations contain 12–18 mg of elemental iron per dose, and most adult preparations contain 60–90 mg of elemental iron per dose.

I. Mechanism of toxicity. Toxicity results from direct corrosive effects and cellular toxicity.

    A. Iron has a direct **corrosive effect** on mucosal tissue and may cause hemorrhagic necrosis and perforation. Fluid loss from the gastrointestinal tract results in severe hypovolemia.

    B. Absorbed iron causes cellular dysfunction, resulting in lactic acidosis and necrosis. The exact mechanism for cellular toxicity is not known.

II. Toxic dose. The acute lethal dose in animal studies is 150–200 mg/kg of elemental iron. The lowest reported lethal dose in a child was 600 mg. Symptoms are unlikely if less than 20 mg/kg of elemental iron has been ingested. Doses between 20–30 mg/kg may produce self-limited vomiting, abdominal pain, and diarrhea. Ingestion of more than 40 mg/kg is considered potentially serious and more than 60 mg/kg potentially lethal.

III. Clinical presentation. The manifestations of poisoning are usually described in 4 stages.

    A. Shortly after ingestion, the corrosive effects of iron cause vomiting and diarrhea, often bloody. Massive fluid or blood loss into the gastrointestinal tract may result in shock, renal failure, and death.

    B. Victims who survive this phase may experience a latent period of apparent improvement over 12 hours.

    C. This may be followed by an abrupt relapse, with coma, shock, seizures, consumptive coagulopathy, hepatic failure, and death. *Yersinia enterocolitica* sepsis may occur.

    D. If the victim survives, scarring from the initial corrosive injury may result in pyloric stricture or other intestinal obstruction.

IV. Diagnosis is based on a history of exposure and the presence of vomiting, diarrhea, hypotension, and other clinical signs. Elevation of the white blood count (> 15,000) or blood glucose (> 150 mg/dL) or visible radiopaque pills on abdominal x-ray also suggest significant ingestion. Serious toxicity is very unlikely if the white count, glucose, and x-ray are normal and there is no spontaneous vomiting or diarrhea.

    A. Specific levels. If the total serum iron level is higher than 450–500 μg/dL, toxicity is likely to develop. Serum levels higher than 800–1000 μg/dL are nearly always associated with severe poisoning. Determine the serum iron level at 4–6 hours after ingestion, and repeat determinations after 8–12 hours to rule out delayed absorption (eg, from a sustained-release tablet or a tablet bezoar). The total iron-binding capacity (TIBC) is unreliable in iron overdose and should not be used to estimate free iron levels.

    B. Other useful laboratory studies. CBC, electrolytes, glucose, BUN, creatinine, liver function tests, abdominal x-ray.

V. Treatment. Patients who have self-limited mild gastrointestinal symptoms or who remain asymptomatic for 6 hours are unlikely to develop serious intoxication. On the other hand, those few with serious ingestion must be promptly and aggressively managed.

    A. Emergency and supportive measures

        1. Maintain the airway and assist ventilation if necessary (see p 4).

        2. Treat shock caused by hemorrhagic gastroenteritis aggressively with intravenous crystalloid fluids (p 15), and replace blood if needed. Patients are often markedly hypovolemic owing to gastrointestinal losses and third-spacing.

        3. Treat coma (p 18), seizures (p 22), and metabolic acidosis (p 30) if they occur.

    B. Specific treatment. For seriously intoxicated victims (eg, shock, severe acidosis, serum iron > 500–600 μg/dL), administer **deferoxamine** (see p 326). Monitor the urine for the characteristic orange or pink-red ("vin rose") color of the chelated deferoxamine-iron complex. Therapy may be stopped when the urine color returns to normal or when the serum iron level decreases to the normal range.

1. The intravenous route is preferred: give 10–15 mg/kg/h by constant infusion; faster rates (up to 45 mg/kg/h) have been reportedly well tolerated in single cases, but rapid boluses usually cause hypotension. The recommended maximum daily dose is 6 g, but larger amounts have been safely given in massive iron overdose.

2. Deferoxamine has also been given intramuscularly (eg, as a test dose in suspected poisonings while awaiting laboratory confirmation); the usual dose is 50 mg/kg, with a maximum of 1 g. However, hypotension can also occur with the intramuscular route, and this route is not recommended.

C. Decontamination (see p 44)

1. **Prehospital.** Induce emesis with syrup of ipecac. Activated charcoal is not effective.

2. **Hospital.**

   a. Induce emesis or perform gastric lavage. Do *not* use phosphate-containing solutions for lavage; these may result in fatal hypernatremia, hyperphosphatemia, and hypocalcemia. Bicarbonate and deferoxamine lavage are of doubtful efficacy. Deferoxamine lavage may enhance toxicity by promoting absorption.

   b. Obtain an abdominal x-ray to determine if radiopaque tablets persist after initial emesis or lavage; if so, perform **whole bowel irrigation** (see p 48).

   c. **Activated charcoal does not adsorb iron** and is not recommended unless other drugs have been ingested.

   d. Massive ingestions may result in tablet concretions or bezoars. Repeated lavage or whole bowel irrigation may remove the tablets, but occasionally endoscopy or even surgical gastrotomy is required.

D. Enhanced elimination

1. Hemodialysis and hemoperfusion are not effective at removing iron but may be necessary to remove deferoxamine-iron complex in patients with renal failure.

2. **Exchange transfusion** is occasionally employed for massive pediatric ingestion but is of questionable efficacy.

ISOCYANATES
Paul D. Blanc, MD, MSPH

ANTIDOTE   IPECAC   LAVAGE   CHARCOAL

Toluene diisocyanate (TDI), methylene diisocyante (MDI), and related chemicals are industrial components in the polymerization of urethane coatings and insulation materials. Most 2-part urethane products contain some amount of one of these chemicals. Methyl isocyanate (the toxin released in the Bhopal, India, tragedy) is a carbamate insecticide precursor; it is not used in urethanes, has actions different from those of the TDI group of chemicals, and is not discussed here (see Table IV–13, p 465).

I. Mechanism of toxicity. Toluene diisocyanate and related isocyanates act as irritants and sensitizers at very low concentrations. The mechanism is poorly understood, but it is thought that they act as haptens. Once a person is sensitized to one isocyanate, cross-reactivity to others may occur.

II. Toxic dose. The ACGIH recommended workplace short-term exposure limit (STEL) for TDI is 0.02 ppm, with a threshold limit value (TLV) of 0.005 ppm as an 8-hour time-weighted average. This exposure limit seeks to prevent acute irritant effects. However, in individuals with prior TDI sensitivity, even this level may be hazardous. The level considered immediately dangerous to life or health (IDLH) is 10 ppm.

III. Clinical presentation
    A. Acute exposure to irritant levels causes skin and upper respiratory tract toxicity. Burning eyes and skin, cough, and wheezing are common. Noncardiogenic pulmonary edema may occur with severe exposure. Symptoms may occur immediately with exposure or may occasionally be delayed several hours.

    B. Low-level chronic exposure may produce dyspnea, wheezing, and other signs and symptoms consistent with asthma. Interstitial lung injury, with radiographic infiltrates and hypoxemia, may occur less commonly.

IV. Diagnosis requires a careful occupational history. Pulmonary function testing may document an obstructive type defect or may be normal. Variable airflow or changing measures of airway reactivity (methacholine or histamine challenge) temporally linked to exposure strongly supports the diagnosis of TDI-induced asthma.
    A. Specific levels. There are no specific blood or urine tests for isocyanates.

        1. Test inhalation challenge to isocyanate is not advised except in experienced laboratories owing to the danger of severe asthma attack.

        2. Isocyanate antibody testing, although useful epidemiologically, is difficult to interpret in an individual patient.

    B. Other useful laboratory studies. Arterial blood gases or oximetry, chest x-ray, pulmonary function tests.

V. Treatment
    A. Emergency and supportive measures

        1. After acute inhalational exposure, maintain the airway (see p 4), give bronchodilators as needed for wheezing (p 9–10), and observe for 8–12 hours for pulmonary edema (p 8).

        2. When airway hyperreactivity has been documented, further exposure to isocyanate is contraindicated. Involve public health or OSHA agencies to determine if other workers are at risk.

    B. Specific drugs and antidotes. There is no specific antidote.

    C. Decontamination after high-level exposure (see p 41)

        1. Inhalation. Remove the victim from exposure, and give supplemental oxygen if available.

        2. Skin and eyes. Remove contaminated clothing (liquid or heavy vapor exposure), and wash exposed skin with copious soap and water. Irrigate exposed eyes with copious saline or tepid water.

    D. Enhanced elimination. There is no role for these procedures.

ISONIAZID (INH)
Christopher R. Brown, MD

ANTIDOTE   IPECAC   LAVAGE   CHARCOAL

Isoniazid (INH), a hydrazide derivative of isonicotinic acid, is the bactericidal drug of choice for tuberculosis. INH is well known for its propensity to cause hepatitis with chronic use. Acute isoniazid overdose is a common cause of drug-induced seizures and metabolic acidosis.

I. Mechanism of toxicity
    A. Acute overdose. Isoniazid produces acute toxic effects by competing with brain pyridoxal 5-phosphate, the active form of vitamin B_6, for the enzyme glutamic acid decarboxylase. This results in lower levels of gamma-aminobutyric acid (GABA), an inhibitory neurotransmitter in the brain, which leads to uninhibited electrical activity manifested as seizures. INH also inhibits the hepatic conversion of lactate to pyruvate, resulting in lactic acidosis.

    B. Chronic toxicity. Peripheral neuritis with chronic use is thought to be related to competition with pyridoxine. The mechanism of chronic hepatic injury and INH-induced systemic lupus erythematosus (SLE) is not discussed here.

II. Toxic dose

   A. Acute ingestion of as little as 1.5 g can produce toxicity. Severe toxicity is common after ingestion of 80–150 mg/kg.

   B. With **chronic use,** 10–20% of patients will develop hepatic toxicity when the dose is 10 mg/kg/d, but less than 2% will develop this toxicity if the dose is 3–5 mg/kg/d. Older persons are more susceptible to chronic toxicity.

III. Clinical presentation

   A. After **acute overdose,** slurred speech, ataxia, coma, and seizures may occur rapidly (usually within 30–60 minutes). Profound anion gap metabolic acidosis (pH 6.8–6.9) often occurs after only 1 or 2 seizures, probably owing to muscle release of lactic acid. This usually clears slowly even after the seizure activity is controlled. Hemolysis may occur in patients with glucose-6-phosphate dehydrogenase (G6PD) deficiency.

   B. Chronic therapeutic INH use may cause peripheral neuritis, hepatitis, hypersensitivity reactions including drug-induced lupus erythematosus, and pyridoxine deficiency.

IV. Diagnosis is usually made by history and clinical presentation. INH should be considered in any patient with acute onset seizures, especially when accompanied by profound metabolic acidosis.

   A. Specific levels. Isoniazid is not usually detected in routine toxicology screening. A 5-mg/kg dose produces a peak INH concentration of 3 mg/L at 1 hour. Serum levels higher than 30 mg/L are associated with acute toxicity.

   B. Other useful laboratory studies. Electrolytes, glucose, BUN, creatinine, liver function tests (chronic toxicity), arterial blood gases.

V. Treatment

   A. Emergency and supportive measures

      1. Maintain the airway and assist ventilation if necessary (see p 4).

      2. Treat coma (p 18), seizures (p 22), and metabolic acidosis (p 30) if they occur. Diazepam, 0.1–0.2 mg/kg IV, is usually effective for treatment of seizures.

   B. Specific drugs and antidotes. Pyridoxine (vitamin B_6) is a specific antidote and usually terminates diazepam-resistant seizures. Administer at least 5-g IV (see p 375) if the amount of INH ingested is not known; if the amount is known, give an equivalent amount in grams of pyridoxine to grams of ingested INH. If no pyridoxine is available, high-dose diazepam (0.3–0.4 mg/kg) may be effective for status epilepticus. Pyridoxine treatment may also hasten the resolution of metabolic acidosis.

   C. Decontamination (see p 44)

      1. Prehospital. Administer activated charcoal, if available. Do **not** induce emesis because of the risk of rapid onset of coma and seizures.

      2. Hospital. Administer activated charcoal and a cathartic. Consider gastric lavage for massive ingestions.

   D. Enhanced elimination. The volume of distribution of INH is 0.6 L/kg, and forced diuresis and dialysis have been reported to be successful. There is probably no role for enhanced elimination because the half-life of INH is relatively short (1–5 hours, depending on acetylator status), and toxicity can usually be easily managed with pyridoxine or diazepam.

ISOPROPYL ALCOHOL
Kent R. Olson, MD

ANTIDOTE   IPECAC   LAVAGE   CHARCOAL

Isopropyl alcohol is widely used as a solvent, an antiseptic, and a disinfectant and is commonly available in the home as a 70% solution (rubbing alcohol). It is often ingested by alcoholics as a cheap substitute for liquor. Unlike the other common alcohol substitutes methanol and ethylene glycol, isopropyl alcohol is not metabolized to highly toxic organic acids.

I. Mechanism of toxicity

A. Isopropyl alcohol is a potent depressant of the central nervous system, and intoxication by ingestion or inhalation may result in coma and respiratory arrest. It is metabolized to acetone (dimethylketone), which may contribute to and prolong central nervous system depression.

B. Very large doses of isopropyl alcohol may cause hypotension secondary to vasodilation and possibly myocardial depression.

C. Isopropyl alcohol is irritating to the gastrointestinal tract and commonly causes gastritis.

II. Toxic dose. Isopropyl alcohol is approximately twice as potent a central nervous system depressant as ethanol.

A. Ingestion. The toxic oral dose is about 0.5–1 mL/kg of rubbing alcohol (70% isopropyl alcohol) but varies depending on individual tolerance and whether any other depressants were ingested. Fatalities have occurred after adult ingestion of 240 mL, but patients with up to 1-L ingestions have recovered with supportive care.

B. Inhalation. The recommended workplace limit (ACGIH TLV-TWA) for isopropyl alcohol vapor is 400 ppm (980 mg/m^3) as an 8-hour time-weighted average. The air level considered immediately dangerous to life or health (IDLH) is 20,000 ppm. Toxicity has been reported in children after isopropyl alcohol sponge baths, probably owing mainly to inhalation as well as skin absorption.

III. Clinical presentation. Intoxication mimics drunkenness from ethanol, with slurred speech, ataxia, and stupor followed in large ingestions by coma, hypotension, and respiratory arrest.

A. Because of the gastric irritant properties of isopropyl alcohol, abdominal pain and vomiting are common, and hematemesis occasionally occurs.

B. Metabolic acidosis may occur but is usually mild. The osmolar gap is usually elevated (see p 30).

C. Isopropyl alcohol is metabolized to **acetone,** which contributes to central nervous system depression and gives a distinct odor to the breath. Acetone is also found in nail polish remover and is widely used as a solvent in industry and chemical laboratories.

IV. Diagnosis is usually based on a history of ingestion and the presence of an elevated osmolar gap, the absence of severe acidosis, and the characteristic smell of isopropyl alcohol or its metabolite acetone.

A. Specific levels. Serum isopropyl alcohol levels are usually available through commercial toxicology laboratories. The serum level may also be estimated by calculating the osmolar gap (see Table I–21, p 30). Isopropyl alcohol levels higher than 150 mg/dL usually cause coma, but patients with levels up to 560 mg/dL have survived with supportive care and dialysis. Serum acetone concentrations may be elevated.

B. Other useful laboratory studies. Electrolytes, glucose, BUN, creatinine, serum osmolality and osmolar gap, arterial blood gases or oximetry.

V. Treatment

A. Emergency and supportive measures

1. Maintain the airway and assist ventilation if necessary (see p 4). Administer supplemental oxygen.

2. Treat coma (p 18), hypotension (p 15), and hypoglycemia (p 32) if they occur.

3. Admit and observe symptomatic patients for at least 6–12 hours.

B. Specific drugs and antidotes. There is no specific antidote. Ethanol therapy is **not** indicated because isopropyl alcohol does not produce a toxic organic acid metabolite.

C. Decontamination (see p 44). Because isopropyl alcohol is rapidly absorbed after ingestion, gastric emptying procedures are not likely to be useful if the ingestion is small (a swallow or two) or if more than 30 minutes has passed. For large ingestions:

1. **Prehospital.** Administer activated charcoal, if available. Do **not** induce emesis because of the risk of rapidly developing coma.
2. **Hospital.** Administer activated charcoal and a cathartic. Although isopropyl alcohol adsorbs poorly to charcoal, approximately 1 g of charcoal will bind 1 mL of 70% alcohol. Consider gastric lavage for very large recent ingestions.

D. **Enhanced elimination**
1. **Hemodialysis** effectively removes isopropyl alcohol and acetone but is rarely indicated because the majority of patients can be managed with supportive care alone. Dialysis is indicated when levels are extremely high (eg, > 500–600 mg/dL) or if hypotension does not respond to fluids and vasopressors.
2. Hemoperfusion, repeat-dose charcoal, and forced diuresis are not effective.

JELLYFISH AND OTHER CNIDARIA
Gerald Joe, PharmD

ANTIDOTE   IPECAC   LAVAGE   CHARCOAL

The large phylum Cnidaria (coelenterates), numbering about 5,000 species, includes **fire coral, Portuguese man-of-war, box jellyfish, sea wasps, sea nettle, and anemones.** Despite considerable morphologic variation, all these organisms have venom contained in microscopic structures like water balloons called nematocysts.

I. **Mechanism of toxicity.** Each nematocyst contains a small ejectable thread soaking in viscous venom. The thread has a barb on the tip and is fired from the nematocyst with enough velocity to pierce human skin. The nematocysts are contained in outer sacs (cnidoblasts) arranged along the tentacles stretched out in the water beneath the body of the jellyfish or along the surface of fire coral and the fingerlike projections of sea anemones. When the cnidoblasts are opened by hydrostatic pressure, physical contact, changes in osmolarity, or chemical stimulants as yet unidentified, they release their nematocysts, which eject the thread and spread venom along and into the skin of the victim. The venom contains numerous chemical components, including neuromuscular toxins, cardiotoxins, hemolysins, dermonecrotoxins, and histaminelike compounds.

II. **Toxic dose.** Each time a nematocyst is opened, all the contained venom is released. The degree of effect will depend on the particular species, the number of nematocysts that successfully discharge venom, the envenomation site, contact time, and individual patient sensitivity. Hundreds of thousands of nematocysts may be discharged with a single exposure.

III. **Clinical presentation**
A. Immediately upon nematocyst discharge, there is stinging, burning pain and a pruritic rash. Depending on the degree of envenomation, there may follow paresthesias, anaphylactoid symptoms, hypotension, muscle spasm, local edema and hemolysis, papular lesions proceeding to pustules and desquamation, chills, fever, nausea, vomiting, abdominal pain, myalgias, arthralgias, headache, anxiety, diaphoresis, dysphonia, ataxia, paralysis, coma, seizures, and cardiac arrhythmias. Lethal outcomes from box jellyfish envenomation are associated with rapid onset of cardiovascular collapse.
B. Potentially severe long-lasting effects include erythema multiforme, keloids, infections, cosmetic tissue damage (fat atrophy, hyperpigmentation), contractures, paresthesias, neuritis, and paralysis.

IV. **Diagnosis** is based on the history and observation of characteristic lines of inflammation along the sites of exposure ("tentacle tracks").
A. **Specific levels.** Specific toxin levels are not available.

   B. Other useful laboratory studies. CBC, electrolytes, glucose, BUN, creatinine, creatine phosphokinase (CPK), urinalysis for hemoglobin.
V. Treatment. Symptomatic care is sufficient for the majority of envenomations, even that of the box jellyfish.
   A. Emergency and supportive measures
      1. Maintain the airway and assist ventilation if necessary (see p 4). Administer supplemental oxygen.
      2. Treat hypotension (p 15), arrhythmias (p 10–14), coma (p 18), and seizures (p 22) if they occur.
   B. Specific drugs and antidotes. Box jellyfish (*Chironex fleckeri*) antivenin from Australia terminates acute pain and cardiovascular symptoms, prevents tissue effects, and can be located by a regional poison control center (see Table I–41, p 53) for use in severe cases. Local marine biologists can help identify indigenous species for planning of specific therapy.
   C. Decontamination. Avoid thrashing about, scratching, scraping, or other mechanical maneuvers that may break open the nematocysts. With double-gloved hands, attempt to wash the affected areas with cold sea or salt water. **Do *not* use fresh water** to wash affected areas because it will cause nematocysts to be instantly discharged. Use vinegar or baking soda as described below.
      The above procedures will not relieve symptoms, but they will allow careful removal of tentacles with double-gloved hands or forceps followed by shaving of the area to remove the undischarged nematocysts.
      1. For most cnidarian envenomations, spray, soak, or flood the affected area with **vinegar** for 30 minutes to disarm nematocysts.
      2. However, for *Chrysaora quinquecirrha* (American sea nettle), *Pelagia noctiluca* (little mauve stinger jellyfish), and *Cyanea captillata* (hair jellyfish), **do *not* apply vinegar** because it may precipitate firing in these species; instead, apply a slurry of **baking soda** for 10 minutes.
   D. Enhanced elimination. These procedures are not applicable.

LEAD
Michael J. Kosnett, MD, MPH

ANTIDOTE

IPECAC

LAVAGE

CHARCOAL

Lead is a soft, malleable metal that is chiefly obtained by primary smelting and refining of natural ores. In the US, one-third of lead production results from secondary smelting of recycled lead scrap. Lead storage batteries account for most commercial use. Lead alloys are used in the production of pipes; cable sheathing; brass, bronze, and steel; ammunition; and solder (predominantly electrical devices and car radiators). Lead compounds are added as pigments, stabilizers, or binders in paints, ceramics, glass, and mortar. Tetraethyl and tetramethyl lead are added as antiknock compounds in some gasolines.
   Although the use of lead in house paint has been curtailed since the 1970s, industrial use of corrosion-resistant, lead-based paint continues, and in all settings high-level exposure may result from renovation, sandblasting, torching, or demolition. Young children are particularly at risk from repeated ingestion of lead-contaminated house dust, yard soil, or paint chips. Lead exposure may also occur from use of lead-glazed ceramics for cooking or eating, or from the consumption of food from lead-soldered cans. Certain folk medicines (eg, the Mexican remedies *azarcon* and *greta*) may contain high amounts of lead salts.
   I. Mechanism of toxicity. The multisystem toxicity of lead is mediated by at least two primary mechanisms: inhibition of enzymatic processes, sometimes as a result of sulfhydryl group binding; and interaction with essential cations, most notably

calcium, zinc, and iron. Pathologic alterations in cellular and mitochondrial membranes, neurotransmitter synthesis and function, heme synthesis, and nucleotide metabolism may occur. The primary organ systems affected are the nervous system, the kidneys, and the reproductive and hematopoietic systems.

II. Toxic dose

A. Dermal absorption is rapid and extensive for alkyl (organic) lead compounds, but minimal for inorganic lead. The LDlo (the lowest dose given over time in one or more divided portions that results in death) for dermal exposure in rabbits to tetraethyl lead is 532 mg/kg. Alkyl compounds are also moderately irritating to the skin.

B. Ingestion. Toxicity is rare after a single exposure, although intoxication has been reported after ingestion of several grams of lead acetate or tetraethyl lead or from lead curtain or fishing weights that remained in the intestinal tract for several days. Absorption from the gastrointestinal tract varies with chemical structure and solubility, and inversely with particle size. Children absorb about 50% of dietary lead, compared with 10% in adults. Low dietary intake of calcium and iron increases lead absorption; coingestion of food decreases bioavailability.

   1. The oral LDlo for lead acetate in dogs is 191 mg/kg and for lead oxide is 1300 mg/kg. Organic lead compounds exhibit greater toxicity; tetraethyl lead has an oral LDlo in rabbits of 19 mg/kg.

   2. The oral dose associated with the lowest observable effect level (LOEL) in humans is uncertain, but in a 21-day chronic ingestion study, 20 μg/kg/day increased the blood lead level from 15 μg/dL to 40 μg/dL with a concomitant increase in erythrocyte protoporphyrin.

   3. Acute human ingestion of 15 g of lead oxide has resulted in death. Ingestion of a single fishing weight or curtain weight has caused encephalopathy and death.

   4. The US EPA recommended maximum contaminant level for lead in drinking water is 20 ppb (parts per billion).

C. Inhalation. The OSHA permissible exposure limit (PEL) for workplace exposure to inorganic lead dusts and fumes is 0.05 mg/m^3 as an 8-hour time-weighted average; and the level considered immediately dangerous to life or health (IDLH) is 700 mg/m^3. The PEL for tetraethyl lead is 0.075 mg/m^3; and the IDLH for tetraethyl lead is 40 mg/m^3.

III. Clinical presentation. The multisystem toxicity of lead presents a spectrum of clinical findings ranging from overt, life-threatening intoxication to subtle, subclinical effects.

A. Acute ingestion of a very large amount of lead (gram quantities) may cause abdominal pain, anemia (usually hemolytic), and toxic hepatitis.

B. Subacute or chronic intoxication is more common than acute poisoning.

   1. Constitutional symptoms include fatigue, malaise, irritability, anorexia, insomnia, weight loss, loss of libido, arthralgias, and myalgias. Hypertension may be associated with lead exposure in susceptible populations.

   2. Gastrointestinal symptoms include nausea, constipation or diarrhea, and crampy abdominal pain (lead colic).

   3. Central nervous system manifestations range from impaired concentration, headache, and diminished visual-motor coordination to overt encephalopathy (a life-threatening emergency characterized by hyperirritability, ataxia, delirium, convulsions, and coma). Chronic low-level exposure in children may result in decreased intelligence and impaired neurobehavioral development, decreased growth, and diminished auditory acuity.

   4. Peripheral motor neuropathy, affecting mainly the upper extremities, can cause severe extensor muscle weakness ("wrist drop").

   5. Hematologic effects include normochromic or microcytic anemia, which may be accompanied by basophilic stippling. Hemolysis may occur.

   6. Nephrotoxic effects include reversible acute tubular dysfunction (including

Fanconi-like aminoaciduria in children), and chronic interstitial fibrosis. Hyperuricemia and gout may occur.

7. **Adverse reproductive outcomes** include diminished or aberrant sperm production, increased rate of miscarriage, decreased gestational age, low birth weight, and impaired neurologic development.

C. **Repeated, intentional inhalation of leaded gasoline** has resulted in ataxia, myoclonic jerking, hyperreflexia, delirium, and convulsions.

IV. **Diagnosis.** Although overt encephalopathy and abdominal colic associated with a suspect activity may readily suggest the diagnosis of severe lead poisoning, the nonspecific symptoms and multisystem signs associated with mild or moderate intoxication may be mistaken for a viral illness or other disorder. Consider lead poisoning in any patient with multisystem findings including abdominal pain, headache, and anemia, and less commonly, motor neuropathy, gout, and renal insufficiency. Consider lead encephalopathy in any child with delirium or convulsions, and chronic lead poisoning in any child with neurobehavioral deficits or developmental delays.

A. **Specific levels.** The **whole blood lead** level is the most useful indicator of lead exposure. Relationships between blood lead levels and clinical findings have generally been based on subacute or chronic exposure and not on transiently high values that may result immediately after acute exposure. In addition, there may be considerable interindividual variability. *Note:* In order to prevent false elevation owing to contamination by the container, blood lead samples must be drawn and stored in lead-free syringes and tubes ("trace metals" tube or royal blue stopper tube containing heparin or EDTA).

1. Blood lead levels are less than 10 μg/dL in populations without occupational or specific environmental exposure. Levels between 10 and 25 μg/dL have been associated with decreased intelligence and impaired neurobehavioral development in children exposed in utero or in early childhood, but these levels are generally without demonstrable toxic effects in adults.

2. Blood lead levels of 25–60 μg/dL may be associated with headache, irritability, difficulty concentrating, slowed reaction time, and other neuropsychiatric effects. Anemia may occur, and subclinical slowing of motor nerve conduction may be detectable.

3. Blood levels of 60–80 μg/dL may be associated with gastrointestinal symptoms and subclinical renal effects.

4. With blood levels in excess of 80 μg/dL, serious overt intoxication may occur, including abdominal pain (lead colic) and nephropathy. Encephalopathy and neuropathy are usually associated with levels over 100 μg/dL.

B. Elevations in **free erythrocyte protoporphyrin (FEP) or zinc protoporphyrin (ZPP)** (> 35 μg/dL) reflect lead-induced inhibition of heme synthesis. Because only actively forming and not mature erythrocytes are affected, elevations will typically lag lead exposure by a few weeks. A high blood lead in the presence of a normal FEP or ZPP therefore suggests very recent exposure. Protoporphyrin elevation is not specific for lead, and may also occur with iron deficiency. Protoporphyrin levels are not sensitive for low-level exposure (blood lead < 30 μg/dL).

C. **Urinary lead excretion** increases and decreases more rapidly than blood lead. Normal urinary lead excretion is less than 50 μg/d. Several empiric protocols that measure 6- or 24-hour urinary lead excretion following EDTA challenge have been developed to identify persons with elevated body lead burdens; however, chelatable lead predominantly reflects lead in soft tissues, which in most cases correlates satisfactorily with blood lead concentration.

D. Noninvasive in vivo **x-ray fluorescence measurement of lead in bone** is an emerging research method that may provide the best index of long-term cumulative lead exposure and total body lead burden.

E. **Other tests.** Nonspecific laboratory findings that support the diagnosis of lead poisoning include anemia (normocytic or microcytic), basophilic stippling of erythrocytes, and increased urinary coproporphyrin and aminolevulinic acid (ALA). Recently ingested lead paint, glazes, chips, or lead weights may be visible on abdominal x-ray.

V. Treatment

A. Emergency and supportive measures

1. Treat seizures (see p 22) and coma (see p 18) if they occur. Provide adequate fluids to maintain urine flow but avoid overhydration, which may aggravate cerebral edema.

2. Patients with increased intracranial pressure may benefit from corticosteroids (eg, dexamethasone, 10 mg IV) and mannitol (1–2 g/kg IV).

B. Specific drugs and antidotes.
Treatment with chelating agents decreases blood lead concentrations and increases urinary excretion. Although chelation has been associated with improvement in symptoms and decreased mortality, controlled clinical trials demonstrating efficacy are lacking, and **treatment recommendations have been largely empiric**.

1. **Encephalopathy.** Administer **calcium EDTA** (see p 335). Some clinicians initiate treatment with a single dose of **BAL** (see p 317), followed 4 hours later by concomitant administration of calcium EDTA and BAL.

2. **Symptomatic intoxication without encephalopathy.** Administer oral **DMSA** (see p 332) or parenteral **calcium EDTA** (see p 335). EDTA is preferred as initial treatment if the patient has severe gastrointestinal toxicity (eg, lead colic).

3. **Asymptomatic children with elevated blood lead levels.** The Centers for Disease Control recommends treatment of children with levels of 45 µg/dL or higher. Use oral **DMSA** (see p 332). There is not yet a consensus on use of chelation for levels less than 45 µg/dL.

4. **Asymptomatic adults.** The usual treatment is removal from exposure and observation. Consider oral DMSA (see p 332) for patients with markedly elevated levels (eg, > 80–100 µg/dL).

5. Although d-penicillamine (see p 366) is an alternative oral treatment, it may be associated with more side effects and less efficient lead diuresis.

C. Decontamination (see p 41)

1. **Acute ingestion.** Because even small items (eg, a paint chip, a sip of lead-containing glaze) may contain several hundred milligrams of lead, gut decontamination is indicated following acute ingestion of virtually any lead-containing substance.

   a. Induce emesis with syrup of ipecac, or perform gastric lavage.

   b. Administer activated charcoal (although efficacy is unknown).

   c. After ingestion of a metallic lead object (fishing or curtain weight), administer activated charcoal and a cathartic.

   d. If lead-containing material is still visible on abdominal x-ray after initial treatment, consider whole bowel irrigation (see p 48), repeated cathartics, or enemas.

2. **Lead-containing buckshot, shrapnel, or bullets** in or adjacent to synovial spaces should be surgically removed if possible, particularly if associated with evidence of systemic lead absorption.

D. Enhanced elimination.
There is no role for dialysis, hemoperfusion, or repeat-dose charcoal.

E. Other required measures

1. Remove the patient from the source of exposure, and institute control measures to prevent repeated intoxication; in addition, other possibly exposed persons should be promptly evaluated.

2. Federal OSHA standards for workers exposed to lead provide specific guidelines for periodic blood lead monitoring and medical surveillance. Under the general industry standard, workers must be removed from exposure if a single blood lead level exceeds 60 µg/dL or if the average of 3 successive monthly levels exceeds 50 µg/dL. In construction workers, re-

moval is required if a single blood lead level exceeds 50 μg/dL. Workers may not return to work until the blood lead level is below 40 μg/dL and any clinical manifestations of toxicity have resolved.

LIONFISH AND OTHER SCORPAENIDAE
Kent R. Olson, MD

ANTIDOTE   IPECAC   LAVAGE   CHARCOAL

The family Scorpaenidae are saltwater fish that are mostly bottom dwellers, noted for their ability to camouflage themselves and disappear into the environment. There are 30 genera and about 300 species, some 30 of which have envenomated humans. Although they were once considered to be only an occupational hazard of commercial fishing, increasing contact with these fish by scuba divers and home aquarists has increased the frequency of envenomations.

I. **Mechanism of toxicity.** Envenomation usually occurs when the fish is being handled or stepped on or when the aquarist has hands in the tank. The dorsal, anal, and pectoral fins are supported by spines that are connected to venom glands. The fish will erect its spines and jab the victim, causing release of venom (and often sloughing of the integumentary sheath of the spine into the wound). The venom of all these organisms is a heat-labile mixture that is not completely characterized.

II. **Toxic dose.** The dose of venom involved in any sting is variable. Interspecies variation in the severity of envenomation is generally the result of the relation between the venom gland and the spines.
   A. **Synanceja** (Australian stonefish) have short, strong spines with the venom gland located near the tip; therefore, large doses of venom are delivered and severe envenomation results.
   B. **Pterois** (lionfish, turkeyfish) have long delicate spines with poorly developed venom glands near the base of the spine and therefore are capable of delivering only small doses of venom.

III. **Clinical presentation.** Envenomation typically produces immediate onset of excruciating, sharp, throbbing, intense pain. In untreated cases, the intensity of pain peaks at 60–90 minutes and may last for 1–2 days.
   A. **Systemic intoxication** typically associated with stonefish envenomation is characterized by the rapid onset of hypotension, tachycardia, cardiac arrhythmias, myocardial ischemia, syncope, diaphoresis, nausea, vomiting, abdominal cramping, dyspnea, pulmonary edema, cyanosis, headache, muscular weakness, and spasticity.
   B. **Local tissue effects** include erythema, ecchymosis, and swelling. Infection may occur owing to retained integumentary sheath. Hyperalgesia, anesthesia, or paresthesias of the affected extremity may occur, and persistent neuropathy has been reported.

IV. **Diagnosis** is usually based on a history of exposure, and the severity of envenomation is usually readily apparent.
   A. **Specific levels.** There are no specific toxin levels available.
   B. **Other useful laboratory studies.** Severe intoxication: electrolytes, glucose, BUN, creatinine, creatine phosphokinase (CPK), urinalysis, ECG monitoring, chest x-ray.

V. **Treatment**
   A. **Emergency and supportive measures**
      1. After severe stonefish envenomation:
         a. Maintain the airway and assist ventilation if needed (see p 4). Administer supplemental oxygen.

      b. Treat hypotension (p 15) and arrhythmias (p 10–14) if they occur.
    2. General wound care:
      a. Clean the wound carefully and remove any visible integumentary sheath. Monitor wounds for development of infection.
      b. Give tetanus prophylaxis if needed.
  B. Specific drugs and antidotes. Immediately immerse the extremity in **hot water** (45 °C or 113 °F) for 30–60 minutes. This should result in prompt relief of pain. For stonefish envenomations, a specific antivenin can be located by a regional poison control center (see Table I–41, p 53), but most of these cases can be successfully managed with hot water immersion and supportive symptomatic care.
  C. Decontamination procedures are not applicable.
  D. Enhanced elimination. There is no role for these procedures.

LITHIUM
Neal L. Benowitz, MD

ANTIDOTE   IPECAC   LAVAGE   CHARCOAL

Lithium is used for the treatment of bipolar depression and other psychiatric disorders and occasionally to boost the white blood cell count in patients with leukopenia. Serious toxicity is most commonly caused by chronic overmedication in patients with renal impairment. Acute overdose, in contrast, is generally less severe.

I. Mechanism of toxicity
  A. Lithium is a cation that enters cells and substitutes for sodium or potassium. Lithium is thought to stabilize cell membranes. With excessive levels, it depresses neural excitation and synaptic transmission.
  B. Pharmacokinetics. Lithium is completely absorbed within 6–8 hours of ingestion. The initial volume of distribution (Vd) is about 0.5 L/kg, with slow entry into tissues and a final Vd of 0.7–0.9 L/kg. Entry into the brain is slow, which explains the delay between peak blood levels and central nervous system effects after acute overdose. Elimination is virtually entirely by the kidney, with a half-life of 14–30 hours.

II. Toxic dose. The usual daily dose of lithium ranges from 300 to 2400 mg/d (8–64 meq/d), and the therapeutic serum lithium level is 0.6–1.2 meq/L. The toxicity of lithium depends on whether the overdose is acute or chronic.
  A. Acute ingestion of 1 meq/kg (40 mg/kg) will produce a blood level at equilibrium of approximately 1.2 meq/L. Acute ingestion of more than 20–30 tablets by an adult would potentially cause serious toxicity.
  B. Chronic intoxication may occur in patients on stable therapeutic doses. Lithium is excreted by the kidney, where it is handled like sodium; any state that causes dehydration, sodium depletion, or excessive sodium reabsorption may lead to increased lithium reabsorption, accumulation, and possibly intoxication. Common states causing lithium retention include acute gastroenteritis, diuretic use, and lithium-induced nephrogenic diabetes insipidus.

III. Clinical presentation. Mild to moderate intoxication results in lethargy, muscular weakness, slurred speech, ataxia, tremor, and myoclonic jerks. Rigidity and extrapyramidal effects may be seen. Severe intoxication may result in agitated delirium, coma, convulsions, and hyperthermia. Recovery is often very slow, and patients may remain confused or obtunded for several days to weeks. The ECG commonly shows T-wave inversions; less commonly, bradycardia and sinus node arrest may occur. The white cell count is often elevated (15–20,000/mm^3).
  A. Acute ingestion may cause initial mild nausea and vomiting, but systemic signs of intoxication are minimal and usually are delayed for several hours

while lithium distributes into tissues. Initially high serum levels fall by 50–70% or more with tissue equilibration.

B. In contrast, patients with **chronic intoxication** usually have already have systemic manifestations on admission, and toxicity may be severe with levels only slightly above therapeutic. Typically, patients with chronic intoxication have elevated BUN and creatinine levels and other evidence of dehydration or renal insufficiency.

C. Nephrogenic diabetes insipidus (see p 33) is a recognized complication of chronic lithium therapy, and may lead to dehydration and hypernatremia.

IV. Diagnosis. Lithium intoxication should be suspected in any patient with a known psychiatric history who is confused, ataxic, or tremulous.

A. Specific levels. The diagnosis is supported by an elevated **lithium** level.

  1. Most hospital clinical laboratories can perform a stat serum lithium concentration. However, the serum lithium level is not an accurate predictor of toxicity.

    a. With chronic poisoning, toxicity may be associated with levels only slightly above the therapeutic range.

    b. On the other hand, peak levels as high as 9.3 meq/L have been reported early after acute ingestion without signs of intoxication, owing to measurement before final tissue distribution.

    c. *Note:* Specimens obtained in a green-top tube (lithium heparin) will give a markedly false elevation of the serum lithium level.

  2. Cerebrospinal fluid lithium levels higher than 0.4 meq/L were associated in one case report with central nervous system toxicity.

B. Other useful laboratory studies. Electrolytes (the anion gap may be narrowed owing to elevated chloride or bicarbonate), glucose, BUN, creatinine, ECG monitoring.

V. Treatment

A. Emergency and supportive measures

  1. In obtunded patients, maintain the airway and assist ventilation if necessary (see p 4). Administer supplemental oxygen.

  2. Treat coma (p 18), seizures (p 22), and hyperthermia (p 20) if they occur.

  3. In dehydrated patients, replace fluid deficits with intravenous crystalloid solutions. Initial treatment should include repletion of sodium and water with 1–2 L of normal saline (children: 10–20 mL/kg). Once fluid deficits are replaced, give hypotonic (eg, half-normal saline) solutions because continued administration of normal saline may lead to hypernatremia, especially in patients with nephrogenic diabetes insipidus.

B. Specific drugs and antidotes. There is no specific antidote. Thiazides and indomethacin have been used for treatment of nephrogenic diabetes insipidus (see p 33).

C. Decontamination (see p 44) measures are appropriate after acute ingestion but not chronic intoxication.

  1. Prehospital. Ipecac-induced emesis may be useful for initial treatment at the scene (eg, children at home) if it can be given within a few minutes of exposure.

  2. Hospital. Induce emesis or perform gastric lavage. Activated charcoal does not adsorb lithium but may be useful if other drug ingestion is suspected.

  3. Whole bowel irrigation (p 48) may enhance gut decontamination, especially in cases involving sustained-release preparations that do not dissolve readily during the lavage procedure.

D. Enhanced elimination. (See p 49) Lithium is excreted exclusively by the kidney. The clearance is about 25% of the glomerular filtration rate and is reduced by sodium depletion or dehydration.

  1. Hemodialysis removes lithium effectively and is indicated for intoxicated patients with seizures or severely abnormal mental status and for patients unable to excrete lithium renally (ie, anephric or anuric patients). Repeated and prolonged dialysis may be necessary because of slow movement of lithium out of the central nervous system.

2. Forced diuresis only slightly increases lithium excretion compared with normal hydration and is not recommended. However, establishing normal urine output may bring the urinary lithium clearance to 25–30 mL/min.

3. Hemoperfusion and repeat-dose charcoal are not effective.

LOMOTIL
Ilene B. Anderson, PharmD

ANTIDOTE   IPECAC   LAVAGE   CHARCOAL

Lomotil is a combination product containing diphenoxylate and atropine that is commonly prescribed for symptomatic treatment of diarrhea (Motofen is another product with similar ingredients). Children are especially sensitive to small doses of Lomotil and may develop delayed toxicity after accidental ingestion.

I. Mechanism of toxicity

  A. Diphenoxylate is an opioid analogue of meperidine. It is metabolized to difenoxin, which has 5 times the antidiarrheal activity of diphenoxylate. Both agents have opioid effects (see p 238) in overdose.

  B. Atropine is an anticholinergic agent (see p 75) that may contribute to lethargy and coma. It also slows drug absorption and may delay the onset of symptoms.

II. Toxic dose. The toxic dose of Lomotil is difficult to predict because of wide individual variability in response to drug effects and promptness of treatment. The lethal dose is unknown, but death in children has been reported after ingestion of **fewer than 5 tablets.**

III. Clinical presentation. Depending on the individual and the time since ingestion, manifestations may be of primarily anticholinergic or opioid intoxication.

  A. Atropine intoxication may occur before, during, or after opioid effects. Anticholinergic effects include: lethargy or agitation, flushed face, dry mucous membranes, mydriasis (dilated pupils), ileus, hyperpyrexia, and tachycardia.

  B. Opioid intoxication produces small pupils, coma, and respiratory arrest, and the onset of these effects is often delayed for several hours after ingestion.

IV. Diagnosis is based on the history and signs of anticholinergic or opioid intoxication.

  A. Specific levels. Specific serum levels are not available.

  B. Other useful laboratory studies. Electrolytes, glucose, arterial blood gases (if respiratory insufficiency is suspected).

V. Treatment

  A. Emergency and supportive measures

    1. Maintain the airway and assist ventilation if necessary (see p 4).

    2. Treat coma (p 18) and hypotension (p 15) if they occur.

    3. Because of the danger of abrupt respiratory arrest, observe all children with Lomotil ingestion in an intensive care unit for 18–24 hours.

  B. Specific drugs and antidotes

    1. Administer **naloxone,** 1–2 mg IV (see p 355), to patients with lethargy, apnea, or coma. Repeated doses of naloxone may be required, because its duration of effect (2–3 hours) is much shorter than that of Lomotil.

    2. There is no evidence that **physostigmine** (see p 370) is beneficial for this overdose, although theoretically it may reverse signs of anticholinergic poisoning.

  C. Decontamination (see p 44)

1. **Prehospital.** Administer activated charcoal, if available. Ipecac-induced emesis may be useful for initial treatment at the scene (eg, children at home) if it can be given within 30 minutes of exposure.

2. **Hospital.** Administer activated charcoal and a cathartic. Gastric emptying is not necessary following a small ingestion if activated charcoal can be given promptly.

D. **Enhanced elimination.** There is no role for these procedures.

LYSERGIC ACID DIETHYLAMIDE (LSD) AND OTHER HALLUCINOGENS
Karl A. Sporer, MD

ANTIDOTE   IPECAC   LAVAGE   CHARCOAL

Patients seeking medical care after self-administering mind-altering substances may have used any of a large variety of chemicals. Several of these agents are discussed elsewhere in this manual (eg, amphetamines [p 66], cocaine [p 138], phencyclidine [p 248], toluene [p 298]). The drugs discussed in this section, LSD and other hallucinogens, have become known in some circles as entactogens ("to touch within"), and several have been widely used for personal experimentation as well as clinically to facilitate psychotherapeutic interviews. Table II–31 lists some of the more common entactogens.

I. **Mechanism of toxicity.** Despite many intriguing theories and much current research, the biochemical mechanism of entactogenesis is not known. LSD and many other agents are thought to alter the activity of serotonin and dopamine in the brain. Central and peripheral sympathetic stimulation may account for some of the side effects such as anxiety, psychosis, dilated pupils, and hyperthermia.

II. **Toxic dose.** The toxic dose is highly variable depending on the agent and the circumstances (Table II–31). In general, entactogenic effects do not appear to be dose-related; therefore, increasing the dose does not intensify the desired effects. Likewise, paranoia or panic attacks may occur with any dose and depend on the surroundings and the patient's current emotional state. On the other hand, hallucinations, visual illusions, and sympathomimetic side effects are dose-related. The toxic dose may be only slightly greater than the therapeutic dose.

III. **Clinical presentation**

A. **Mild to moderate intoxication**

1. The person experiencing a "bad trip" is conscious, coherent, and oriented but is anxious and fearful and may display paranoid or bizarre reasoning. The patient may also be tearful, combative, or self-destructive. Delayed intermittent "flashbacks" may occur after the acute effects have worn off and are usually precipitated by use of another mind-altering drug.

2. The person with dose-related sympathomimetic side effects may also exhibit tachycardia, mydriasis (dilated pupils), diaphoresis, bruxism, short attention span, tremor, hyperreflexia, hypertension, and fever.

B. **Life-threatening toxicity**

1. This results from intense sympathomimetic stimulation and includes seizures, severe hyperthermia, hypertension, and cardiac arrhythmias. Hyperthermic patients are usually obtunded, agitated or thrashing about, diaphoretic, and hyperreflexic. Untreated, hyperthermia may result in hypotension, coagulopathy, rhabdomyolysis, and multiple organ failure (see p 20). Hyperthermia has been associated with LSD, MDA, MDMA, and PMA.

TABLE II–31. EXAMPLES OF HALLUCINOGENS AND ENTACTOGENS

Drug or Compound	Common Name	Comments
5-Hydroxy-N,N-dimethyltryptamine	Bufotenine	From skin secretions of the toad *Bufo vulgaris*.
N,N-dimethyltryptamine	DMT	"Businessman's trip": short duration (30–60 minutes).
2,5-Dimethoxy-4-bromo-amphetamine[a]	DOB	Potent ergotlike vascular spasm may result in ischemia, gangrene.
2,5-Dimethoxy-4-methyl-amphetamine[a]	DOM, STP	Potent sympathomimetic.
4,9-Dihydro-7-methoxy-1-methyl-3-pyrido(3,4)-indole	Harmaline	South American drink yage or ayahuasca.
Lysergic acid diethylamide	LSD, acid	Potent hallucinogen. Average dose 50–150 μg.
n-Methyl-1-(1,3-benzodioxol-5-yl)-2-butanamine	MBDB	Nearly pure entactogen without hallucinosis or sympathomimetic stimulation.
3,4-Methylenedioxy-amphetamine[a]	MDA	Potent sympathomimetic. Several hyperthermic deaths reported.
3–4-Methylenedioxy-methamphetamine[a]	MDMA, ecstasy, Adam	Sympathomimetic; hyperthermia reported.
3,4-Methylenedioxy-n-ethylamphetamine[a]	MDE, Eve	
3,4,5-Trimethoxyphenethylamine	Mescaline	Derived from peyote cactus.
3-Methoxy-4,5-methylene-dioxyallylbenzene	Myristicin, nutmeg	
p-Methoxyamphetamine[a]	PMA	
4-Phosphoryloxy-N-N-dimethyltryptamine	Psilocybin	From *Psilocybe* mushrooms.

[a]Amphetamine derivatives. See also p 66.

2. Use of 2,5-dimethoxy-4-bromoamphetamine (DOB) has resulted in ergotlike vascular spasm, circulatory insufficiency, and gangrene (see pp 66 and 158).

IV. Diagnosis is based on a history of use and the presence of signs of sympathetic stimulation. Diagnosis of hyperthermia requires a high level of suspicion and use of a thermometer that accurately measures core temperature (rectal, tympanic membrane, or esophageal probe).

A. Specific levels. Serum drug levels are neither widely available nor clinically useful in emergency management. The amphetamine derivatives (DOB, STP, MDA, MDMA, etc) will cross-react in screening procedures for amphetamine class drugs. However, LSD and the other nonamphetamine hallucinogens listed in Table II–31 are not identified on routine toxicology screening.

B. Other useful laboratory studies. Electrolytes, glucose, BUN, creatinine. In hyperthermic patients: obtain prothrombin time, creatine phosphokinase (CPK), urinalysis dipstick for occult blood (myoglobinuria will be positive).

V. Treatment

A. Emergency and supportive measures

1. For the patient with a "bad trip" or panic reaction, provide gentle reassurance and relaxation techniques in a quiet environment. Treat agitation (see p 23) or severe anxiety states with diazepam (see p 327) or midazolam (p 353). Butyrophenones such as haloperidol (p 343) or droperidol are useful despite a small theoretic risk of lowering the seizure threshold.

2. Treat seizures (p 22), hyperthermia (p 20), rhabdomyolysis (p 25), hypertension (p 17), and cardiac arrhythmias (p 14) if they occur.

B. Specific drugs and antidotes. There is no specific antidote. Sedating doses of **diazepam** (2–10 mg) may alleviate anxiety, and hypnotic doses (10–20 mg) can induce sleep for the duration of the "trip" (usually 4–10 hours).

C. Decontamination (see p 44). Most of these drugs are taken orally in small doses.

1. **Prehospital.** Administer activated charcoal, if available. In general, do **not** induce emesis, because it is relatively ineffective and is likely to aggravate psychologic distress. Emesis might be performed after a recent massive ingestion if there is no charcoal available and hospital transport will take more than 30 minutes.

2. **Hospital.** Administer activated charcoal and a cathartic. There is no need for gastric lavage, unless massive ingestion is suspected or the person is unable or unwilling to ingest the charcoal.

D. Enhanced elimination. These procedures are not useful. Although urinary acidification may increase the urine concentration of some agents, it does not significantly enhance total body elimination, and may aggravate myoglobinuric renal failure.

MAGNESIUM
Kathryn H. Meier, PharmD

ANTIDOTE   IPECAC   LAVAGE   CHARCOAL

Magnesium (Mg) is a divalent cation required for a variety of enzymatic reactions involving protein synthesis and carbohydrate metabolism. It is also an essential ion for proper neuromuscular functioning. Oral magnesium is widely available in over-the-counter antacids (eg, Maalox, Mylanta) and carthartics (milk of magnesia, magnesium citrate). Intravenous magnesium is used to treat toxemia of pregnancy, polymorphous ventricular tachycardia, refractory ventricular arrhythmias, and rarely, bronchospasm.

I. Mechanism of toxicity
A. Elevated serum magnesium concentrations act as a central nervous system depressant and block neuromuscular transmission, perhaps by inhibiting acetylcholine release at the motor endplate.
B. Hypermagnesemia amplifies the response to neuromuscular blockers.
C. Large doses of orally administered magnesium cause diarrhea. Repeated or excessive doses of cathartics can cause serious fluid and electrolyte abnormalities.

II. Toxic dose.
Only about 30% of orally administered magnesium is absorbed from the gastrointestinal tract, and excess magnesium is usually rapidly excreted by the kidneys. Hypermagnesemia rarely occurs after acute or chronic overexposure except in patients with renal insufficiency or massive overdose.
A. Commonly available antacids (eg, Maalox, Mylanta, others) contain 12.5–37.5 meq of magnesium per 15 mL (one tablespoon), milk of magnesia contains about 40 meq per 15 mL, and magnesium sulfate contains 8 meq per g.
B. Ingestion of 200 g of magnesium sulfate (1600 meq magnesium) caused coma in a young woman with normal renal function.

III. Clinical presentation.
Moderate toxicity may cause nausea, vomiting, weakness, and cutaneous flushing. Larger doses can cause cardiac conduction abnormalities, hypotension, severe muscle weakness, and lethargy. Very high levels can cause coma, respiratory arrest, and asystole (see Table II–32).

IV. Diagnosis
should be suspected in a patient with renal insufficiency who presents with weakness or hypotonia and a history of using magnesium-containing antacids or cathartics.
A. Specific levels. Serum magnesium concentration is usually rapidly available. The normal range is 1.5–2.2 meq/L. Therapeutic levels for treatment of toxemia of pregnancy (eclampsia) are 2.5–5 meq/L.
B. Other useful laboratory studies. Electrolytes, BUN, creatinine, serum osmolality and osmolar gap (magnesium may elevate the osmolar gap), calcium, ECG.

V. Treatment
A. Emergency and supportive measures
   1. Maintain the airway and assist ventilation if necessary (see p 44).
   2. Replace fluid and electrolyte losses caused by excessive catharsis.
   3. Treat hypotension with intravenous fluids and dopamine (see p 15).
B. Specific drugs and antidotes. There is no specific antidote. Administration of intravenous **calcium** (see p 323) may temporarily alleviate respiratory depression.
C. Decontamination (see p 44)
   1. Prehospital. Ipecac-induced emesis may be useful for initial treatment at the scene (eg, children at home) if it can be given within a few minutes of exposure.
   2. Hospital. Consider gastric lavage for large recent ingestions. Do **not** administer a cathartic. Activated charcoal is not effective.
D. Enhanced elimination

TABLE II–32. MAGNESIUM POISONING

Magnesium Serum Levels (meq/L)	Symptoms
> 3	Nausea, vomiting, weakness, cutaneous flushing
> 5	ECG changes—prolonged PR, QRS, QT intervals
7–10	Hypotension, loss of deep tendon reflexes, sedation
> 10	Muscle paralysis, respiratory arrest, hypotension, arrhythmias
> 14	Death from respiratory arrest or asystole

1. **Hemodialysis** rapidly removes magnesium and is the only route of elimination in anuric patients.
2. Hemoperfusion and repeat-dose charcoal are not effective.

MANGANESE
Paul D. Blanc, MD, MSPH

Manganese intoxication is generally caused by chronic rather than acute exposure. Sources of exposure are almost universally industrial—mining, metal working, smelting, foundries, and welding. Recent studies also suggest a possible link between an organic manganese fungicide (maneb) and chronic neurologic toxicity.

I. **Mechanism of toxicity.** The precise mechanism is not known. The central nervous system is the target organ, and enzymatic inhibition leading to neurotransmitter imbalance is suspected.

II. **Toxic dose.** The primary route of exposure is inhalation; inorganic manganese is poorly absorbed from the gastrointestinal tract. The OSHA workplace permissible exposure limit (PEL) for manganese dusts is 5 mg/m^3. The air level considered to be immediately dangerous to life or health (IDLH) is 10,000 ppm.

III. **Clinical presentation.** Acute high-level manganese inhalation can produce an irritant-type pneumonitis (see p 176). More typically, toxicity occurs after chronic exposure to low levels over months or years. The patient usually presents with an effective psychiatric disorder, frequently misdiagnosed as schizophrenia or atypical psychosis. Organic signs of neurologic toxicity, such as parkinsonism or other extrapyramidal movement disorders, usually appear later, some time after a primarily psychiatric presentation.

IV. **Diagnosis** depends on a thorough occupational and psychiatric history.
   A. **Specific levels.** Testing of whole blood, serum, or urine may be performed, but the results should be interpreted with caution, as they may not correlate with clinical effects.
   1. Normal serum manganese concentrations are usually less than 1.2 µg/L.
   2. Elevated urine manganese concentrations (> 25 µg/L) may confirm recent acute exposure. Chelation challenge does not have a role in diagnosis.
   3. Hair and nail levels are not useful.
   B. **Other useful laboratory studies.** Arterial blood gases or oximetry, chest x-ray (after acute, heavy, symptomatic inhalation exposure).

V. **Treatment**
   A. **Emergency and supportive measures**
   1. **Acute inhalation.** Administer supplemental oxygen. Treat bronchospasm (see p 9–10) and noncardiogenic pulmonary edema (see p 8) if they occur.
   2. **Chronic intoxication.** Psychiatric and neurologic effects are treated with the usual psychiatric and antiparkinsonian drugs.
   B. **Specific drugs and antidotes.** EDTA and other chelators have **not** been proved effective after chronic neurologic damage has occurred. The efficacy of chelators early after acute exposure has not been studied.
   C. **Decontamination** (see p 41)
   1. **Acute inhalation.** Remove victim from exposure and give supplemental oxygen, if available.
   2. **Ingestion.** Because inorganic manganese is so poorly absorbed from the gastrointestinal tract, gut decontamination is probably not necessary. For massive ingestions, particularly of organic compounds (eg, Maneb), gastric lavage and activated charcoal may be appropriate but have not been studied.

D. Enhanced elimination. There is no known role for dialysis or hemoperfusion.

MARIJUANA
Neil L. Benowitz, MD

ANTIDOTE   IPECAC   LAVAGE   CHARCOAL

Marijuana consists of the leaves and flowering parts of the plant *Cannabis sativa* and is usually smoked in cigarettes ("joints" or "reefers") or pipes or added to food (usually cookies or brownies). Resin from the plant may be dried and compressed into blocks called hashish. Marijuana contains a number of cannabinoids; the primary psychoactive one is delta-9-tetrahydrocannabinol (THC). THC is also available in capsule form as an experimental treatment for emesis associated with cancer chemotherapy and for glaucoma.

I. **Mechanism of toxicity.** THC may have stimulant, sedative, or hallucinogenic actions depending on the dose and time after consumption. Both catecholamine release (resulting in tachycardia) and inhibition of sympathetic reflexes (resulting in orthostatic hypotension) may be observed.

II. **Toxic dose.** Typical marijuana cigarettes contain 1–3% THC, but more potent varieties may contain up to 15% THC. Hashish contains 3–6% and hashish oil 30–50% THC. Toxicity is dose-related, but there is much individual variability, influenced in part by prior experience and degree of tolerance.

III. **Clinical presentation**

A. **Subjective effects** after smoking a marijuana cigarette include euphoria, palpitations, heightened sensory awareness, and altered time perception followed after about 30 minutes by sedation. More severe intoxication may result in impaired short-term memory, depersonalization, visual hallucinations, and acute paranoid psychosis. Occasionally, even with low doses of THC, subjective effects may precipitate a panic reaction.

B. **Physical findings** may include tachycardia, orthostatic hypotension, conjunctival injection, incoordination, slurred speech, and ataxia. Stupor with pallor, conjunctival injection, fine tremor, and ataxia have been observed in children after eating marijuana cookies.

C. **Other health problems** include salmonellosis and pulmonary aspergillosis from use of contaminated marijuana. Marijuana may be contaminated by paraquat, but the latter is destroyed by pyrolysis and there have been no reports of paraquat toxicity from smoking marijuana.

D. **Intravenous use** of marijuana extract or hash oil may cause dyspnea, abdominal pain, fever, shock, disseminated intravascular coagulation, acute renal failure, and death.

IV. **Diagnosis** is usually based on the history and typical findings such as tachycardia and conjunctival injection combined with evidence of altered mood or cognitive function.

A. **Specific levels.** Blood levels are not commonly available. Cannabinoid metabolites may be detected in the urine by enzyme immunoassay for up to several days after single acute exposure or weeks after chronic THC exposure. Urine levels do not correlate with degree of intoxication or functional impairment.

B. **Other useful laboratory studies.** Electrolytes, glucose.

V. **Treatment**

A. **Emergency and supportive measures**

1. Most psychologic disturbances may be managed by simple reassurance, possibly with adjunctive use of diazepam (see p 327) or midazolam (p 353).

2. Sinus tachycardia usually does not require treatment but if necessary may be controlled with beta blockers such as propranolol (p 373).

3. Orthostatic hypotension responds to head-down position and intravenous fluids.

B. Specific drugs and antidotes. There is no specific antidote.

C. Decontamination after ingestion (see p 44)

1. Prehospital. Administer activated charcoal, if available. Ipecac-induced emesis may be useful for initial treatment at the scene (eg, children at home) if it can be given within a few minutes of exposure.

2. Hospital. Administer activated charcoal and a cathartic. Gastric emptying is not necessary if activated charcoal can be given promptly.

D. Enhanced elimination. These procedures are not effective owing to the large volume of distribution of cannabinoids.

MERCURY
Michael J. Kosnett, MD, MPH

| ANTIDOTE | IPECAC | LAVAGE | CHARCOAL |

Mercury (Hg) is a naturally occurring metal that is mined chiefly as HgS in cinnabar ore. It is converted to three primary forms, each with a distinct toxicology: elemental (metallic) mercury (Hg^0), inorganic mercury salts (eg, mercuric chloride, $HgCl_2$), and organic (alkyl) mercury (eg, methylmercury). Approximately one-third of commercial mercury use is in the manufacture of chlorine and caustic soda; other major uses include electrical equipment, thermometers and other measuring and control instruments, dental amalgam, paints and pigments, and gold mining and extracting. Previous use in pharmaceuticals and biocides has sharply declined, although mercuric chloride is still commonly used as a stool fixative, and Mercurochrome and thimerosal are still used as topical antiseptics. Aquatic organisms can convert inorganic mercury into methylmercury, with resulting bioaccumulation in large carnivorous fish such as swordfish.

I. Mechanism of toxicity. Mercury reacts with sulfhydryl (SH) groups, resulting in enzyme inhibition and pathologic alteration of cellular membranes.

A. Elemental and methylmercury are particularly toxic to the central nervous system. Metallic mercury vapor is also a pulmonary irritant. Methylmercury is teratogenic.

B. Inorganic mercuric salts are corrosive to the skin, eyes, and gastrointestinal tract, and are nephrotoxic.

II. Toxic dose. The pattern and severity of toxicity are highly dependent on the form of mercury and the route of exposure, mostly because of different pharmacokinetic profiles. Chronic exposure to any form may result in toxicity. See Table II–33 for a summary of absorption and toxicity.

A. Elemental (metallic) mercury is a highly volatile liquid at room temperature.

1. Hg^0 vapor is rapidly absorbed by the lungs and distributed to the central nervous system. Airborne exposure to 28 mg/m³ is considered immediately dangerous to life or health (IDLH), and chemical pneumonitis may occur at levels in excess of 1 mg/m³. The recommended workplace limit (ACGIH TLV-TWA) is 0.05 mg/m³ as an 8-hour time-weighted average; however, recent data suggest that subclinical effects on the central nervous system and kidneys may occur below this level. The US Agency for Toxic Substances and Disease Registry (ATSDR) has proposed a minimal risk level for chronic inhalation of 0.00006 mg/m³.

2. Liquid metallic mercury is poorly absorbed from the gastrointestinal tract, and acute ingestion has been associated with poisoning only in the presence of abnormal gut motility that markedly delays normal fecal elimination, or after peritoneal contamination.

B. Inorganic mercuric salts. The acute lethal oral dose of mercuric chloride is

TABLE II–33. SUMMARY OF ABSORPTION AND TOXICITY OF MERCURY COMPOUNDS

	Absorption		Toxicity	
Form	Oral	Inhalation	Neurologic	Renal
Elemental (metallic) mercury				
Hg^0 liquid	Poor	NA	Rare	Rare
Hg^0 vapor	NA	Good	Likely	Possible
Inorganic mercuric salts				
Hg^{2+}	Good	Rare but possible	Rare	Likely
Organic (alkyl) mercury				
RHg^+	Good	Rare but possible	Likely	Possible

approximately 1–4 g. Severe toxicity and death have been reported after use of peritoneal lavage solutions containing mercuric chloride concentrations of 0.2–0.8%.

  C. **Organic mercury** antiseptics undergo limited skin penetration; however, in rare cases, such as topical application to an infected omphalocele, intoxication has resulted. Oral absorption is significant and may also pose a hazard. Methylmercury is well absorbed after inhalation, ingestion, and probably dermal exposure. Ingestion of 10–60 mg/kg may be lethal, and chronic daily ingestion of 10 µg/kg may be associated with adverse neurologic and reproductive effects. The US Environmental Protection Agency (EPA) reference dose (RfD), the daily lifetime dose believed to be without potential hazard, is 0.3 µg/kg/d.

III. **Clinical presentation**
  A. **Acute inhalation of high concentrations of metallic mercury vapor** may cause severe chemical pneumonitis and noncardiogenic pulmonary edema. Acute gingivostomatitis may also occur.
  B. **Chronic intoxication from inhalation of mercury vapor** produces a classic triad of tremor, neuropsychiatric disturbances, and gingivostomatitis.
    1. Early stages feature a fine intention tremor of the fingers, but involvement of the face and progression to choreiform movements of the limbs may occur.
    2. Neuropsychiatric manifestations include fatigue, insomnia, anorexia, and memory loss. There may be an insidous change in mood to shyness, withdrawal, and depression, combined with explosive irritability and frequent blushing ("erethism").
    3. Subclinical changes in peripheral nerve function and renal function have been reported, but frank neuropathy and nephropathy are rare.
    4. Acrodynia, a rare idiosyncratic reaction to chronic mercury exposure, occurs mainly in children and has the following features: pain in the extremities, often accompanied by pinkish discoloration and desquamation ("pink disease"); hypertension; profuse sweating; anorexia, insomnia, irritability and/or apathy; and a miliarial rash.
  C. **Acute ingestion of inorganic mercuric salts,** particularly mercuric chloride, causes abrupt onset of hemorrhagic gastroenteritis and abdominal pain. Intestinal necrosis, shock, and death may ensue. Acute oliguric renal failure from acute tubular necrosis may occur within days. Chronic exposure may result in central nervous system toxicity.
  D. **Organic mercury compounds,** particularly short-chain alkyl compounds such as methylmercury, primarily affect the CNS, causing paresthesias, ataxia, dysarthria, hearing impairment, and progressive constriction of the visual fields. Symptoms first become apparent after several weeks or months.
    1. Ethylmercury compounds may also cause gastroenteritis.
    2. Phenylmercury compounds produce a pattern of toxicity intermediate between alkyl and inorganic mercury.

     3. Methylmercury is a potent teratogen, and perinatal exposure has caused mental retardation and a cerebral palsy–type syndrome in offspring.

IV. Diagnosis depends on integration of characteristic findings with a history of known or potential exposure, and presence of elevated mercury blood levels or urinary excretion.

    A. Specific levels. Elemental and inorganic mercury follow a biphasic elimination rate (initially rapid, then slow), and both urinary and fecal excretion occur. The urinary elimination half-time is approximately 40 days.

       1. Metallic and inorganic mercury. Whole blood, and preferably urine mercury, levels are useful in confirming exposure. In most people without occupational exposure, whole blood Hg is less than 2 μg/dL and urine Hg is less than 10 μg/L. Overt neurologic effects have occurred in persons with chronic urine Hg levels greater than 100–200 μg/L. In patients with acute inorganic mercury poisoning resulting in gastroenteritis and acute tubular necrosis, blood Hg levels are often greater than 50 μg/dL.

       2. Organic mercury. Methylmercury undergoes biliary excretion and enterohepatic recirculation, with 90% eventually excreted in the feces; as a result, urine levels are not useful. Whole blood Hg levels greater than 20 μg/dL have been associated with symptoms. The blood mercury half-life is 50–70 days. Hair levels have been used to document remote exposure.

    B. Other useful laboratory studies. Electrolytes, glucose, BUN, creatinine, liver transaminases, urinalysis; chest x-ray and arterial blood gases (if pneumonitis suspected). Urinary markers of early nephrotoxicity (microalbuminuria, retinol binding protein, β_2-microglobulin, N-acetylglucosaminidase) may aid detection of early adverse effects.

V. Treatment

    A. Emergency and supportive measures

       1. Inhalation. Observe closely for several hours for development of acute pneumonitis and pulmonary edema (see p 8), and give supplemental oxygen if indicated.

       2. Mercuric salt ingestion. Anticipate severe gastroenteritis and treat shock aggressively with intravenous fluid replacement (see p 15). Vigorous hydration may also help maintain urine output. Acute renal failure is usually reversible, but hemodialysis may be required for 1–2 weeks.

       3. Organic mercury ingestion. Provide symptomatic supportive care. Limited data suggest that oral neostigmine may improve motor strength in patients with moderate to severe chronic intoxication.

    B. Specific drugs and antidotes

       1. Metallic (elemental) mercury. In acute or chronic poisoning, oral **DMSA** (see p 332) may enhance urinary Hg excretion (although its effect on clinical outcome has not been fully studied). Although penicillamine (see p 366) is an alternative oral treatment, it may be associated with more side effects and less efficient Hg excretion.

       2. Inorganic mercury salts. Treatment with intramuscular **BAL** (see p 317), if begun within minutes to a few hours after ingestion, may reduce or avert severe renal injury. Because prompt intervention is necessary, do not delay treatment while waiting for specific laboratory confirmation. Oral **DMSA** (see p 332) is also effective, but its absorption may be limited by gastroenteritis and shock, and it is more appropriately used as a follow-up to BAL treatment.

       3. Organic mercury. In methylmercury intoxication, limited data suggest that oral **DMSA** (see p 332) may be effective in decreasing Hg levels in tissues, including the brain.

       4. Because BAL may redistribute mercury to the brain from other tissue sites, it should not be used in poisoning by metallic or organic mercury, as the brain is a key target organ.

    C. Decontamination (see p 41–49)

       1. Inhalation

a. Immediately remove victim from exposure and give supplemental oxygen, if needed.

b. Even minute indoor spills (eg, 1 mL) of metallic mercury can result in hazardous chronic airborne levels. Cover the spill with powdered sulfur, and carefully clean up and discard all residue and contaminated carpeting, porous furniture, and permeable floor covering. Do *not* use a home vacuum cleaner, as this may disperse the liquid mercury, increasing its airborne concentration. For large spills, professional cleanup with self-contained vacuum systems is recommended.

2. **Ingestion of metallic mercury.** In healthy persons, metallic mercury passes through the intestinal tract with minimal absorption, and there is no need for gut decontamination. With extremely large ingestions, or in patients with abnormally diminished bowel motility or intestinal perforation, there is a risk of chronic intoxication. Multiple-dose cathartics, whole bowel irrigation (see p 48), or even surgical removal may be necessary, depending on x-ray evidence of mercury retention or elevated blood or urine Hg levels.

3. **Ingestion of inorganic mercuric salts**

   a. **Prehospital.** Administer activated charcoal, if available. Do *not* induce emesis because of the risk of serious corrosive injury.

   b. **Hospital.** Perform gastric lavage. Administer activated charcoal, although it is of uncertain benefit.

   c. Arrange for endoscopic examination if corrosive injury is suspected.

4. **Ingestion of organic mercury.** After acute ingestion, perform gastric lavage and administer activated charcoal. Immediately stop breast feeding, but continue to express and discard milk, as some data suggest this may accelerate reduction of blood Hg levels.

D. **Enhanced elimination**

1. There is no role for dialysis, hemoperfusion, or repeat-dose charcoal in removing metallic or inorganic mercury. However, dialysis may be required for supportive treatment of renal failure, and it may slightly enhance removal of the mercury-chelator complex in patients with renal failure (hemodialysis clearance of the mercury-BAL complex is about 5 mL/min).

2. In patients with chronic methylmercury intoxication, repeated oral administration of an experimental polythiol resin was effective in enhancing Hg elimination by interrupting enterohepatic recirculation.

METALDEHYDE
Gerald Joe, PharmD

ANTIDOTE   IPECAC   LAVAGE   CHARCOAL

Metaldehyde is widely used in the USA as a snail and slug poison. In Europe, it is also used as a solid fuel for small heaters. The pellets are often mistaken for cereal or candy. Common commercial products containing metaldehyde (2–4%) include Cory's Slug and Snail Death, Deadline for Slugs and Snails, and Bug-Geta Snail and Slug Pellets.

I. **Mechanism of toxicity.** The mechanism of toxicity is not well understood. Metaldehyde, like paraldehyde, is a polymer of acetaldehyde, and depolymerization to form acetaldehyde may account for some of its toxic effects. Further metabolism to acetone bodies may contribute to metabolic acidosis.

II. **Toxic dose.** Ingestion of 100–150 mg/kg may cause myoclonus and convulsions, and ingestion of more than 400 mg/kg is potentially lethal. Death occurred in a child after ingestion of 3 g.

III. **Clinical presentation.** Symptoms usually begin within 1–3 hours after ingestion.

A. Small ingestions (5–10 mg/kg) cause salivation, facial flushing, vomiting, abdominal cramps, diarrhea, and fever.

B. Larger doses may produce irritability, ataxia, drowsiness, myoclonus, opisthotonus, convulsions, and coma. Rhabdomyolysis and hyperthermia may result from seizures or excessive muscle activity. Liver and kidney damage have been reported.

IV. Diagnosis is based on a history of ingestion and clinical presentation. Ask about containers in the garage or planting shed; metaldehyde is frequently packaged in brightly colored cardboard boxes similar to cereal containers.

  A. Specific levels. Serum levels are not generally available.

  B. Other useful laboratory studies. Electrolytes, glucose, BUN, creatinine, osmolar gap (may be elevated), liver enzymes. If rhabdomyolysis suspected: urine dipstick for occult blood (myoglobin is positive), serum creatine phosphokinase (CPK).

V. Treatment

  A. Emergency and supportive measures

    1. Maintain the airway and assist ventilation if necessary (see p 4).

    2. Treat coma (p 18) and seizures (p 22) if they occur. Paraldehyde should **not** be used to treat seizures because of its chemical similarity to metaldehyde.

    3. Treat fluid loss from vomiting or diarrhea with intravenous crystalloid fluids (p 15).

    4. Monitor asymptomatic patients for at least 4–6 hours after ingestion.

  B. Specific drugs and antidotes. There is no specific antidote.

  C. Decontamination (see p 44)

    1. Prehospital. Administer activated charcoal, if available. Ipecac-induced emesis may be useful for initial treatment at the scene (eg, children at home) if it can be given immediately after exposure, but may be dangerous if given later because of the risk of sudden onset of seizures.

    2. Hospital. Administer activated charcoal and a cathartic. Gastric emptying is not necessary if activated charcoal can be given promptly.

  D. Enhanced elimination. There is no apparent benefit from dialysis, hemoperfusion, or forced diuresis. Repeat-dose charcoal has not been studied.

METAL FUME FEVER
Paul D. Blanc, MD, MSPH

ANTIDOTE   IPECAC   LAVAGE   CHARCOAL

Metal fume fever is an acute febrile illness associated with the inhalation of respirable particles of zinc oxide. Although metal fume fever has also been invoked as a generic effect of exposure to numerous metal oxides (copper, cadmium, iron, magnesium, manganese), there is little evidence to support this (except for magnesium). Metal fume fever usually occurs in workplace settings involving welding, melting, or flame-cutting galvanized metal or in brass foundry operations.

  I. Mechanism of toxicity. Metal fume fever results from inhalation of zinc oxide (neither ingestion nor parenteral administration can induce the illness). The mechanism is uncertain, but may be cytokine-mediated. It does not involve sensitization, and can occur with the first exposure.

  II. Toxic dose. The toxic dose is variable. Resistance to the condition develops after a few days of exposure but wears off rapidly when exposure ceases. The ACGIH recommended workplace exposure limit (TLV-TWA) for zinc oxide fumes is 5 mg/m^3 as an 8-hour time-weighted average, which is intended to prevent metal fume fever in most exposed workers.

  III. Clinical presentation. Symptoms begin 4–8 hours after exposure, when the victim develops fever, malaise, myalgias, and headache. The white blood cell count may be elevated (12,000–16,000). The chest x-ray is usually normal. Typically, all symptoms resolve spontaneously within 24–36 hours.

Pulmonary infiltrates and hypoxemia **are not consistent** with pure metal fume fever, and if present suggest possible heavy metal pneumonitis resulting from cadmium or other toxic inhalations associated with metal-working and foundry operations (eg, phosgene, nitrogen oxides).

IV. **Diagnosis.** A history of welding, especially with galvanized metal, and typical symptoms and signs are sufficient to make the diagnosis.

    A. **Specific levels.** There are no specific tests to diagnose or exclude metal fume fever. Blood or urine zinc determinations do not have a role in clinical diagnosis of the syndrome.

    B. **Other useful laboratory studies.** CBC, arterial blood gases or oximetry, chest x-ray.

V. **Treatment**

    A. **Emergency and supportive measures**

        1. Administer supplemental oxygen, and give bronchodilators if there is wheezing (see p 9–10). If hypoxemia or wheezing is present, consider other toxic inhalations (see p 176).

        2. Provide symptomatic care (eg, acetaminophen) as needed; symptoms are self-limited.

    B. **Specific drugs and antidotes.** There is no specific antidote.

    C. **Decontamination** is not necessary; by the time symptoms develop, the exposure has usually been over for several hours.

    D. **Enhanced elimination.** There is no role for these procedures.

METHANOL
Ilene B. Anderson, PharmD

ANTIDOTE   IPECAC   LAVAGE   CHARCOAL

Methanol (wood alcohol) is a common ingredient in many solvents, windshield-washing solutions, duplicating fluids, and paint removers. It is sometimes used as an ethanol substitute by alcoholics. Although methanol itself produces mainly inebriation, its metabolic products may cause metabolic acidosis, blindness, and death after a characteristic latent period of 6–30 hours.

  I. **Mechanism of toxicity.** Methanol is slowly metabolized by alcohol dehydrogenase to formaldehyde and subsequently by aldehyde dehydrogenase to formic acid (formate). Systemic acidosis is caused by the formic acid as well as by lactic acid, while blindness is caused primarily by formate. Both ethanol and methanol compete for the enzyme alcohol dehydrogenase; the preference of this enzyme for metabolizing ethanol forms the basis for ethanol therapy in methanol poisonings.

  II. **Toxic dose.** The fatal oral dose of methanol is estimated to be 30–240 mL (20–150 g). The minimum toxic dose is approximately 100 mg/kg. Elevated serum methanol levels have been reported after extensive dermal exposure and concentrated inhalation. The ACGIH recommended workplace exposure limit (TLV-TWA) for inhalation is 200 ppm as an 8-hour time-weighted average, and the level considered immediately dangerous to life or health (IDLH) is 25,000 ppm.

III. **Clinical presentation**

    A. **In the first few hours** after ingestion, methanol-intoxicated patients present with inebriation and gastritis. Acidosis is not usually present because metabolism to toxic products has not yet occurred. There may be a noticeable elevation in the osmolar gap (see p 30); an osmolar gap of as little as 10 mosm/L is consistent with toxic concentrations of methanol.

    B. **After a latent period** of up to 30 hours, severe anion gap metabolic acidosis, visual disturbances, blindness, seizures, coma, and death may occur. Patients describe the visual disturbance as haziness or "like standing in a snowfield." Fundoscopic examination may reveal optic disc hyperemia, venous engorgement, or papilledema. The latent period is longer when ethanol has been ingested concurrently with methanol.

IV. **Diagnosis** is usually based on the history, symptoms, and laboratory findings because stat methanol levels are rarely available. Calculation of the osmolar and anion gaps (see p 30) can be used to estimate the methanol level and to predict the severity of the ingestion. A large anion gap not accounted for by elevated lactate suggests possible methanol (or ethylene glycol) poisoning, because the anion gap in these cases is mostly nonlactate.

A. **Specific levels**
1. **Serum methanol** levels higher than 20 mg/dL should be considered toxic, and levels higher than 40 mg/dL should be considered very serious. Following the latent period, a low or nondetectable methanol level does not rule out a serious intoxication in a symptomatic patient because all the methanol may already have been metabolized to formate.
2. Elevated **serum formate** concentrations may confirm the diagnosis and are a better measure of toxicity, but formate levels are not yet widely available. Formate is not osmotically active and therefore will not result in an increased osmolar gap.

B. **Other useful laboratory studies.** Electrolytes, glucose, BUN, creatinine, serum osmolality and osmolar gap, arterial blood gases, ethanol level, lactate level.

V. **Treatment**

A. **Emergency and supportive measures**
1. Maintain the airway and assist ventilation if necessary (see p 14).
2. Treat coma (p 18) and seizures (p 22) if they occur.
3. Treat metabolic acidosis with intravenous sodium bicarbonate (p 30). Correction of acidosis should be guided by arterial blood gases.

B. **Specific drugs and antidotes**
1. **Ethanol.** Start an oral or intravenous infusion of ethanol (see p 339) to saturate the enzyme alcohol dehydrogenase and prevent the formation of methanol's toxic metabolites. Ethanol therapy is indicated in patients with the following:
   a. A history of a significant methanol ingestion, when methanol serum levels are not immediately available and the osmolar gap is greater than 5 mosm/L.
   b. Metabolic acidosis and an osmolar gap greater than 5–10 mosm/L not accounted for by ethanol.
   c. Methanol blood concentration greater than 20 mg/dL.
2. **Folic acid** (see p 341) may enhance the conversion of formate to carbon dioxide and water. A reasonable dose is 50 mg IV every 4 hours.
3. An experimental drug, 4-methylpyrazole, inhibits alcohol dehydrogenase and prevents methanol metabolism but is not yet available in the USA.

C. **Decontamination** (see p 44)
1. **Prehospital.** Ipecac-induced emesis may be useful for initial treatment at the scene (eg, children at home) if it can be given within a few minutes of exposure.
2. **Hospital.** Perform gastric lavage. Activated charcoal has not been shown to efficiently adsorb methanol in vivo. In addition, charcoal may delay the absorption of orally administered ethanol.

D. **Enhanced elimination.** Hemodialysis rapidly removes both methanol (half-life reduced to 3–6 hours) and formate. The indications for dialysis are suspected methanol poisoning with significant metabolic acidosis, an osmolar gap greater than 10 mosm/L, or a measured serum methanol concentration greater than 40 mg/dL. Dialysis should be continued until the methanol concentration is less than 20 mg/dL. **Note:** The ethanol infusion must be increased during dialysis (see Ethanol, p 339).

METHEMOGLOBINEMIA
Paul D. Blanc, MD, MSPH

ANTIDOTE   IPECAC   LAVAGE   CHARCOAL

Methemoglobin is an oxidized form of hemoglobin. Many oxidant chemicals and drugs are capable of inducing methemoglobinemia: nitrites and nitrates, bromates and chlorates, aniline derivatives, antimalarial agents, dapsone, sulfonamides, local anesthetics, and numerous others (Table II–34). Occupational risk groups include chemical and munitions workers. An important environmental source for methemoglobinemia in infants is nitrate-contaminated well water. Amyl and butyl nitrate are often abused for their alleged sexual enhancement properties. Oxides of nitrogen and other oxidant combustion products make smoke inhalation an important potential cause of methemoglobinemia.

I. **Mechanism of toxicity**
   A. Methemoglobin inducers act by oxidizing ferrous (Fe^{2+}) to ferric (Fe^{3+}) hemoglobin. This abnormal hemoglobin is incapable of carrying oxygen, inducing a functional anemia. In addition, the shape of the oxygen-hemoglobin dissociation curve is altered, aggravating cellular hypoxia.
   B. Methemoglobinemia does not directly cause hemolysis; however, many oxidizing agents that induce methemoglobinemia may also cause hemolysis through either hemoglobin (Heinz body) or cell membrane effects, particularly in patients with low tolerance for oxidative stress (eg, those with glucose-6-phosphate dehydrogenase [G6PD] deficiency).

II. **Toxic dose.** The ingested dose or inhaled air level of toxin required to induce methemoglobinemia is highly variable. Neonates and persons with congenital methemoglobin reductase deficiency or G6PD deficiency have an impaired ability to regenerate normal hemoglobin and are therefore more likely to accumulate methemoglobin after oxidant exposure. Concomitant hemolysis suggests either heavy oxidant exposure or increased cell vulnerability.

III. **Clinical presentation.** The severity of symptoms usually correlates with measured methemoglobin level (Table II–35).
   A. Symptoms and signs are caused by decreased blood oxygen content and cellular hypoxia and are nonspecific: headache, dizziness, and nausea, progressing to dyspnea, confusion, seizures, and coma. Even at low levels, skin discoloration ("chocolate cyanosis"), especially of the nails, lips, and ears, is striking.
   B. Usually, mild methemoglobinemia (< 15–20%) is well-tolerated and will resolve spontaneously. Continued metabolism of oxidant compounds from a long-acting parent compound (eg, dapsone) may lead to prolonged effects (2–3 days).

TABLE II–34. SELECTED AGENTS CAPABLE OF INDUCING METHEMOGLOBINEMIA

Local anesthetics	Analgesics	Miscellaneous
Benzocaine	Phenazopyridine	Aminophenol
Lidocaine	Phenacetin	Aniline dyes
Antimicrobials	**Nitrites and nitrates**	Bromates
Chloroquine	Amyl nitrite	Chlorates
Dapsone	Butyl nitrite	Metoclopramide
Primaquine	Isobutyl nitrite	Nitrobenzene
Sulfonamides	Sodium nitrite	Nitrogen oxides
		Nitroglycerin

TABLE II–35. CORRELATION OF SYMPTOMS WITH METHEMOGLOBIN LEVELS

Methemoglobin Level	Typical Symptoms
< 15%	Usually asymptomatic
15–20%	Cyanosis, mild symptoms
20–45%	Marked cyanosis, moderate symptoms
45–70%	Severe cyanosis, severe symptoms
> 70%	Usually lethal

IV. **Diagnosis.** The patient with mild to moderate methemoglobinemia appears markedly cyanotic yet may be relatively asymptomatic. The arterial oxygen partial pressure (P_{O2}) is normal. The diagnosis is suggested by the finding of "chocolate brown" blood (put a drop of blood on filter paper and compare with normal blood), which is usually apparent when the methemoglobin level exceeds 15%. Differential diagnosis includes other causes of cellular hypoxia (eg, carbon monoxide, cyanide, hydrogen sulfide) and sulfhemoglobinemia.

    A. **Specific levels.** The co-oximeter type of arterial blood gas analyzer will directly measure oxygen saturation and methemoglobin saturation. ***Note:*** Sulfhemoglobin and the antidote methylene blue both produce erroneously high levels on the co-oximeter: a dose of 2 mg/kg methylene blue gives a false-positive methemoglobin of approximately 15%.

        1. The routine arterial blood gas machine measures the serum P_{O2} (which is normal) and calculates a falsely normal oxygen saturation.

        2. Pulse oximetry is ***not*** reliable: it will appear deceptively near-normal in a patient with severe methemoglobinemia, and falsely desaturated in a patient who has been given methylene blue.

    B. **Other useful laboratory studies.** Electrolytes, glucose. If hemolysis suspected: CBC, haptoglobin, peripheral smear, urinalysis dipstick for occult blood (free hemoglobin is positive).

V. **Treatment**

    A. **Emergency and supportive measures**

        1. Maintain the airway and assist ventilation if necessary (see p 4). Administer supplemental oxygen.

        2. Usually, mild methemoglobinemia (< 15–20%) will resolve spontaneously and requires no intervention.

    B. **Specific drugs and antidotes**

        1. **Methylene blue** (see p 351) is indicated in the symptomatic patient with methemoglobin levels higher than 20% or when even minimal compromise of oxygen-carrying capacity is potentially harmful (eg, preexisting anemia, congestive heart failure, angina pectoris, etc). Give methylene blue, 1–2 mg/kg (0.1–0.2 mL/kg of 1% solution) over several minutes. ***Caution:*** Methylene blue can slightly worsen methemoglobinemia when given in excessive amounts; in patients with G6PD deficiency, it may cause hemolysis.

        2. Ascorbic acid, which can reverse methemoglobin by an alternate metabolic pathway, is of minimal use acutely because of its slow action.

    C. **Decontamination** (see p 41–49)

        1. **Inhalation.** Remove victim from exposure and give supplemental oxygen, if available.

        2. **Skin.** Remove contaminated clothing, and wash exposed skin with soap and water.

        3. **Ingestion** (see p 44)

            a. **Prehospital.** Administer activated charcoal, if available. Ipecac-induced emesis may be useful for initial treatment at the scene (eg, children at home) if it can be given within a few minutes of exposure.

    b. Hospital. Administer activated charcoal and a cathartic. Gastric emptying is not necessary if activated charcoal can be given promptly.

D. Enhanced elimination (see p 49)

  1. In patients with severe intoxication, if methylene blue is contraindicated (eg, G6PD deficiency) or has not been effective, **exchange transfusion** may rarely be necessary.

  2. Hyperbaric oxygen is theoretically capable of supplying sufficient oxygen independent of hemoglobin to be useful in extremely serious cases that do not respond rapidly to antidotal treatment.

  3. Repeat-dose activated charcoal enhances the elimination of dapsone.

METHYL BROMIDE
Delia A. Dempsey, MS, MD

ANTIDOTE   IPECAC   LAVAGE   CHARCOAL

Methyl bromide is an odorless, colorless lethal gas used as an insecticidal fumigant on soil, perishable foods, and in buildings. It also serves as an alkylating agent in the chemical industry. Prior to World War II, liquid methyl bromide was used as a refrigerant and in some fire extinguishers. Although its predominant present use is agricultural, urban use for structural pest control has been steadily increasing. The building is evacuated, covered with a giant tarp, and sealed; and the gas is introduced. Afterward, the tarp is removed, and the building is ventilated and then tested for residual methyl bromide before reoccupation.

    Methyl bromide gas has poor warning properties, so the lacrimator chloropicrin (2%) is usually added. Methyl bromide is 3 times heavier than air and may accumulate in low-lying areas. Also, it may condense to a liquid at cold temperatures (38.5 °F, 3.6 °C), then vaporize when temperatures rise.

I. Mechanism of toxicity

  A. Methyl bromide is a potent alkylating agent and irreversibly alkylates DNA, glutathione, and numerous proteins. Its special affinity for sulfhydryl groups leads to enzyme inactivation. *In vitro* studies show inhibition of glucose metabolism and phosphate transfer. Animal data clearly indicate that its toxicity does not result from dissociation into methyl alcohol and bromide ion.

  B. NIOSH considers methyl bromide a potential occupational carcinogen.

II. Toxic dose

  A. Inhalation is the most important route of exposure. The ACGIH recommended workplace exposure limit (TLV-TWA) in air is 5 ppm as an 8-hour time-weighted average. Toxic effects are generally seen at levels of 200 ppm. The air level considered immediately dangerous to life or health (IDLH) is 2000 ppm.

  B. Skin absorption may occur. Methyl bromide may penetrate clothing and some protective gear. Retention of the gas in clothing and rubber boots can be a source of prolonged percutaneous exposure.

III. Clinical presentation

  A. Acute irritant effects are limited, and lethal exposures can occur without warning if chlorpicrin has not been added. Chlorpicrin is probably responsible for most reports of eye, mucous membrane, and upper respiratory irritation after low-level exposures. Moderate skin exposure can result in dermatitis and, in severe cases, chemical burns.

  B. Acute systemic effects include malaise, visual disturbances, headache, nausea, vomiting, tremor, seizures, and coma. There may be a 6- to 48-hour prodrome of nausea, vomiting, and other symptoms before the onset of intractable seizures and coma. Death may be caused by fulminant respiratory failure with noncardiogenic pulmonary edema or complications of status epilepticus. Sublethal exposure may result in flulike symptoms, respiratory complaints, or chronic effects.

    C. Chronic neurologic sequelae can result from chronic exposure or a sublethal acute exposure. A wide spectrum of neurologic and psychiatric problems may occur that may take months or years to resolve, or may be irreversible. Reported sequelae include delirium, dementia, psychoneurosis, psychosis, visual disturbances, vertigo, aphasia, ataxia, peripheral neuropathy, extrapyramidal symptoms, myoclonic jerking, tremors, and seizures.

IV. Diagnosis is based primarily on a history of exposure to the compound and typical symptoms.

    A. Specific levels. Methylation of tissues releases free bromide ion (see Bromide, p 110). Endogenous serum bromide does not usually exceed 4 mg/L (0.05 meq/L). Although elevated bromide concentrations may indicate exposure, they do not correlate with clinical severity after acute methyl bromide poisoning, and levels of 40–400 mg/L (0.5–5 meq/L) have been reported with both lethal and nonlethal exposures. Moreover, commonly used assays (eg, gold chloride spectrophotometric method) are not sensitive enough to accurately determine bromide levels lower than 50 mg/L (0.6 meq/L), which means that methyl bromide poisoning is not necessarily ruled out by negative test results.

    B. Other useful laboratory studies. Electrolytes (falsely elevated chloride is seen with some methods: 1 meq bromide = 1.5 meq chloride), glucose, BUN, creatinine. If respiratory distress: arterial blood gases or oximetry, chest x-ray.

V. Treatment

    A. Emergency and supportive measures

        1. Administer supplemental oxygen, and treat bronchospasm (p 9–10), pulmonary edema (p 8), seizures (p 22), and coma (p 18) if they occur. Seizures are often intractable, and may require induction of barbiturate coma with a short-acting agent such as pentobarbital (p 367); consult a neurologist as soon as possible.

        2. Monitor patients for a minimum of 6–12 hours to detect development of delayed symptoms, including seizures and noncardiogenic pulmonary edema.

    B. Specific drugs and antidotes. Theoretically, *N*-acetylcysteine (NAC, p 311) or dimercaprol (BAL, p 317) can offer a reactive sulfhydryl group to bind free methyl bromide, although neither agent has been critically tested. If either is used, it should be given as soon as possible after exposure.

    C. Decontamination. Properly trained personnel should use self-contained breathing apparatus and chemical protective clothing before entering contaminated areas. The absence of irritant effects from chloropicrin does not guarantee that it is safe to enter without protection.

        1. Remove victim from exposure and administer supplemental oxygen, if available.

        2. If exposed to liquid methyl bromide, remove contaminated clothing and wash affected skin with soap and water. Irrigate exposed eyes with copious water or saline.

    D. Enhanced elimination. There is no role for these procedures.

METHYLENE CHLORIDE
Diane Liu, MD, MPH

ANTIDOTE   IPECAC   LAVAGE   CHARCOAL

Methylene chloride (dichloromethane) is widely used in paint and varnish removers and as a solvent in degreasing operations; it is found in some Christmas tree lights and magic trick sets. It is metabolized to carbon monoxide in vivo, and may produce phosgene, chlorine, or hydrogen chloride upon combustion. It was considered to be the least toxic of all the chlorinated hydrocarbon solvents prior to its implication as a suspected human carcinogen.

    I. Mechanism of toxicity. Methylene chloride, like other chlorinated hydrocarbon solvents, is an irritant to mucous membranes, defats the skin epithelium, is a direct central nervous system depressant, and may sensitize the myocardium to arrhythmogenic effects of catecholamines.

A. Carbon monoxide (CO) is generated in vivo during metabolism by the mixed-function oxidases in the liver. The contribution of CO to methylene chloride intoxication is unknown.

B. Methylene chloride is a **suspected human carcinogen.**

II. Toxic dose. Toxicity may occur after inhalation or ingestion.

A. Inhalation. OSHA considers methylene chloride a potential human carcinogen and has no established permissible exposure limit (PEL). The ACGIH workplace exposure threshold limit value (TLV-TWA) is 50 ppm for an 8-hour shift, which may result in a carboxyhemoglobin level of 3–4%. The air level considered immediately dangerous to life or health (IDLH) is 5000 ppm.

B. Ingestion. The acute oral toxic dose is approximately 0.5–5 mL/kg.

III. Clinical presentation

A. Inhalation is the most common route of exposure and results in mucous membrane and skin irritation, nausea, vomiting, and headache. Severe exposures may lead to pulmonary edema, cardiac arrhythmias, and central nervous system depression with respiratory arrest.

B. Ingestion can cause corrosive gastrointestinal injury and systemic intoxication.

C. Extensive **skin exposure** can cause significant burns and systemic symptoms owing to skin absorption.

D. Chronic exposure can cause bone marrow, hepatic, and renal toxicity.

IV. Diagnosis is based on a history of exposure and clinical presentation.

A. Specific levels

1. Carboxyhemoglobin levels should be obtained, although they may not correlate with the severity of the intoxication.

2. Expired air and blood levels of **methylene chloride** may be obtained but are not useful in clinical management.

B. Other useful laboratory studies. CBC, electrolytes, glucose, BUN, creatinine, liver transaminases, ECG monitoring.

V. Treatment

A. Emergency and supportive measures

1. Maintain the airway and assist ventilation if necessary (see p 4).

2. Administer supplemental oxygen, and treat coma (p 18) and pulmonary edema (p 8) if they occur.

3. Monitor the ECG for at least 4–6 hours, and treat arrhythmias (p 14) if they occur. Avoid the use of epinephrine, which may aggravate cardiac arrhythmias. Tachyarrhythmias caused by myocardial sensitization may be treated with **propranolol** (see p 373), 1–2 mg IV, or **esmolol** (see p 338), 25–100 μg/kg/min IV.

4. If corrosive injury is suspected after ingestion, consult a gastroenterologist regarding possible endoscopy.

B. Specific drugs and antidotes. Administer 100% **oxygen** by tight-fitting mask or endotracheal tube if the carboxyhemoglobin level is elevated.

C. Decontamination (see p 41)

1. Inhalation. Remove the victim from exposure and give supplemental oxygen, if available.

2. Skin and eyes. Remove contaminated clothing, and wash exposed skin with soap and water. Irrigate exposed eyes with copious saline or tap water.

3. Ingestion (see p 44)

a. Prehospital. Administer activated charcoal, if available. Do *not* induce emesis because of the risk of rapid central nervous system depression.

b. Hospital. Perform gastric lavage (if large, recent ingestion), and administer activated charcoal and a cathartic. The effectiveness of charcoal is not known.

D. Enhanced elimination. There is no documented efficacy for repeat-dose activated charcoal, hemodialysis, hemoperfusion, or hyperbaric oxygen.

MONOAMINE OXIDASE INHIBITORS
Neal L. Benowitz, MD

ANTIDOTE   IPECAC   LAVAGE   CHARCOAL

Most monoamine oxidase (MAO) inhibitors are used in treating severe depression; procarbazine is a cancer chemotherapeutic drug. Available drugs in this class include furazolidone (Furoxone), isocarboxazid (Marplan), nialamide (Niamid), pargyline (Eutonyl), phenelzine (Nardil), procarbazine (Matulane), and tranylcypromine (Parnate). Serious toxicity from MAO inhibitors occurs either with overdose or owing to interactions with certain other drugs or foods (Table II–36). Selegiline (Eldepryl), a MAO type B inhibitor, is not generally associated with the same toxicity or drug interactions with the other MAO inhibitors (which act on MAO type A), although there have been reports of adverse interactions with meperidine.

I. Mechanism of toxicity. MAO inhibitors irreversibly inactivate MAO, an enzyme responsible for degradation of catecholamines within neurons in the central nervous system. MAO is also found in the liver and the intestinal wall, where it metabolizes tyramine and therefore limits its absorption by the systemic circulation.

    A. Toxicity results from release of excessive neuronal stores of vasoactive amines, inhibition of metabolism of catecholamines or interacting drugs, or absorption of large amounts of dietary tyramine (which in turn releases catecholamines from neurons).

    B. In addition, severe rigidity and hyperthermia may occur when patients receiving MAO inhibitors use therapeutic doses of meperidine (Demerol), dextromethorphan, fluoxetine (Prozac), paroxetine (Paxil), sertraline (Zoloft), or tryptophan; the mechanism is unknown but may be related to inhibition of serotonin metabolism in the central nervous system, resulting in "serotonin syndrome" (see p 21).

II. Toxic dose. MAO inhibitors have a low therapeutic index. Acute ingestion of 2–3 mg/kg or more should be considered potentially life-threatening. Serious drug or food interactions may occur in patients receiving therapeutic doses of MAO inhibitors. *Note:* Because of irreversible MAO inhibition, adverse drug interactions may occur for up to 2 weeks after discontinuing MAO inhibitors. Interactions may also occur when MAO inhibitors are started within 10 days of stopping fluoxetine, owing to the long half-life of fluoxetine.

III. Clinical presentation. Symptoms may be delayed 6–24 hours after acute overdose, but occur rapidly following ingestion of interacting drugs or foods in a patient on chronic MAO inhibitor therapy. Because of irreversible inactivation of MAO,

TABLE II–36. INTERACTIONS WITH MONOAMINE OXIDASE INHIBITORS[a]

Drugs		Foods
Amphetamines	Metaraminol	Beer
Buspirone	Methyldopa	Broad bean pods and Fava beans
Clomipramine	Methylphenidate	Cheese (natural or aged)
Cocaine	Paroxetine	Chicken liver
Dextromethorphan	Phenylephrine	Pickled herring
Ephedrine	Phenylpropanolamine	Smoked, pickled, or aged meats
Fluoxetine	Reserpine	Snails
Guanethidine	Sertraline	Spoiled or bacterially contaminated foods
L-Dopa	Trazodone	Summer sausage
LSD (lysergic acid diethylamide)	Tryptophan	Wine (red)
MDMA		Yeast (dietary supplement and Marmite)
Meperidine (Demerol)		

[a]Possible interactions, based on case reports or pharmacologic considerations.

toxic effects (and the potential for drug or food interactions) may persist for several days.

A. Anxiety, restlessness, flushing, headache, tremor, myoclonus, hyperreflexia, sweating, shivering, tachypnea, tachycardia, and moderate hypertension are common with mild intoxication.

B. Severe intoxication may result in severe hypertension (which may be complicated by intracranial hemorrhage), delirium, hyperthermia, and eventually cardiovascular collapse and multisystem failure.

C. Hypotension, particularly when upright (orthostatic hypotension), is seen with therapeutic dosing and also may occur with overdose.

IV. Diagnosis is based on clinical features of sympathomimetic drug intoxication with a history of MAO inhibitor use, particularly with use of drugs or foods known to interact. Serotonin syndrome (see p 21) is suspected when the patient has myoclonic jerking, hyperreflexia, diaphoresis, and hyperthermia.

  A. Specific levels. Specific drug levels are not available.

  B. Other useful laboratory studies. Electrolytes, glucose, BUN, creatinine, creatine phosphokinase (CPK), ECG and ECG monitoring. If intracranial hemorrhage suspected, CT head scan.

V. Treatment

  A. Emergency and supportive measures

  1. Maintain the airway and assist ventilation if necessary (see p 4). Administer supplemental oxygen.

  2. Treat hypertension (p 17), hypotension (p 15), coma (p 18), seizures (p 22), and hyperthermia (p 20) if they occur.

  3. Continuously monitor temperature, other vital signs, and ECG for a minimum of 6 hours in asymptomatic patients, and admit all symptomatic patients for continuous monitoring for 24 hours.

  B. Specific drugs and antidotes

  1. Since the hypertension is catecholamine-mediated, alpha-adrenergic blockers (eg, phentolamine, p 369) or combined alpha- and beta-adrenergic blockers (eg, labetalol, p 347) are particularly useful.

  2. Serotonin syndrome should be treated with sedation and cooling. Anecdotal reports suggest possible benefit with methysergide (Sansert), 2 mg PO every 6 hours for 3 doses, or cyproheptadine (Periactin), 4 mg PO every hour for 3 doses, presumably because of their serotonin-antagonist activity.

  C. Decontamination (see p 44)

  1. Prehospital. Administer activated charcoal, if available. Ipecac-induced emesis may be useful for initial treatment at the scene (eg, children at home) if it can be given within a few minutes of an acute overdose. However, it should not be used for patients with suspected food or drug interaction because of the risk of aggravating hypertension.

  2. Hospital. Administer activated charcoal and a cathartic. Perform gastric lavage for suspected large overdose.

  D. Enhanced elimination. Dialysis and hemoperfusion are not effective. Repeat-dose activated charcoal has not been studied.

MUSHROOMS
Kent R. Olson, MD

ANTIDOTE   IPECAC   LAVAGE   CHARCOAL

There are more than 5000 varieties of mushrooms in the USA, about 100 of which are potentially toxic. The majority of toxic mushrooms cause mild to moderate self-limited gastroenteritis. A few species may cause severe or even fatal reactions. The major categories of poisonous mushrooms are described in Table II–37. *Amanita phalloides* and other amatoxin-containing mushrooms are discussed on p 225.

TABLE II–37. CLASSIFICATION OF MUSHROOM TOXICITY[a]

Toxins	Mushrooms	Onset	Symptoms and Signs
Amatoxins	*Amanita phalloides, A ocreata, A verna, A virosa,* some *Lepiota* and *Galerina* species.	6–12 h	Vomiting, diarrhea, abdominal cramps, hepatic failure.
Monomethylhydrazine	*Gyrometra (Helvella) esculenta,* others.	6–12 h	Vomiting, diarrhea, weakness, seizures, hemolysis, hepatitis, methemoglobinemia.
Muscarine	*Clitocybe dealbata, C cerusata, Inocybe, Omphalotus olearius.*	0.5–2 h	Salivation, sweating, vomiting, diarrhea, miosis.
Coprine	*Coprinus armamentarius, Clitocybe clavipes.*	30 min	Disulfiramlike reaction with alcohol may occur up to 5 days after ingesting fungi.
Ibotenic acid, muscimol	*Amanita muscaria, A pantherina,* others.	0.5–2 h	Muscular jerking, anticholinergic syndrome, hallucinations.
Orellanine	*Cortinarius orellanus,* other *Cortinarius* spp.	1–12 days	Acute renal failure (tubulointerstitial nephritis).
Psilocybin	*Psilocybe cubensis,* others.	0.5–1 h	Hallucinations.
Gastrointestinal irritants	Many species.	0.5–2 h	Vomiting, diarrhea.

[a]Modified and reproduced, with permission, from Becker CE et al: Diagnosis and treatment of *Amanita phalloides*-type mushroom poisoning: Use of thioctic acid. *West J Med* 1976;**125**:100.

I. **Mechanism of toxicity.** The various mechanisms thought responsible for poisoning are listed in Table II–37. The majority of toxic incidents are caused by gastrointestinal irritants that produce vomiting and diarrhea shortly after ingestion.

II. **Toxic dose.** This is not known. The amount of toxin varies considerably between members of the same species, depending on local geography and weather conditions. In most cases, the exact amount of toxic mushroom ingested is unknown because the victim has unwittingly added a toxic species to a meal of edible fungi.

III. **Clinical presentation.** The various clinical presentations are described in Table II–37. In most cases, the onset of vomiting and diarrhea is rapid. A delay in onset of more than 6–12 hours suggests amatoxin, monomethylhydrazine, or orellanine poisoning.

IV. **Diagnosis** may be difficult because the victim may not realize that the illness has been caused by mushrooms, especially if symptoms are delayed 12 or more hours after ingestion. If leftover mushrooms are available, obtain assistance from a mycologist through a local university or mycologic society. However, note that the mushrooms brought for identification may not be the same ones that were eaten.

   A. **Specific levels.** Specific toxin levels are not available.

   B. **Other useful laboratory studies.** Electrolytes, glucose, BUN, creatinine, liver transaminases, and prothrombin time (PT).

V. **Treatment**

   A. **Emergency and supportive measures**

      1. Treat hypotension from gastroenteritis with intravenous crystalloid solutions (see p 15) and supine positioning.

      2. Monitor patients for 12–24 hours for delayed-onset gastroenteritis associated with amatoxin or monomethylhydrazine poisoning.

      3. For suspected *Cortinarius spp* ingestion, monitor renal function for 1–2 weeks.

   B. **Specific drugs and antidotes**

      1. For **monoethylhydrazine** poisoning, give pyridoxine, 20–30 mg/kg IV (see p 375) for seizures; treat methemoglobinemia with methylene blue, 1 mg/kg IV (p 351).

    2. For **muscarine** intoxication, atropine, 0.01–0.03 mg/kg IV (p 315), may alleviate cholinergic symptoms.

    3. Ibotenic acid–induced or **muscimol-induced** anticholinergic symptoms may improve with physostigmine (p 370).

    4. Treat **amatoxin-type** poisoning as described below.

C. Decontamination (see p 44)

    1. Prehospital. Administer activated charcoal, if available. Ipecac-induced emesis may be useful for initial treatment at the scene (eg, children at home) if it can be given within a few minutes of exposure.

    2. Hospital. Administer activated charcoal and a cathartic. Gastric emptying is not necessary if activated charcoal can be given promptly.

D. Enhanced elimination. There is no accepted role for enhanced removal procedures.

MUSHROOMS, AMATOXIN-TYPE
Kent R. Olson, MD

ANTIDOTE   IPECAC   LAVAGE   CHARCOAL

Amatoxins, (α-amanitin, β-amanitin, others) are a group of highly toxic peptides found in several species of mushrooms, including *Amanita phalloides, Amanita virosa, Amanita ocreata, Amanita verna, Galerina autumnalis, Galerina marginata,* and some species of *Lepiota.* These mushrooms are often picked and eaten by amateur foragers who have misidentified them as an edible species.

  I. Mechanism of toxicity. Amatoxins are highly stable and resistant to heat and are not removed by any form of cooking. They are thought to act by inhibiting cellular protein synthesis by interfering with RNA polymerase.

    A. Absorption of amatoxins (and phalloidins) by intestinal cells causes cell death and sloughing after a delay of 8–12 hours.

    B. Absorption by the liver and kidneys results in severe hepatic necrosis and renal failure.

 II. Toxic dose. Amatoxins are among the most potent toxins known; the minimum lethal dose is about 0.1 mg/kg. One *Amanita* cap may contain 10–15 mg. In contrast, *Galerina* species contain far less toxin; 15–20 caps would be a fatal dose for an adult.

III. Clinical presentation. The onset of symptoms is characteristically delayed 8–12 hours or more after ingestion. Death occurring within the first 1–2 days usually results from massive fluid loss owing to gastroenteritis, while death occurring later usually results from hepatic failure.

    A. Gastroenteritis. Initially, vomiting is accompanied by severe abdominal cramps and explosive watery diarrhea. Severe fluid losses can occur rapidly, and some patients die of shock within 24 hours.

    B. Hepatic failure. Those who survive the gastroenteritis phase may appear to improve for 1–2 days before the onset of hepatic failure. Hepatic transaminase levels often exceed 10,000 units then fall rapidly, and the bilirubin and prothrombin time steadily rise. Hepatic encephalopathy, metabolic acidosis, and hypoglycemia are grave prognostic signs and usually predict a fatal outcome.

IV. Diagnosis is usually based on a history of wild mushroom ingestion and the characteristic delay of 8–12 hours before onset of severe gastroenteritis (see also monomethylhydrazine-type mushrooms, p 223). However, if a variety of mushrooms has been eaten, stomach upset may occur much earlier owing to a different toxic species, making diagnosis of amatoxin poisoning more difficult.

    Any available mushroom specimens that may have been ingested should be examined by a mycologist. Pieces of mushroom retrieved from the emesis or even mushroom spores found on microscopic examination may provide clues to the ingested species.

A. Specific levels

   1. A radioimmunoassay has been developed for amatoxins but is not widely available. The toxin is rapidly bound in the body within the first several hours after ingestion, and amatoxins are generally not detectable in the serum or urine more than 24 hours after exposure.

   2. A qualitative test (the Meixner test) may determine the presence of amatoxins in mushroom specimens. A single drop of concentrated hydrochloric acid is added to dried juice from the mushroom cap that has been dripped onto newspaper or other unrefined paper; a blue color suggests the presence of amatoxins. ***Caution:*** This test should not be used to determine edibility of mushroom specimens!

B. Other useful laboratory studies. Electrolytes, glucose, BUN, creatinine, liver transaminases, bilirubin, prothrombin time (PT).

V. Treatment. The mortality rate may be higher than 60% if the patient is not treated for severe fluid losses, but is probably less than 10–15% with intensive supportive care.

A. Emergency and supportive measures

   1. Maintain the airway and assist ventilation if necessary (see p 4). Administer supplemental oxygen.

   2. Treat fluid and electrolyte losses aggressively, because massive fluid losses may cause circulatory collapse. Administer normal saline or other crystalloid solution, 10- to 20-mL/kg boluses, with monitoring of central venous pressure or even pulmonary artery pressure (p 15) to guide fluid therapy.

   3. Provide vigorous supportive care for hepatic failure (p 37); orthotopic **liver transplantation** may be lifesaving in patients who develop encephalopathy.

B. Specific drugs and antidotes. There is no proved effective antidote for amatoxin poisoning, although many popular therapies have been promoted and are still widely used. Animal studies suggest that early treatment with penicillin, silibinin, or cimetidine may partially protect against hepatic injury. Consult a medical toxicologist or a regional poison control center (see Table I–41, p 53) for further information.

C. Decontamination (see p 44)

   1. Prehospital. Administer activated charcoal, if available. Ipecac-induced emesis may be useful for initial treatment at the scene (eg, children at home) if it can be given within a few minutes of exposure.

   2. Hospital. Administer activated charcoal. Gastric lavage may not remove mushroom pieces.

D. Enhanced elimination. There is no proved role for forced diuresis, hemoperfusion, or hemodialysis in the removal of amatoxins.

   1. Repeat-dose activated charcoal may trap small quantities of amatoxin undergoing enterohepatic recirculation.

   2. Cannulation of the bile duct and removal of bile have been effective in dog studies.

NAPHTHALENE AND PARADICHLOROBENZENE
Mark J. Galbo, MS

ANTIDOTE   IPECAC   LAVAGE   CHARCOAL

Naphthalene and paradichlorobenzene are common ingredients in diaper pail and toilet bowl deodorizers and mothballs. Both compounds have a similar pungent odor and clear to white crystalline substances, and are therefore difficult to distinguish visually. Naphthalene is no longer commonly used because it has been largely replaced by the far less toxic paradichlorobenzene.

I. Mechanism of toxicity. Both compounds cause gastrointestinal upset, and both may cause central nervous system stimulation. In addition, naphthalene may produce hemolysis, especially in patients with glucose-6-phosphate dehydrogenase (G6PD) deficiency.

II. Toxic dose

    A. Naphthalene. As little as one mothball containing naphthalene (250–500 mg) may produce hemolysis in a patient with G6PD deficiency. The amount necessary to produce lethargy or seizures is not known but may be as little as 1–2 g (4–8 mothballs).

    B. Paradichlorobenzene is much less toxic than naphthalene; up to 20-g ingestions have been well-tolerated in adults. The oral LD_{50} for paradichlorobenzene in rats is 2.5–3.2 g/kg.

III. Clinical presentation. Acute ingestion usually causes prompt nausea and vomiting. Both compounds are volatile, and inhalation of vapors may cause eye, nose, and throat irritation.

    A. Naphthalene. Agitation, lethargy, and seizures may occur with naphthalene ingestion. In patients with G6PD deficiency, naphthalene ingestion may cause acute hemolysis.

    B. Paradichlorobenzene ingestions are virtually always innocuous. Serious poisoning in animals is reported to cause tremors and hepatic necrosis. Paradichlorobenzene decomposes to hydrochloric acid, which may explain some of its irritant effects.

IV. Diagnosis is usually based on a history of ingestion and the characteristic "mothball" smell around the mouth and in the vomitus. Differentiation between naphthalene and paradichlorobenzene by odor or color is difficult. Paradichlorobenzene is reportedly more rapidly soluble in turpentine.

    A. Specific levels. Serum levels are not available.

    B. Other useful laboratory studies. CBC. If hemolysis suspected: haptoglobin, free hemoglobin, urine dipstick for occult blood (positive with hemoglobinuria).

V. Treatment

    A. Emergency and supportive measures

        1. Maintain the airway and assist ventilation if necessary (see p 4).

        2. Treat coma (p 18) and seizures (p 22) if they occur.

        3. Treat hemolysis and resulting hemoglobinuria, if they occur, by intravenous hydration and urinary alkalinization (see Rhabdomyolysis, p 25).

    B. Specific drugs and antidotes. There is no specific antidote.

    C. Decontamination (see p 44)

        1. Naphthalene

            a. Prehospital. Administer activated charcoal, if available. Ipecac-induced emesis may be useful for initial treatment at the scene (eg, children at home) if it can be given immediately after exposure. Do not administer milk, fats, or oils, which may enhance absorption.

            b. Hospital. Administer activated charcoal and a cathartic. Gastric emptying is not necessary if activated charcoal can be given promptly.

        2. Paradichlorobenzene. Gut emptying and charcoal are not necessary unless a massive dose has been ingested.

        3. Inhalation. Either agent: remove victim from exposure; fresh air is all that is required.

    D. Enhanced elimination. There is no role for these procedures.

NICOTINE
Neal L. Benowitz, MD

ANTIDOTE   IPECAC   LAVAGE   CHARCOAL

Nicotine poisoning may occur in children after they ingest tobacco or drink saliva expectorated by a tobacco chewer (which is often collected in a can or other containers);

in children or adults after accidental or suicidal ingestion of nicotine-containing pesticides (such as Black Leaf 40, which contains 40% nicotine sulfate); and occasionally after cutaneous exposure to nicotine, such as in tobacco harvesters. Nicotine chewing gum (Nicorette) and transdermal delivery formulations (Habitrol, Nicoderm, Nicotrol, Prostep) are widely available as adjunctive therapy for smoking cessation.

I. **Mechanism of toxicity.** Nicotine binds to nicotinic cholinergic receptors, resulting initially, via actions on ganglia, in predominantly sympathetic nervous stimulation. With higher doses, parasympathetic stimulation and then ganglionic and neuromuscular blockage may occur. Direct effects on the brain may also result in vomiting and seizures.

II. **Toxic dose.** Owing to presystemic metabolism and spontaneous vomiting, which limit absorption, the bioavailability of nicotine that is swallowed is about 30–40%. Rapid absorption of 2–5 mg can cause nausea and vomiting, particularly in a person who does not habitually use tobacco. Absorption of 40–60 mg in an adult is said to be lethal, although this dose spread throughout the day is not unusual in a cigarette smoker.

   A. **Tobacco.** Cigarette tobacco contains about 1.5% nicotine, or 10–15 mg of nicotine per cigarette. Moist snuff is also about 1.5% nicotine; most containers hold 30 g of tobacco. Chewing tobacco contains 2.5–8% nicotine. In a child, ingestion of 1 cigarette or 3 butts should be considered potentially toxic, although serious poisoning from ingestion of cigarettes is very uncommon.

   B. **Nicotine gum** contains 2 mg per piece in the USA and 4 mg in Canada and Europe, but owing to its slow absorption and high degree of presystemic metabolism, nicotine intoxication from these products is uncommon.

   C. **Transdermal nicotine patches** deliver an average of 5–22 mg of nicotine over the 16–24 hours of intended application, depending on the brand and size. Transdermal patches may produce intoxication in light smokers or in nonsmokers, particularly children to whom a used patch inadvertently sticks. Ingestion of a discarded patch may also potentially produce poisoning.

III. **Clinical presentation.** Nicotine intoxication commonly causes dizziness, nausea, vomiting, pallor, and diaphoresis. Abdominal pain, salivation, lacrimation, and diarrhea may be noted. Pupils may be dilated or constricted. Confusion, agitation, lethargy, and convulsions are seen with severe poisonings. Initial tachycardia and hypertension may be followed by bradycardia and hypotension. Respiratory muscle weakness with respiratory arrest is the most likely cause of death.

   Symptoms usually begin within 15 minutes after acute liquid nicotine exposure and resolve in 1 or 2 hours, although more prolonged symptoms may be seen with higher doses or cutaneous exposure, the latter owing to continued absorption from the skin. Delayed onset and prolonged symptoms may also be seen with nicotine gum or transdermal patches.

IV. **Diagnosis** is suggested by vomiting, pallor, and diaphoresis, although these symptoms are nonspecific. The diagnosis is usually made by a history of tobacco, insecticide, or therapeutic nicotine product exposure. Nicotine poisoning should be considered in a small child with unexplained vomiting whose parents consume tobacco.

   A. **Specific levels.** Nicotine is detected in urine screens, but because it is so commonly present, it will not be reported unless specifically requested. Serum levels can be performed but are not useful in acute management.

   B. **Other useful laboratory studies.** Electrolytes, glucose, arterial blood gases or oximetry.

V. **Treatment**

   A. **Emergency and supportive measures**

      1. Maintain the airway and assist ventilation if necessary (see p 4). Administer supplemental oxygen.

      2. Treat seizures (p 22), coma (p 18), hypotension (p 15), hypertension (p 17), and arrhythmias (p 10–14) if they occur.

      3. Observe for at least 4–6 hours to rule out delayed toxicity, especially after skin exposure. For ingestion of intact gum tablets or transdermal patches, observe for a longer period (up to 12–24 hours).

B. Specific drugs and antidotes

1. **Mecamylamine (Inversine)** is a specific antagonist of nicotine actions; however, it is available only in tablets, a form not suitable for a patient who is vomiting, convulsing, or hypotensive.
2. Signs of muscarinic stimulation (bradycardia, salivation, wheezing, etc), if they occur, may respond to **atropine** (see p 315).

C. Decontamination (see p 41). *Caution:* Rescuers should wear appropriate skin protective gear when treating patients with oral or skin exposure to liquid nicotine.

1. **Skin and eyes.** Remove all contaminated clothing and wash exposed skin with copious soap and water. Irrigate exposed eyes with copious saline or water.
2. **Ingestion** (see p 44). For asymptomatic small quantity cigarette ingestions, no gut decontamination is necessary.
   a. **Prehospital.** Administer activated charcoal, if available. Do *not* induce emesis because of the risk of abrupt onset of seizures.
   b. **Hospital.** Administer activated charcoal and a cathartic. Consider gastric lavage for large recent ingestion of liquid nicotine.
   c. For ingestion of transdermal patches or large amounts of gum, consider repeated doses of charcoal and whole bowel irrigation (see p 48).

D. Enhanced elimination. These procedures are not likely to be useful because the endogenous clearance of nicotine is high, its half-life is relatively short (2 hours), and the volume of distribution is large.

NITRATES AND NITRITES
Neal L. Benowitz, MD

ANTIDOTE   IPECAC   LAVAGE   CHARCOAL

Organic nitrates (eg, nitroglycerin, isosorbide dinitrate, isosorbide mononitrate) are widely used as vasodilators for the treatment of ischemic heart disease and heart failure. Organic nitrates such as nitroglycerin are also used in explosives. Bismuth subnitrate, ammonium nitrate, and silver nitrate are used in antidiarrheal, diuretic, and topical burn medications, respectively. Sodium and potassium nitrate and nitrite are used in preserving cured foods and may also occur in high concentrations in some well water. Butyl, amyl, ethyl, and isobutyl nitrite are often sold as "room deodorizers" or "liquid incense" and are inhaled for abuse purposes.

I. **Mechanism of toxicity.** Nitrates and nitrites both cause vasodilation, which can result in hypotension.
   A. **Nitrates** relax veins at lower doses and arteries at higher doses. Nitrates may be converted into nitrites in the gastrointestinal tract, especially in infants.
   B. **Nitrites** are potent oxidizing agents. Oxidation of hemoglobin by nitrites may result in methemoglobinemia (see p 217), which hinders oxygen-carrying capacity and oxygen delivery. Many organic nitrites (eg, amyl nitrite, butyl nitrite) are volatile and may be inhaled.

II. **Toxic dose.** In the quantities found in food, nitrates and nitrites are generally not toxic; however, infants may develop methemoglobinemia after ingestion of sausages or well water because they readily convert nitrate to nitrite and because their hemoglobin is more susceptible to oxidation compared with that of adults.
   A. **Nitrates.** The estimated adult lethal oral dose of nitroglycerin is 200–1200 mg. Hypotension occurs at low doses, but massive doses are required to produce methemoglobinemia.
   B. **Nitrites.** Ingestion of as little as 15 mL of butyl nitrite produced 40% methemoglobinemia in an adult. The estimated adult lethal oral dose of sodium nitrite is 1 g.

III. Clinical presentation. Headache, skin flushing, and orthostatic hypotension with reflex tachycardia are the most common adverse effects of nitrates and nitrites and occur commonly even with therapeutic doses of organic nitrates.

    A. Hypotension may aggravate or produce symptoms of cardiac ischemia or cerebrovascular disease and may even cause seizures. However, fatalities from hypotension are rare.

    B. Workers or patients regularly exposed to nitrates may develop tolerance and may suffer **angina** or **myocardial infarction** owing to rebound coronary vasoconstriction upon sudden withdrawal of the drug.

    C. Methemoglobinemia (see p 217) is most common after nitrite exposure; the skin is cyanotic, even at levels low enough to be otherwise asymptomatic (eg, 15%).

IV. Diagnosis is suggested by hypotension with reflex tachycardia and headache. Methemoglobinemia of 15% or more may be diagnosed by noting a chocolate brown coloration of the blood when it is dripped onto filter paper.

    A. Specific levels. Serum levels are not commercially available.

        1. With the use of a nitrite dipstick (normally used to detect bacteria in urine), nitrite can be detected in the serum of patients intoxicated by butyl nitrite.

        2. The Kodak Ektachem analyzer may report an increased total CO_2 (HCO_3), 0.6 meq/L for each mmol/L of nitrate, in the presence of serum nitrates.

    B. Other useful laboratory studies. Electrolytes, glucose, arterial blood gases or oximetry, methemoglobin concentration, ECG and ECG monitoring.

V. Treatment

    A. Emergency and supportive measures

        1. Maintain the airway and assist ventilation if necessary (see p 4). Administer supplemental oxygen.

        2. Treat hypotension with supine positioning, intravenous crystalloid fluids, and low-dose pressors if needed (see p 15).

        3. Monitor vital signs and ECG for 4–6 hours.

    B. Specific drugs and antidotes. Symptomatic methemoglobinemia may be treated with **methylene blue** (see p 351).

    C. Decontamination (see p 41)

        1. Inhalation. Remove victim from exposure and administer supplemental oxygen, if available.

        2. Skin and eyes. Remove contaminated clothing and wash with copious soap and water. Irrigate exposed eyes with water or saline.

        3. Ingestion (see p 44)

            a. Prehospital. Administer activated charcoal, if available. Ipecac-induced emesis may be useful for initial treatment at the scene (eg, children at home) if it can be given within a few minutes of exposure.

            b. Hospital. Administer activated charcoal and a cathartic. Gastric emptying is not necessary for small ingestions if activated charcoal can be given promptly.

    D. Enhanced elimination. Hemodialysis and hemoperfusion are not effective. Severe methemoglobinemia in infants not responsive to methylene blue therapy may require **exchange transfusion.**

NITROGEN OXIDES
Kent R. Olson, MD

ANTIDOTE   IPECAC   LAVAGE   CHARCOAL

Nitrogen oxides (nitric oxide, nitrogen dioxide) are dangerous chemical gases commonly released from nitrous or nitric acid, from reactions between nitric acid and organic materials, and from burning of nitrocellulose and many other products. Exposure to nitrogen oxides occurs in electric arc welding, electroplating, and engraving. Nitrogen oxides are found in engine exhaust, and they are produced when stored grain with a high nitrite content ferments in storage silos.

I. **Mechanism of toxicity.** Nitrogen oxides are irritant gases with relatively low water solubility. Slow accumulation and hydration to nitric acid in the alveoli results in delayed onset of chemical pneumonitis. In addition, nitrogen oxides can oxidize hemoglobin to methemoglobin.

II. **Toxic dose.** The ACGIH-recommended workplace exposure limit (threshold limit value; TLV) for nitric oxide is 25 ppm, and for nitrogen dioxide it is 3 ppm as 8-hour time-weighted averages. The air levels considered immediately dangerous to life or health (IDLH) are 100 ppm and 50 ppm, respectively.

III. **Clinical presentation.** Because of the poor water solubility of nitrogen oxides, there is very little upper respiratory irritation at low levels (< 10 ppm nitrogen dioxide), and allowing prolonged exposure with no warning symptoms other than mild cough or nausea. With more concentrated exposures, upper respiratory symptoms such as burning eyes, sore throat, and painful brassy cough may occur.

   A. After a delay of up to 24 hours, chemical pneumonia may develop, with progressive cough, tachypnea, hypoxemia, and pulmonary edema. The onset may be more rapid after exposure to higher concentrations.

   B. Following recovery from acute chemical pneumonia and after chronic low-level exposure to nitrogen oxides, permanent restrictive and obstructive lung disease from bronchiolar damage may become evident.

   C. Methemoglobinemia has (see p 217) been described in victims exposed to nitrogen oxides in smoke during major structural fires.

IV. **Diagnosis** is based on a history of exposure, if known. Because of the potential for delayed effects, all patients with significant smoke inhalation should be observed for several hours.

   A. **Specific levels.** There are no specific blood levels.

   B. **Other useful laboratory studies.** Arterial blood gases or oximetry, methemoglobin level, chest x-ray, pulmonary function tests.

V. **Treatment**

   A. **Emergency and supportive measures**

      1. Observe closely for signs of upper airway obstruction, and intubate the trachea and assist ventilation if necessary (see p 13). Administer humidified supplemental oxygen.

      2. Observe symptomatic victims for a minimum of 24 hours after exposure and treat chemical pneumonia and noncardiogenic pulmonary edema (see p 8) if they occur.

   B. **Specific drugs and antidotes**

      1. Administration of corticosteroids has been recommended, but there is no convincing evidence that they can improve nitrogen oxide–induced chemical pneumonia or pulmonary edema or prevent chronic bronchitis.

      2. Treat methemoglobinemia with **methylene blue** (see p 351).

   C. **Decontamination** (see p 41). Rescuers should wear self-contained breathing apparatus, and if there is the potential for high-level gas exposure or exposure to liquid nitric acid, chemical protective clothing.

      1. **Inhalation.** Remove victim from exposure immediately and give supplemental oxygen, if available.

      2. **Skin and eyes.** Remove any wet clothing, and flush exposed skin with water. Irrigate exposed eyes with copious water or saline.

   D. **Enhanced elimination.** There is no role for enhanced elimination procedures.

NITROPRUSSIDE
Neal L. Benowitz, MD

ANTIDOTE   IPECAC   LAVAGE   CHARCOAL

Sodium nitroprusside is a short-acting parenterally administered vasodilator used to treat severe hypertension and cardiac failure. It is also used to induce hypotension for certain surgical procedures. Toxicity may occur with acute high-dose nitroprusside treatment or with prolonged infusions.

I. **Mechanism of toxicity.** Nitroprusside is rapidly hydrolyzed and releases free cyanide, which is normally quickly converted to thiocyanate by rhodanase enzymes in the liver and blood vessels.

   A. **Acute cyanide poisoning** (see p 145) may occur with short-term high-dose nitroprusside infusions (eg, > 10–15 μg/kg/min for 1 hour or longer).

   B. **Thiocyanate** is eliminated by the kidney and may accumulate in patients with renal insufficiency, especially after prolonged infusions.

II. **Toxic dose.** The toxic dose depends on renal function and the rate of infusion.

   A. **Cyanide** poisoning is uncommon at nitroprusside infusion rates of less than 8–10 μg/kg/min, but has been reported after infusion of 4 μg/kg/min for 3 hours.

   B. **Thiocyanate** toxicity does not occur with acute brief use in persons with normal renal function, but may result from prolonged infusions (eg, > 3 μg/kg/min for 48 hours or longer), especially in persons with renal insufficiency (with rates as low as 1 μg/kg/min).

III. **Clinical presentation.** The most common adverse effect of nitroprusside is hypotension, which is often accompanied by reflex tachycardia.

   A. **Cyanide** poisoning is accompanied by headache, hyperventilation, anxiety, agitation, seizures, and metabolic acidosis. The ECG may reveal ischemic patterns.

   B. **Thiocyanate** poisoning causes somnolence, confusion, delirium, tremor, and hyperreflexia. Seizures and coma may rarely occur with severe toxicity.

   C. Methemoglobinemia occurs rarely and is usually mild.

IV. **Diagnosis.** Lactic acidosis, coma, or seizures after short-term high-dose nitroprusside infusion should suggest cyanide poisoning, while confusion or delirium developing gradually after several days of continuous use should suggest thiocyanate poisoning.

   A. **Specific levels. Cyanide** levels may be obtained but are not usually available rapidly enough to guide treatment when cyanide poisoning is suspected. Cyanide levels may not accurately reflect toxicity because of simultaneous production of methemoglobin, which binds some of the cyanide. Cyanide levels greater than 1 mg/L usually produce a demonstrable lactic acidosis. **Thiocyanate** levels higher than 50–100 mg/L may cause delirium and somnolence.

   B. **Other useful laboratory studies.** Electrolytes, glucose, BUN, creatinine, serum lactate, ECG, arterial blood gases and measured arterial and venous oxygen saturation (see Cyanide, p 145), methemoglobin level.

V. **Treatment**

   A. **Emergency and supportive measures**

      1. Maintain the airway and assist ventilation if necessary (see p 4). Administer supplemental oxygen.

      2. For hypotension, stop the infusion immediately and administer intravenous fluids or even pressors if necessary (p 15).

   B. **Specific drugs and antidotes.** If cyanide poisoning is suspected, administer **sodium thiosulfate** (see p 376). Sodium nitrite treatment may aggravate hypotension and should not be used. **Hydroxocobalamin** (see p 344), 25 mg/h IV infusion, is sometimes coadministered with high-dose nitroprusside as prophylaxis against cyanide toxicity.

   C. **Decontamination.** These procedures are not relevant because the drug is administered only parenterally.

   D. **Enhanced elimination.** Nitroprusside and cyanide are both metabolized rapidly, so there is no need to consider enhanced elimination for these. Hemodialysis may accelerate **thiocyanate** elimination and is especially useful in patients with renal failure.

NITROUS OXIDE
Charles E. Becker, MD

ANTIDOTE   IPECAC   LAVAGE   CHARCOAL

Nitrous oxide, or laughing gas, is used as a general anesthetic agent and as a propellant in many commercial products such as whipped cream or cooking oil spray. Nitorus oxide is used by up to 50% of US dentists, in many cases without adequate scavenging equipment. Abuse of nitrous oxide is not uncommon in the medical and dental professions.

I. Mechanism of toxicity

    A. Acute toxicity following exposure to nitrous oxide is mainly caused by asphyxia if adequate oxygen is not supplied with the gas.

    B. Chronic toxicity to the hematologic and nervous systems is believed to be secondary to the selective inactivation of vitamin B_{12}. Adverse reproductive outcome has been reported in workers chronically exposed to nitrous oxide.

II. Toxic dose. The toxic dose is not established. Chronic occupational exposure to 2000 ppm nitrous oxide produced asymptomatic but measurable depression of vitamin B_{12} in dentists. The ACGIH recommended workplace exposure limit (TLV-TWA) is 50 ppm (91 mg/m^3) as an 8-hour time-weighted average.

III. Clinical presentation

    A. Signs of **acute toxicity** are related to **asphyxia.** These include headache, dizziness, confusion, syncope, seizures, and cardiac arrhythmias. Interstitial emphysema and pneumomediastinum have been reported following forceful inhalation from a pressurized whipped cream dispenser.

    B. Chronic nitrous oxide abuse may produce megaloblastic anemia, thrombocytopenia, leukopenia, peripheral neuropathy, and myelopathy, similar to effects of vitamin B_{12} deficiency.

IV. Diagnosis is based on a history of exposure and clinical presentation with evidence of asphyxia and an empty can or tank or with manifestations of chronic vitamin B_{12} deficiency but with normal vitamin B_{12} levels.

    A. Specific levels. Specific levels are not generally available and are unreliable owing to off-gassing.

    B. Other useful laboratory studies. CBC, platelet count, vitamin B_{12}.

V. Treatment

    A. Emergency and supportive measures

        1. Maintain the airway and assist ventilation if necessary (see p 4). Administer high-flow supplemental oxygen.

        2. After significant asphyxia, anticipate and treat coma (p 18), seizures (p 22), and cardiac arrhythmias (p 10–14).

    B. Specific drugs and antidotes. There is no specific antidote. Chronic effects may resolve over 2–3 months after discontinuing exposure.

    C. Decontamination. Remove victim from exposure and give supplemental oxygen, if available.

    D. Enhanced elimination. These procedures are not effective.

NONSTEROIDAL ANTI-INFLAMMATORY DRUGS
Kathryn H. Keller, PharmD

ANTIDOTE   IPECAC   LAVAGE   CHARCOAL

The nonsteroidal anti-inflammatory drugs (NSAIDs) are a chemically diverse group of agents that share similar pharmacologic properties and are widely used for control of

TABLE II–38. COMMON NSAIDs

Drug	Maximum Daily Adult Dose (mg)	Half-Life (h)	Comments
Carboxylic acids			
Diclofenac	195	2	
Fenoprofen	3200	3	Acute renal failure
Ibuprofen	3200	2.5	Massive overdose may cause coma, renal failure, metabolic acidosis, and cardiorespiratory depression.
Indomethacin	200	3–11	
Ketoprofen	300	2–4	
Meclofenamate	400	3	
Mefenamic acid	750	3	Seizures, twitching
Naproxen	1500	10–20	
Sulindac	400	7	
Suprofen	800	2–4	
Tolmetin	2000	5–6	
Enolic acids			
Oxyphenbutazone	600	27–64	Seizures, acidosis
Phenylbutazone	600	75	Seizures, acidosis
Piroxicam	20	45–50	Seizures, coma

pain and inflammation (Table II–38). Overdose by most of the agents in this group usually produces only mild gastrointestinal upset. However, toxicity may be severe following overdose with **oxyphenbutazone, phenylbutazone, mefenamic acid, piroxicam,** or **diflunisal.**

I. **Mechanism of toxicity.** NSAIDs produce their pharmacologic and most toxicologic effects by inhibiting the enzyme cyclooxygenase; this results in decreased production of prostaglandins and decreased pain and inflammation. Central nervous system, hemodynamic, pulmonary, and hepatic dysfunction also occur with some agents, but the relationship to prostaglandin production remains uncertain. Prostaglandins are also involved in maintaining the integrity of the gastric mucosa and regulating renal blood flow; thus, acute or chronic intoxication may affect these organs.

II. **Toxic dose.** Human data are insufficient to establish a reliable correlation between amount ingested, plasma concentrations, and clinical toxic effects. Generally, significant symptoms occur after ingestion of more than 5–10 times the usual therapeutic dose.

III. **Clinical presentation.** In general, patients with NSAID overdose are asymptomatic or have mild gastrointestinal upset (nausea, vomiting, abdominal pain, sometimes hematemesis). Occasionally patients exhibit drowsiness, lethargy, ataxia, nystagmus, tinnitus, and disorientation.

A. With the more toxic agents **oxyphenbutazone, phenylbutazone, mefenamic acid,** or **piroxicam** and with massive **ibuprofen** overdose, seizures, coma, renal failure, and cardiorespiratory arrest may occur. Hepatic dysfunction, hypoprothrombinemia, and metabolic acidosis are also commonly reported.

B. **Diflunisal** overdose produces toxicity resembling salicylate poisoning (see p 277).

IV. **Diagnosis** is usually based primarily on a history of ingestion of NSAIDs, because symptoms are mild and nonspecific and quantitative levels are not usually available.

A. Specific levels are not usually readily available and do not contribute to clinical management.

B. Other useful laboratory studies. CBC, electrolytes, glucose, BUN, creatinine, liver transaminases, prothrombin time (PT), urinalysis.

V. Treatment

A. Emergency and supportive measures

1. Maintain the airway and assist ventilation if necessary (see p 4). Administer supplemental oxygen.
2. Treat seizures (p 22), coma (p 18), and hypotension (p 15) if they occur.
3. Antacids may be used for mild gastrointestinal upset. Replace fluid losses with intravenous crystalloid solutions.

B. Specific drugs and antidotes. There is no antidote. Vitamin K (see p 377) may be used for patients with elevated prothrombin time (PT) caused by hypoprothrombinemia.

C. Decontamination (see p 44)

1. **Prehospital.** Administer activated charcoal, if available. Ipecac-induced emesis may be useful for initial treatment at the scene (eg, children at home) if it can be given within a few minutes of exposure.
2. **Hospital.** Administer activated charcoal and a cathartic. Gastric emptying is not necessary for most ingestions if activated charcoal can be given promptly. Consider gastric lavage for massive overdoses.

D. Enhanced elimination. NSAIDs are highly protein-bound and extensively metabolized. Thus, hemodialysis, peritoneal dialysis, and forced diuresis are not likely to be effective.

1. **Charcoal hemoperfusion** may be effective for **phenylbutazone** overdose, although there are limited clinical data to support its use.
2. There are no data on the use of repeat-dose activated charcoal therapy.

NONTOXIC OR MINIMALLY TOXIC HOUSEHOLD PRODUCTS
Ilene B. Anderson, PharmD

| ANTIDOTE | IPECAC | LAVAGE | CHARCOAL |

There are a variety of products commonly found around home that have little or no toxicity after typical accidental exposures (Tables II–39, II–40, and II–41). Treatment is rarely required after small to moderate acute ingestions because the products contain no toxic materials, the concentrations of toxic ingredients are minimal, or the construction or packaging of the product is such that a significant dose is very unlikely. Some water or other liquid may be given to dilute the taste or texture of the product.

TABLE II–39. NONTOXIC PRODUCTS[a]

Air fresheners	Cat food	Cyanoacrylate glues
Allergan Clean-n-Soak	Caulk	Cyclamate
Aluminum foil	Charcoal	Deodorants
Antiperspirants	Charcoal briquettes	Desiccants
Antrol Ant Killer Formula II (boric acid 2%)	Cigarette ashes	Diaperene Baby Wash Cloths
	Cigarette filter tips (unsmoked)	Diapers, disposable
Ashes, wood/fireplace	Clay	Dyprotex Diaper Rash Pads
Baby Magic Baby Lotion	Cold packs (for large ingestions, see Nitrates, p 229)	Elmer's Glue
Baby Wipes		Erasers
Ball-point pen ink	Crayola Markers	Etch-A-Sketch
Calamine lotion	Crayons	Eye makeup
Candles	Crazy Glue	Felt-tip markers and pens

Fingernail polish
Florever, Oasis
Fly Control Trap attractant
Glade Plug-In's
Glitter
Glow stick/jewelry
Gum
Gypsum
Incense
Indelible markers
Ink (w/out aniline dyes)
Kitty litter
Lipstick
Magic markers
Makeup
Mascara
Massengil Disposable Douche
Matches (< 3 paper books)
Mylar balloons

Newspaper
Nox-Ich
Nutrasweet
PAAS Easter egg dyes (after
    1980)
Pencils (contain graphite, not
    lead)
Photographs
Plastic
Playdoh
Putty
Renuzit Air Freshener
Rouge
Rust
Saccharin (Sweet 'n Lo)
Sheetrock
Shoe polish
Silica gel
Silly putty

Soil
Spackle
Stamp pad Ink
Starch
Stick-em Glue Traps
Styrofoam
Sunscreen products
Suntan lotions
Superglue
Teething rings (fluid may have
    bacterial growth)
Thermometers (elemental
    mercury or phthalates/alcohol)
Watercolor paints
Windex Glass Cleaner with
    Ammonia-D (for large inges-
    tion, see Isopropyl alcohol,
    p 193)
Zinc oxide ointment

[a]These items are virtually nontoxic in small to moderate exposures. However, the taste or texture of the product may result in mild stomach upset. In addition, some of the products may cause a foreign body effect or choking hazard, depending on the size of the product and the age of the child.

TABLE II–40. MILD GASTROINTESTINAL IRRITANTS[a]

A & D Ointment
Ajax Cleanser
Antacids
Antibiotic ointments
Aosept Disinfectant Solution
    (3% hydrogen peroxide)
Baby Magic Baby Bath
Baby Magic Baby Shampoo
Baby oil (if aspirated, see p 178)
Bar soap
Bath oil beads
Bath oils (if aspirated, see p 178)
Bleach (household, less than 6%
    hypochlorite)
Body lotions and creams
Boston Cleaner
Bubble bath
Bubbles
Caldesene Medicated Ointment
Carbamide peroxide 6.5%
Chalk (calcium carbonate)
Clorox Liquid Bleach
Clotrimazole cream
Comet Cleanser
Cortaid Cream
Corticosteroids
Cortisporin Otic
Cyalume Lightstick
Dawn Dishwashing Liquid
Debrox Drops
Desenex Ointment
Desitin Diaper Rash Ointment
Dishwashing liquid soaps (not
    electric dishwashing type)
Fabric softeners

Fantastik All Purpose Cleaner
Fertilizers (nitrogen, phosphoric
    acid, and potash)
Formula 409 All Purpose Cleaner
Glory rug cleaner
Hair conditioners
Hair shampoos
Hand soaps
Head and Shoulders shampoo
Hydrocortisone cream
Hydrogen peroxide 3%
Ivory Bar Soap
Joy dishwashing soap
Kaolin
Lactaid
Lanolin
Latex paint
Liquid soaps
Lotrimin Cream
Lubricating oils (if aspirated; see
    p 178)
Lysol Deodorizing Cleaner
Lysol Disinfectant Spray (70%
    ethanol, if large ingestion, see
    p 160)
Maalox antacid
Mineral oil (if aspirated, see
    p 178)
Miracle-Gro Plant Food
Motor oil (if aspirated, see p 178)
Mr. Clean
Murine Ear Drops
Murphys' Oil Soap
Mylanta antacid
Mylicon Drops

Neosporin Ointment
Neutrogena Soap
Nystatin Cream
Palmolive Dishwashing Detergent
Polysporin Ointment
Prednisone
Preparation H Ointment
Preparation H Suppository
Pre-wash Soil and Stain Remover
Purex Liquid Bleach
Resolve carpet cleaner
Rolaids antacids
Schultz Liquid Plant Food
Shaving cream
Shout Laundry Soil and Stain
    Remover
Simethicone
Simple Green
Soft Scrub
Spic and Span
Spray and Wash
Steroid creams
Stick-em Glue Traps
Tinactin
Triphasil
Tums antacids
Vaseline Petroleum Jelly
Wisk
Woolite Rug Cleaner

[a]The items in this list usually have little or no effect in small ingestions. In moderate to large ingestions, gastrointestinal effects such as diarrhea, constipation, stomach cramps, or vomiting may occur. The effects are usually mild and rarely require medical intervention.

TABLE II–41. OTHER LOW-TOXICITY PRODUCTS[a]

Products	Comments
Holiday hazards	
Angel hair	Finely spun glass. Dermal or ocular irritation or corneal abrasion is possible.
Bubble lights	May contain a tiny amount of methylene chloride.
Christmas tree ornaments	Can cause foreign body effect or choking hazard. Antique or foreign-made ornaments may be decorated with lead-based paint.
Christmas tree preservatives	Homemade solutions may contain aspirin, bleach, or sugar. Commercial products usually contain only concentrated sugar solution.
Easter egg dyes	Most of these contain nontoxic dyes. Most also contain sodium bicarbonate or sodium chloride, which can cause hypernatremia if a large amount is ingested (see Sodium, p 33)
Fireplace crystals	May contain salts of copper, selenium, arsenic, and antimony. Small amounts can cause irritation to the mouth or stomach. (Larger ingestions could conceivably result in heavy metal poisoning; see specific heavy metal).
Halloween candy	Tampering rarely occurs. X-ray of candy provides a false sense of security; although it may reveal radiopaque glass or metallic objects, most poisons are radiolucent. Prudent approach is to discard candy or food items that are not commercially packaged or if the package is damaged.
Snow scenes	The "snow" is comprised of insoluble particles of calcium carbonate that are not toxic. The fluid may have bacterial growth.
Snow sprays	Sprays may contain hydrocarbon solvent vehicle. Inhalation may cause headache and nausea. Once dried, the snow is not toxic.
Household pesticides	
Black Flag Ant and Roach Spray Black Flag Ant and Roach Spray, Formula B Ortho Ant, Roach and Spider Killer Ovitrol Plus Flea Spray with Precor Raid Ant and Roach Killer	Numerous formulations, some contain hydrocarbon solvents, others are water-based. Pesticides used may include pyrethrins, organophosphates, or carbamates, but generally low potency and in concentrations less than 1.5%. The risk of pesticide poisoning is very low unless intentional misuse results in massive exposure. Major potential toxicity is related to inhalation of the hydrocarbon solvent.
Black Flag Ant Trap Black Flag Ant Trap, Formula II Combat Ant Control System Ortho Ant Killer Bait Raid ant controller Raid ant traps	Most of these ant traps contain less than 1% pesticide, and the remainder is a nontoxic attractant. Poisoning is very unlikely from ingestion of the contents of one trap.
Roundup Herbicide	Contains glyphosate, which has produced dermatitis with skin exposure. Ingestion results in gastrointestinal upset, but not serious systemic toxicity.
Miscellaneous	
Birth control pills (Ortho-Novum, Lo-Ovral, etc)	Birth control pills contain varying amounts of estrogens and progesterones. In excessive amounts these may cause stomach upset, and in females (even prepubertal) may cause transient vaginal spotting.
Capsaicin sprays (eg, Cobra, Halt)	These self-defense sprays contain capsaicin, the main ingredient in chili peppers. Exposure causes intense mucous membrane irritation and burning sensation.

(continued)

TABLE II–41. OTHER LOW-TOXICITY PRODUCTS[a] (CONTINUED)

Products	Comments
Fire extinguishers	The 2 common types contain sodium bicarbonate (white powder) or monoammonium phosphate (yellow powder). Small ingestions result in little to no effect. Mucous membrane irritation is common. Major risk is pneumonitis after extensive inhalation.
Fluorescent light bulbs	Contain inert gases and a nontoxic powder that may be irritating to mucous membranes.
Respiratory irritants	
Aerosol products with hydrocarbon propellants Baby powders Caldesene powder Desenex powder Spray starch	These products have little or no toxicity when ingested. However, if aspirated into the lungs, they can cause an inflammatory pneumonitis.

[a]These products may contain small amounts of potentially toxic ingredients, but rarely cause problems because of the small concentrations or conditions of exposure.

OPIATES AND OPIOIDS
Kent R. Olson, MD

ANTIDOTE   IPECAC   LAVAGE   CHARCOAL

Opiates are a group of naturally occurring compounds derived from the juice of the poppy *Papaver somniferum*. Morphine is the classic opiate derivative used widely in medicine; heroin (diacetylmorphine) is a well-known, highly addictive street narcotic. The term *opioids* refers to these and other derivatives of naturally occurring opium (eg, morphine, heroin, codeine, hydrocodone) as well as new, totally synthetic opiate analogues (eg, fentanyl, butorphanol, meperidine, methadone; Table II–42). A wide variety of prescription medications contain opioids, often in combination with aspirin or acetaminophen. Dextromethorphan (see p 153) is an opioid derivative with potent antitussive but no analgesic or addictive properties.

I. **Mechanism of toxicity.** In general, opioids share the ability to stimulate a number of specific opiate receptors in the central nervous system, causing sedation and respiratory depression. Death results from respiratory failure, usually as a result of apnea or pulmonary aspiration of gastric contents. In addition, acute noncardiogenic pulmonary edema may occur by unknown mechanisms.

II. **Toxic dose.** The toxic dose varies widely depending on the specific compound, the route and rate of administration, and tolerance to the effects of the drug as a result of chronic use. Some newer fentanyl derivatives have a potency up to 2000 times that of morphine. The duration of effect and elimination half-lives of the opioids also vary greatly (Table II–42).

III. **Clinical presentation**

A. **With mild or moderate overdose,** lethargy is common. The pupils are usually small, often "pinpoint" size. Blood pressure and pulse rate are decreased, bowel sounds are diminished, and the muscles are usually flaccid.

B. **With higher doses,** coma is accompanied by respiratory depression, and apnea often results in sudden death. Noncardiogenic pulmonary edema may occur, often after resuscitation and administration of the opiate antagonist naloxone.

C. **Seizures** are not common after opioid overdose but occur occasionally with certain compounds (eg, meperidine, propoxyphene, dextromethorphan). Seizures may occur in renally compromised patients receiving repeated doses of meperidine, owing to accumulation of the metabolite normeperidine.

D. Some newer synthetic opioids have mixed agonist and antagonist effects with unpredictable results in overdose.

IV. Diagnosis is simple when typical manifestations of opiate intoxication are present (pinpoint pupils, respiratory and CNS depression) and the patient quickly awakens after administration of naloxone. Signs of intravenous drug abuse (eg, needle track marks) may be present.

   A. Specific levels are not usually performed because of poor correlation with clinical effects. Qualitative screening of the urine is an effective way to confirm recent use. Fentanyl derivatives and some other synthetic opioids are not detected by routine toxicologic screens.

   B. Other useful laboratory studies. Electrolytes, glucose, arterial blood gases or oximetry, chest x-ray, stat serum acetaminophen or salicylate levels (if ingested overdose was a combination product).

V. Treatment

   A. Emergency and supportive measures
   1. Maintain the airway and assist ventilation if necessary (see p 4). Administer supplemental oxygen.
   2. Treat coma (p 18), seizures (p 22), hypotension (p 15), and noncardiogenic pulmonary edema (p 8) if they occur.

   B. Specific drugs and antidotes. Naloxone (p 355) is a specific opioid antagonist with no agonist properties of its own; huge doses may be given safely.
   1. Administer naloxone, 0.4–2 mg IV. Repeat dose every 2–3 minutes if there is no response, up to a total dose of 10–20 mg if opioid overdose is strongly suspected.
   2. *Caution:* The duration of effect of naloxone (2–3 hours) is shorter than that of many opioids. Therefore, do not release the patient who has awakened after naloxone treatment until at least 3–4 hours have passed since the last dose of naloxone. In general, if naloxone was required to reverse opioid-

TABLE II–42. COMMON OPIATES AND OPOIDS[a]

Drug	Type of Activity	Usual Dose[a] (mg)	Elimination Half-Life (h)	Duration of Analgesia (h)
Morphine	Agonist	10	3	4–5
Hydromorphone	Agonist	1.5	2.5	4–5
Methadone	Agonist	10	35	4–6
Heroin[b]	Agonist	4	(b)	3–4
Meperidine	Agonist	100	3	2–4
Fentanyl	Agonist	0.2	4	1–2
Codeine	Agonist	60	3	3–4
Oxycodone	Agonist	4.5	4	3–4
Propoxyphene	Agonist	100	15	4–5
Pentazocine	Mixed	50	3	3–4
Nalbuphine	Mixed	10	3.5	3–6
Butorphanol	Mixed	2	3	3–4
Naloxone	Antagonist	1–2	1	NA

[a]Usual dose: Dose equivalent to 10 mg of morphine.
[b]Rapidly hydrolyzed to morphine.

induced coma, it is safer to admit the patient for at least 6–12 hours of observation.

  C. Decontamination (see p 44)

    1. Prehospital. Administer activated charcoal, if available. Ipecac-induced emesis may be useful for initial treatment at the scene (eg, children at home) if it can be given within a few minutes of exposure, but caution should be exercised because of the potential for developing progressive lethargy and coma.

    2. Hospital. Administer activated charcoal and a cathartic. Gastric emptying is not necessary if activated charcoal can be given promptly.

  D. Enhanced elimination. Because of the very large volumes of distribution of the opioids, and the availability of an effective antidotal treatment, there is no role for enhanced elimination procedures.

ORGANOPHOSPHATES
Olga F. Woo, PharmD

ANTIDOTE   IPECAC   LAVAGE   CHARCOAL

Organophosphates are widely used pesticides that may cause acute or chronic poisonings after accidental or suicidal exposure. Poisonings are particularly common in rural areas and third-world countries where potent organophosphates are widely available. Organophosphates often contain solvents such as toluene or xylene that can themselves produce toxic effects in an overdose.

  I. Mechanism of toxicity

    A. Organophosphates and their potent sulfoxidation ("-oxon") derivatives inhibit the enzyme acetylcholinesterase, allowing the accumulation of excessive acetylcholine at muscarinic receptors (cholinergic effector cells), at nicotinic receptors (skeletal neuromuscular junctions and autonomic ganglia), and in the central nervous system (CNS).

    B. Organophosphates are well absorbed by inhalation and ingestion and through the skin. Some organophosphates (eg, disulfoton, fenthion, others) are highly lipophilic and are stored in fat tissue, which may lead to delayed and persistent toxicity for several days after exposure.

  II. Toxic dose. There is a wide spectrum of relative potency of organophosphates (Table II–43). The degree of intoxication is also affected by the rate of exposure (acute versus chronic), by the ongoing metabolic degradation and elimination of the organophosphate, and by the rate of metabolism to its more toxic "-oxon" derivative. Some agents, including the highly toxic "nerve gases" developed for chemical warfare, are direct and powerful inhibitors of cholinesterase.

  III. Clinical presentation. Signs and symptoms of acute organophosphate poisoning usually occur within 1–2 hours of exposure but may be delayed up to several hours, especially after skin exposure. Clinical manifestations may be classified into muscarinic, nicotinic, and CNS effects. In addition, chemical pneumonitis (see p 178) may occur if a product containing a hydrocarbon solvent is aspirated into the lungs.

    A. Muscarinic manifestations include vomiting, diarrhea, abdominal cramping, bronchospasm, miosis, bradycardia, and excessive salivation and sweating. Severe diaphoresis can actually lead to dehydration with systemic hypovolemia, resulting in shock.

    B. Nicotinic effects include muscle fasciculations, tremor, and weakness. Death is usually caused by respiratory muscle paralysis. Blood pressure and pulse rate may be increased because of nicotinic effects or decreased because of muscarinic effects.

TABLE II–43. RELATIVE TOXICITIES OF ORGANOPHOSPHATES

Low toxicity (LD$_{50}$ > 1000 mg/kg)[a]

Bromophos (3750–8000 mg/kg)	Primiphos-methyl (>2000)
Etrimfos (1800)	Propylthiopyrophosphate (2710–5010)
Iodofenphos (2100) (jodfenphos)	Temephos (4204–10,000)
Malathion (1000–2800)	Tetrachlorvinphos (4000–5000)
Phoxim (2000)	

Moderate toxicity (LD$_{50}$ > 50–1000 mg/kg)

Acephate (700–950 mg/kg)	Isoxathion (180–242)
Bensulide (271–1470)	Leptophos (52.8)
Chlorpyrifos (96–270)	Methyl trithion
Crotoxyphos (53)	Naled (250)
Cyanophos (580–610)	Oxydemeton-methyl (30–75)
Cythioate (160)	Oxydeprofos (105)
DEF (200)	Phencapton (182)
Demeton-S-methyl (180)	Phenthoate (440)
Diazinon (300–400)	Phosalone (120)
Dichlofenthion (270)	Phosmet (147–316)
Dichlorvos (DDVP) (50)	Pirimiphos-ethyl
Dimethoate (255 –310)	Profenofos (358)
Edifenphos (100–260)	Propetamphos (119)
EPBP (274)	Pyrazophos (151–778)
Ethion (21–208)	Pyridaphenthion (769–850)
Ethoprop (61.5)	Quinalphos (71)
Fenitrothion (800)	Sulprofos (150)
Fenthion (250)	Thiometon (120–130)
Formothion (365–500)	Triazophos (57–59)
Heptenophos (96–121)	Tribufos (348–712)
IBP (Kitacin) (490)	Trichlorfon (250)
Heptenophos (96–121)	

High toxicity (LD$_{50}$ < 50 mg/kg)[a]

Azinphos-methyl (10 mg/kg)	Isofenphos (20 mg/kg)
Bomyl (31)	Isofluorphate
Carbophenothion (6.8–36.9)	Mephosfolan (8.9)
Chlorfenvinphos (10–39)	Methamidophos (20)
Chlormephos (7)	Methidathion (44)
Coumaphos (16–41)	Mevinphos (3–12)
Cyanofenphos (43.7)	Monocrotophos (8–23)
Demeton (2.5–6)	Parathion (2)
Dialifor (43–53)	Phorate (2–4)
Dicrotophos (17–22)	Phosfolan (8.9)
Disulfoton (4)	Phosphamidon (17–30)
EPN (26)	Prothoate (8)
Famphur (35)	Schradan (9)
Fenamiphos (3)	Sulfotep (10)
Fenophosphon (37.5)	Terbufos (4.5–9)
Fensulfothion (2)	Tetraethylpyrophosphate (1.2–2)
Fonofos (8–17.5)	Triorthocresylphosphate

[a]Based on oral LD$_{50}$ values in the rat.

    C. Central nervous system poisoning may cause agitation, seizures, and coma.

    D. Some organophosphates may cause a delayed, often permanent peripheral neuropathy. An **"intermediate syndrome"** has also been described, characterized by recurrent muscle weakness occurring within several days of the exposure. It may be associated with inadequate pralidoxime therapy.

IV. Diagnosis is based on the history of exposure and the presence of characteristic muscarinic, nicotinic, and CNS manifestations. There is frequently a solvent odor, and some describe a garliclike odor of the organophosphate.

A. **Specific levels.** Laboratory confirmation may be obtained by measuring decreases in the plasma pseudocholinesterase (PChE) and red blood cell acetylcholinesterase (AChE) activities. *Note:* Because of wide interindividual variability, significant depression of enzyme activity may occur but still fall within the "normal" range.

1. The AChE activity provides a more reliable measure of the toxic effect; a 25% or greater depression in activity from baseline generally indicates true exposure.

2. PChE activity is a sensitive indicator of exposure but is not as reliable as AChE activity (PChE may be depressed owing to genetic deficiency, medical illness, or chronic organophosphate exposure). PChE activity usually recovers within weeks after exposure, whereas AChE recovery may take several months.

B. **Other useful laboratory studies.** Electrolytes, glucose, BUN, creatinine, liver transaminases, arterial blood gases or oximetry, ECG monitoring, chest x-ray.

V. **Treatment**

A. **Emergency and supportive measures**

1. Maintain the airway and assist ventilation if necessary (see p 4). Pay careful attention to respiratory muscle weakness; sudden respiratory arrest may occur. If intubation is required, note potential interactions between neuromuscular blockers and organophosphates (see p 357). Administer supplemental oxygen.

2. Treat hydrocarbon pneumonitis (p 8), seizures (p 22), and coma (p 18) if they occur.

3. Observe patients for at least 6–8 hours to rule out delayed-onset symptoms resulting from skin absorption.

B. **Specific drugs and antidotes.** Specific treatment includes the antimuscarinic agent **atropine** and the enzyme reactivator **pralidoxime.**

1. Give **atropine,** 0.5–2 mg IV initially (see p 315), repeated frequently as needed. Large cumulative doses of atropine (up to 100 mg or more) may occasionally be required in severe cases. The most clinically important indication for continued atropine administration is persistent wheezing or bronchorrhea. Atropine will reverse muscarinic but not nicotinic effects.

2. **Pralidoxime** (2-PAM, Protopam; see p 371) is a specific antidote that acts to regenerate the enzyme activity at all affected sites (muscarinic, nicotinic, and probably CNS), and it should be given immediately to reverse muscular weakness and fasciculations: 1–2 g initial bolus dose (20–40 mg/kg in children) IV over 5–10 minutes, followed by a continuous infusion (see p 371). Pralidoxime is most effective if started within the first 24 hours of the exposure prior to irreversible phosphorylation of the enzyme, but may still be effective if given late, particularly after exposure to highly lipid soluble compounds.

C. **Decontamination** (see p 41). *Note:* Rescuers must wear chemical protective clothing and gloves when handling a grossly contaminated victim. If there is heavy liquid contamination with a solvent such as xylene or toluene, clothing removal and victim decontamination should be carried out outdoors or in a room with high-flow ventilation.

1. **Skin.** Remove all contaminated clothing and wash exposed areas with soap and water, including the hair and under the nails. Irrigate exposed eyes with copious tepid water or saline.

2. **Ingestion** (see p 44)

   a. **Prehospital.** Administer activated charcoal, if available. Ipecac-induced emesis may be useful for initial treatment at the scene (eg, children at home) if it can be given within a few minutes of exposure, although caution is advised because of the potential for rapid onset of symptoms.

   b. **Hospital.** Administer activated charcoal and a cathartic (cathartics are not necessary if the patient already has diarrhea). Perform gastric lavage for large recent ingestions.

D. Enhanced elimination. Dialysis and hemoperfusion are not generally indicated because of the large volume of distribution of organophosphates and the effectiveness of the specific therapy described above.

OXALIC ACID
Kent R. Olson, MD

ANTIDOTE   IPECAC   LAVAGE   CHARCOAL

Oxalic acid and oxalates are used as bleaches, metal cleaners, and rust removers and in chemical synthesis and leather tanning. Soluble and insoluble oxalate salts are found in several species of plants.

I. Mechanism of toxicity
  A. Oxalic acid solutions are highly irritating and corrosive. Ingestion and absorption of oxalate cause acute hypocalcemia resulting from precipitation of the insoluble calcium oxalate salt. Calcium oxalate crystals may then deposit in the brain, heart, kidneys, and other sites, causing serious systemic damage.
  B. Insoluble calcium oxalate salt found in dieffenbachia and similar plants is not absorbed but causes local mucous membrane irritation.
II. Toxic dose. Ingestion of 5–15 g of oxalic acid has caused death. The recommended workplace limit (ACGIH TLV-TWA) for oxalic acid vapor is 1 mg/m^3 as an 8-hour time-weighted average.
III. Clinical presentation. Toxicity may occur as a result of skin or eye contact, inhalation, or ingestion.
  A. Acute skin or eye contact causes irritation and burning, which may lead to serious corrosive injury if the exposure and concentration are high.
  B. Inhalation may cause sore throat, cough, and wheezing. Large exposures may lead to chemical pneumonitis or pulmonary edema.
  C. Ingestion of soluble oxalates may result in weakness, tetany, convulsions, and cardiac arrest owing to profound hypocalcemia. The QT interval may be prolonged, and variable conduction defects may occur. Oxalate crystals may be found on urinalysis. Insoluble oxalate crystals are not absorbed but can cause irritation and swelling in the oropharynx and esophagus.
IV. Diagnosis is based on a history of exposure and evidence of local or systemic effects or oxalate crystalluria.
  A. Specific levels. Serum oxalate levels are not available.
  B. Other useful laboratory studies. Electrolytes, glucose, BUN, creatinine, calcium, ECG monitoring, urinalysis.
V. Treatment
  A. Emergency and supportive measures
    1. Protect the airway (see p 2), which may become acutely swollen and obstructed after significant ingestion or inhalation. Administer supplemental oxygen, and assist ventilation if necessary (p 4).
    2. Treat coma (p 18), seizures (p 22), and arrhythmias (p 10–14) if they occur.
    3. Monitor the ECG and vital signs for at least 6 hours after significant exposure, and admit symptomatic patients to an intensive care unit.
  B. Specific drugs and antidotes. Administer 10% **calcium solution** (chloride or gluconate) to counteract symptomatic hypocalcemia.
  C. Decontamination (see p 41)
    1. **Insoluble oxalates** in plants: Flush exposed areas. For ingestions, dilute with plain water; do not induce emesis or give charcoal.
    2. **Oxalic acid or strong commercial oxalate solutions.** Immediately flush with copious water. Do ***not*** induce vomiting because of the risk of aggravat-

ing corrosive injury; instead, give water to dilute, and on arrival in hospital perform gastric lavage (see p 45).

3. **Plants containing soluble oxalates.** Induce emesis with syrup of ipecac (see p 44) if it can be administered within a few minutes of the ingestion. In hospital, consider gastric lavage.

4. Precipitate ingested oxalate in the stomach by administering calcium (chloride or gluconate, 1–2 g; or calcium carbonate [Tums], several tablets) orally or via gastric tube.

5. The effectiveness of activated charcoal is unknown.

D. **Enhanced elimination.** Maintain high-volume urine flow (3–5 mL/kg/h) to help prevent calcium oxalate precipitation in the tubules. Oxalate is removed by hemodialysis, but the indications for this treatment are not established.

PARALDEHYDE
Timothy McCarthy, PharmD

ANTIDOTE   IPECAC   LAVAGE   CHARCOAL

Paraldehyde is a cyclic trimer of acetaldehyde. Although it has been largely replaced by newer agents, paraldehyde was widely used in the past as an anticonvulsant, a sedative-hypnotic, and an anesthetic. It has a characteristic penetrating odor and a disagreeable taste. It is incompatible with plastic and must be stored and administered in glass containers only. It rapidly decomposes to acetaldehyde and acetic acid upon exposure to light and air.

I. **Mechanism of toxicity.** Paraldehyde is a potent CNS depressant. It is a strong irritant to intestinal mucosa, especially if it has partially decomposed to acetic acid. If the produce has developed a brown discoloration or the pungent smell of acetic acid, it should **not** be used.

II. **Toxic dose.** The typical therapeutic dose of paraldehyde for control of seizures or alcohol withdrawal is 5–10 mL IM or PO or 0.1–0.2 mL/kg IV every 4–6 hours. Deaths have been reported after a rectal dose of only 12 mL (undecomposed paraldehyde) and an oral dose of 25 mL. However, survival has been reported after ingestion of 125 mL. Coingestion of alcohol or other depressant drugs increases the risk of serious toxicity.

III. **Clinical presentation.** Peak effects are usually seen within 30–60 minutes after ingestion but may be delayed up to 2–3 hours after rectal administration. Lethargy, stupor, and coma are common. Gastritis, often hemorrhagic, may occur. Metabolic acidosis with an elevated anion gap may be a result of acetic acid or may be a manifestation of starvation-type ketoacidosis in a patient with paraldehyde-induced gastritis. Severe leukocytosis (> 30,000), hypercoagulability, tachycardia, hypotension, tachypnea, right ventricular failure, and pulmonary edema have been reported.

IV. **Diagnosis** is based on a history of exposure and is suggested by the typical pungent odor on the breath, metabolic acidosis, and altered mental status.

A. **Specific levels.** Serum levels are not routinely available. The anticonvulsant therapeutic level is approximately 200 mg/L; serum levels higher than 500 mg/L are often associated with death.

B. **Other useful laboratory studies.** Electrolytes, glucose, arterial blood gases or oximetry.

V. **Treatment**

A. **Emergency and supportive measures**

1. Maintain the airway and assist ventilation if necessary (see p 4). Administer supplemental oxygen.

2. Treat coma (p 18), hypotension (p 15), metabolic acidosis (p 30), and pulmonary edema (p 8) if they occur.

B. Specific drugs and antidotes. There is no specific antidote.

C. Decontamination (see p 44)

1. **Prehospital.** Administer activated charcoal, if available. Do **not** induce emesis because paraldehyde is mildly corrosive and because of the risk of abrupt decline in mental status.

2. **Hospital.** Administer activated charcoal and a cathartic. Consider gastric lavage for large recent ingestion.

D. Enhanced elimination. The volume of distribution is 0.9 L/kg, making paraldehyde accessible to enhanced elimination procedures. However, there are few data to support use of extracorporeal methods of enhanced elimination.

PARAQUAT AND DIQUAT
Kent R. Olson, MD

ANTIDOTE   IPECAC   LAVAGE   CHARCOAL

Paraquat and diquat are dipyridyl herbicides used primarily for weed control. Paraquat has also been used for large-scale control of illegal marijuana growing. Solutions available for home use are generally extremely dilute (0.2%), whereas commercial preparations may contain up to 21% paraquat. Weedol is a granular formulation containing a 2.5% mixture of paraquat and diquat salts.

I. **Mechanisms of toxicity**

A. **Paraquat** is a strong cation in aqueous solution, and concentrated solutions (20–24%) may cause corrosive injury when applied to the skin or ingested. After absorption, paraquat is selectively taken up and concentrated by pulmonary alveolar cells over several days. Lipid peroxidation then results in cell necrosis and proliferation of fibrous connective tissue, leading to pulmonary fibrosis. Although paraquat is poorly absorbed through intact skin, it is probably absorbed across abraded skin and fatalities have been reported following skin application.

B. **Diquat** is also corrosive in concentrated solutions. Unlike paraquat, diquat does not cause pulmonary fibrosis. Instead, it causes gastrointestinal fluid sequestration, renal failure, and cerebral and brain stem hemorrhagic infarctions.

II. **Toxic dose.** Paraquat and diquat are both extremely toxic, although diquat is less toxic than paraquat.

A. **Paraquat.** Ingestion of as little as 2–4 g, or 10–20 mL of concentrated 20% paraquat solution, has resulted in death. With ingestion of 60 mL or more, the onset of toxicity and death is more rapid.

1. If food is present in the stomach, it may bind paraquat, preventing its absorption and reducing its toxicity.

2. Once applied to plants or soil, paraquat is rapidly bound and is not likely to . be toxic. When burned, it is combusted and does not produce poisoning.

B. **Diquat.** The animal LD_{50} is approximately 400 mg/kg. Survival has been reported after ingestion of 60 g (300 mL of a 20% solution) of diquat.

III. **Clinical presentation**

A. **Paraquat.** After ingestion of concentrated solutions, there is pain and swelling in the mouth and throat and oral ulcerations may be visible. Nausea, vomiting, and abdominal pain are common. Renal failure develops over 3–5 days, and progressive pulmonary fibrosis occurs over 10–15 days, with death from irreversible pulmonary fibrosis. With ingestion of more than 60 mL of concentrated solution, death may occur within 24 hours owing to massive gastroenteritis, corrosive esophageal injury, pulmonary edema, and cardiogenic shock.

B. **Diquat.** Corrosive injury may also occur with concentrated solutions. Severe gastroenteritis may cause massive fluid and electrolyte loss and renal failure.

Pulmonary toxicity has not been reported, but cerebral and brain stem hemor-rhagic infarctions may occur.

IV. Diagnosis is based on a history of ingestion and the presence of gastroenteritis and oral burns. The oral mucosal burns may have the appearance of a pseudomembrane on the soft palate, sometimes confused with diphtheria.

A. Specific levels

1. Paraquat. Prognosis may be correlated with specific paraquat serum levels. These may be obtained free of charge 24 hours a day from ICI Americas, Inc; telephone 1-(800)-327-8633. Paraquat levels associated with a high likelihood of death are 2 mg/L at 4 hours, 0.9 mg/L at 6 hours, and 0.1 mg/L at 24 hours after ingestion.

2. Diquat. Levels are not readily available.

B. Other useful laboratory studies. Electrolytes, glucose, BUN, creatinine, liver transaminases, urinalysis, arterial blood gases or oximetry, chest x-ray.

V. Treatment

A. Emergency and supportive measures. For paraquat poisoning, contact ICI Americas, Inc, 24 hours a day at 1-(800)-327-8633 for assistance with treatment.

1. Maintain the airway and assist ventilation if necessary (see p 4).

2. Avoid excessive oxygen administration in patients with paraquat poison-ing, as this may aggravate lipid peroxidation reactions in the lungs. Treat significant hypoxemia with supplemental oxygen, but use only the lowest oxygen concentration necessary to achieve a P_{O_2} of about 60 mm.

3. Treat fluid and electrolyte imbalance caused by gastroenteritis with intrave-nous crystalloid solutions.

B. Specific drugs and antidotes. There is no specific antidote.

C. Decontamination (see p 41)

1. Skin and eyes. Remove all contaminated clothing, and wash exposed skin with soap and water. Irrigate exposed eyes with copious saline or water.

2. Ingestion (see p 44)

a. Prehospital. Administer activated charcoal, if available. Ingestion of any food or even plain dirt may afford some protection if other adsorbents are not immediately available. Ipecac-induced emesis may be useful for ini-tial treatment at the scene (eg, children at home) if it can be given within a few minutes of exposure. Note that many commercial solutions contain an added emetic agent.

b. Hospital. Administer activated charcoal and a cathartic. Perform gastric lavage. Various clays, such as bentonite and fuller's earth, adsorb para-quat and diquat but are probably no more effective than charcoal.

D. Enhanced elimination. (see p 49) Although the volume of distribution of para-quat is relatively large (2.8 L/kg) and little paraquat is actually removed, some recommend repeated and prolonged hemoperfusion (every day for 8 hours) in an attempt to limit transfer of paraquat from tissues to the lung. Increased sur-vival has been reported with this technique, although no controlled studies have been performed. One recent study suggests that hemoperfusion is effec-tive only if initiated within 4 hours of the ingestion. Hemodialysis and forced diuresis are not effective.

PENTACHLOROPHENOL AND DINITROPHENOL
Delia A. Dempsey, MS, MD

ANTIDOTE   IPECAC   LAVAGE   CHARCOAL

Pentachlorophenol (Penchlor, Chlorophen, Pentachlorofenol, Penta, Pentanol, Pen-tachlorophenate, PCP, others) is a chlorinated aromatic hydrocarbon widely used as a fungicide, as well as an herbicide and defoliant. It is applied to wood, leather, burlap, twine, and rope to prevent fungal rot and decay. It is used predominantly in wood preservation and in the paper industry. Sodium pentachlorophenol is an ingredient in some paints.

Dinitrophenol (Dinoseb, DNP, Dinitrobutylphenol, and analogs Disophenol, Dinitrocresol) is an insecticide, herbicide, fungicide, and chemical intermediary and is used in some explosives, dyes, and photographic chemicals. It has also been taken orally for weight reduction but is banned for this use. Its structure and toxicity are similar to those of pentachlorophenol.

I. **Mechanism of toxicity**
   A. Pentachlorophenol and dinitrophenol, like salicylate, uncouple oxidative phosphorylation in the mitochondria. Substrates are metabolized but the energy produced is dissipated as heat instead of producing adenosine triphosphate (ATP). The basal metabolic rate increases, placing increased demands on the cardiorespiratory system. Excess lactic acid results from nonmitochondrial ATP production.
   B. Dinitrophenol may oxidize hemoglobin to methemoglobin (see p 217).
   C. In animal studies, pentachlorophenol is mutagenic, teratogenic, and carcinogenic. DNP is teratogenic and may be weakly carcinogenic.

II. **Toxic dose.** These agents are readily absorbed through the skin, lungs, and gastrointestinal tract.
   A. **Inhalation.** The air level of pentachlorophenol considered immediately dangerous to life or health (IDLH) is 150 mg/m^3. The ACGIH recommended workplace air exposure limit (TLV-TWA) is 0.5 mg/m^3 as an 8-hour time-weighted average.
   B. **Skin.** This is the main route associated with accidental poisoning. An epidemic of moderate intoxication occurred in a neonatal nursery after diapers were inadvertently washed in 23% sodium pentachlorophenate.
   C. **Ingestion.** The minimum lethal oral dose of pentachlorophenol for humans is not known, but death occurred after ingestion of 2 g. Ingestion of 1–3 g of dinitrophenol is considered lethal.

III. **Clinical presentation.** The toxic manifestations of pentachlorophenol and dinitrophenol are nearly identical. Profuse sweating, fever, tachypnea, and tachycardia are universally reported in serious poisonings.
   A. **Acute exposure** causes irritation of the skin, eyes, and upper respiratory tract. Systemic absorption may cause headache, vomiting, weakness, and lethargy. Profound sweating, hyperthermia, tachycardia, tachypnea, convulsions, and coma are associated with severe or fatal poisonings. Pulmonary edema may occur. Death is usually caused by cardiovascular collapse or hyperthermia. After death an extremely rapid onset of rigor mortis is frequently reported. Dinitrophenol may also induce methemoglobinemia, liver and kidney failure, and yellow-stained skin.
   B. **Chronic exposure** may present in a similar manner, and in addition may cause weight loss, gastrointestinal disturbances, fevers and night sweats, weakness, flulike symptoms, contact dermatitis, and aplastic anemia (rare). Cataracts and glaucoma have been associated with DNP.

IV. **Diagnosis** is based on history of exposure and clinical findings, and should be suspected in patients with fever, metabolic acidosis, diaphoresis, and tachypnea.
   A. **Specific levels.** Blood levels are not readily available; levels higher than 1 mg/L indicate excessive exposure. Death has been reported with pentachlorophenol levels about 40 mg/L, and toxicity was reported with a DNP level of 10 mg/L.
   B. **Other useful laboratory studies.** CBC, electrolytes, glucose, BUN, creatinine, creatine phosphokinase (CPK), liver transaminases, amylase, urine dipstick for occult blood (positive with hemolysis or rhabdomyolysis), arterial blood gases, methemoglobin level, chest x-ray.

V. **Treatment**
   A. **Emergency and supportive measures**
      1. Maintain the airway and assist ventilation if necessary (see p 4).
      2. Treat coma (p 18), seizures (p 22), hypotension (p 15), or hyperthermia

(p 20) if they occur. Dehydration from tachypnea, fever, and sweating is common and may require large volume fluid replacement.

3. Monitor asymptomatic patients for at least 6 hours after exposure.
4. Do **not** use salicylates or anticholinergic agents, as these may worsen hyperthermia.

B. Specific drugs and antidotes. There is no specific antidote. Treat **methemoglobinemia** with methylene blue (see p 351).

C. Decontamination (see p 41)

1. **Inhalation.** Remove the victim from exposure and administer supplemental oxygen, if available.
2. **Skin and eyes.** Remove contaminated clothing and store in a plastic bag; wash exposed areas thoroughly with soap and copious water. Irrigate exposed eyes with copious saline or tepid water. Rescuers should wear appropriate protective clothing and respirators to avoid exposure.
3. **Ingestion** (see p 44)
   a. **Prehospital.** Administer activated charcoal, if available. Do not induce vomiting, because of the risk of seizures.
   b. **Hospital.** Place a gastric tube and immediately administer a dose of activated charcoal, then perform gastric lavage. Following lavage, administer activated charcoal and a cathartic. For small ingestions, charcoal may be given without gut emptying.

D. Enhanced elimination. There is no evidence that enhanced elimination procedures are effective.

PHENCYCLIDINE (PCP)
Evan T. Wythe, MD

ANTIDOTE   IPECAC   LAVAGE   CHARCOAL

Phencyclidine (PCP) is a dissociative anesthetic agent with properties similar to those of ketamine. It was previously marketed for veterinary use, and it became popular as an inexpensive street drug in the late 1960s. PCP is commonly smoked, but may also be snorted, ingested, or injected, and it is frequently substituted for or added to other illicit psychoactive drugs such as THC (tetrahydrocannabinol, marijuana), mescaline, or LSD. PCP is known by a variety of street names, including "peace pill," "angel dust," "hog," "goon," "animal tranquilizer," and "krystal."

I. **Mechanism of toxicity.** PCP is a dissociative anesthetic that produces generalized loss of pain perception with little or no depression of airway reflexes or ventilation. It also has CNS-stimulant, anticholinergic, dopaminergic, opioid, and alpha-adrenergic activity.

II. **Toxic dose.** In tablet form the usual street dose is 1–6 mg, which results in hallucinations, euphoria, and disinhibition. Ingestion of 6–10 mg causes toxic psychosis and signs of sympathomimetic stimulation. Acute ingestion of 150–200 mg has resulted in death. Smoking PCP produces rapid onset of effects and thus may be an easier route for users to titrate to the desired level of intoxication.

III. **Clinical presentation.** Clinical effects may be seen within minutes of smoking PCP, and can last 24 hours or longer depending on the dose.

A. **Mild intoxication** causes lethargy, euphoria, hallucinations, and occasionally bizarre or violent behavior. Patients may abruptly swing between quiet catatonia and loud or agitated behavior. Vertical and horizontal nystagmus are prominent.

B. **Severe intoxication** produces signs of adrenergic hyperactivity, including hypertension, rigidity, localized dystonic reactions, hyperthermia, tachycardia, diaphoresis, convulsions, and coma. The pupils are sometimes paradoxically small. **Death** may occur as a result of self-destructive behavior or as a complication of hyperthermia (eg, rhabdomyolysis, renal failure, coagulopathy, brain damage).

IV. Diagnosis is suggested by the presence of rapidly fluctuating behavior, vertical nystagmus, and signs of sympathomimetic excess.

A. Specific levels
1. Specific serum PCP levels are not readily available, nor do they correlate reliably with the degree of intoxication. Levels of 30–100 ng/mL have been associated with toxic psychosis.
2. Qualitative urine screening for PCP is widely available. PCP analogues may not appear on routine screening, although they can cross-react in some immunologic assays.

B. Other useful laboratory studies.
Electrolytes, glucose, BUN, creatinine, creatine phosphokinase (CPK), urinalysis dipstick for occult blood (positive with myoglobinuria).

V. Treatment
A. Emergency and supportive measures
1. Maintain the airway and assist ventilation if necessary (see p 4).
2. Treat coma (p 18), seizures (p 22), hypertension (p 17), hyperthermia (p 20), and rhabdomyolysis (p 25) if they occur.
3. Agitated behavior (p 23) may respond to limiting sensory stimulation but may require sedation with haloperidol (see p 343), midazolam (see p 353), or diazepam (see p 327). Do *not* use physostigmine.
4. Monitor temperature and other vital signs for a minimum of 6 hours, and admit all patients with hyperthermia or other evidence of significant intoxication.

B. Specific drugs and antidotes.
There is no specific antidote.

C. Decontamination.
No decontamination measures are necessary after smoking or injecting PCP. For ingestion (see p 44):
1. **Prehospital.** Administer activated charcoal, if available. Ipecac-induced emesis may be useful for initial treatment of children at home if it can be given within a few minutes of exposure.
2. **Hospital.** Administer activated charcoal and a cathartic. Gastric emptying is not necessary if activated charcoal can be given promptly.

D. Enhanced elimination.
Because of its large volume of distribution, PCP is not effectively removed by dialysis, hemoperfusion, or other enhanced removal procedures.
1. Repeat-dose activated charcoal has not been studied but might marginally increase elimination by adsorbing PCP partitioned into the acidic stomach fluid. Continuous nasogastric suction has also been proposed for removal of gastric-partitioned PCP.
2. Although urinary acidification increases the urinary concentration of PCP, there is no evidence that this significantly enhances elimination; and it may be dangerous because urinary acidification may aggravate myoglobinuric renal failure.

PHENOL AND RELATED COMPOUNDS
Olga F. Woo, PharmD

ANTIDOTE   IPECAC   LAVAGE   CHARCOAL

Phenol (carbolic acid) was introduced into household use as a potent germicidal agent but has limited use today because less toxic compounds have replaced it. **Hexachlorophene** is a chlorinated biphenol that was widely used as a topical antiseptic and preoperative scrub until recently, when its adverse neurologic effects were recognized. Other phenolic compounds include **creosote, creosol, hydroquinone, euge-**

nol, dinitrophenol, and **pentachlorophenol.** Pentachlorophenol and dinitrophenol toxicity is discussed on p 246.

I. **Mechanism of toxicity.** Phenol denatures protein and penetrates tissues well. It is a potent irritant that may cause corrosive injury to the eyes, skin, and respiratory tract. Systemic absorption causes central nervous system (CNS) stimulation. The mechanism of CNS intoxication is not known. Some phenolic compounds (eg, dinitrophenol and hydroquinone) may induce **methemoglobinemia** (see p 217).

II. **Toxic dose.** The minimum toxic and lethal doses have not been well established. Phenol is well absorbed by inhalation, skin application, and ingestion.

    A. **Inhalation.** The ACGIH recommended workplace exposure limit (TLV-TWA) is 5 ppm as an 8-hour time-weighted average. The level considered immediately dangerous to life or health (IDLH) is 100 ppm.

    B. **Skin application.** Death has occurred in infants from repeated dermal applications of small doses (one infant died after a 2% solution of phenol was applied for 11 hours on the umbilicus under a closed bandage).

    C. **Ingestion.** Deaths have occurred after adult ingestions of 1–32 g of phenol; however, survival after ingestion of 45–65 g has been reported. As little as 50–500 mg has been reported as fatal in infants.

    D. **Pharmacokinetics.** Phenol is rapidly absorbed by all routes. Elimination half-life is 0.5–4.5 hours.

III. **Clinical presentation.** Toxicity may result from inhalation, skin or eye exposure, or ingestion.

    A. **Inhalation.** Vapors of phenol may cause respiratory tract irritation and chemical pneumonia. Smoking of clove cigarettes (clove oil contains the phenol derivative eugenol) may cause severe tracheobronchitis.

    B. **Skin and eyes.** Topical exposure to the skin may produce a deep white patch that turns red, then stains the skin brown. This lesion is often relatively painless. Eye irritation and severe corneal damage may occur if concentrated liquids are spilled into the eye.

    C. **Ingestion** usually causes vomiting and diarrhea, and diffuse corrosive gastrointestinal tract injury may occur. Systemic absorption may cause agitation, confusion, seizures, coma, hypotension, arrhythmias, and respiratory arrest.

IV. **Diagnosis** is based on a history of exposure, the presence of a characteristic odor, and painless white skin burns.

    A. **Specific levels.** Normal urine phenol levels are less than 20 mg/L. Urine phenol levels may be elevated in workers exposed to benzene, and after use of phenol-containing throat lozenges and mouthwashes.

    B. **Other useful laboratory studies.** CBC, electrolytes, glucose, BUN, creatinine, ECG. After hydroquinone exposure: methemoglobin level.

V. **Treatment**

    A. **Emergency and supportive measures**

        1. Maintain the airway and assist ventilation if necessary (see p 4).

        2. Treat coma (p 18), seizures (p 22), hypotension (p 15), and arrhythmias (p 10–44) if they occur.

        3. If corrosive injury to the gastrointestinal tract is suspected, consult a gastroenterologist for possible endoscopy.

    B. **Specific drugs and antidotes.** No specific antidote is available. If **methemoglobinemia** occurs, administer methylene blue (see p 351).

    C. **Decontamination** (see p 41)

        1. **Inhalation.** Remove victim from exposure and administer supplemental oxygen, if available.

        2. **Skin and eyes.** Remove contaminated clothing and wash exposed skin with soapy water or, if available, mineral oil, olive oil, or petroleum jelly. Immediately flush exposed eyes with copious tepid water or saline.

        3. **Ingestion** (see p 44)

            a. **Prehospital.** Do *not* induce emesis, because phenol is corrosive and may induce seizures. Administer activated charcoal, if available.

            b. **Hospital.** Administer activated charcoal and a cathartic, orally or by gastric tube. Consider gastric lavage for large ingestions.

D. **Enhanced elimination.** Enhanced removal methods are generally not effective because of the large volume of distribution of these lipid soluble compounds. Hexachlorophene is excreted in the bile, and repeat-dose activated charcoal (see p 52) may possibly be effective in increasing its clearance from the gut.

PHENOTHIAZINES AND OTHER ANTIPSYCHOTIC DRUGS
Neal L. Benowitz, MD

ANTIDOTE   IPECAC   LAVAGE   CHARCOAL

Phenothiazines, butyrophenones, and other related drugs are widely used to treat psychosis and agitated depression. In addition, some of these drugs (eg, prochlorperazine, promethazine, droperidol) are used as antiemetic agents. Suicidal overdose is common, but because of the high toxic-therapeutic ratio, acute overdose seldom results in death. Table II–44 describes available antipsychotic agents.

I. **Mechanism of toxicity.** A variety of pharmacologic effects are responsible for toxicity involving primarily the cardiovascular and central nervous systems.

A. **Cardiovascular** effects. anticholinergic effects produce tachycardia. Alpha-adrenergic blockade causes orthostatic hypotension. With very large overdoses of some agents, quinidinelike membrane-depressant effects on the heart may occur.

B. **Central nervous system** effects. Centrally mediated sedation and anticholinergic effects contribute to CNS depression. Alpha-adrenergic blockade causes small pupils, despite anticholinergic effects on other systems. Extrapyramidal dystonic reactions are relatively common with therapeutic doses and are probably caused by central dopamine receptor blockade. The seizure threshold may be lowered by unknown mechanisms. Temperature regulation is also disturbed, resulting in poikilothermy.

II. **Toxic dose.** Extrapyramidal reactions, anticholinergic side effects, and orthostatic hypotension are often seen with therapeutic doses. Tolerance to the sedating effects of the antipsychotics is well-described, and patients on chronic therapy may tolerate much larger doses than other persons.

A. Typical daily doses are given in Table II–43.

B. The toxic dose after acute ingestion is highly variable. Serious CNS depression and hypotension may occur after ingestion of 200–1000 mg of chlorpromazine in children or 3–5 g in adults.

III. **Clinical presentation.** Major toxicity is manifested in the cardiovascular and central nervous systems.

A. **Mild intoxication** causes sedation, small pupils, and orthostatic hypotension. Anticholinergic manifestations include dry mouth, absence of sweating, tachycardia, and urinary retention.

B. **Severe intoxication** may cause coma, seizures, and respiratory arrest. The ECG usually shows QT interval prolongation and occasionally QRS prolongation (particularly with thioridazine [Mellaril]). Hypothermia or hyperthermia may occur.

C. **Extrapyramidal** dystonic side effects of therapeutic doses include torticollis, jaw muscle spasm, oculogyric crisis, rigidity, bradykinesia, and pill-rolling tremor.

D. Patients on chronic antipsychotic medication may develop the **neuroleptic malignant syndrome** (see p 20) characterized by rigidity, hyperthermia, sweating, lactic acidosis, and rhabdomyolysis.

IV. **Diagnosis** is based on a history of ingestion and is suggested by the findings of sedation, small pupils, hypotension, and QT interval prolongation. Dystonias in children should always suggest the possibility of antipsychotic exposure, often as a result of intentional administration by parents. Phenothiazines are occasionally visible on plain abdominal x-rays (see Table I–34).

TABLE II–44. COMMON PHENOTHIAZINES AND OTHER ANTIPSYCHOTIC DRUGS

Drug	Type[a]	Equivalent Dose (mg)	Usual Adult Daily Dose (mg)	Toxicity[b]
Chlorpromazine	P	100	200–2000	E, A, H
Chlorprothixene	T	100	75–200	E
Clozapine	D	100	100–900	A, H
Ethopropazine	P	50	50–400	A, H
Fluphenazine	P	2	2.5–20	E, A
Haloperidol	B	2	1–100	E
Loxapine	D	15	60–100	E
Mesoridazine	P	50	150–400	A, H
Molindone	O	10	50–225	E
Perphenazine	P	10	10–30	E
Prochlorperazine[c]	P	15	15–40	E
Promethazine[c]	P	25	25–200	A, E
Thioridazine	P	100	150–300	A, H
Thiothixene	T	5	5–60	E
Trifluoperazine	P	5	1–40	E
Trimethobenzamide[c]	O	250	600–1000	A, E

[a]P = Phenothiazine; T = Thiothixine; B = Butyrophenone; D = Dibenzodiazepine; O = Other.
[b]E = Extrapyramidal reactions; A = Anticholinergic effects; H = Hypotension.
[c]Used primarily as an antiemetic.

> **A. Specific levels.** Quantitative blood levels are not routinely available and do not help in diagnosis or treatment. Qualitative screening may easily detect phenothiazines in urine or gastric juice, but butyrophenones such as haloperidol are usually not included in toxicologic screens (see Table I–29, p 38).
>
> **B. Other useful laboratory studies.** Electrolytes, glucose, BUN, creatinine, creatine phosphokinase (CPK), arterial blood gases or oximetry, abdominal x-ray (to look for radiopaque pills), chest x-ray.

V. Treatment
A. Emergency and supportive measures
1. Maintain the airway and assist ventilation if necessary (see p 4). Administer supplemental oxygen.
2. Treat coma (p 18), seizures (p 22), hypotension (p 15), and hyperthermia (p 20) if they occur.
3. Monitor vital signs and ECG for at least 6 hours, and admit the patient for at least 24 hours if there are signs of significant intoxication. Children with antipsychotic intoxication should be evaluated for possible intentional abuse.

B. Specific drugs and antidotes. There is no specific antidote.
1. **Dystonic reactions.** Give **diphenhydramine,** 0.5–1 mg/kg IM or IV (see p 331).
2. **QRS interval prolongation.** Treat quinidinelike cardiotoxic effects with **bicarbonate,** 1–2 meq/kg IV (see p 318).

C. Decontamination (see p 44)
1. **Prehospital.** Administer activated charcoal, if available. Ipecac-induced emesis may be useful for initial treatment at the scene (eg, children at home) if it can be given within a few minutes of exposure.
2. **Hospital.** Administer activated charcoal and a cathartic. Gastric emptying is not necessary if activated charcoal can be given promptly.

D. Enhanced elimination. Owing to extensive tissue distribution and large volumes of distribution, these drugs are not effectively removed by dialysis or hemoperfusion. Repeat-dose activated charcoal has not been evaluated.

PHENYLPROPANOLAMINE AND RELATED DECONGESTANTS
Neal L. Benowitz, MD

ANTIDOTE   IPECAC   LAVAGE   CHARCOAL

Phenylpropanolamine (PPA), phenylephrine, ephedrine, and pseudoephedrine are sympathomimetic drugs widely available in nonprescription nasal decongestants and cold preparations. These remedies usually also contain antihistamines and cough suppressants. PPA is also widely used as an appetite suppressant. Combinations of nonprescription sympathomimetics and caffeine are sometimes sold on the underground market as amphetamine or cocaine substitutes.

I. Mechanism of toxicity. All these agents stimulate the adrenergic system, with variable effects on alpha- and beta-adrenergic receptors depending on the compound.

    A. PPA and phenylephrine are direct alpha-adrenergic agonists. In addition, PPA produces mild β_1-adrenergic stimulation and acts in part indirectly by enhancing norepinephrine release.

    B. Ephedrine and pseudoephedrine have both direct and indirect alpha- and beta-adrenergic activity but clinically produce more beta-adrenergic stimulation than PPA or phenylephrine.

II. Toxic dose. Table II–45 lists the usual therapeutic doses of each agent. Patients developing autonomic insufficiency and those taking monoamine oxidase (MAO) inhibitors (see p 222) may be extraordinarily sensitive to these and other sympathomimetic drugs, developing severe hypertension after ingestion of even subtherapeutic doses.

    A. PPA, phenylephrine, and ephedrine have low toxic:therapeutic ratios, with toxicity often occurring after ingestion of just 2–3 times the therapeutic dose.

    B. Pseudoephedrine is slightly less toxic, with symptoms occurring after 4–5 times the usual therapeutic dose.

III. Clinical presentation. The time course of intoxication by these drugs is usually brief, with resolution within 4–6 hours (unless sustained-release preparations are involved). The major toxic effect of these drugs is **hypertension,** which may lead to headache, confusion, seizures, and intracranial hemorrhage.

    A. Intracranial hemorrhage may occur in normal, healthy young persons after what might appear to be only modest elevation of the blood pressure (ie, 170/110 mm Hg) and is often associated with focal neurologic deficits, coma, or seizures.

    B. Bradycardia or atrioventricular block is common in patients with moderate to severe hypertension associated with PPA and phenylephrine, owing to the baroreceptor reflex response to hypertension. The presence of drugs such as antihistamines or caffeine prevents reflex bradycardia and may enhance the hypertensive effects of PPA and phenylephrine.

    C. Myocardial infarction and diffuse myocardial necrosis have been associated with PPA intoxication.

IV. Diagnosis is usually based on a history of excessive ingestion of diet pills or decongestant medications and the presence of hypertension. Bradycardia or AV block suggests PPA or phenylephrine. Severe headache, focal neurologic deficits, or coma should raise the possibility of intracerebral hemorrhage.

    A. Specific levels. Serum drug levels are not generally available and do not alter treatment. Urine toxicology screens may be reported as positive for amphetamine because of the presence of these drugs.

TABLE II–45. COMMON OVER-THE-COUNTER SYMPATHOMIMETIC DRUGS

Drug	Major Effects[a]	Usual Daily Adult Dose (mg)	Usual Daily Pediatric Dose (mg/kg)
Ephedrine	β, α	100–200	2–3
Phenylephrine	α	40–60	0.5–1
Phenylpropanolamine	α	100–150	1–2
Pseudoephedrine	β, α	180–360	3–5

[a] α = alpha-adrenergic; β = beta-adrenergic.

    B. Other useful laboratory studies. Electrolytes, glucose, BUN, creatinine, creatine phosphokinase (CPK) with MB band fractions, ECG and ECG monitoring, CT head scan if intracranial hemorrhage suspected.

V. Treatment

  A. Emergency and supportive measures

    1. Maintain the airway and assist ventilation if necessary (see p 4). Administer supplemental oxygen.

    2. Treat hypertension aggressively (p 17 and **B,** below). Treat seizures (p 22) and ventricular tachyarrhythmias (p 14) if they occur. Do *not* treat reflex bradycardia, except indirectly by lowering blood pressure.

    3. Monitor the vital signs and ECG for a minimum of 4–6 hours after exposure, and longer if a sustained-release preparation has been ingested.

  B. Specific drugs and antidotes

    1. **Hypertension.** Treat hypertension if the diastolic pressure is higher than 100–105 mm Hg, especially in a patient with no prior history of hypertension. If there is computed tomographic or obvious clinical evidence of intracranial hemorrhage, lower the diastolic pressure cautiously, to no lower than 90 mm Hg, and consult a neurosurgeon immediately.

      a. Use a vasodilator such as **phentolamine** (p 369) or **nitroprusside** (p 362).

      b. *Caution:* Do *not* use beta blockers alone to treat hypertension without first giving a vasodilator; paradoxic worsening of the hypertension may result.

      c. Many patients have moderate orthostatic variation in the blood pressure; therefore, for immediate partial relief of severe hypertension, try placing the patient in an upright position.

    2. **Arrhythmias**

      a. Tachyarrhythmias usually respond to low-dose **propranolol** (p 373) or **esmolol** (p 338).

      b. *Caution:* Do *not* treat AV block or sinus bradycardia associated with hypertension; increasing the heart rate with atropine may abolish this reflex response that serves to limit hypertension, resulting in worsening elevation of the blood pressure.

  C. Decontamination (see p 44)

    1. **Prehospital.** Administer activated charcoal, if available. Ipecac-induced emesis may be useful for initial treatment at the scene (eg, children at home) if it can be given within a few minutes of exposure. However, it should not be used later because of the risk of aggravating hypertension.

    2. **Hospital.** Administer activated charcoal and a cathartic. Gastric emptying is not necessary if activated charcoal can be given promptly.

  D. Enhanced elimination. Dialysis and hemoperfusion are not effective. Urinary acidification may enhance elimination of PPA, ephedrine, and pseudoephedrine, but may also aggravate myoglobin deposition in the kidney if the patient has rhabdomyolysis.

PHENYTOIN
Kathryn H. Keller, PharmD

ANTIDOTE   IPECAC   LAVAGE   CHARCOAL

Phenytoin is used orally for the prevention of grand mal and psychomotor seizures. Intravenous phenytoin is used to treat status epilepticus and occasionally as an antiarrhythmic agent (see p 370). Oral formulations include suspensions, capsules, and tablet preparations. The brand Dilantin Kapseals exhibits delayed absorption characteristics not usually shared by generic products.

I. **Mechanism of toxicity.** Toxicity may be caused by the phenytoin itself or by the propylene glycol diluent used in parenteral preparations.
  A. **Phenytoin** alters neuronal ion fluxes, increasing refractory periods and decreasing repetitive neuronal firing. It is also known to increase brain concentrations of gamma aminobutyric acid (GABA). Toxic levels usually cause central nervous system depression.
  B. The **propylene glycol** diluent in parenteral preparations may cause myocardial depression and cardiac arrest when infused rapidly (> 40–50 mg/min [0.5–1 mg/kg/min]). The mechanism is not known.

II. **Toxic dose.** The minimum acute toxic oral overdose is approximately 20 mg/kg. Because phenytoin exhibits dose-dependent elimination kinetics, accidental intoxication can easily occur in patients on chronic therapy owing to drug interactions or slight dosage adjustments.

III. **Clinical presentation.** Toxicity caused by phenytoin may be associated with acute oral overdose or chronic accidental overmedication. In acute oral overdose, absorption and peak effects may be delayed.
  A. **Mild to moderate intoxication** commonly causes nystagmus, ataxia, and dysarthria. Nausea, vomiting, diplopia, hyperglycemia, agitation, and irritability have also been reported.
  B. **Severe intoxication** can cause stupor, coma, and respiratory arrest. Although seizures have been reported, literature reports are unconvincing; seizures in a phenytoin-intoxicated patient should prompt a search for other causes (eg, anoxia, hyperthermia, other drug overdose).
  C. **Rapid IV injection,** usually at rates exceeding 50 mg/min, can cause profound hypotension, bradycardia, or cardiac arrest. Cardiac toxicity does not occur with oral overdose.

IV. **Diagnosis** is based on a history of ingestion or is suspected in any epileptic patient with altered mental status or ataxia.
  A. **Specific levels.** Serum phenytoin concentrations are generally available in all hospital clinical laboratories. Obtain repeated blood samples because slow absorption may result in delayed peak levels. The therapeutic concentration range is 10–20 mg/L.
    1. Above 20 mg/L, nystagmus is common. Above 30 mg/L, ataxia, slurred speech, and tremor are common. With levels higher than 40 mg/L, lethargy, confusion, and stupor ensue. Survival has been reported in 3 patients with levels above 100 mg/L.
    2. Because phenytoin is protein-bound, patients with renal failure or hypoalbuminemia may experience toxicity at lower serum levels. Free (unbound) serum phenytoin levels are not routinely available.
  B. **Other useful laboratory studies.** Electrolytes, glucose, BUN, creatinine, serum albumin, ECG monitoring (during IV infusion).

V. **Treatment**
  A. **Emergency and supportive measures**
    1. Maintain the airway and assist ventilation if necessary (see p 4). Administer supplemental oxygen.
    2. Treat stupor and coma (p 18) if they occur. Protect the patient from self-injury caused by ataxia.

    3. If seizures occur, consider an alternative diagnosis and treat with other usual anticonvulsants (p 22).

    4. If hypotension occurs with intravenous phenytoin administration, immediately stop the infusion and administer intravenous fluids and pressors (p 15) if necessary.

  B. Specific drugs and antidotes. There is no specific antidote.

  C. Decontamination (see p 44)

    1. Prehospital. Administer activated charcoal, if available. Ipecac-induced emesis may be useful for initial treatment at the scene (eg, children at home) if it can be given within a few minutes of exposure.

    2. Hospital. Administer activated charcoal and a cathartic. Gastric emptying is not necessary if activated charcoal can be given promptly.

  D. Enhanced elimination. Repeat-dose activated charcoal (see p 52) may enhance phenytoin elimination. There is no role for diuresis, dialysis, or hemoperfusion.

PHOSGENE
John Balmes, MD

ANTIDOTE   IPECAC   LAVAGE   CHARCOAL

Phosgene was originally manufactured as a war gas. It is now used in the manufacture of dyes, resins, and pesticides. It is also commonly produced when chlorinated compounds are burned, such as in a fire, or in the process of welding metal that has been cleaned with chlorinated solvents.

  I. Mechanism of toxicity. Phosgene is an irritant. However, because it is poorly water-soluble, in lower concentrations it does not cause immediate upper airway or skin irritation. Thus, an exposed individual may inhale phosgene deeply into the lungs for prolonged periods, where it is slowly hydrolyzed to hydrochloric acid. This results in necrosis and inflammation of the small airways and alveoli that may lead to noncardiogenic pulmonary edema.

  II. Toxic dose. The ACGIH recommended workplace exposure limit (TLV-TWA) is 0.1 ppm as an 8-hour time-weighted average. The level considered immediately dangerous to life or health (IDLH) is 2 ppm. Exposure to 50 ppm may be rapidly fatal.

  III. Clinical presentation. Exposure to moderate concentrations of phosgene causes mild cough and minimal mucous membrane irritation. After an asymptomatic interval of 30 minutes to 8 hours (depending on the duration and concentration of exposure), the victim develops dyspnea and hypoxemia. Pulmonary edema may be delayed up to 24 hours. Permanent pulmonary impairment may be a sequela of serious exposure.

  IV. Diagnosis is based on a history of exposure and the clinical presentation. Many other toxic gases may cause delayed-onset pulmonary edema (see p 176).

    A. Specific levels. There are no specific blood or urine levels.

    B. Other useful laboratory studies. Chest x-ray, arterial blood gases or oximetry.

  V. Treatment

    A. Emergency and supportive measures

      1. Maintain the airway and assist ventilation if necessary (see p 4). Administer supplemental oxygen, and treat noncardiogenic pulmonary edema (see p 8) if it occurs.

      2. Monitor the patient for at least 12–24 hours after exposure because of the potential for delayed-onset pulmonary edema.

    B. Specific drugs and antidotes. There is no specific antidote.

    C. Decontamination. Remove the victim from exposure and give supplemental oxygen, if available. Rescuers should wear self-contained breathing apparatus.

    D. Enhanced elimination. These procedures are not effective.

PHOSPHINE
Diane Liu, MD, MPH

Phosphine is a colorless gas that is heavier than air. It has a characteristic fishy or garliclike odor. It has been used for fumigation and it is a serious potential hazard in operations producing metal phosphides, where phosphine can be released in the chemical reaction of water and metal alloys. Workers at risk include metal refiners, acetylene workers, fire fighters, pest-control operators, and those in the semiconductor industry.

I. **Mechanism of toxicity.** Phosphine is a highly toxic gas, especially to organs of high oxygen flow and demand such as the lungs, brain, kidneys, heart, and liver. The pathophysiologic action of phosphine is not clearly understood.

II. **Toxic dose.** The ACGIH recommended workplace exposure limit (TLV-TWA) is 0.3 ppm, much lower than the minimal detectable (fishy odor) concentration of 1–3 ppm. Hence, the odor threshold does not provide sufficient warning of dangerous concentrations. A level of 200 ppm is considered immediately dangerous to life or health (IDLH).

Chronic exposure to sublethal concentrations for extended periods may produce toxic symptoms.

III. **Clinical presentation.** Toxicity occurs following inhalation exposure and is characterized by severe pulmonary irritation, cough, dyspnea, headache, dizziness, lethargy, and stupor. Seizures, gastroenteritis, and renal and hepatic toxicity may also occur. The onset of symptoms is usually rapid, although delayed onset of pulmonary edema and focal myocardial necrosis has been described.

IV. **Diagnosis** is based on a history of exposure to the agent. *Caution:* Pulmonary edema may have a delayed onset, and initial respiratory symptoms may be mild or absent.

   A. **Specific levels.** Plasma phosphine levels are not clinically useful. Chronic low-level exposure to phosphine may be identified through blood and urine phosphorus levels, although this procedure is not well established.

   B. **Other useful laboratory studies.** BUN, creatinine, liver transaminases, arterial blood gases, chest x-ray, ECG.

V. **Treatment**

   A. **Emergency and supportive measures**

   1. Maintain the airway and assist ventilation if necessary (see p 4). Administer supplemental oxygen, and treat noncardiogenic pulmonary edema (p 8) if it occurs.

   2. Treat seizures (p 22) and hypotension (p 15) if they occur.

   3. Patients with a history of significant phosphine inhalation should be admitted and observed for 48–72 hours for delayed onset of pulmonary edema.

   B. **Specific drugs and antidotes.** There is no specific antidote.

   C. **Decontamination.** Immediately remove the victim from exposure and administer supplemental oxygen, if available.

   D. **Enhanced elimination.** Dialysis and hemoperfusion have not been shown to be useful in hastening elimination of phosphine.

PHOSPHORUS
Kent R. Olson, MD

There are 2 naturally occurring types of elemental phosphorus: red and white-yellow. **Red phosphorus** is not absorbed and is essentially nontoxic. In contrast, **white** or **yellow phosphorus** is a highly toxic cellular poison. Although no longer a component of matches, white phosphorus is still used in the manufacture of fireworks and fertilizer and as a rodenticide.

I. Mechanism of toxicity

A. Phosphorus is highly corrosive and is also a general cellular poison. Cardiovascular collapse occurring after ingestion probably results not only from fluid loss owing to vomiting and diarrhea but also from direct toxicity on the heart and vascular tone.

B. White-yellow phosphorus spontaneously combusts in air to yield phosphorus oxide, a highly irritating fume.

II. Toxic dose

A. **Ingestion.** The fatal oral dose of white-yellow phosphorus is approximately 1 mg/kg. Deaths have been reported after ingestion of as little as 15 mg.

B. **Inhalation.** The recommended workplace limit (ACGIH TLV-TWA) for white-yellow phosphorus is 0.1 mg/m^3 (0.02 ppm) as an 8-hour time-weighted average.

III. Clinical presentation

A. **Acute inhalation** may cause conjunctivitis, mucous membrane irritation, cough, wheezing, chemical pneumonitis, and noncardiogenic pulmonary edema. **Chronic inhalation** of phosphorus (over at least 10 months) may result in mandibular necrosis ("phossy jaw").

B. **Skin or eye contact** may cause severe dermal or ocular burns.

C. **Acute ingestion** may cause gastrointestinal burns, severe vomiting, and diarrhea with "smoking" stools. Systemic effects include headache, confusion, seizures, coma, arrhythmias, and shock. Metabolic derangements may occur, including hypocalcemia and hyperphosphatemia (or hypophosphatemia). If the victim survives, hepatic or renal failure may occur after 4–8 days.

IV. Diagnosis is based on a history of exposure and the clinical presentation. Smoking stools caused by spontaneous combustion of elemental phosphorus suggests phosphorus ingestion.

A. **Specific levels.** Because serum phosphorus may be elevated, depressed, or normal, it is not a useful test for diagnosis or estimation of severity.

B. **Other useful laboratory studies.** BUN, creatinine, liver transaminases, urinalysis, arterial blood gases or oximetry, chest x-ray (acute inhalation).

V. Treatment

A. **Emergency and supportive measures**

1. After inhalation, observe closely for signs of upper airway injury and perform endotracheal intubation and assist ventilation if necessary (see p 4). Administer supplemental oxygen. Treat bronchospasm (p 9–10) and pulmonary edema (p 8) if they occur.

2. Treat fluid losses from gastroenteritis with aggressive intravenous crystalloid fluid replacement.

3. Consider endoscopy if oral, esophageal, or gastric burns are suspected (p 126).

B. **Specific drugs and antidotes.** There is no specific antidote.

C. **Decontamination** (see p 41). Rescuers should wear appropriate protective gear to prevent accidental exposure.

1. **Inhalation.** Remove the victim from exposure and give supplemental oxygen, if available.

2. **Skin and eyes.** Remove contaminated clothing and wash exposed areas with soap and water. Irrigate exposed eyes with copious tepid water or saline. Covering exposed areas may help prevent spontaneous combustion of white-yellow phosphorus.

3. **Ingestion** (see p 44)

a. **Prehospital.** Administer activated charcoal, if available (although there is no evidence that it adsorbs phosphorus). Do **not** induce emesis because of the potential for corrosive injury.

b. **Hospital.** Perform careful gastric lavage. Administer activated charcoal (although there is no evidence that it adsorbs phosphorus).

D. **Enhanced elimination.** There is no effective method of enhanced elimination.

PLANTS AND HERBS
Olga F. Woo, PharmD

| ANTIDOTE | IPECAC | LAVAGE | CHARCOAL |

Plant ingestions are second only to drugs as the most common poisoning exposure in children. Fortunately, serious poisoning or death is extremely rare because the quantity of toxin ingested is small. During the past 2 decades, public interest in natural foods and traditional medical remedies and in "herbal highs" has resulted in increasing use of herbal products. Unfortunately, there is little consumer awareness of the potential harm from some herbal preparations. Besides toxicity from natural products contained in some medicinal plants, "herbal" or "traditional" preparations may sometimes actually contain allopathic drugs such as phenylbutazone, corticosteroids, salicylates, ephedrine, or toxic metal salts such as mercury or lead.

I. **Mechanism of toxicity.** Table II–46 is a list of potentially toxic plants, categorized in groups 1, 2a, 2b, and 3.
    A. **Group 1** plants contain systemically active poisons that may cause serious intoxication.
    B. **Group 2a** plants contain insoluble calcium oxalate crystals that cause burning pain and swelling of mucous membranes.
    C. **Group 2b** plants contain soluble oxalate salts (sodium or potassium) that can produce acute hypocalcemia, renal injury, and other organ damage secondary to precipitation of calcium oxalate crystals in various organs (see p 243). Mucous membrane irritation and gastroenteritis may also occur.
    D. **Group 3** plants contain various chemical agents that generally produce only mild to moderate gastrointestinal irritation after ingestion or dermatitis after skin contact.

II. **Toxic dose**
    A. **Plants.** The amount of toxin ingested is usually unknown. Concentrations of the toxic agent may vary depending on the plant part, the season, and soil conditions. In general, childhood ingestion of a few leaves or petals from even group 1 plants results in little or no toxicity because of the small amount of toxin absorbed.
    B. **Herbs.** Herbal teas and medications often contain only minute, "homeopathic" amounts of the toxin, in which case toxicity might occur only after chronic overuse or massive acute overdose.

III. **Clinical presentation**
    A. **Group 1.** The presentation depends upon the active toxic agent (Table II–46). In most cases, vomiting, abdominal pain, and diarrhea occur within 60–90 minutes of a significant ingestion. With some toxins (eg, ricin), severe gastroenteritis may result in massive fluid and electrolyte loss.
    B. **Group 2a.** Insoluble calcium oxalate crystals cause immediate burning prickly pain upon contact with mucous membranes. Swelling of the lips, tongue, and pharynx may occur, and in rare cases glottic edema may result in airway obstruction. Symptoms usually resolve within a few hours.
    C. **Group 2b.** Soluble oxalates may be absorbed into the circulation, where they precipitate with calcium, resulting in acute hypocalcemia and multiple-organ injury, including renal tubular necrosis.
    D. **Group 3.** Skin or mucous membrane irritation may occur, although it is less severe than with group 2 plants. Vomiting and diarrhea are common but are usually mild and self-limited. Fluid and electrolyte imbalance caused by severe gastroenteritis is rare.

IV. **Diagnosis** is usually based on a history of exposure and suspected when plant material is seen in vomitus. Identification of the plant is essential to proper treatment. Because common names sometimes refer to more than one plant, it is preferable to confirm the botanical name. If in doubt about the plant identification, take the specimen to a local nursery, florist, or college botany department.

TABLE II–46. POISONOUS PLANTS AND HERBS

Common Name	Botanical Name	Toxic Group	Remarks
Acorn	*Quercus* spp	3	Tannin; irritant
Akee	*Blighia sapida*	1	Hypoglycemica and hepato-toxicity
Almond, bitter	*Prunus* spp	1	Cyanogenic glycosides (see p 145)
Aloe vera	*Aloe vera*	3	Hypersensitivity; skin irritant
Amaryllis	*Hippeastrum equestre*	3	
American bittersweet	*Celastrus scandens*	3	
American ivy	*Parthenocissus* spp	2b	Soluble oxalates (see p 243)
Angel's trumpet	*Brugmansia arborea*	1, 3	Anticholinergic alkaloids (see p 75)
Anthurium	*Anthurium* spp	2a	Calcium oxalate crystals (see text)
Apple (seeds)	*Malus domestica*	1	Cyanogenic glycosides (see p 145)
Apricot (chewed pits)	*Prunus* spp	1	Cyanogenic glycosides (see p 145)
Arrowhead vine	*Syngonium podophyllum*	2a	Calcium oxalate crystals (see text)
Asparagus fern	*Asparagus plumosus*	3	
Autumn crocus	*Colchicum autumnale*	1	Colchicine (see p 141)
Avocado (leaves)	*Avocado*	1	Unknown toxin
Azalea	*Azalea* spp	1	Andromedotoxin: hypotension, AV block, arrhythmias; lethargy
Azalea	*Rhododendron* genus	1	Andromedotoxin: hypotension, bradycardia, AV block; lethargy
Bahia	*Bahia oppositifolia*	1	Cyanogenic glycosides (see p 145)
Baneberry	*Actaea* spp	3	Irritant oil protoanemonin: severe gastroenteritis
Barbados nut; purging nut	*Jatropha* spp	1	Phytotoxins: severe gastroenteritis
Barberry	*Berberis* spp	3	
Beech	*Fagus sylvatica*	3	Saponins
Begonia	*Begonia rex*	2a	Calcium oxalate crystals (see text)
Belladonna	*Atropa belladonna*	1	Atropine (see p 75)
Bellyache bush	*Jatropha* spp	1	Phytotoxins: severe gastroenteritis
Be-still tree	*Thevetia peruviana*	1	Cardiac glycosides (see p 124)
Birch (bark, leaves)	*Betula* spp	1,3	Methyl salicylate, irritant oils
Bird of paradise	*Poinciana gillesi*	3	
Black cohosh	*Cimicifuga* spp	3	
Black locust	*Robinia pseudoacacia*	1	Phytotoxins: severe gastroenteritis
Black nightshade	*Hyoscyamus* spp	1	Anticholinergic alkaloids (see p 75)
Black snakeroot	*Zigadenus* spp	1	Similar to veratramine: hypotension, bradycardia, lethargy
Bleeding heart	*Dicentra*	3	
Bloodroot	*Sanguinaria canadensis*	3	
Blue cohosh	*Caulophyllum thalictroides*	1,3	Cytisine: similar to nicotine (see p 227)
Boston ivy	*Parthenocissus* spp	2b	Soluble oxalates (see p 243)
Boxwood; box plant	*Buxus* spp	3	

TABLE II-46. POISONOUS PLANTS AND HERBS (CONTINUED)

Common Name	Botanical Name	Toxic Group	Remarks
Broom; scotch broom	*Cytisus* spp	1, 3	Cytisine: similar to nicotine (see p 227); sparteine: cardiotoxic; sparteione: diuretic, oxytoxic
Buckeye	*Aesculus* spp	1, 3	Coumarin glycosides (see p 143)
Buckthorn; tullidora	*Karwinskia humboltiana*	1	Chronic ingestion may cause ascending paralysis
Buckthorn	*Rhamnus* spp	3	Anthraquinone cathartic
Bunchberry	*Cornus canadensis*	3	
Burdock root	*Arctium minus*	1, 3	Anticholinergic alkaloids (see p 75)
Burning bush	*Euonymus* spp	3	
Buttercups	*Ranunculus* spp	3	Irritant oil protoanemonin
Cactus (thorn)	*Cactus*	3	Cellulitis, abscess may result
Caladium	*Caladium* spp	2a	Calcium oxalate crystals (see text)
Caladium	*Xanthosoma* spp	2a	Calcium oxalate crystals (see text)
California geranium	*Senecio* spp	1	Hepatotoxic pyrrolizidine alkaloids
California privet	*Ligustrum* spp	3	
Calla lily	*Zantedeschia* spp	2a	Calcium oxalate crystals (see text)
Cannabis	*Cannabis sativa*	1	Mild hallucinogen
Caraway	*Carum carvi*	3	When used as herbal medication
Cardinal flower	*Lobelia* spp	1	Lobeline: nicotinelike alkaloid (see p 227)
Carnation	*Dianthus caryophyllus*	3	
Carolina allspice	*Calycanthus* spp	1	Strychninelike alkaloid
Cascara	*Rhamnus* spp	3	Anthraquinone cathartic
Cassava	*Manihot esculenta*	1	Cyanogenic glycosides (see p 145)
Castor bean	*Ricinus communis*	1	Phytotoxins: severe gastroenteritis
Catnip	*Nepeta cataria*	1, 3	Mild hallucinogen
Century plant	*Agave americana*	3	Thorns can cause cellulitis
Chamomile	*Chamomilla recucita*	3	Highly antigenic
Cherry (chewed pits)	*Prunus* spp	1	Cyanogenic glycosides (see p 145)
Chili pepper	*Capsicum* spp	3	Irritant to skin, eyes, mucous membranes
Chinaberry	*Melia azedarach*	1, 3	Severe fatal gastroenteritis reported; contains convulsant
Christmas rose	*Helleborus niger*	1, 3	Similar to cardiac glycosides (see p 124)
Chrysanthemum; mum	*Chrysanthemum* spp	3	Pyrethrins (see p 269)
Coffeeberry	*Rhamnus* spp	3	Anthraquinone cathartic
Cola nut; gotu kola	*Cola* spp	1	Caffeine, theobromin
Comfrey	*Symphytum officinale*	1, 3	Irritant tannin and hepatotoxic pyrrolizidine alkaloids
Conquer root	*Exogonium purga*	3	

(*continued*)

TABLE II–46. POISONOUS PLANTS AND HERBS (CONTINUED)

Common Name	Botanical Name	Toxic Group	Remarks
Coral bean	Sophora secundiflora	1	Cytisine: similar to nicotine (see p 227)
Coral berry	Symphoricarpos spp	3	
Coriaria	Coriaria myrtifolia	1	Contains convulsant agent
Cotoneaster	Cotoneaster	1, 3	Cyanogenic glycosides (see p 145)
Coyotillo	Karwinskia humboldtiana	1	Chronic ingestion may cause ascending paralysis
Creeping charlie	Glecoma hederacea	1, 3	Volatile oils; mild stimulant
Crown of thorns	Euphorbia spp	3	
Cyclamen	Cyclamen	3	
Daffodil (bulb)	Narcissus spp	3	
Daphne	Daphne spp	1, 3	Bark: coumarin glycosides (see p 143) berries: blisters
Deadly nightshade	Atropa belladonna	1	Atropine (see p 75)
Death camas	Zigadenus spp	1	Similar to veratramine: hypotension, bradycardia, lethargy
Devils ivy	Scindapsus aureus	2a	Calcium oxalate crystals (see text)
Dogbane	Apocynum spp	1	Cardiac glycosides (see p 124)
Dolls-eyes	Actaea spp	3	Irritant oil protoanemonin: severe gastroenteritis
Dragon root	Arisaema spp	2a	Calcium oxalate crystals (see text)
Dumbcane	Dieffenbachia spp	2a	Calcium oxalate crystals (see text)
Dusty miller	Senecio spp	1	Hepatotoxic pyrrolizidine alkaloids
Elderberry	Sambucus	1	Unripe berries contain cyanogenic glycosides (see p 145)
Elephant's ear; taro	Alocasia spp	2a	Calcium oxalate crystals (see text)
Elephant's ear	Colocasia spp	2a	Calcium oxalate crystals (see text)
Elephant's ear	Philodendron spp	2a	Calcium oxalate crystals (see text)
English ivy; heart ivy	Hedera helix	3	Saponins
English laurel	Prunus laurocerasus	1	Cyanogenic glycosides (see p 145)
Ergot	Claviceps spp	1	Ergot alkaloids (see p 158)
Eucalyptus	Eucalyptus	3	Irritant oils
False hellebore	Veratrum spp	1, 3	Veratramine: hypotension, AV block, arrhythmias; seizures
Fava bean	Vicia faba	1	Hemolytic anemia in G6PD-deficient persons
Ficus (sap)	Ficus benjamina	3	
Firethorn	Pyracantha	3	
Fool's parsley	Conilium maculatum	1	Coniline: nicotinelike alkaloid (see p 227)
Four o'clock	Mirabilis jalapa	3	Seeds have hallucinogenic effects
Foxglove	Digitalis purpurea	1	Cardiac glycosides (see p 124)

TABLE II–46. POISONOUS PLANTS AND HERBS (CONTINUED)

Common Name	Botanical Name	Toxic Group	Remarks
Glacier ivy	*Hedera glacier*	3	Saponins
Glory pea	*Sesbania* spp	3	Saponins
Goldenrod; rayless	*Haplopappus heterophyllus*	1	Higher alcohol tremetol: CNS depression
Golden chain	*Labumum anagyroides*	1	Cytisine: similar to nicotine (see p 227)
Golden seal	*Hydrastis* spp	1, 3	Fatalities reported after use as herbal tea
Gordolobo	*Senecio* spp	1	Hepatotoxic pyrrolizidine alkaloids
Grindelia	*Grindelia* spp	1	Balsamic resin: renal, cardiac toxicity
Groundsel	*Senecio* spp	1	Hepatotoxic pyrrolizidine alkaloids
Guaiac	*Guaiacum officinale*	3	
Harmaline	*Banisteriopsis* spp	1	Harmaline: hallucinogen (see p 204)
Harmel; Syrian rue	*Peganum harmala*	1	Harmaline: hallucinogen (see p 204)
Heart leaf	*Philodendron* spp	2a	Calcium oxalate crystals (see text)
Heath	*Ericaceae* family	1, 3	Andromedotoxin: hypotension, AV block, arrhythmias; lethargy
Heliotrope	*Heliotropium* spp	1	Pyrrolizidine alkaloids: hepatotoxicity
Hemlock; poison hemlock	*Conium maculatum*	1	Coniine: nicotinelike alkaloid (see p 227)
Henbane; black henbane	*Hyoscyamus* spp	1	Anticholinergic alkaloids (see p 75)
Holly (berry)	*Ilex aquifolium*	3	
Honeysuckle	*Caprifoliaceae family*	3	Red berries contain toxin
Hops	*Humulus lupulus*	1	Sedative
Horse chestnut	*Aesculus* spp	1,3	Coumarin glycosides (see p 143)
Hyacinth	*Hyacinthus*	3	
Hydrangea	*Hydrangea* spp	1, 3	Cyanogenic glycosides (see p 145)
Indian currant	*Symphoricarpos* spp	3	
Indian tobacco	*Lobelia* spp	1	Lobeline: nicotinelike alkaloid (see p 227)
Inkberry	*Phytolacca americana*	3	If absorbed may cause hemolysis; cooked berries edible
Iris	*Iris*	3	
Ivy bush; sheepkill	*Kalmia* spp	1	Andromedotoxin: hypotension, AV block, arrhythmias; lethargy
Jack-in-the-pulpit	*Arisaema* spp	2a	Calcium oxalate crystals (see text)
Jalap	*Exogonium purga*	3	
Jequirity bean	*Abrus precatorius*	1	Phytotoxin abrin: severe fatal gastroenteritis reported
Jerusalem cherry (unripe berry)	*Solanum pseudocapsicum*	1, 3	Solanine and anticholinergic alkaloids (see p 75)
Jessamine	*Gelsemium sempervirens*	1	Alkaloids similar to strychnine (see p 290)

(*continued*)

TABLE II–46. POISONOUS PLANTS AND HERBS (CONTINUED)

Common Name	Botanical Name	Toxic Group	Remarks
Jessamine, Carolina	*Gelsemium sempervirens*	1	Alkaloids similar to strychnine (see p 290)
Jessamine, day or night	*Cestrum* spp	1, 3	Solanine and anticholinergic alkaloids (see p 75)
Jessamine, yellow	*Gelsemium sempervirens*	1	Alkaloids similar to strychnine (see p 290)
Jetbead	*Rhodotypos scandens*	1	Cyanogenic glycosides (see p 145)
Jetberry bush	*Rhodotypos scandens*	1	Cyanogenic glycosides (see p 145)
Jimmyweed	*Haplopappus heterophyllus*	1	Higher alcohol tremetol: CNS depression
Jimsonweed	*Brugmansia arborea*	1, 3	Anticholinergic alkaloids (see p 75)
Jimsonweed; thornapple	*Datura stramonium*	1	Anticholinergic alkaloids (see p 75)
Juniper	*Juniperus macropoda*	1, 3	Hallucinogen (see p 204)
Kava-kava	*Piper methysticum*	1	Mild hallucinogen (see p 204)
Kentucky coffee tree	*Gymnocladus dioica*	1	Cytisine: similar to nicotine (see p 227)
Khat; chat	*Catha edulis*	1	Mild hallucinogen and stimulant
Labrador tea	*Ledum* spp	1	Andromedotoxin: hypotension, AV block, arrhythmias; lethargy
Lantana	*Lantana camara*	1	Hepatotoxic in animals; ingestion of unripe berries may cause cardiovascular collapse and death
Larkspur	*Delphinium*	1	Cardiotoxic delphinine: arrhythmias, AV block
Licorice root	*Glycyrrhiza lepidata*	1, 3	Hypokalemia after chronic use
Lily of the Nile	*Agapanthus*	3	Burning sensation when ingested
Lily-of-the-valley	*Convallaria majalis*	1	Cardiac glycosides (see p 124)
Lily-of-the-valley shrub	*Pieris japonica*	1	Andromedotoxin: hypotension, AV block, arrhythmias; lethargy
Mandrake	*Mandragora officinarum*	1	Anticholinergic alkaloids (see p 75)
Mandrake	*Podophyllum peltatum*	1, 3	Oil is keratolytic, irritant; hypotension, seizures reported after ingestion of resin; ripe fruit nontoxic
Marble queen	*Scindapsus aureus*	2a	Calcium oxalate crystals (see text)
Marijuana	*Cannabis sativa*	1	Mild hallucinogen
Marsh marigold	*Caltha palustris*	3	Irritant oil protoanemonin
Mate	*Ilex paraguayensis*	1, 3	Irritant tannins; caffeine
Mayapple	*Podophyllum peltatum*	1, 3	Oil is keratolytic, irritant; hypotension, seizures reported
Meadow crocus	*Colchicum autumnale*	1	Colchicine (see p 141)
Mescal bean	*Sophora secundiflora*	1	Cytisine: similar to nicotine (see p 227)
Mescal button	*Lophophora williamsii*	1	Mescaline: hallucinogen (see p 204)

TABLE II–46. POISONOUS PLANTS AND HERBS (CONTINUED)

Common Name	Botanical Name	Toxic Group	Remarks
Milkweed	*Asclepias* spp	3	Galitoxin: fatal poisonings in livestock
Mistletoe, American	*Phoradendron flavescens*	1, 3	Cardiotoxic phoratoxin: potential pressor effects
Mistletoe, European	*Viscum album*	1	Cardiotoxic viscotoxin; vasoconstrictor
Mock azalea	*Menziesia ferruginea*	1	Andromedotoxin: hypotension, AV block, arrythmias; lethargy
Monkshood	*Aconitum napellus*	1	Aconitine: hypotension, AV block, arrhythmias; seizures
Moonseed	*Menispermaceae*	1	Contains convulsant agent
Mormon tea	*Ephedra viridis*	1	Sympathomimetic (see p 253)
Morning glory	*Ipomoea violacea*	1	Seeds are hallucinogenic (see p 204)
Mountain laurel	*Kalmia* spp	1	Andromedotoxin: hypotension, AV block, arrhythmias; lethargy
Nectarine (chewed pits)	*Prunus* spp	1	Cyanogenic glycosides (see p 145)
Nephthytis	*Syngonium podophyllum*	2a	Calcium oxalate crystals (see text)
Nightshade	*Solanum* spp	1, 3	Solanine and anticholinergic alkaloids (see p 75)
Nightshade, black	*Hyoscyamus* spp	1	Anticholinergic alkaloids (see p 75)
Nightshade, deadly	*Atropa belladonna*	1	Atropine (see p 75)
Nutmeg	*Myristica fragrans*	1	Hallucinogen (see p 204)
Oakleaf ivy	*Toxicodendron* spp	3	Urushiol oleoresin contact dermatitis (*Rhus* dermatitis)
Oleander	*Nerium oleander*	1	Cardiac glycosides (see p 124)
Oleander, yellow	*Thevetia peruviana*	1	Cardiac glycosides (see p 124)
Pampus grass	*Cortaderia selloana*	1	Cyanogenic glycosides (see p 145)
Paraguay tea	*Ilex paraguayensis*	1, 3	Irritant tannins; caffeine
Peach (chewed pits)	*Prunus* spp	1	Cyanogenic glycosides (see p 145)
Pear (chewed seeds)	*Prunus* spp	1	Cyanogenic glycosides (see p 145)
Pennyroyal (oil)	*Mentha pulegium*	1	Hepatotoxic cyclic ketone; seizures reported
Periwinkle	*Vinca*	1	*Vinca* alkaloids
Periwinkle, rose	*Catharanthus roseus*	1	Hallucinogen (see p 204)
Peyote; mescal	*Lophophora williamsii*	1	Mescaline: hallucinogen (see p 204)
Pheasant's-eye	*Adonis* spp	1	Cardiac glycosides (see p 124)
Pigeonberry	*Duranta repens*	3	Saponins
Pigeonberry	*Phytolacca americana*	3	If absorbed may cause hemolysis; cooked berries edible
Plum (chewed pits)	*Prunus* spp	1	Cyanogenic glycosides (see p 145)
Poinsettia	*Euphorbia* spp	3	
Poison ivy	*Toxicodendron* spp	3	Urushiol oleoresin contact dermatitis (*Rhus* dermatitis) *(continued)*

TABLE II–46. POISONOUS PLANTS AND HERBS (CONTINUED)

Common Name	Botanical Name	Toxic Group	Remarks
Poison oak	*Toxicodendron* spp	3	Urushiol oleoresin contact dermatitis (*Rhus* dermatitis)
Poison sumac	*Toxicodendron* spp	3	Urushiol oleoresin contact dermatitis (*Rhus* dermatitis)
Poison vine	*Toxicodendron* spp	3	Urushiol oleoresin contact dermatitis (*Rhus* dermatitis)
Pokeweed (unripe berries)	*Phytolacca americana*	3	If absorbed may cause hemolysis; cooked berries edible
Potato (unripe)	*Solanum* spp	1, 3	Solanine and anticholinergic alkaloids (see p 75)
Pothos; yellow pothos	*Scindapsus aureus*	2a	Calcium oxalate crystals (see text)
Prickly poppy	*Argemone mexicana*	1	Narcotic-analgesic, smoked as euphoriant
Pride-of-Madeira	*Echium* spp	1	Pyrrolizidine alkaloids: hepatotoxicity
Privet; common privet	*Ligustrum* spp	3	
Purslane	*Portulaca oleracea*	2b	Soluble oxalates (see p 243)
Pyracantha	*Pyracantha*	3	
Ragwort, tansy	*Senecio* spp	1	Hepatotoxic pyrrolizidine alkaloids
Rattlebox	*Sesbania* spp	3	Saponins
Rattlebox; bush tea	*Crotalaria* spp	1	Pyrrolizidine alkaloids: hepatotoxicity
Rattlebox, purple	*Daubentonia* spp	3	
Rhododendron	*Rhododendron* genus	1	Andromedotoxin: hypotension, bradycardia, AV block; lethargy
Rhubarb	*Rheum rhaponticum*	2b	Soluble oxalates (see p 243)
Rosary pea; rosary bean	*Abrus precatorius*	1	Phytotoxin abrin: severe fatal gastroenteritis reported
Rose periwinkle	*Catharanthus roseus*	1	Hallucinogen (see p 204)
Rustyleaf	*Menziesia ferruginea*	1	Andromedotoxin: hypotension, AV block, arrhythmias; lethargy
Sassafras	*Sassafras albidium*	1	Hepatocarcinogenic
Scotch broom	*Cytisus scoparins*	1, 3	Cytisine: gastrointestinal, nicotinic effects; spartei-ine: cardiotoxic; sparteione: diuretic, oxytoxic
Shamrock	*Oxalis* spp	2b	Soluble oxalates (see p 243)
Skunk cabbage	*Symplocarpus foetidus*	2a	Calcium oxalate crystals (see text)
Skunk cabbage	*Veratrum* spp	1, 3	Veratramine: hypotension, AV block, arrhythmias; seizures
Sky-flower	*Duranta repens*	3	Saponins
Snakeroot	*Rauwolfia serpentina*	1	Antihypertensive reserpine tranquilizer
Snowberry	*Symphoricarpos* spp	3	
Sorrel; soursob	*Oxalis* spp	2b	Soluble oxalates (see p 243)
Spathiphyllum	*Spathiphyllum*	2a	Calcium oxalate crystals (see text)
Spindle tree	*Euonymous* spp	3	
Split leaf	*Philodendron* spp	2a	Calcium oxalate crystals (see text)
Sprengeri fern	*Asparagus densiflorus*	3	

TABLE II–46. POISONOUS PLANTS AND HERBS (CONTINUED)

Common Name	Botanical Name	Toxic Group	Remarks
Squill	*Scilla*	1	Cardiac glycosides (see p 124)
Squill	*Urginea maritima*	1	Cardiac glycosides (see p 124)
Star-of-Bethlehem	*Ornithogalum* spp	1	Cardiac glycosides (see p 124)
String of pearls/beads	*Senecio* spp	1	Hepatotoxic pyrrolizidine alkaloids
Strychnine	*Strychnos nux-vomica*	1	Strychnine (see p 290)
Sweet clover	*Melilotus* spp	1	Coumarin glycosides (see p 143)
Sweet pea	*Lathyrus odoratus*	1	Neuropathy (lathyrism) after chronic use
Swiss cheese plant	*Monstera friedrichsthali*	2a	Calcium oxalate crystals (see text)
Tobacco	*Nicotiana* spp	1	Nicotine (see p 227)
Tomato (leaves)	*Lycopersicon esculentum*	1	Solanine: sympathomimetic; bradycardia
Tonka bean	*Dipteryx odorata*	1	Coumarin glycosides (see p 143)
Toyon (leaves)	*Heteromeles arbutifolia*	1	Cyanogenic glycosides (see p 145)
Tulip (bulb)	*Tulipa*	3	
Tung tree; candle nut	*Aleurites* spp	1, 3	Phytotoxins, saponins
Turbina	*Turbina corymbosa*	1	Hallucinogen (see p 204)
T'u-san-chi	*Gynura segetum*	1	Hepatotoxic pyrrolizidine alkaloids
Umbrella plant	*Cyperus alternifolius*	1	See essential oils (p 115)
Uva-ursi	*Arctostaphylos uvo-ursi*	1, 3	Hydroquinone: berries edible
Valerian	*Valeriana officinalis*	1	Valerine alkaloids: used as mild tranquilizer
Walnut (green shells)	*Juglans*	1	Moldy parts contain convulsant mycotoxins
Water hemlock	*Cicuta maculata*	1	Cicutoxin: seizures; vomiting; diaphoresis, salivation
Wild calla	*Calla palustris*	2a	Calcium oxalate crystals (see text)
Wild onion	*Zigadenus* spp	1	Similar to veratramine: hypotension, bradycardia, lethargy
Windflower	*Anemone*	3	Irritant oil protoanemonin
Wisteria	*Wisteria*	3	Severe gastroenteritis
Woodruff	*Galium odoratum*	1	Coumarin glycosides (see p 143)
Wood rose	*Ipomoea violacea*	1	Seeds are hallucinogenic (see p 204)
Wood rose	*Merremia tuberosa*	1	Seeds are hallucinogenic
Wormwood	*Artemesia absinthium*	1	See essential oils (p 115); smoked as relaxant
Yarrow	*Achillea millefolium*	3	Prepared as a tea
Yellow oleander	*Thevetia peruviana*	1	Cardiac glycosides (see p 124)
Yew	*Taxus*	1	Taxine: similar to cardiac glycosides (see p 124); seizures
Yohimbine	*Corynanthe yohimbe*	1	Aphrodisiac; mild hallucinogen; α_2-blocker

    A. Specific levels. Serum toxin levels are not available for most plant toxins. In selected cases, laboratory analyses for therapeutic drugs may be used (eg, digoxin assay for oleander glycosides).

    B. Other useful laboratory studies. For patients with gastroenteritis: CBC, electrolytes, glucose, BUN, creatinine, urinalysis. If hepatotoxicity suspected: liver transaminases and prothrombin time (PT).

V. Treatment. Most ingestions cause no symptoms or only mild gastroenteritis, and patients recover quickly with supportive care.

    A. Emergency and supportive measures

        1. Maintain the airway and assist ventilation if necessary (see p 4). Administer supplemental oxygen.

        2. Treat coma (p 18), seizures (p 22), arrhythmias (p 10–14), and hypotension (p 15) if they occur.

        3. Replace fluid losses caused by gastroenteritis with intravenous crystalloid solutions.

    B. Specific drugs and antidotes. There are few effective antidotes. See the "Remarks" column in Table II–46 for specific information or referral to additional discussion elsewhere in Section II.

    C. Decontamination (see p 44)

        1. Group 1 and group 2b plants

            a. Prehospital. Administer activated charcoal, if available. Ipecac-induced emesis may be useful for initial treatment at the scene (eg, children at home) if it can be given within a few minutes of exposure.

            b. Hospital. Administer activated charcoal and a cathartic. Gastric emptying is not necessary if activated charcoal can be given promptly.

        2. Group 2a and group 3 plants

            a. Wash the affected areas with plain water and give water or milk to drink.

            b. Do **not** induce emesis, because of potential aggravation of irritant effects. Gastric lavage and activated charcoal are not necessary.

    D. Enhanced elimination. These procedures are not generally effective.

POLYCHLORINATED BIPHENYLS (PCBs)
Diane Liu, MD, MPH

ANTIDOTE   IPECAC   LAVAGE   CHARCOAL

Polychlorinated biphenyls (PCBs) are a group of chlorinated hydrocarbon compounds that are widely used as high-temperature insulators for transformers and other electric equipment and are also found in carbonless copy papers and some inks and paints. Since 1974, all uses in the US are confined to closed systems. Most PCB poisonings are chronic occupational exposures, with delayed-onset symptoms being the first indication that an exposure has occurred. In 1977, the Environmental Protection Agency banned further manufacturing of PCBs because they are suspected carcinogens.

    I. Mechanism of toxicity. PCBs are irritating to mucous membranes. When burned, PCBs may produce highly toxic polychlorinated dibenzodioxins (PCDDs) and polychlorinated dibenzofurans (PCDFs; see p 154). It is difficult to establish the specific effects of PCB intoxication because PCBs are nearly always contaminated with small amounts of these compounds. PCBs, and particularly the PCDD and PCDF contaminants, are mutagenic and teratogenic and are considered potential human carcinogens.

    II. Toxic dose. PCBs are well absorbed by all routes (skin, inhalation, ingestion) and are widely distributed in fat; bioaccumulation occurs even with low-level exposure.

        A. Inhalation. PCBs are mildly irritating to the skin at airborne levels of 0.1 mg/m^3 and very irritating at 10 mg/m^3. The recommended workplace limits (ACGIH

TLV-TWA) are 0.5 mg/m^3 (for PCBs with 54% chlorine) and 1 mg/m^3 (for PCBs with 42% chlorine) as 8-hour time-weighted averages. The air levels considered immediately dangerous to life or health (IDLH) are 5 mg/m^3 and 10 mg/m^3, respectively.

B. Ingestion. Acute toxicity after ingestion is unlikely; the oral LD$_{50}$ is 1–10 g/kg.

III. Clinical presentation

    A. Acute PCB exposure may cause skin, eye, nose, and throat irritation.

    B. Chronic exposure may cause **chloracne** (cystic acneiform lesions predominantly found on the posterior neck, axillas, and upper back); the onset is usually 6 weeks or longer after exposure. Skin pigmentation and porphyria may occur. Elevation of hepatic transaminases may occur, although the significance is unclear.

IV. Diagnosis is usually based on a history of exposure and the presence of chloracne or elevated hepatic transaminases.

    A. Specific levels. PCB serum and fat levels are poorly correlated with health effects. Serum PCB concentrations are usually less than 20 µg/L; higher levels may indicate exposure but not necessarily toxicity.

    B. Other useful laboratory studies. BUN, creatinine, liver enzymes.

V. Treatment

    A. Emergency and supportive measures

        1. Treat bronchospasm (see p 9–10) if it occurs.

        2. Monitor for elevated hepatic enzymes; chloracne; and nonspecific eye, gastrointestinal, and neurologic symptoms.

    B. Specific drugs and antidotes. There is no specific antidote.

    C. Decontamination (see p 41)

        1. Inhalation. Remove the victim from exposure and give supplemental oxygen, if available.

        2. Skin and eyes. Remove contaminated clothing and wash exposed skin with soap and water. Irrigate exposed eyes with copious tepid water or saline.

        3. Ingestion (see p 44)

            a. Prehospital. Administer activated charcoal, if available. Ipecac-induced emesis may be useful for initial treatment if it can be given within a few minutes of exposure.

            b. Hospital. Administer activated charcoal and a cathartic. Gastric emptying is not necessary if activated charcoal can be given promptly.

    D. Enhanced elimination. There is no role for dialysis, hemoperfusion, or repeat-dose charcoal. Lipid-clearing drugs (eg, clofibrate and resins) have been suggested, but insufficient data exist to recommend them.

PYRETHRINS AND PYRETHROIDS
Olga F. Woo, PharmD

ANTIDOTE   IPECAC   LAVAGE   CHARCOAL

Pyrethrins are naturally occurring insecticides derived from the chrysanthemum plant. Pyrethroids (Table II–47) are synthetically derived compounds. Acute human poisoning from exposure to these insecticides is rare; however, inhalation frequently causes upper airway irritation and hypersensitivity reactions. Piperonyl butoxide is added to these compounds to prolong their activity by inhibiting mixed oxidase enzymes in the liver that metabolize the pyrethrins. Common pyrethrin-containing pediculicides are A-200, Triple-X, and RID.

    I. Mechanism of toxicity. In insects, pyrethrins and pyrethroids rapidly cause death by paralyzing the nervous system through disruption of the membrane ion transport system in nerve axons, and pyrethroids prolong sodium influx and also may

TABLE II–47. PYRETHROIDS

Allethrin	Decamethrin	Furamethrin
Barthrin	Deltamethrin	Permethrin
Bioallethrin	Fenothrin	Phthalthrin
Bioresmethrin	Fenpropanate	Resmethrin
Cypermethrin	Fenvalerate	Tetramethrin

block inhibitory pathways. Mammals are generally able to metabolize these compounds rapidly and thereby render them harmless.

II. **Toxic dose.** The toxic oral dose in mammals is greater than 100–1000 mg/kg, and the potentially lethal acute oral dose is 10–100 g. Pyrethrins are not well absorbed across the skin or from the gastrointestinal tract. They have been used for many years as oral anthelmintic agents with minimum adverse effects other than mild gastrointestinal upset.

   A. **Chinese chalk** contains 37.6 mg of deltamethrin per chalk. Ingestion of a single chalk is generally considered nontoxic. There is one report of seizures in a young woman who ingested 30 mL of 2.5% deltamethrin (750 mg).

   B. A 45-year-old man died after ingesting beans cooked in 10% **cypermethrin.**

III. **Clinical presentation.** Toxicity to humans is primarily associated with hypersensitivity reactions and direct irritant effects rather than from any pharmacologic property.

   A. **Anaphylactic** reactions including bronchospasm, oropharyngeal edema, and shock may occur in hypersensitive individuals.

   B. **Inhalation** of these compounds may precipitate wheezing in asthmatics. Inhalation or pulmonary aspiration may also cause a hypersensitivity pneumonitis.

   C. **Skin** exposure may cause burning, tingling, numbness, and erythema.

   D. **Eyes.** Accidental eye exposure during scalp application of A-200 Pyrinate has caused corneal injury including keratitis and denudation. The cause is uncertain, but may be related to the surfactant (Triton-X) contained in the product.

   E. **Ingestion.** With large ingestions (200–500 mL of concentrated solution), the central nervous system may be affected, resulting in seizures, coma, or respiratory arrest.

IV. **Diagnosis** is based on a history of exposure. There are no characteristic clinical symptoms or laboratory tests that are specific for identifying these compounds.

   A. **Specific levels.** These compounds are rapidly metabolized in the body, and methods for determining the parent compound are not routinely available.

   B. **Other useful laboratory studies.** Electrolytes, glucose, arterial blood gases or oximetry.

V. **Treatment**

   A. **Emergency and supportive measures**

      1. Treat bronchospasm (see p 9–10) or anaphylaxis (see p 26) if they occur.

      2. Observe patients with a history of a large ingestion for at least 4–6 hours for any signs of central nervous system depression or seizures.

   B. **Specific drugs and antidotes.** There is no specific antidote.

   C. **Decontamination** (see p 41)

      1. **Inhalation.** Remove victim from exposure and give supplemental oxygen, if available.

      2. **Skin.** Wash with copious soap and water. Topical application of vitamin E in vegetable oil was reported anecdotally to relieve paresthesias.

      3. **Eyes.** Irrigate with copious water. After irrigation, perform a fluorescein examination and refer to an ophthalmologist if there is evidence of corneal injury.

      4. **Ingestion** (see p 44). In the majority of cases, a subtoxic dose has been ingested and no decontamination is necessary. However, after a large ingestion of Chinese chalk or a concentrated solution:

         a. **Prehospital.** Administer activated charcoal, if available. Ipecac-induced emesis may be useful for initial treatment at the scene (eg, children at home) if it can be given within a few minutes of exposure. **Caution:** Most commercial products contain a hydrocarbon solvent that may cause chemical pneumonitis if aspirated.

    b. Hospital. Administer activated charcoal and a cathartic. Gastric lavage is not necessary if activated charcoal can be given promptly.

D. Enhanced elimination. These compounds are rapidly metabolized by the body, and extracorporeal methods of elimination would not be expected to enhance their elimination.

QUINIDINE AND OTHER TYPE Ia ANTIARRHYTHMIC DRUGS
Neal L. Benowitz, MD

ANTIDOTE   IPECAC   LAVAGE   CHARCOAL

Quinidine, procainamide (Pronestyl), and disopyramide (Norpace) are type Ia antiarrhythmic agents. Quinidine and procainamide are commonly used for suppression of acute and chronic supraventricular and ventricular arrhythmias. Disopyramide is used for ventricular arrhythmias. All 3 agents have a low toxic:therapeutic ratio and may produce fatal intoxication (Table II–48).

I. Mechanism of toxicity. Type Ia agents depress the fast sodium-dependent channel, slowing phase zero of the cardiac action potential. At high concentrations, this results in reduced myocardial contractility and excitability, and severe depression of cardiac conduction velocity. Repolarization is also delayed, resulting in a prolonged QT interval that may be associated with polymorphic ventricular tachycardia (torsades des pointes; see Fig I–5, p 15).

    Quinidine and disopyramide also have anticholinergic activity; quinidine has alpha-adrenergic receptor-blocking activity, and procainamide has ganglionic- and neuromuscular-blocking activity.

II. Toxic dose. Acute adult ingestion of 1 g of quinidine, 5 g of procainamide, or 1 g of disopyramide, and any ingestion in children, should be considered potentially lethal.

III. Clinical presentation. The primary manifestations of toxicity involve the cardiovascular and central nervous systems.

    A. Cardiotoxic effects of the type Ia agents include sinus bradycardia; sinus node arrest or asystole; PR, QRS, or QT interval prolongation; sinus tachycardia (caused by anticholinergic effects); polymorphous ventricular tachycardia (torsades des pointes); and depressed myocardial contractility, which, along with alpha-adrenergic or ganglionic blockade, may result in hypotension and occasionally pulmonary edema.

    B. Central nervous system toxicity. Quinidine and disopyramide can cause anticholinergic effects such as dry mouth, dilated pupils, and delirium. All type Ia agents can produce seizures, coma, and respiratory arrest.

TABLE II–48. TYPE Ia ANTIARRHYTHMIC DRUGS

Drug	Serum Half-Life (h)	Usual Adult Daily Dose (mg)	Therapeutic Serum Levels (mg/L)	Major Toxicity[a]
Quinidine	6	1000–2000	2–4	S, B, V, H
Disopyramide	7	400–800	2–4	B, V, H
Procainamide	4	1000–4000	4–10	B, V, H
NAPA[b]	10	N/A	15–25	H

[a]S = seizures; B = bradycardia; V = ventricular tachycardia; H = hypotension.
[b]NAPA = N-acetylprocainamide, an active metabolite of procainamide.

    C. **Other effects.** Quinidine commonly causes nausea, vomiting, and diarrhea after acute ingestion and, especially with chronic doses, cinchonism (tinnitus, vertigo, deafness, visual disturbances). Procainamide may cause gastrointestinal upset and, with chronic therapy, a lupuslike syndrome.

IV. **Diagnosis** is based on a history of exposure and typical cardiotoxic features such as QRS and QT interval prolongation, AV block, or polymorphous ventricular tachycardia.

    A. **Specific levels.** Rapid serum levels are generally available for each agent. Serious toxicity with these drugs usually occurs only with levels above the therapeutic range; however, some complications, such as QT prolongation and polymorphous ventricular tachycardia, may occur at therapeutic levels.

        1. Methods for detecting quinidine may vary in specificity, with some also measuring metabolites and contaminants.

        2. Procainamide has an active metabolite, *N*-acetylprocainamide (NAPA); with therapeutic procainamide dosing, NAPA levels can range up to 15 mg/L.

    B. **Other useful laboratory studies.** Electrolytes, glucose, BUN, creatinine, arterial blood gases or oximetry, ECG monitoring.

V. **Treatment**

    A. **Emergency and supportive measures**

        1. Maintain the airway and assist ventilation if necessary (see p 4).

        2. Treat hypotension (p 15), arrhythmias (p 10–14), coma (p 18), and seizures (p 22) if they occur.

        3. Treat recurrent ventricular tachycardia with lidocaine, phenytoin, or overdrive pacing (p 14). Do *not* use other type Ia or type Ic agents, as they may worsen cardiac toxicity.

        4. Continuously monitor vital signs and ECG for a minimum of 6 hours, and admit symptomatic patients until the ECG returns to normal.

    B. **Specific drugs and antidotes.** Treat cardiotoxic effects such as wide QRS interval or hypotension with **hypertonic sodium bicarbonate** (see p 318), 1–2 meq/kg rapid IV bolus, repeated every 5–10 minutes and as needed. Markedly impaired conduction or high-degree atrioventricular block unresponsive to bicarbonate therapy is an indication for insertion of a cardiac pacemaker.

    C. **Decontamination** (see p 44)

        1. **Prehospital.** Administer activated charcoal, if available. Do *not* induce emesis because of the risk of abrupt onset of seizures and coma.

        2. **Hospital.** Administer activated charcoal and a cathartic. Consider gastric lavage for large ingestions.

    D. **Enhanced elimination** (see p 49)

        1. **Quinidine** has a very large volume of distribution, and therefore it is not effectively removed by dialysis. Acidification of the urine may enhance excretion, but this is not recommended because it may aggravate cardiac toxicity.

        2. **Disopyramide, procainamide,** and *N*-acetylprocainamide (NAPA) have smaller volumes of distribution and are effectively removed by hemoperfusion or dialysis.

        3. The efficacy of repeat-dose activated charcoal has not been studied for the type Ia agents.

QUININE
Neal L. Benowitz, MD

ANTIDOTE   IPECAC   LAVAGE   CHARCOAL

Quinine is an optical isomer of quinidine. Quinine was once widely used for the treatment of malaria and is still occasionally used for chloroquine-resistant cases, but it is now prescribed primarily for the treatment of nocturnal muscle cramps. It has also been used as an abortifacient.

I. Mechanism of toxicity. The mechanism of quinine toxicity is believed to be similar to that of quinidine (see p 271); however, quinine is a much less potent cardiotoxin. Quinine also has toxic effects on the retina that can result in blindness. At one time, vasoconstriction of retinal arterioles resulting in retinal ischemia was thought to be the cause of blindness; however, recent evidence indicates a direct toxic effect on photoreceptor and ganglion cells.

II. Toxic dose. Quinine sulfate is available in capsules and tablets containing 130–325 mg. The minimum toxic dose is approximately 3–4 g in adults; 1 g has been fatal in a child.

III. Clinical presentation. Toxic effects involve the cardiovascular and central nervous systems, the eyes, and other organ systems.

A. Mild intoxication produces nausea, vomiting, and cinchonism (tinnitus, deafness, vertigo, headache, and visual disturbances).

B. Severe intoxication may cause ataxia, obtundation, convulsions, coma, and respiratory arrest. With massive intoxication, quinidinelike cardiotoxicity (hypotension, QRS and QT interval prolongation, AV block, and ventricular arrhythmias) may be fatal.

C. Retinal toxicity occurs 9–10 hours after ingestion and includes blurred vision, impaired color perception, constriction of visual fields, and blindness. The pupils are often fixed and dilated. Funduscopy may reveal retinal artery spasm, disk pallor, and macular edema. Although gradual recovery occurs, many patients are left with permanent visual impairment.

D. Other toxic effects of quinine include hypokalemia, hypoglycemia, hemolysis (in patients with glucose-6-phosphate dehydrogenase [G6PD] deficiency), and congenital malformations when used in pregnancy.

IV. Diagnosis is based on a history of ingestion and the presence of cinchonism and visual disturbances. Quinidinelike cardiotoxic effects may or may not be present.

A. Specific levels. Serum quinine levels can be measured by the same assay as for quinidine, as long as quinidine is not present. Plasma quinine levels above 10 mg/L have been associated with visual impairment; 87% of patients with levels above 20 mg/L reported blindness. Levels above 16 mg/L have been associated with cardiac toxicity.

B. Other useful laboratory studies. CBC, electrolytes, glucose, BUN, creatinine, arterial blood gases or oximetry, ECG monitoring.

V. Treatment

A. Emergency and supportive measures

1. Maintain the airway and assist ventilation if necessary (see p 4).
2. Treat coma (p 18), seizures (p 22), hypotension (p 15), and arrhythmias (p 10–14) if they occur.
3. Avoid type Ia and type Ic antiarrhythmic drugs; they may worsen cardiotoxicity.
4. Continuously monitor vital signs and the ECG for at least 6 hours after ingestion, and admit symptomatic patients to an intensive care unit.

B. Specific drugs and antidotes

1. Treat cardiotoxicity with **hypertonic sodium bicarbonate** (see p 318), 1–2 meq/kg rapid IV bolus.
2. Stellate ganglion block has previously been recommended for quinine-induced blindness, the rationale being to increase retinal blood flow. However, recent evidence indicates that this treatment is not effective and the procedure may have serious complications.

C. Decontamination (see p 44)

1. **Prehospital.** Administer activated charcoal, if available. Do **not** induce emesis because of the risk of abrupt onset of seizures or coma.
2. **Hospital.** Administer activated charcoal and a cathartic. Consider gastric lavage for large ingestions.

D. Enhanced elimination. Because of extensive tissue distribution (volume of distribution is 3 L/kg), dialysis and hemoperfusion procedures are ineffective.

Acidification of the urine may slightly increase renal excretion but does not significantly alter the overall elimination rate and may aggravate cardiotoxicity.

RADIATION (IONIZING)*
Evan T. Wythe, MD

ANTIDOTE   IPECAC   LAVAGE   CHARCOAL

Ionizing radiation exposure is a rare but potentially challenging complication of the nuclear age. Dependence on nuclear energy, and the expanded use of radioactive isotopes in industry and medicine, increase the possibility of accidental exposures. Radiation may be generated from a variety of sources. **Particle-emitting** radiation sources may produce beta and alpha particles, neutrons, protons, and positrons. **Electromagnetic** radiation that can cause ionization includes gamma rays and x-rays (magnetic fields, microwaves, radio waves, and ultrasound are examples of *nonionizing* electromagnetic radiation).

Management of a radiation accident depends on whether the victim has been **contaminated** or only **irradiated**. Irradiated victims pose no threat to health care providers and may be managed with no special precautions. On the other hand, contaminated victims must be decontaminated in order to prevent spread of radioactive materials to others and the environment.

I. **Mechanism of toxicity**
   A. Radiation impairs biologic function by ionizing atoms and breaking chemical bonds, resulting in the intracellular formation of highly reactive free radicals that damage cell walls, organelles, and DNA. Affected cells are either killed or inhibited in division. Cells with a high turnover rate (eg, bone marrow, epithelial coverings such as skin, gastrointestinal tract, and pulmonary system) are more sensitive to radiation.
   B. Radiation also causes a poorly understood inflammatory response and microvascular effects after moderately high doses (eg, 600 rads).
   C. Radiation effects may be deterministic or stochastic. **Deterministic** effects are associated with a threshold dose and usually occur within an acute time frame (within a year). **Stochastic** effects have no known threshold and may occur after a latency period of years (eg, cancer).

II. **Toxic dose.** Various terms are used to describe radiation dose: R (roentgen), rad (radiation absorbed dose), and rem (radiation equivalent, man). Rad is the unit of radiation dose commonly referred to in exposures, whereas rem is useful in describing dose-equivalent biologic damage. For practical purposes, these units can be considered interchangeable.
   A. **Toxicity thresholds**
      1. **Acute effects.** Exposure to more than 75 rads causes nausea and vomiting. Exposure to more than 400 rads is potentially lethal without medical intervention. Brief exposure to 5000 rads or more usually causes death within minutes to hours.
      2. **Carcinogenesis.** Radiation protection organizations have not agreed upon a threshold dose for stochastic effects such as cancer.
   B. **Recommended exposure limits**
      1. **Exposure to the general population.** The National Council on Radiation Protection (NCRP) recommends a maximum of 0.5 rem per year.
      2. **Occupational exposure to x-rays.** The federal government has set standards for such exposures: 5 rem/year to the total body, gonads, or blood forming organs; 75 rem/year to the hands or feet. A single chest x-ray re-

*Special thanks to Fun H. Fong, MD, FACEP, of the Oak Ridge Institute for Science and Education, for his assistance in reviewing and revising this material.

sults in a radiation exposure of about 15 millirem (0.015 rem) to the patient, and about 0.006 millirem to nearby health care personnel (at a distance of 160 cm). A head CT scan gives about 1 rad to the head; an abdominal CT scan may give as much as 2–5 rad to the area of concern.

3. Radiation during pregnancy. Established guidelines vary but generally recommend a maximum exposure of no more than 50 millirem per month (NCRP). Exposure to the ovaries and fetus from a routine abdominal (KUB) film may be as high as 146 millirem; from a chest x-ray, the dose is about 15 millirem.

4. Exposure guidelines for emergency health care personnel. To save a life, the NCRP recommended maximum exposure for a rescuer is 50 rem whole body exposure.

III. Clinical presentation

A. The acute radiation syndrome (ARS) consists of a constellation of symptoms and signs indicative of systemic radiation injury. It is often described in four stages (prodrome, latency, manifest illness, and recovery). The onset and severity of each stage of radiation poisoning are determined largely by the dose.

1. The prodromal stage may include nausea, vomiting, abdominal cramps, and diarrhea. Severe exposures are associated with diaphoresis, disorientation, fever, ataxia, coma, shock, and death.
2. During the latent stage, there may be an improvement in symptoms. The duration of this stage may be short or absent with massive exposures.
3. The manifest illness stage is characterized by multiple organ system involvement, particularly bone marrow suppression, which may lead to sepsis and death.
4. The recovery phase may be accompanied by hair loss, disfiguring burns, and scars.

B. Gastrointestinal system. Exposure to 100 R or more usually produces nausea, vomiting, abdominal cramps, and diarrhea within a few hours. After exposure to 600 rads or more, loss of integrity of the GI mucosal layer leads to denudation and severe necrotic gastroenteritis, which may lead to marked dehydration and death within a few days. Doses of 1500 rads are thought to completely destroy GI stem cells.

C. Central nervous system. With exposures of several thousand rads, confusion and stupor may occur, followed within minutes to hours by ataxia, convulsions, coma, and death. In animal models of massive exposure, a phenomenon known as "early transient incapacitation" occurs.

D. Bone marrow depression may be subclinical but apparent on a CBC after exposure to as little as 25 rads. Immunocompromise usually follows exposure to more than 100 rads.

1. Early neutropenia is caused by margination; the true nadir occurs at about 30 days, or as soon as 14 days after severe exposure. Neutropenia is the most significant factor in septicemia.
2. Thrombocytopenia is usually not evident for 2 weeks or more after exposure.
3. The lymphocyte count is of great prognostic importance and usually reaches a nadir within 48 hours of serious exposure; a count of less than 300–500 lymphocytes/mm^3 during this period indicates a poor prognosis, while 1200/mm^3 or more suggests likely survival.

E. Other complications of high-dose acute radiation syndrome include multisystem organ failure, veno-occlusive disease of the liver, interstitial pneumonitis, renal failure, tissue fibrosis, skin burns, and hair loss.

IV. Diagnosis depends on the history of exposure. The potential for contamination should be assessed by determining the type of radionuclide involved and the potential route(s) of exposure.

A. Specific levels

1. **Detection.** Depending on the circumstances, the presence of radionuclides may be verified by one or more of the following devices: survey meters with

either pancake or alpha probes; whole body counts; chest counts; or nuclear medicine cameras.

   2. Biologic specimens. Nasopharyngeal swabs, wound bandages, and clothing articles (particularly shoes) may be collected for radionuclide analysis. Collection of urine and feces for 24–72 hours may assist in estimation of an internal dose. Serum levels of radioactive materials are not generally available or clinically useful.

   B. Other useful laboratory studies. CBC (repeat every 6 hours), electrolytes, glucose, BUN, creatinine, urinalysis. Immediately draw lymphocytes for HLA typing in case bone marrow transplant is required later.

V. Treatment. For expert assistance in evaluation and treatment of victims and on-scene management, immediately contact the **Radiation Emergency Assistance Center & Training Site (REAC/TS): telephone (615) 576-3131 or (615) 481-1000.** REAC/TS is operated for the US Department of Energy by the Oak Ridge Associated Universities, and assistance is available 24 hours a day. Also contact the local state agency responsible for radiation safety.

   A. Emergency and supportive measures. Depending on the risk to rescuers, treatment of serious medical problems takes precedence over radiologic concerns. If there is a potential for contamination of rescuers and equipment, appropriate radiation response protocols should be implemented, and rescuers should wear protective clothing and respirators. If the exposure was to electromagnetic radiation only, the victim is not contaminating and does not pose a risk to downstream personnel.

   1. Maintain the airway and assist ventilation if necessary (see p 4).

   2. Treat coma (p 18) and seizures (p 22) if they occur.

   3. Replace fluid losses from gastroenteritis with intravenous crystalloid solutions (see p 15).

   4. Treat leukopenia and resulting infections as needed. Immunosuppressed patients require reverse isolation and appropriate broad-spectrum antibiotic therapy.

   B. Specific drugs and antidotes. Chelating agents or pharmacologic blocking drugs may be useful in cases of ingestion or inhalation of certain biologically active radioactive materials, if they are given before or shortly after exposure (Table II–49). Contact REAC/TS (see above) for specific advice on use of these agents.

   C. Decontamination (p 41–49)

   1. Exposure to particle-emitting solid or liquids. The victim is potentially highly contaminating to rescuers, transport vehicles, and attending health personnel.

   a. Remove the victim from exposure, and if condition permits, remove all contaminated clothing and wash the victim with soap and water.

   b. All clothing and cleansing water must be saved and properly disposed of.

   c. Rescuers should wear protective clothing and respiratory gear to avoid contamination. At the hospital, measures must be taken to prevent contamination of facilities and personnel.

   d. Induce emesis or perform gastric lavage (see p 44–45) if radioactive material has been ingested. Administer activated charcoal (see p 47), although its effectiveness is unknown. Certain other adsorbent materials may be effective (see Table II–49).

   e. Contact REAC/TS (see above) and the state radiologic health department for further advice. In some exposures, unusually aggressive steps may be needed (eg, lung lavage for significant inhalation of plutonium).

   2. Electromagnetic radiation exposure. The patient is not radioactive and does not pose a contamination threat. There is no need for decontamination once the patient has been removed from the source of exposure, unless electromagnetic radiation emitter fragments are embedded in body tissues.

   D. Enhanced elimination. Chelating agents and forced diuresis may be useful for certain exposures (Table II–49).

TABLE II–49. CHELATING AND BLOCKING AGENTS FOR SOME RADIATION EXPOSURES[a]

Radionuclide	Chelating or Blocking Agents
Cesium-137	Prussian blue (ferric hexacyanoferrate). Adsorbs cesium in the GI tract, and may also enhance elimination. Dose: 500 mg PO 6 times daily in 100–200 mL of water.
Iodine-131	Potassium iodide. Dilutes radioactive iodine and blocks thyroid iodine uptake. Dose: 300 mg PO immediately, then 130 mg PO daily.
	Perchlorate, 200 mg PO, then 100 mg every 5 h, has also been recommended.
Plutonium-239	DTPA (diethylenetriamine pentaacetic acid). Chelator. Dose: 1 g in 250 mL D5W IV over 30–60 min daily. Wounds: Irrigate with 1 g DTPA in 250 mL water.
	EDTA (see p 335) may also be effective if DTPA is not immediately available.
	Aluminum-containing antacids may bind plutonium in GI tract.
Strontium-90	Alginate or aluminum hydroxide-containing antacids. May reduce intestinal absorption of strontium. Dose: 10 g, then 1 g 4 times daily.
	Barium sulfate may also reduce Sr absorption. Dose: 100 g in 250 mL water PO.
	Calcium gluconate may dilute the effect of strontium. Dose: 2 g in 500 mL PO or IV.
	Ammonium chloride is a demineralizing agent. Dose: 3 g PO 3 times daily.
Tritium	Forced fluids, diuretics, (?) hemodialysis. Water dilutes tritium, enhances urinary excretion.
Uranium-233, -235, -238	Sodium bicarbonate. Forms a carbonate complex with uranyl ion, which is then eliminated in the urine. Dose: 100 meq in 500 mL D5W by slow constant IV infusion.
	Aluminum-containing antacids may help prevent uranium absorption.

[a]References: Bhattacharyya ANL et al: Methods of treatment. Pages 27–36 in: *Radiation Protection Dosimetry.* Gerber GB, Thomas RG (editors). Vol. 41, No. 1 (1992); and Ricks RC: *Hospital Emergency Department Management of Radiation Accidents.* Oak Ridge Associated Universities, 1984.

SALICYLATES
Susan Kim, PharmD

ANTIDOTE   IPECAC   LAVAGE   CHARCOAL

Salicylates are widely used for their analgesic and anti-inflammatory properties. They are found in a variety of prescription and over-the-counter analgesics, cold preparations, and topical keratolytic products (methyl salicylate), and even Pepto-Bismol (bismuth subsalicylate). Before the introduction of child-resistant containers, salicylate overdose was one of the leading causes of accidental death in children. Two distinct syndromes of intoxication may occur, depending on whether the exposure is **acute** or **chronic.**

I. **Mechanism of toxicity.** Salicylates have a variety of toxic effects.
    A. Central stimulation of the respiratory center results in hyperventilation, leading to respiratory alkalosis and compensatory metabolic acidosis and contributing to dehydration.
    B. Intracellular effects include uncoupling of oxidative phosphorylation and interruption of glucose and fatty acid metabolism.
    C. The mechanism by which cerebral and pulmonary edema occur is not known but may be related to alteration in capillary integrity.
    D. Salicylates alter platelet function and may also prolong the prothrombin time.

II. **Toxic dose.** The average therapeutic single dose is 10 mg/kg, and the usual daily therapeutic dose is 40–60 mg/kg/d. Each tablet of aspirin contains 325–650 mg of acetylsalicylic acid. One teaspoon of concentrated **oil of wintergreen** contains 5 g of methyl salicylate, equivalent to about 7.5 g of aspirin.

   A. Acute ingestion of 150–200 mg/kg will produce mild intoxication; severe intoxication is likely after acute ingestion of 300–500 mg/kg.
   B. Chronic intoxication may occur with ingestion of more than 100 mg/kg/d for 2 or more days.
III. Clinical presentation. Patients may become intoxicated following acute accidental or suicidal overdose or as a result of chronic repeated overmedication for several days.
   A. Acute ingestion. Vomiting occurs shortly after ingestion, followed by hyperpnea, tinnitus, and lethargy. Mixed respiratory alkalemia and metabolic acidosis are apparent when arterial blood gases are determined. With severe intoxication, coma, seizures, hypoglycemia, hyperthermia, and pulmonary edema may occur. Death is caused by central nervous system failure and cardiovascular collapse.
   B. Chronic intoxication. Victims are usually young children or confused elderly. The diagnosis is often overlooked because the presentation is nonspecific; confusion, dehydration, and metabolic acidosis are often attributed to sepsis, pneumonia, or gastroenteritis. However, morbidity and mortality rates are much higher than after acute overdose. Cerebral and pulmonary edema are more common than with acute intoxication, and severe poisoning occurs at lower salicylate levels.
IV. Diagnosis is not difficult if there is a history of acute ingestion, accompanied by typical signs and symptoms. In the absence of a history of overdose, diagnosis is suggested by the characteristic arterial blood gases, which reveal a mixed respiratory alkalemia and metabolic acidosis.
   A. Specific levels. Obtain stat and serial serum salicylate concentrations. Systemic acidemia increases brain salicylate concentration, worsening toxicity.
       1. Acute ingestion. Salicylate levels are plotted on the nomogram (Figure II–2) to estimate expected toxicity. Single determinations are *not* sufficient because of the possibility of prolonged or delayed absorption from sustained-release tablets or a tablet mass or bezoar (especially after massive ingestion). Many toxicologists have abandoned dependence on the nomogram to determine toxicity.
       2. Chronic intoxication. Intoxication correlates poorly with serum levels, and the nomogram cannot be used to predict toxicity. Chronic therapeutic concentrations in arthritis patients range from 100 to 300 mg/L (10–30 mg/dL). A level greater than 600 mg/L (60 mg/dL) accompanied by acidosis and altered mental status is considered very serious.
   B. Other useful laboratory studies. Electrolytes (anion gap calculation), glucose, BUN, creatinine, prothrombin time (PT), arterial blood gases, chest x-ray.
V. Treatment
   A. Emergency and supportive measures
       1. Maintain the airway and assist ventilation if necessary (see p 4). Administer supplemental oxygen. Obtain serial arterial blood gases and chest x-rays to observe for pulmonary edema (more common with chronic or severe intoxication).
       2. Treat coma (p 18), seizures (p 22), pulmonary edema (p 18), and hyperthermia (p 20) if they occur.
       3. Treat metabolic acidosis with intravenous sodium bicarbonate (p 318). Do *not* allow the serum pH to fall below 7.4.
       4. Replace fluid and electrolyte deficits caused by vomiting and hyperventilation with intravenous crystalloid solutions. Be cautious with fluid therapy, because excessive fluid administration may contribute to pulmonary edema.
       5. Monitor asymptomatic patients for a minimum of 6 hours (longer if an enteric-coated preparation or a massive overdose has been ingested and there is suspicion of a tablet bezoar). Admit symptomatic patients to an intensive care unit.
   B. Specific drugs and antidotes. There is no specific antidote for salicylate in-

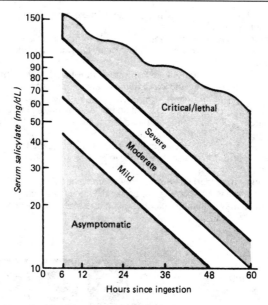

Figure II–2. Nomogram for determining severity of salicylate intoxication. Absorption kinetics assume acute (single) ingestion of non–enteric-coated preparation. (Redrawn and reproduced, with permission, from Done AK: Salicylate intoxication: Significance of measurement of salicylate in blood in cases of acute ingestion. *Pediatrics* 1960;**26**:800.)

toxication. **Sodium bicarbonate** is frequently given both to prevent acidemia and to promote salicylate elimination by the kidneys (see **D**, below).

C. Decontamination (see p 44). Decontamination is not necessary for patients with chronic intoxication.

1. **Prehospital.** Administer activated charcoal, if available. Ipecac-induced emesis may be useful for initial treatment of children at home if it can be given within 30 minutes of exposure.

2. **Hospital.** Administer activated charcoal and a cathartic orally or by gastric tube. Gastric lavage is not necessary after small ingestions (ie, < 200–300 mg/kg) if activated charcoal is given promptly.

3. *Note:* With very large ingestions of salicylate (eg, 30–60 g), very large doses of activated charcoal (300–600 g) are theoretically necessary to adsorb all the salicylate and prevent desorption. In such cases, the charcoal may be given in several 25- to 50-g doses at 3- to 5-hour intervals. Charcoal should be continued until the serum salicylate levels are clearly falling.

D. Enhanced elimination (see p 49)

1. **Urinary alkalinization** is effective in enhancing urinary excretion of salicylate, although often difficult to achieve in dehydrated or critically ill patients.

   a. Add 100 meq of sodium bicarbonate to 1 L of 5% dextrose in quarter normal saline, and infuse intravenously at 200 mL/h (3–4 mL/kg/h). If the patient is dehydrated, start with a bolus of 10–20 mL/kg. Fluid and bicarbonate administration is potentially dangerous in patients at high risk for pulmonary edema (eg, chronic intoxication).

   b. Unless renal failure is present, also add potassium, 30–40 meq, to each liter of intravenous fluids (potassium depletion inhibits alkalinization).

   c. Alkalemia is not a contraindication to bicarbonate therapy, considering that patients often have a significant base deficit in spite of the elevated serum pH.

2. **Hemodialysis** is very effective in rapidly removing salicylate and correcting acid-base and fluid abnormalities. Indications for hemodialysis are as follows:

   a. Patients with acute ingestion and serum levels higher than 1200 mg/L (120 mg/dL), or with severe acidosis and other manifestations of intoxication.

   b. Patients with chronic intoxication with serum levels higher than 600 mg/L (60 mg/dL) accompanied by acidosis, confusion, or lethargy, especially if the patient is elderly or debilitated.

   c. Any patient with severe manifestations of intoxication.

3. **Hemoperfusion** is also very effective but does not correct acid-base or fluid disturbances.

4. **Repeat-dose activated charcoal** therapy effectively reduces the serum salicylate half-life, but it is not as rapidly effective as dialysis, and frequent stooling may contribute to dehydration and electrolyte disturbances.

SCORPIONS
Gerald Joe, PharmD

ANTIDOTE   IPECAC   LAVAGE   CHARCOAL

The order Scorpionida contains several families, genera, and species of scorpions. All have paired venom glands in a bulbous segment called the telson, located just anterior to a stinger on the end of the 6 terminal segments of the abdomen (often called a tail).

The only dangerous species in the USA is the *Centruroides exilicauda (formerly C sculpturatus)*, the bark scorpion. The most serious envenomations are usually reported in children under age 10 years. This scorpion is found primarily in the arid southwestern USA but has been found as a stowaway in cargo as far north as Michigan.

Other dangerous scorpions are found in Mexico (*Centruroides* species), Brazil (*Tityus* species), India (*Buthus* species), and north Africa and the eastern Mediterranean (*Leiurus* species).

I. **Mechanism of toxicity.** The scorpion grasps the skin with its anterior pincers, arches its pseudoabdomen, and stabs with the stinger. Stings also result from stepping on the stinger. The venom of *C exilicauda* contains numerous digestive enzymes (eg, hyaluronidase, phospholipase) and also several neurotoxins. Alteration in sodium channel flow results in excessive stimulation at neuromuscular junctions and the autonomic nervous system.

II. **Toxic dose.** Variable amounts of venom from none to the complete contents of the telson may be ejected through the stinger.

III. **Clinical presentation**

   A. **Common scorpion stings.** Most stings result only in local, immediate, burning pain. Some local tissue inflammation and occasionally local paresthesias may occur. Symptoms usually resolve within several hours. This represents the typical scorpion sting seen in the USA.

   B. **Dangerous scorpion stings.** In some victims, especially children under age 10 years, systemic symptoms occur, including weakness, restlessness, diaphoresis, diplopia, nystagmus, roving eye movements, hyperexcitability, muscle fasciculations, opisthotonos, priapism, salivation, slurred speech, hypertension, tachycardia, and, rarely, convulsions, paralysis, and respiratory arrest. Pulmonary edema, cardiovascular collapse, and death have been reported, as well as coagulopathies, disseminated intravascular coagulation, pancreatitis, and renal failure with hemoglobinuria and jaundice. In nonfatal cases, recovery usually occurs within 12-36 hours.

IV. Diagnosis. Either the patient saw the scorpion, or the clinician must recognize the symptoms. In the case of *Centruroides* stings, tapping on the sting site usually produces severe pain ("tap test").

    A. Specific levels. Serum toxin levels are not available.

    B. Other useful laboratory studies. None are needed for minor envenomations. For severe envenomations, obtain CBC, electrolytes, glucose, BUN, creatinine, coagulation profile, arterial blood gases.

V. Treatment. The majority of even *Centruroides* stings can be managed with symptomatic care at home, consisting of oral analgesics and cool compresses or intermittent ice packs.

    A. Emergency and supportive measures

        1. For severe envenomations, maintain the airway and assist ventilation if necessary (see p 4). Administer supplemental oxygen.

        2. Treat hypertension (p 17), tachycardia (p 13), and convulsions (p 22) if they occur.

        3. Do *not* overtreat with excessive sedation.

        4. Clean the wound and provide tetanus prophylaxis if indicated.

        5. Do *not* immerse the injured extremity in ice or perform local incision or suction.

    B. Specific drugs and antidotes. Some **antivenins** have been produced, but none are approved for human use. In selected cases, they can be located by a regional poison control center (see Table I–41, p 53).

    C. Decontamination. These procedures are not applicable.

    D. Enhanced elimination. These procedures are not applicable.

SEDATIVE-HYPNOTIC AGENTS
Evan T. Wythe, MD

ANTIDOTE   IPECAC   LAVAGE   CHARCOAL

Sedative-hypnotic agents are widely used for the treatment of anxiety and insomnia. As a group they are one of the most frequently prescribed medications. Barbiturates (see p 93), benzodiazepines (p 97), antihistamines (p 78), and anticholinergic agents (p 75) are discussed elsewhere in this book. In this section are listed some of the less commonly used hypnotic agents.

  I. Mechanism of toxicity. The exact mechanism of action and the pharmacokinetics vary for each agent. The major toxic effect that causes serious poisoning or death is central nervous system depression resulting in coma, respiratory arrest, and pulmonary aspiration of gastric contents.

 II. Toxic dose. The toxic dose varies considerably between drugs and also depends largely on individual tolerance and the presence of other drugs such as alcohol (Table II–50). For most of these drugs, ingestion of 3–5 times the usual hypnotic dose results in coma. However, coingestion of alcohol or other drugs may cause coma after smaller ingestions, while individuals chronically using large doses of these drugs may tolerate much higher acute doses.

 III. Clinical presentation. Overdose with any of these drugs may cause drowsiness, ataxia, nystagmus, stupor, coma, and respiratory arrest. Deep coma may result in absent reflexes, fixed pupils, and depressed or absent electroencephalographic (EEG) activity. Hypothermia is common. Most agents also slow gastric motility and decrease muscle tone. Hypotension with large overdose is caused primarily by depression of cardiac contractility, and to a lesser extent, loss of venous tone.

    A. Chloral hydrate is metabolized to trichloroethanol, which also has CNS-

TABLE II–50. COMMON SEDATIVE-HYPNOTIC AGENTS[a]

Drug	Usual Adult Oral Hypnotic Dose (mg)	Approximate Lethal Dose (g)	Toxic Concentration (mg/L)	Usual Half-Life[b] (h)
Buspirone	5–20	Unknown	—	2–3
Chloral hydrate	500–1000	5–10	> 20	5–10
Ethchlorvynol[c]	500–1000	5–10	> 10	10–20
Glutethimide	250–500	10–20	> 10	10–40
Meprobamate	600–1200	10–20	> 60	8–12
Methaqualone	150–250	3–8	> 5	10–40
Methyprylon	200–400	5–10	> 10	3–6

[a]See also benzodiazepines (p 97), barbiturates (p 93), paraldehyde (p 244), antihistamines (p 78), and anticholinergic agents (p 75).
[b]Half-life in overdose may be considerably longer.
[c]Toxic concentration is measured as trichloroethanol.

depressant activity. Trichloroethanol may also sensitize the myocardium to the effects of catecholamines, resulting in cardiac arrhythmias.

B. Buspirone may cause nausea, vomiting, drowsiness, and miosis. There are no reported deaths.

C. Ethchlorvynol has a pungent odor sometimes described as pearlike, and gastric fluid often has a pink or green color depending on the capsule form (200- and 500-mg are red; 750-mg is green).

D. Glutethimide often produces mydriasis (dilated pupils) and other anticholinergic side effects, and patients may exhibit prolonged and cyclic or fluctuating coma. It is sometimes taken in combination with codeine ("loads"), which may produce opioid effects.

E. Meprobamate has been reported to form tablet concretions in large overdose, occasionally requiring surgical removal. Hypotension is more common with this agent than with other sedative-hypnotics.

F. Methaqualone is unusual among sedative-hypnotic agents in frequently causing muscular hypertonicity, clonus, and hyperreflexia.

IV. Diagnosis is usually based on a history of ingestion, because clinical manifestations are fairly nonspecific. Hypothermia and deep coma may cause the patient to appear to be dead; thus, careful evaluation should precede the diagnosis of brain death. Chloral hydrate is radiopaque and may be visible on plain abdominal x-rays.

  A. Specific levels and qualitative urine screening are usually available through commercial toxicology laboratories.

   1. Drug levels do not always correlate with severity of intoxication, especially in patients who have tolerance to the drug or who have also ingested other drugs or alcohol. In addition, early after ingestion blood levels may not reflect brain concentrations.

   2. Some agents (chloral hydrate, glutethimide) have active metabolites, levels of which may correlate better with the state of intoxication.

  B. Other useful laboratory studies. Electrolytes, glucose, serum ethanol, BUN, creatinine, arterial blood gases, chest x-ray.

V. Treatment

  A. Emergency and supportive measures

   1. Maintain the airway and assist ventilation if necessary (see p 4). Administer supplemental oxygen.

   2. Treat coma (p 18), hypothermia (p 19), hypotension (p 15), and pulmonary edema (p 8) if they occur.

   3. Monitor patients for at least 6 hours after ingestion, because delayed ab-

sorption may occur. Patients with chloral hydrate ingestion should be monitored at least 18–24 hours because of the risk of cardiac arrhythmias. Tachyarrhythmias caused by myocardial sensitization may be treated with **propranolol** (see p 373), 1–2 mg IV, or **esmolol** (see p 338), 25–100 µg/kg/min IV.

B. Specific drugs and antidotes. Flumazenil (see p 340) is a specific antagonist of benzodiazepine receptors. It does not appear to cross-react with other sedative agents.

C. Decontamination (see p 44)

1. **Prehospital.** Administer activated charcoal, if available. Ipecac-induced emesis may be useful for initial treatment (eg, children at home) if it can be given within a few minutes of exposure.

2. **Hospital.** Administer activated charcoal and a cathartic. Gastric emptying is not necessary if activated charcoal can be given promptly; however, consider gastric lavage for massive ingestions.

3. If a gastric tablet mass (concretion, bezoar) is suspected because of sustained coma or sustained high serum drug levels, obtain a plain abdominal x-ray or perform a contrast material swallow x-ray to attempt to identify a mass. Repeat-dose charcoal (p 52), whole gut lavage (p 48), or even surgical removal may be necessary.

D. Enhanced elimination. Because of extensive tissue distribution, dialysis and hemoperfusion are not very effective for most of the drugs in this group.

1. Repeat-dose charcoal may enhance elimination of glutethimide (which undergoes enterohepatic recirculation) and meprobamate, although no studies have been performed to document this.

2. Meprobamate has a relatively small volume of distribution (0.75 L/kg), and hemoperfusion is indicated for deep coma complicated by intractable hypotension.

3. Resin hemoperfusion has been reported to be partially effective for ethchlorvynol overdose.

SELENIUM
Janet Weiss, MD

ANTIDOTE   IPECAC   LAVAGE   CHARCOAL

Selenium is a trace metal considered an essential element in the human diet, with multiple roles in metabolic chemistry. It is present as selenocysteine at the active site of glutathione peroxidase, and has an important antioxidant function. Excessive selenium absorption can cause acute and chronic toxicity. Selenium is used in the electronics industry in rectifiers, photoelectric cells, and solar batteries; in glass, rubber, steel, and ceramic manufacturing; and in some paints, inks, varnishes, fungicides, and insecticides. **Selenious acid** is used in gun blueing solutions. Food sources of selenium include plants, grains, seafood (especially shrimp), meat, and milk products. Geographic concentration of selenium resulting from environmental factors has been reported. Self-medication with selenium-containing supplements and excessive use of selenium-containing shampoos have caused toxicity.

I. Mechanism of toxicity. Elemental selenium is not well absorbed and poses no significant risk. Other forms of selenium are better absorbed by the skin, lungs, and gastrointestinal tract. Organic selenium compounds (selenomethionine) are more bioavailable, while inorganic selenite and selenate are less well absorbed. Once absorbed, selenium may have a variety of toxic effects, including inhibition of sulfhydryl enzymes and displacement of sulfur in certain tissues.

A. Hydrogen selenide (selenium hydride) is a highly irritating gas produced by acid reaction with metal selenides.

   B. Selenious acid is a corrosive agent with systemic toxic effects. Selenium
   oxide is converted to selenious acid on contact with water and is highly toxic.
II. Toxic dose
   A. Ingestion. Little is known about the oral toxic dose because there are few reports of poisoning. Coingestion of vitamin C may reduce selenite to elemental
   selenium and decrease its absorption.
   1. **Acute overdose.** The oral mean lethal dose of selenite salts in the dog is
      about 4 mg/kg. Ingestion of 1–5 mg/kg sodium selenite in 5 adults caused
      moderate reversible toxicity. Ingestion of as little as 20 mL of gun blueing
      solution (2% selenious acid) has been fatal.
   2. **Chronic ingestion.** The recommended nutritional daily intake is 50–200
      µg/d. The drinking water maximum contaminant level (MCL) is 10 µg/L.
      Chronic ingestion of 3–6 mg/d has been associated with toxicity.
   B. Inhalation. The recommended workplace limit (ACGIH TLV-TWA) for hydrogen selenide is 0.05 ppm as an 8-hour time-weighted average; and the level
   immediately dangerous to life or health (IDLH) is 2 ppm (Table II–51).
III. Clinical presentation
   A. Acute inhalation of hydrogen selenide may cause burning eyes and throat,
   metallic taste, coughing, wheezing, chemical pneumonitis, and noncardiogenic
   pulmonary edema.
   B. Skin irritation is common after direct exposure.
   C. Acute ingestion may cause vomiting, hypersalivation, garlicky odor on the
   breath, esophageal burns, and metabolic acidosis. Hypotension, hemo-
   concentration, coma, convulsions, and prolonged QT intervals and T-wave
   changes may occur. Hepatic dysfunction has been reported. **Death** has occurred after small ingestions of selenious acid in gun blueing solutions.
   D. Chronic ingestion of large quantities of selenium has been associated with
   reddish discoloration and loss of hair and nails, polyneuritis, fatigue, irritability,
   garlicky breath, elevation of hepatic transaminases, dermatitis, nausea, and
   vomiting. Animal studies suggest that chronic excessive selenium exposure is
   embryotoxic and teratogenic, causes hepatic cirrhosis, and may be carcinogenic.
   E. Chronic inhalation of hydrogen selenide may cause nausea, vomiting,
   chronic diarrhea, abdominal pain, bitter taste, garlicky breath, dizziness, fatigue, conjunctivitis, dental caries, and impaired pulmonary function.
IV. Diagnosis is difficult without a history of exposure but should be suspected in a
   patient with hair and nail loss or discoloration and other characteristic symptoms.
   A. Specific levels. Selenium can be measured in the blood, hair, and urine.
   1. On a normal diet, whole blood selenium levels range from 0.1 to 0.2 mg/L.
      One patient with chronic intoxication after ingestion of 31 mg/d had a whole
      blood selenium of 0.53 mg/L.
   2. Average hair levels are up to 0.5 ppm. The relationship between hair and
      tissue concentrations is not well understood.
   3. Urinary concentrations reflect dietary intake. Overexposure should be con-
      sidered when urinary excretion exceeds 600–1000 µg/d.
   B. Other useful laboratory studies. Electrolytes, glucose, BUN, creatinine, liver

TABLE II–51. TOXIC LEVELS OF SELENIUM COMPOUNDS

Selenium Compound	TLV[a]	Level Immediately Dangerous to Life or Health (IDLH)
Hydrogen selenide (selenium hydride)	0.05 ppm	2 ppm
Selenium compounds, general	0.2 mg/m³	100 mg/m³
Selenium hexafluoride	0.05 ppm	5 ppm

[a]TLV = ACGIH recommended exposure limit as an 8-hour time-weighted average (TLV-TWA).

transaminases, ECG. After inhalation exposure, obtain arterial blood gases or oximetry, and chest x-ray.

V. Treatment

A. Emergency and supportive measures

1. Maintain the airway and assist ventilation if necessary (see p 4). Administer supplemental oxygen.
2. Treat coma (p 18), convulsions (p 22), bronchospasm (p 9–10), and pulmonary edema (p 8) if they occur.
3. Observe for at least 6 hours after exposure.
4. After ingestion of selenious acid, consider endoscopy to rule out esophageal or gastric corrosive injury.

B. Specific drugs and antidotes.
There is no established specific antidote. Although chelation with EDTA (p 335) and dimercaprol (BAL, p 317) has been studied in animals, their use is not supported in humans. N-acteylcysteine (NAC, p 311) may have therapeutic value, but further studies are needed. High-dose vitamin C (several g daily) has produced equivocal results.

C. Decontamination (see p 41)

1. **Inhalation.** Immediately remove the victim from exposure and give supplemental oxygen, if available.
2. **Skin and eyes.** Remove contaminated clothing and wash exposed skin with soap and copious water. Irrigate exposed eyes with copious tepid water or saline.
3. **Ingestion** (see p 44)
   a. **Prehospital.** Administer activated charcoal, if available. Do not administer ipecac or induce emesis because of risk of corrosive injury and potential for abrupt onset of seizures.
   b. **Hospital.** If tablets, solids, or a large quantity of liquid (more than 1–2 oz) has been ingested, perform gastric lavage, and administer activated charcoal and a cathartic. (Gastric lavage may not be effective after ingestion of small amounts of liquid or delayed presentation.)
   c. In vitro experiments indicate that vitamin C can reduce selenium salts to elemental selenium, which is poorly absorbed. Its use has not been studied in vivo, but oral or nasogastric administration of several grams of ascorbic acid is probably reasonable.

D. Enhanced elimination.
There is no known role for any enhanced removal procedure.

SNAKEBITE
Evan T. Wythe, MD

ANTIDOTE   IPECAC   LAVAGE   CHARCOAL

Of the 14 families of snakes, 5 are poisonous (Table II–52). The annual incidence of snakebite in the USA is 3–4 bites per 100,000 population. Clinically significant morbidity occurs in less than 60%, and only about 20 deaths are reported each year. Rattlesnake bite is the most common envenomation in the USA, and the victim is often a young, intoxicated male who was teasing or trying to capture the snake. Snakes strike accurately to about one-third their body length, with a maximum striking distance of a few feet.

I. **Mechanism of toxicity.** Snake venoms are complex mixtures of 50 or more components that function to immobilize, kill, and predigest prey. These substances produce local "digestive" effects as well as neurotoxic and other systemic effects. The relative predominance of digestive or neurotoxic venom components depends on the species of the snake and geographic variables.

II. **Toxic dose.** The potency of the venom and the amount of venom injected vary

TABLE II–52. EXAMPLES OF POISONOUS SNAKES

Family and Genera	Common Name	Comments
Colubridae		
Lampropeltis	King snake	Human envenomation difficult because of small mouth
Heterodon	Hognose	and small fixed fangs in the rear of the mouth. May cause
Coluber	Racer	severe systemic coagulopathy.
Dispholidus	Boomslang	
Crotalidae		
Crotalus	Rattlesnake	Most common envenomation in USA. Long rotating
Agkistrodon	Copperhead, cottonmouth	fangs in the front of the mouth. Heat-sensing facial pits
Bothrops	Fer-de-lance	(hence the name "pit vipers").
Elapidae		
Micrurus	Coral snake	Human envenomation difficult because of small mouth
Naja	Cobra	and small fixed fangs in rear of mouth. Neurotoxicity
Bungarus	Krait	usually predominates.
Dendroaspis	Mamba	
Hydrophidae	Sea snakes	Also have small rear-located fangs.
Viperidae		
Bitis	Puff adder, gaboon viper	Long rotating fangs in the front of the mouth, but no
Cerastes	Cleopatra's asp	heat-sensing facial pits.
Echis	Saw-scaled viper	

considerably. About 20% of all snake strikes are "dry" bites in which there is no envenomation.

III. **Clinical presentation.** The most common snake envenomations in the USA are rattlesnake (Crotalidae) bites. Bites from common North American Elapidae (eg, coral snake) and Colubridae (eg, king snake) are also discussed here. For bites from other, exotic snakes, contact a regional poison control center (see Table I–41, p 53) for specific consultation.

A. **Crotalidae.** Fang marks may look like puncture wounds or lacerations, the latter resulting from a glancing blow by the snake or sudden movement by the victim. The fangs often penetrate only a few millimeters but occasionally enter deeper tissue spaces or veins.

1. **Local effects.** Within minutes of envenomation, stinging, burning pain begins and progressive proximal swelling, erythema, petechiae, ecchymosis, and hemorrhagic blebs develop over the next several hours. The limb may swell to twice its normal size within the first few hours. Hypovolemic shock and local compartment syndrome may occur secondary to fluid and blood sequestration in injured areas.

2. **Systemic effects** may include nausea and vomiting, weakness, muscle fasciculations, diaphoresis, perioral and peripheral parasthesias, a rubbery or minty taste, thrombocytopenia, and coagulopathy. Circulating vasodilatory compounds may contribute to hypotension. Pulmonary edema and cardiovascular collapse have been reported.

3. **Mojave rattlesnake** (*Crotalus scutulatus scutulatus*) bites deserve special consideration and caution, because neurologic signs and symptoms of envenomation may be delayed and there is often little swelling or evidence of tissue digestion. The onset of muscle weakness, ptosis, and respiratory arrest may occur several hours after envenomation. Facial and laryngeal edema have also been reported.

B. **Elapidae.** Coral snake envenomation is rare because of the snake's small mouth and fangs. The snake must hold on and "chew" the extremity for several seconds or more to work its rear fangs into the skin.

       1. Local effects. There is usually minimal swelling and inflammation around the fang marks. Local paresthesias may occur.

       2. Systemic effects. Systemic symptoms may be delayed 12 hours or more. Nausea and vomiting, euphoria, confusion, diplopia, dysarthria, muscle fasciculations, generalized muscle weakness, and respiratory arrest may occur.

  C. Colubridae. These small-mouthed rear-fanged snakes must also hang onto their victims and "chew" the venom into the skin before significant envenomation can occur.

       1. Local effects. There is usually little local reaction other than mild pain and paresthesias, although swelling of the extremity may occur.

       2. Systemic effects. The most serious effect of envenomation is systemic coagulopathy, which can be fatal.

IV. Diagnosis. Correct diagnosis and treatment depend on proper identification of the offending snake, especially if there are more than one indigenous poisonous species or an exotic snake is involved.

  A. Determine whether the bite was by an indigenous (wild) species or an exotic zoo animal or illegally imported pet. (The owner of an illegal pet snake may be reluctant to admit this for fear of fines or confiscation.) Envenomation occurring during the fall and winter months (October–March) when snakes usually hibernate is not likely to be caused by a wild species.

  B. If the snake is available, attempt to have it identified by a herpetologist. *Caution:* Be careful not to handle a "dead" snake; accidental envenomation may still occur up to several hours after death.

  C. Specific levels. These tests are not applicable.

  D. Other useful laboratory studies. CBC, platelet count, prothrombin time (PT), fibrin split products, fibrinogen, blood type and screen, creatine phosphokinase (CPK), urine dipstick for occult blood (positive with free myoglobin or hemoglobin). If compromised respiratory function suspected: serial arterial blood gases.

V. Treatment

  A. Emergency and supportive measures. Regardless of the species, prepare for both local and systemic manifestations. Monitor patients closely for at least 3–4 hours after typical crotalid bite and for at least 12–24 hours after *C scutulatus scutulatus* or elapid bites.

    1. Local effects

      a. Monitor local swelling at least hourly with measurements of limb girth, the presence and extent of local ecchymosis, and assessment of circulation.

      b. Obtain consultation with an experienced surgeon for management of serious wound complications. Do not perform fasciotomy unless compartment syndrome is documented with tissue compartment pressure monitoring.

      c. Provide tetanus prophylaxis if needed.

      d. Administer broad spectrum antibiotics if there are signs of infection.

    2. Systemic effects

      a. Monitor for respiratory muscle weakness. Maintain the airway and assist ventilation if necessary (see p 4). Administer supplemental oxygen.

      b. Treat severe coagulopathy with fresh-frozen plasma (and antivenin; see below). Treat hypotension with intravenous crystalloid fluids (p 15) and rhabdomyolysis (p 25) with fluids and sodium bicarbonate.

  B. Specific drugs and antidotes. For patients with documented envenomation, be prepared to administer specific **antivenin**. Virtually all local and systemic manifestations of envenomation improve after antivenin administration. *Caution:* Life-threatening anaphylactic reactions may occur with antivenin administration, even after a negative skin test.

    1. For **rattlesnake** and other **Crotalidae** envenomations, the presence of fang marks, limb swelling, ecchymosis, and severe pain at the bite site are considered minimal indications for **polyvalent Crotalidae antivenin** (see p 312). Progressive systemic manifestations such as generalized fasciculations, coagulopathy, and muscle weakness are indications for prompt and aggressive treatment. For Mojave rattlesnake bite, the decision to administer antivenin is more difficult because there are few local signs of toxicity.

   2. For **coral snake** envenomation, consult a regional poison control center (see Table I–41, p 53) or an experienced herpetologist to determine the advisability of *Micrurus fulvius* antivenin (see p 314). In general, if there is evidence of coagulopathy or neurologic toxicity, administer antivenin.
   3. For **Colubridae** envenomations, there are no antivenins available.
   4. For **other exotic snakes,** consult a regional poison control center (see Table I–41, p 53) for assistance in diagnosis, location of specific antivenin, and indications for administration.

C. **Decontamination.** First-aid measures are generally ineffective and may cause additional tissue damage.
   1. Remain calm, remove the victim to at least 20 feet from the snake, wash the area with soap and water, and remove any constricting clothing or jewelry. Do *not* apply ice to the site.
   2. Loosely splint or immobilize the extremity near heart level. *Do **not** apply a tourniquet.*
   3. Do *not* make cuts over the bite site. If performed within 15 minutes, **suction** over the fang marks (ie, with a Sawyer extractor) may remove some venom but this should not delay transport to a hospital.

D. **Enhanced elimination.** Dialysis, hemoperfusion, and charcoal administration are not applicable.

SPIDERS
Karl A. Sporer, MD

ANTIDOTE   IPECAC   LAVAGE   CHARCOAL

Most of the more than 50,000 species of spiders in the USA possess poison glands connected to fangs in the large, paired, jawlike structures known as chelicerae. However, only a very few spiders have fangs long and tough enough to pierce human skin. In the USA, these include *Latrodectus* (black widow), *Loxosceles* (brown recluse spider), *Phidippus* (jumping spider), and *tarantulas* (a common name given to many large spiders). Tarantulas rarely cause significant envenomation but produce a painful bite because of their large size. Spiders not common to North America are not discussed here.

   Latrodectus species (black widow) are ubiquitous in the continental US, and the female can cause serious envenomations, with rare fatalities. They are usually encountered in the summer months while gardening or moving firewood, or during house repairs. The spider has a body size of 1–2 cm and is characteristically shiny black with a red hourglass shape on its bulbous abdomen. It makes coarse, irregular webs in dimly lit locations.

   Loxosceles species (brown recluse) are found mainly in the central and southeastern US (Missouri, Kansas, Arkansas, and Tennessee), but have been identified nationwide. The spider's nocturnal hunting habits and reclusive temperament result in infrequent contact with humans; most encounters occur at outdoor woodpiles or in basements. The spider is 1–3 cm in length, light to dark brown in color, with a characteristic violin- or fiddle-shaped marking on its cephalothorax (back).

I. **Mechanism of toxicity.** Spiders use their hollow fangs (chelicerae) to inject their venoms, which contain various protein and polypeptide toxins that are poorly characterized but appear to be designed to induce rapid paralysis of the insect victim and to aid in digestion.

A. *Latrodectus* (black widow) spider venom contains alpha-latrotoxin. This extremely potent toxin binds to specific synaptic membrane receptor proteins and causes opening of nonspecific cation channels, leading to an increased influx of calcium, indiscriminate release of acetylcholine, and excessive stimulation of the motor endplate.

B. *Loxosceles* (brown spiders) and *Phidippus* (jumping spiders) toxins contain a variety of digestive enzymes such as collagenases, proteases, and phospholipases. Loxosceles venom also contains sphingomyelinase D, which is cytotoxic and chemotactically attracts white blood cells to the bite site, and also has a role in producing systemic symptoms such as hemolysis.

II. Toxic dose. Spider venoms are generally extremely potent toxins (far more potent than most snake venoms), but the delivered dose is extremely small. The size of the victim is an important variable.

III. Clinical presentation. Manifestations of envenomation are quite different depending on the species.

A. *Latrodectus* (black widow) inflicts a bite that can range from mild erythema to a target lesion with a central punctate site with central blanching and an outer erythematous ring.

1. The bite is often initially unnoticed but becomes painful within 30–120 minutes. By 3–4 hours, painful cramping and muscle fasciculations occur in the involved extremity. This cramping progresses toward the chest, back, or abdomen, producing boardlike rigidity, weakness, dyspnea, headache, and paresthesias. Black widow envenomation may mimic myocardial infarction or an acute surgical abdomen. Symptoms often persist for 1–2 days.

2. Additional common symptoms may include hypertension, regional diaphoresis, restlessness, nausea, vomiting, and tachycardia.

3. Other less common symptoms include leukocytosis, fever, delirium, arrhythmias, and paresthesias. Rarely, hypertensive crisis or respiratory arrest may occur within 4–6 hours after severe envenomation, mainly in very young or very old victims.

B. *Loxosceles* syndrome is often called "loxoscelism" or "necrotic arachnidism."

1. Envenomation usually produces a painful burning sensation at the bite site within 10 minutes. Over the next 1–12 hours, a "bull's-eye" lesion forms, consisting of a central vesicle (which may be hemorrhagic) surrounded by a blanched ring enclosed by a ring of ecchymosis. The entire lesion can range from 1 to 5 cm in diameter. Over the next 24–72 hours, an indolent necrotic ulcer develops that may persist for a month or more.

2. Systemic illness may occur in the first 24–48 hours and does not necessarily correlate with the severity of the ulcer. Systemic manifestations include fever, chills, malaise, nausea, and myalgias. Rarely, intravascular hemolysis and disseminated intravascular coagulopathy may occur.

C. *Phidippus.* Many necrotic spider bites in the USA are probably caused by *Phidippus* species, which inflicts a painful bite, resulting in localized wheals, rashes, ecchymosis, and pruritus that are occasionally complicated by arthralgias, myalgias, headache, fever, nausea, vomiting, and hypotension. The duration of effects is generally no more than 1–4 days, and death is very rare.

IV. Diagnosis is most commonly made based on the characteristic clinical presentation. Bite marks of all spiders but the tarantulas are usually too small to be easily visualized, and victims often do not recall feeling the bite or seeing the spider.

Besides *Loxosceles* and *Phidippus,* many arthropods and insects may also produce small puncture wounds, pain, itching, redness, swelling, and even necrotic ulcers, so the offending animal often cannot be precisely identified unless it was captured or seen by the victim.

A. **Specific levels.** Serum toxin levels are not currently available. In the future, diagnostic serologic tests may be useful in diagnosing the specific responsible spider.

B. **Other useful laboratory studies**

1. ***Latrodectus:*** electrolytes, calcium, glucose, creatine phosphokinase (CPK), ECG (for chest pain).
2. ***Loxosceles:*** CBC, platelets, BUN, creatinine. If hemolysis suspected: haptoglobin, urine dipstick for occult blood (positive with free hemoglobin); repeat daily for 1–2 days.

V. Treatment
A. Emergency and supportive measures
1. **General**
   a. Cleanse the wound and apply cool compresses or intermittent ice packs. Treat infection if it occurs.
   b. Give tetanus prophylaxis if indicated.
2. ***Latrodectus* envenomation**
   a. Monitor victims for at least 6–8 hours.
   b. Maintain the airway and assist ventilation if necessary (see p 4), and treat severe hypertension (p 17) if it occurs.
3. ***Loxosceles* or *Phidippus* envenomation.**
   a. Do not excise or debride aggressively on initial evaluation.
   b. Admit patients with systemic symptoms and monitor for hemolysis, renal failure, and other complications.

B. Specific drugs and antidotes
1. ***Latrodectus***
   a. Muscle cramping may be treated with **intravenous calcium** (p 323) or muscle relaxants such as **methocarbamol** (p 350).
   b. Most patients will also require opioids such as **morphine** (p 354) and often are admitted for 24–48 hours for pain control.
   c. Equine-derived antivenin (**Antivenin *Latrodectus mactans;*** see p 313) is rapidly effective, but rarely used because symptomatic therapy is usually adequate and because of the small risk of anaphylaxis. It may still be indicated for seriously ill, elderly, or pediatric patients who do not respond to conventional therapy for hypertension, muscle cramping, or respiratory distress and for pregnant victims threatening premature labor.
2. ***Loxosceles.*** Therapy for necrotic arachnidism has been difficult to evaluate because of the inherent difficulty of accurate diagnosis.
   a. ***Dapsone*** has shown some promise in reducing the severity of necrotic ulcers, presumably because it is an effective inhibitor of polymorphonuclear (pmn) leukocytes, but there is not enough evidence to recommend its routine use.
   b. Steroids are usually recommended for hemolysis.
   c. A goat-derived antivenin has been studied, but is not FDA-approved or commercially available.

C. Decontamination.
These measures are not applicable. There is no proved value in the sometimes popular early excision of *Loxosceles* bites to prevent necrotic ulcer formation.

D. Enhanced elimination.
These procedures are not applicable.

STRYCHNINE
Neal L. Benowitz, MD

ANTIDOTE IPECAC LAVAGE CHARCOAL

Strychnine is an alkaloid derived from the seeds of a tree, *Strychnos nux-vomica.* At one time, strychnine was an ingredient in a variety of over-the-counter tonics and laxatives. Today, strychnine is no longer used in any pharmaceuticals. Instead, it is used primarily as a rodenticide and is sometimes found as an adulterant in illicit drugs such as cocaine or heroin.

I. **Mechanism of toxicity.** Strychnine competitively antagonizes glycine, an inhibitory neurotransmitter released by postsynaptic inhibitory neurons in the spinal cord. This causes increased neuronal excitability, which results in generalized seizurelike contraction of skeletal muscles. Simultaneous contraction of opposing flexor and extensor muscles causes severe muscle injury, with rhabdomyolysis, myoglobinuria, and, in some cases, acute renal failure.

II. **Toxic dose.** It is difficult to establish a toxic dose, although 16 mg was fatal in an adult in one case. Because life-threatening clinical manifestations can occur rapidly and because management decisions are based on clinical findings rather than on a history of ingested amount, any dose of strychnine should be considered life-threatening.

III. **Clinical presentation.** Symptoms and signs usually develop within 15–30 minutes of ingestion, and may last several hours (the serum elimination half-life of strychnine was 10 hours in one reported overdose).

   A. Muscular stiffness and painful cramps precede generalized muscle contractions and opisthotonos. The face may be drawn into a forced grimace ("sardonic grin," or *risus sardonicus*). Muscle contractions are intermittent and are easily triggered by emotional or physical stimuli. Repeated and prolonged muscle contractions often result in hyperthermia, rhabdomyolysis, myoglobinuria, and renal failure.

   B. The muscle contractions may resemble the tonic phase of a grand mal seizure, but strychnine does not cause true seizures and the patient is awake and painfully aware of the contractions.

   C. Victims may also experience hyperacusis, hyperalgesia, and increased visual stimulation. Sudden noises or other sensory input may trigger muscle contractions.

   D. Death is usually caused by respiratory arrest owing to intense contraction of the respiratory muscles. Death may also be secondary to hyperthermia or rhabdomyolysis and renal failure.

IV. **Diagnosis** is based on a history of ingestion of a rodenticide or recent intravenous drug abuse and the presence of seizurelike generalized muscle contractions, often accompanied by hyperthermia, lactic acidosis, and rhabdomyolysis (with myoglobinuria and elevated serum creatine phosphokinase [CPK]). In the differential diagnosis (see Table I–15, p 24), one should consider other causes of generalized muscle rigidity such as black widow spider bite (p 288), neuroleptic malignant syndrome (p 20), or tetanus (see p 293).

   A. **Specific levels.** Strychnine can be measured in the gastric fluid, urine, or blood. The toxic serum concentration is reported to be 1 mg/L, although in general, blood levels do not correlate well with the severity of toxicity.

   B. **Other useful laboratory studies.** Electrolytes, BUN, creatinine, creatine phosphokinase (CPK), arterial blood gases or oximetry, urine test for occult blood (positive in the presence of urine myoglobinuria).

V. **Treatment**

   A. **Emergency and supportive measures**

   1. Maintain the airway and assist ventilation if necessary (see p 4).

   2. Treat hyperthermia (p 20), metabolic acidosis (p 30), and rhabdomyolysis (p 25) if they occur.

   3. Limit external stimuli such as noise, light, and touch.

   4. **Treat muscle spasms** aggressively:

      a. Administer **diazepam** (see p 327), 0.1–0.2 mg/kg IV, or **midazolam** (p 353), 0.05–0.1 mg/kg IV, to patients with mild muscle contractions. Give **morphine** (p 354) for pain relief. *Note:* These agents may impair respiratory drive.

      b. In more severe cases, use **pancuronium** (p 357), 0.06–0.1 mg/kg IV, to produce complete neuromuscular paralysis. *Caution:* Neuromuscular paralysis will cause respiratory arrest; patients will need endotracheal intubation (p 3) and assisted ventilation (p 7).

   B. **Specific drugs and antidotes.** There is no specific antidote.

C. Decontamination (see p 44)

    1. Prehospital. Administer activated charcoal, if available. Do **not** induce emesis because of the risk of aggravating muscle spasms.

    2. Hospital. Administer activated charcoal and a cathartic orally or by gastric tube. Gastric lavage is not necessary for small ingestions if activated charcoal can be given promptly.

D. Enhanced elimination. Symptoms usually abate within several hours, and can be managed effectively with intensive supportive care, so there is little to be gained from accelerated drug removal by dialysis or hemoperfusion. The use of repeat-dose activated charcoal has not been studied.

SULFUR DIOXIDE
John Balmes, MD

ANTIDOTE   IPECAC   LAVAGE   CHARCOAL

Sulfur dioxide is a colorless, nonflammable gas formed by the burning of materials that contain sulfur. It is a major air pollutant from automobiles, smelters, and plants burning soft coal or oils high in sulfur content. It is soluble in water to form caustic sulfurous acid, which may be oxidized to sulfuric acid; both are components of acid rain. Occupational exposures to sulfur dioxide occur in ore and metal refining, chemical manufacturing, and wood pulp treatment and in its use as a disinfectant, refrigerant, and dried food preservative.

I. Mechanism of toxicity. Sulfur dioxide is an irritant because it rapidly forms sulfurous acid on contact with moist mucous membranes. Most effects occur in the upper respiratory tract because 90% of inhaled sulfur dioxide is rapidly deposited there, but with very large exposures sufficient gas reaches the lower airways to cause chemical pneumonitis and pulmonary edema.

II. Toxic dose. The sharp odor or taste of sulfur dioxide is noticed at 3–5 ppm. Throat and conjunctival irritation begin at 8–12 ppm and are severe at 50 ppm. The ACGIH recommended workplace permissible limit (TLV-TWA) is 2 ppm as an 8-hour time-weighted average, and the air level considered immediately dangerous to life or health (IDLH) is 100 ppm.

III. Clinical presentation

A. Acute exposure causes burning of the eyes, nose, and throat; lacrimation; and cough. Laryngospasm may occur. Wheezing may be seen in normal subjects as well as asthmatics. Chemical bronchitis is not uncommon. With a very high-level exposure, chemical pneumonitis and noncardiogenic pulmonary edema may occur.

B. Asthma and chronic bronchitis may be exacerbated.

C. Sulfhemoglobinemia has been reported owing to absorption of sulfur.

D. Frostbite injury to the skin may occur from exposure to liquid sulfur dioxide.

IV. Diagnosis is based on a history of exposure and the presence of upper airway and mucous membrane irritation. Symptoms usually occur rapidly following exposure.

A. Specific levels. Blood levels are not available. Urinary sulfate excretion holds future promise as an indicator of exposure.

B. Other useful laboratory studies. Arterial blood gases or oximetry, chest x-ray, spirometry or peak expiratory flow rate.

V. Treatment

A. Emergency and supportive measures

    1. Remain alert for progressive upper airway edema or obstruction, and be prepared to intubate the trachea and assist ventilation if necessary (see p 3).

    2. Administer humidified oxygen, treat wheezing with bronchodilators (p 9–10), and observe for at least 4–6 hours for development of pulmonary edema (p 8).

B. Specific drugs and antidotes. There is no specific antidote.

C. Decontamination

    1. Inhalation. Remove victim from exposure and give supplemental oxygen, if available.

    2. Skin and eyes. Wash exposed skin and eyes with copious tepid water or saline. Treat frostbite injury as for thermal burns.

D. Enhanced elimination. There is no role for these procedures.

TETANUS
Karl A. Sporer, MD

ANTIDOTE   IPECAC   LAVAGE   CHARCOAL

Tetanus is a rare disease in the USA, with fewer than 50 cases reported annually. It is caused by an exotoxin produced by *Clostridium tetani,* an anaerobic, spore-forming, gram-positive rod found widely in soil and in the gastrointestinal tract. Tetanus is typically seen in older persons (especially older women), recent immigrants, and intravenous drug users who have not maintained adequate tetanus immunization.

I. Mechanism of toxicity. The growth of *tetani* in a wound under anaerobic conditions produces the toxin tetanospasmin. The toxin enters the myoneural junction of alpha motor neurons and travels via retrograde axonal transport to the synapse. There it blocks the release of the presynaptic inhibitory neurotransmitters γ-aminobutyric acid (GABA) and glycine, causing intense muscular spasms.

II. Toxic dose. Tetanospasmin is an extremely potent toxin. Fatal tetanus can result from a minor puncture wound in a susceptible individual.

III. Clinical presentation. The incubation period between the initial wound and development of symptoms averages 1–2 weeks (range 2–56 days). The wound is not apparent in about 5% of cases. Wound cultures are positive for *C tetani* only about one-third of the time.

    A. The most common initial complaint is pain and stiffness of the jaw, progressing to trismus, *risus sardonicus,* and opisthotonos over several days. Uncontrollable and painful reflex spasms involving all muscle groups are precipitated by minimal stimuli and can result in fractures, rhabdomyolysis, hyperpyrexia, and asphyxia. The patient remains awake during the spasms. In survivors, the spasms may persist for days or weeks.

    B. A syndrome of sympathetic hyperactivity often accompanies the muscular manifestations, with hypertension, tachycardia, arrhythmias, and diaphoresis.

    C. Neonatal tetanus occurs frequently in developing countries, owing to inadequate maternal immunity and poor hygiene, especially around the necrotic umbilical stump. Localized tetanus has been reported, involving rigidity and spasm only in the affected limb. Cephalic tetanus is uncommonly associated with head wounds and involves primarily the cranial nerves.

IV. Diagnosis is based on the finding of characteristic muscle spasms in an awake person with a wound and an inadequate immunization history. Strychnine poisoning (p 290) produces identical muscle spasms and should be considered in the differential diagnosis. Other considerations include hypocalcemia and dystonic reactions.

    A. Specific levels. There are no specific toxin assays. A serum antibody level of 0.01 IU/mL or greater suggests prior immunity and makes the diagnosis less likely.

    B. Other useful laboratory studies. Electrolytes, glucose, calcium, BUN, creatinine, creatine phosphokinase (CPK), arterial blood gases, urine dipstick for occult blood (positive with myoglobinuria). A diagnostic electromyographic pattern has been described but is not commonly used.

V. Treatment

   A. Emergency and supportive measures

     1. Maintain the airway and assist ventilation if necessary (see p 4).

     2. Treat hyperthermia (p 22), arrhythmias (p 10–14), metabolic acidosis (p 30), and rhabdomyolysis (p 327) if they occur.

     3. Limit external stimuli such as noise, light, and touch.

     4. **Treat muscle spasms** aggressively:

       a. Administer **diazepam** (see p 327), 0.1–0.2 mg/kg IV, or **midazolam** (p 353), 0.05–0.1 mg/kg IV, to patients with mild muscle contractions. Give **morphine** (see p 354) for pain relief. *Note:* These agents may impair respiratory drive.

       b. In more severe cases, use **pancuronium** (p 357), 0.06–0.1 mg/kg IV, to produce complete neuromuscular paralysis. *Caution:* Neuromuscular paralysis will cause respiratory arrest; patients will need endotracheal intubation (p 3) and assisted ventilation (p 7).

   B. Specific drugs and antidotes

     1. **Human tetanus immune globulin (TIG),** 3000–5000 IU administered IM, will neutralize circulating toxin but has no effect on toxin already fixed to neurons. TIG should be given as early as possible to a patient with suspected tetanus, and to persons with a fresh wound but possibly inadequate prior immunization.

     2. **Prevention** can be ensured by an adequate immunization series with tetanus toxoid in childhood and repeated boosters at 10-year intervals. Survival of tetanus may not protect against future exposures, because the small amount of toxin required to cause disease is inadequate to confer immunity.

   C. Decontamination. Thoroughly debride and irrigate the wound, and administer appropriate antibiotics (penicillin is adequate for *C tetani*).

   D. Enhanced elimination. There is no role for these procedures.

THALLIUM
Kent R. Olson, MD

ANTIDOTE   IPECAC   LAVAGE   CHARCOAL

Thallium is a soft metal that quickly oxidizes upon exposure to air. It is a minor constituent in a variety of ores and is commonly found in flue dusts. The metal itself finds little use, but thallium salts are widely used in industry and chemical analysis; example of uses include the manufacture of optical lenses, photoelectric cells, and costume jewelry. It is no longer used in the USA as a depilatory or a rodenticide because of its high human toxicity.

   I. Mechanism of toxicity. The mechanism of thallium toxicity is not entirely known. It appears to affect the mitochondria and a variety of enzyme systems, resulting in generalized cellular poisoning. Thallium metabolism has some similarities to that of potassium, and it may inhibit potassium flux across membranes. Some thallium salts are well absorbed across intact skin.

   II. Toxic dose. The minimum lethal dose of thallium salts is probably 12–15 mg/kg, although toxicity varies widely depending on the compound, and there are reports of death after adult ingestion of as little as 200 mg. The more water-soluble salts (eg, thallous acetate, thallic chloride) are slightly more toxic than the less soluble forms (thallic oxide, thallous iodide).

   III. Clinical presentation. Symptoms do not occur immediately but usually within 12–14 hours after ingestion.

     A. Acute effects include abdominal pain, vomiting, and diarrhea (with hemorrhage). Shock may result from massive fluid or blood loss. Within 2–3 days, delirium, seizures, and coma may occur.

B. Chronic effects. Chronic neurologic toxicity includes muscle weakness and atrophy, chorea, and peripheral neuropathy. Hair loss and nail dystrophy (Mees' lines) may appear after 2–4 weeks.

IV. Diagnosis may be made from a history of acute exposure and the presence of severe gastroenteritis, but in chronic exposures toxicity may not be suspected until alopecia or nail dystrophy occurs.

    A. Specific levels. Urinary thallium is normally less than 1.5 µg/L. Concentrations greater than 100 µg/L are considered toxic. Blood and hair thallium levels are not reliable measures of exposure.

    B. Other useful laboratory studies. CBC, electrolytes, glucose, BUN, creatinine, hepatic transaminases.

V. Treatment

    A. Emergency and supportive measures

        1. Maintain the airway and assist ventilation if necessary (see p 4).

        2. Treat seizures (p 22) and coma (p 18) if they occur.

        3. Treat gastroenteritis with aggressive intravenous replacement of fluids (and blood, if needed). Use pressors only if shock does not respond to fluid therapy (p 15).

    B. Specific drugs and antidotes. There is currently no recommended specific treatment in the USA.

        1. Prussian blue (ferric ferrocyanide) is believed to enhance removal of thallium from tissues and increase renal and fecal elimination; however, it is not available for use in the USA, and charcoal is probably equally effective at enhancing fecal elimination.

        2. BAL (see p 317) and other chelators have been tried with varying success.

    C. Decontamination (see p 44)

        1. Prehospital. Administer activated charcoal, if available. Ipecac-induced emesis may be useful for initial treatment at the scene (eg, children at home) if it can be given within a few minutes of exposure.

        2. Hospital. Administer activated charcoal and a cathartic. Consider gastric lavage for large recent ingestion.

    D. Enhanced elimination. Repeat-dose activated charcoal may enhance fecal elimination by binding thallium secreted into the gut lumen or via the biliary system, interrupting enterohepatic or enteroenteric recirculation. Forced diuresis, dialysis, and hemoperfusion are of no proved benefit.

THEOPHYLLINE
Kent R. Olson, MD

ANTIDOTE   IPECAC   LAVAGE   CHARCOAL

Theophylline is a methylxanthine widely used for the treatment of asthma. Intravenous infusions of aminophylline, the ethylenediamine salt of theophylline, are used to treat bronchospasm, congestive heart failure, and neonatal apnea. Theophylline is most commonly used orally in sustained-release preparations (eg, Theo-Dur, Slo-Phyllin, Theobid, many others).

I. Mechanism of toxicity

    A. The exact mechanism of toxicity is not known. Theophylline is known to inhibit phosphodiesterase at high levels, increasing intracellular cyclic adenosine monophosphate (cAMP). It also is known to release endogenous catecholamines at therapeutic concentrations and may itself stimulate beta-adrenergic receptors. It also is an antagonist of adenosine receptors.

    B. Pharmacokinetics. The normal elimination half-life is 4–6 hours; this may be doubled by illnesses or interacting drugs that slow hepatic metabolism, such as liver disease, congestive heart failure, influenza, erythromycin, or cimetidine, and may increase to as much as 20 hours after overdose.

II. Toxic dose. An acute single dose of 8–10 mg/kg will produce a therapeutic level of 15–20 mg/L. Acute oral overdose of more than 50 mg/kg may potentially result in a level above 100 mg/L and significant toxicity.

III. Clinical presentation. Two distinct syndromes of intoxication may occur, depending on whether the exposure is **acute** or **chronic**.

A. Acute single overdose is usually a result of a suicide attempt or accidental childhood ingestion but may also be caused by accidental or iatrogenic misuse (therapeutic overdose).

1. Usual manifestations include vomiting (sometimes with hematemesis), tremor, anxiety, and tachycardia. Metabolic effects include pronounced hypokalemia, hypophosphatemia, hyperglycemia, and metabolic acidosis.

2. With serum levels above 100 mg/L, hypotension, ventricular arrhythmias, and seizures are common; status epilepticus is frequently resistant to anti-convulsant drugs.

3. Seizures and other manifestations of severe toxicity may be delayed 12–16 hours or more after ingestion, in part owing to delayed absorption of drug from sustained-release preparations.

B. Chronic intoxication occurs when excessive doses are administered repeatedly over 24 hours or longer, or when intercurrent illness or an interacting drug interferes with hepatic metabolism of theophylline. The usual victims are very young infants or elderly patients.

1. Vomiting may occur but is not as common as in acute overdose. Tachycardia is common, but hypotension is rare. Metabolic effects such as hypokalemia and hyperglycemia do not occur.

2. Seizures are commonly associated with levels of 40–60 mg/L, and have been reported with levels as low as 20 mg/L.

IV. Diagnosis is based on a history of ingestion or the presence of tremor, tachycardia, and other manifestations in a patient known to be on theophylline. Hypokalemia strongly suggests acute overdose rather than chronic intoxication.

A. Specific levels. Serum theophylline levels are essential for diagnosis and determination of emergency treatment. After acute oral overdose, obtain repeated levels every 2–4 hours; single determinations are not sufficient, because continued absorption from sustained-release preparations may result in peak levels 12–16 hours or longer after ingestion.

1. Levels less than 90–100 mg/L after acute overdose are not usually associated with severe symptoms such as seizures or ventricular arrhythmias.

2. However, with chronic intoxication, severe toxicity may occur with levels of 40–60 mg/L.

Note: Acute caffeine overdose (see p 112) will cause a similar clinical picture and will produce falsely elevated theophylline concentrations with most commercial immunoassays.

B. Other useful laboratory studies. Electrolytes, glucose, BUN, creatinine, hepatic function tests, ECG monitoring.

V. Treatment

A. Emergency and supportive measures

1. Maintain the airway and assist ventilation if necessary (see p 4).

2. Treat seizures (p 22), arrhythmias (p 10–14), and hypotension (p 15) if they occur. Tachyarrhythmias and hypotension are best treated with a beta-adrenergic agent (see **B.,** below).

3. Hypokalemia is caused by intracellular movement of potassium and does not reflect significant total body deficit; it usually resolves spontaneously without aggressive treatment.

4. Monitor vital signs, ECG, and serial theophylline levels for at least 16–18 hours after a significant oral overdose.

B. Specific drugs and antidotes. Hypotension, tachycardia, and ventricular arrhythmias are caused primarily by excessive beta-adrenergic stimulation. Treat with low-dose **propranolol** (see p 373), 0.01–0.03 mg/kg IV, or **esmolol** (see p 338), 25–50 µg/kg/min. Use beta blockers cautiously in patients with a prior history of asthma or wheezing.

C. Decontamination (see p 44)

1. **Prehospital.** Administer activated charcoal, if available. Ipecac-induced emesis may be useful for initial treatment at the scene (eg, children at home) if it can be given within a few minutes of exposure.

2. **Hospital.** Administer activated charcoal and a cathartic. Gastric emptying is not necessary for small ingestions if activated charcoal can be given promptly.

3. Undissolved sustained-release tablets may not be removed with even the largest (40F) gastric tube. For significant ingestions, consider the following special techniques:

   a. Administer repeated doses of activated charcoal (p 52).

   b. Perform whole bowel irrigation (p 48).

D. Enhanced elimination. (see p 49) Theophylline has a small volume of distribution (0.5 L/kg) and is efficiently removed by dialysis, charcoal hemoperfusion, or repeat-dose activated charcoal.

1. **Hemoperfusion** should be performed if the patient is in status epilepticus or if the serum theophylline concentration is greater than 100 mg/L. **Hemodialysis** is not as effective but may be used if hemoperfusion is not readily available.

2. **Repeat-dose activated charcoal** (see p 49) is not as effective as hemoperfusion but may be used for stable patients with levels below 100 mg/L.

THYROID HORMONE
Kent R. Olson, MD

| ANTIDOTE | IPECAC | LAVAGE | CHARCOAL |

Thyroid hormone is available as synthetic triiodothyronine (T_3, liothyronine), synthetic tetraiodothyronine (T_4, levothyroxine), or natural dessicated animal thyroid (containing both T_3 and T_4; Table II–53). Despite concern over the potentially life-threatening manifestations of thyrotoxicosis, serious toxicity rarely occurs after acute thyroid hormone ingestion.

I. Mechanism of toxicity. Thyroid hormone stimulates the cardiovascular, gastrointestinal, and neurologic systems, presumably by potentiating adrenergic activity. The effects of T_3 overdose are manifested within the first 6 hours following an ingestion. In contrast, symptoms of T_4 overdose may be delayed 2–5 days after ingestion while metabolic conversion to T_3 occurs.

II. Toxic dose

A. An acute ingestion of more than 3 mg of **levothyroxine** (T_4) or 0.75 mg of **triiodothyronine** (T_3) is considered potentially toxic. An adult has survived an ingestion of 48 g of unspecified thyroid tablets; a 15-month-old child had moderate symptoms after ingesting 1.5 g of desiccated thyroid.

B. Euthyroid persons and children appear to have a high tolerance to the effects of an acute overdose. Patients with preexisting cardiac disease and those with chronic overmedication have a lower threshold of toxicity. Sudden deaths have been reported following chronic thyroid hormone abuse in healthy adults.

III. Clinical presentation. The effects of an acute T_4 overdose may not be evident for several days because of delay for metabolism to more active T_3.

A. Mild to moderate intoxication may cause sinus tachycardia, elevated temperature, diarrhea, vomiting, headache, anxiety, agitation, psychosis, and confusion.

TABLE II–53. DOSAGE EQUIVALENTS OF THYROID HORMONE

Thyroid USP	65 mg (1 gr)
l-Thyroxine (T_4)	0.1 mg (100 µg)
1-Triiodothyronine (T_3)	0.025 mg (25 µg)

    B. Severe toxicity may include supraventricular tachycardia, hyperthermia, and hypotension. There is one case report of a seizure following acute overdose.

IV. Diagnosis is based on a history of ingestion and signs and symptoms of increased sympathetic activity.

    A. Specific levels. Obtain total serum T_3 and T_4 levels (T_3RIA and T_4RIA) and T_3 resin uptake (T_3RU) approximately 2–6 hours after an acute ingestion; repeat over the following 5–7 days. There is a reasonable qualitative relationship between the presence of elevated levels and the presence of symptoms.

    B. Other useful laboratory studies. Electrolytes, glucose, BUN, creatinine, ECG monitoring.

V. Treatment

    A. Emergency and supportive measures

        1. Maintain the airway and assist ventilation if necessary (see p 4).

        2. Treat seizures (p 22), hyperthermia (p 20), hypotension (p 15), and arrhythmias (p 13–14) if they occur.

        3. Repeated examinations over several days are necessary after T_4 or combined ingestions, because serious symptoms may be delayed.

        4. Most patients will suffer no serious toxicity or will recover with simple supportive care.

    B. Specific drugs and antidotes

        1. Treat serious tachyarrhythmias with **propranolol** (see p 373), 0.01–0.1 mg/kg IV repeated every 2–5 minutes to desired effect, or **esmolol** (see p 338), 25–100 µg/kg/min IV. Simple sinus tachycardia may be treated with oral propranolol, 0.1–0.5 mg/kg every 4–6 hours.

        2. Peripheral metabolic conversion of T_4 to T_3 can be partially inhibited by **propylthiouracil,** 6–10 mg/kg/d (maximum 1 g) divided into 3 oral doses, for 5–7 days.

    C. Decontamination (see p 44)

        1. Prehospital. Administer activated charcoal, if available. Ipecac-induced emesis may be useful for initial treatment at the scene (eg, children at home) if it can be given within a few minutes of exposure.

        2. Hospital. Administer activated charcoal and a cathartic. Gastric emptying is not necessary following small ingestions if activated charcoal can be given promptly.

    D. Enhanced elimination. Diuresis and hemodialysis are not useful because thyroid hormones are extensively protein-bound. Charcoal hemoperfusion may be effective, but limited data are available. Exchange transfusion has been performed in children and adults, but data on its efficacy are limited.

TOLUENE AND XYLENE
Janet Weiss, MD

ANTIDOTE   IPECAC   LAVAGE   CHARCOAL

Toluene (methylbenzene) and xylene (dimethylbenzene, xylol) are very common aromatic solvents widely used in glues, inks, dyes, lacquers, varnishes, paints, paint removers, pesticides, cleaners, and degreasers. The largest source of exposure to toluene is in the production and use of gasoline. Toluene is also frequently abused intentionally by inhaling paints containing toluene to induce a "sniffer's high."

I. Mechanism of toxicity. Toluene and xylene cause generalized central nervous system depression. Like other aromatic hydrocarbons, they may sensitize the myocardium to the arrhythmogenic effects of catecholamines. They are mild mucous membrane irritants affecting the eyes, respiratory, and gastrointestinal tracts. Pulmonary aspiration can cause a hydrocarbon pneumonitis (see p 178). Chronic abuse of toluene can cause diffuse CNS demyelination, renal tubular damage, and myopathy.

II. Toxic dose
  A. Ingestion. There is little information concerning the toxic dose by ingestion, although as little as 15–20 mL of toluene is reported to cause serious toxicity. Whether this reflects the risk for aspiration chemical pneumonitis rather than true systemic toxicity is not known.
  B. Inhalation. The recommended workplace limits (ACGIH TLV-TWA) are 50 ppm for toluene and 100 ppm for xylene, as 8-hour time-weighted averages, with a "skin" notation indicating the potential for appreciable skin absorption. The air levels considered immediately dangerous to life or health (IDLH) are 2000 ppm for toluene and 10,000 ppm for xylene.

III. Clinical presentation. Toxicity may be a result of ingestion, pulmonary aspiration, or inhalation.
  A. Ingestion of toluene or xylene may cause vomiting and diarrhea, and if pulmonary aspiration occurs, chemical pneumonitis. Systemic absorption may result in CNS depression.
  B. Inhalation produces euphoria, dizziness, headache, nausea, and weakness. Exposure to high concentrations may rapidly cause delirium, coma, pulmonary edema, respiratory arrest, and death. Arrhythmias may occasionally occur due to cardiac sensitization.
  C. Chronic exposure to toluene may cause permanent CNS impairment, including tremors, ataxia, cerebellar and cerebral atrophy, and cognitive and neurobehavioral abnormalities. Myopathy, hypokalemia, and renal tubular acidosis are also common. Animal studies suggest that toluene may cause adverse reproductive effects.

IV. Diagnosis is based on a history of exposure and typical manifestations of acute CNS effects such as euphoria or "drunkenness." After acute ingestion, pulmonary aspiration is suggested by coughing, choking, tachypnea, or wheezing, and is confirmed by chest x-ray.
  A. Specific levels. In acute symptomatic exposures, toluene or xylene may be detectable in blood drawn with a gas-tight syringe but usually only for a few hours. The metabolites hippuric acid (toluene) and methylhippuric acid (xylene) are excreted in the urine and can be used to document exposure, but urine levels do not correlate with systemic effects.
  B. Other useful laboratory studies. Electrolytes, glucose, BUN, creatinine, liver transaminases, creatine phosphokinase (CPK), urinalysis.

V. Treatment
  A. Emergency and supportive measures
    1. Maintain the airway and assist ventilation if necessary (see p 4). Administer supplemental oxygen, and monitor arterial blood gases and chest x-rays.
      a. If the patient is coughing or dyspneic, aspiration chemical pneumonia is likely. Treat as for hydrocarbon pneumonia (see p 178).
      b. If the patient remains asymptomatic after a 6-hour observation period, chemical pneumonia is unlikely and further observation or chest x-ray is not needed.
    2. Treat coma (p 18), arrhythmias (p 14), and bronchospasm (p 9–10) if they occur. *Caution:* Epinephrine and other sympathomimetic amines can provoke or aggravate cardiac arrhythmias. Tachyarrhythmias may be treated with **propranolol** (p 373), 1–2 mg IV, or **esmolol** (p 338), 25–100 µg/kg/min IV.

B. Specific drugs and antidotes. There is no specific antidote.

C. Decontamination. Rescuers should treat heavily contaminated victims in a well-ventilated area or should use self-contained breathing apparatus or other appropriate respiratory protection, as well as chemical-resistant clothing and gloves.

  1. Inhalation. Remove the victim from exposure and give supplemental oxygen, if available.

  2. Skin and eyes. Remove contaminated clothes and wash exposed skin with soap and water. Irrigate exposed eyes with copious tepid water or saline.

  3. Ingestion (see p 44)

   a. Prehospital. Administer activated charcoal, if available. Do **not** induce emesis because of the risk of rapidly progressive CNS depression.

   b. Hospital. Administer activated charcoal and a cathartic. Consider gastric lavage for large ingestions (> 1–2 oz) if it can be performed within 30 minutes of ingestion.

D. Enhanced elimination. There is no role for enhanced elimination.

TRICHLOROETHANE AND TRICHLOROETHYLENE
Diane Liu, MD, MPH

ANTIDOTE   IPECAC   LAVAGE   CHARCOAL

Trichloroethane and trichloroethylene are widely used solvents found as ingredients in many products including typewriter correction fluid ("white-out"), color film cleaners, insecticides, spot removers, fabric cleaning solutions, adhesives, and paint removers. They are used extensively in industry as degreasers. Trichloroethane is available in 2 isomeric forms, 1,1,2- and 1,1,1-, with the latter (methyl chloroform) being the most common.

I. Mechanism of toxicity

  A. Trichloroethane and trichloroethylene act as respiratory and central nervous system depressants and skin and mucous membrane irritants. They have rapid anesthetic action, and both were used for this purpose medically until the advent of safer agents.

  B. Trichloroethane, trichloroethylene, and their metabolite trichloroethanol may sensitize the myocardium to the arrhythmogenic effects of catecholamines.

  C. Trichloroethylene or a metabolite may act to inhibit acetaldehyde dehydrogenase, blocking the metabolism of ethanol and causing "degreaser's flush."

  D. NIOSH considers 1,1,2-trichloroethane and trichloroethylene possible carcinogens.

II. Toxic dose

  A. Trichloroethane. The acute lethal oral dose to humans is reportedly between 0.5–5 mL/kg. The recommended workplace limits (ACGIH TLV-TWA) in air for the 1,1,1- and 1,1,2- isomers are 350 and 10 ppm, respectively, and the air levels considered immediately dangerous to life or health (IDLH) are 1000 and 500 ppm, respectively. Anesthetic levels are in the range of 10,000–26,000 ppm. The odor is detectable by a majority of people at 500 ppm, but olfactory fatigue commonly occurs.

  B. Trichloroethylene. The acute lethal oral dose is reported to be approximately 3–5 mL/kg. The recommended workplace limit (ACGIH TLV-TWA) is 50 ppm, and the air level considered immediately dangerous to life or health (IDLH) is 1000 ppm.

III. Clinical presentation. Toxicity may be a result of inhalation, skin contact, or ingestion.

  A. Inhalation or ingestion may cause nausea, euphoria, ataxia, dizziness, agitation, and lethargy, and if intoxication is significant, respiratory arrest, seizures, and coma. Hypotension and cardiac arrhythmias may occur. With severe overdose, renal and hepatic injury may be apparent 1–2 days after exposure.

B. Local effects of exposure to liquid or vapors include irritation of the eyes, nose, and throat. Prolonged skin contact can cause defatting and dermatitis.

C. Ingestion. Aspiration into the tracheobronchial tree may result in hydrocarbon pneumonia (see p 178).

D. Degreaser's flush. Workers exposed to these vapors may have acute flushing and orthostatic hypotension if they ingest alcohol, owing to a disulfiramlike effect (see Disulfiram, p 155).

IV. Diagnosis is based on a history of exposure and typical symptoms. Addictive inhalational abuse of typewriter correction fluid suggests trichloroethylene poisoning.

A. Specific levels

1. Although trichloroethane can be measured in expired air, blood, and urine, levels are not routinely rapidly available and are not needed for evaluation or treatment. Confirmation of exposure might be possible by detecting the metabolite trichloroethanol in the blood or urine. Hospital laboratory methods are not usually sensitive to these amounts.

2. Breath analysis is becoming more widely used for workplace exposure control, and serial measurements may allow for estimation of the amount absorbed. Expired air is collected in a plastic bag and analyzed by infrared or gas chromatography.

B. Other useful laboratory studies. Electrolytes, glucose, BUN, creatinine, liver transaminases, arterial blood gases, ECG monitoring.

V. Treatment

A. Emergency and supportive measures

1. Maintain the airway and assist ventilation if necessary (see p 4). Administer supplemental oxygen, and treat hydrocarbon aspiration pneumonitis (p 178) if it occurs.

2. Treat seizures (p 22), coma (p 18), and arrhythmias (p 14) if they occur. *Caution:* Avoid the use of epinephrine or other sympathomimetic amines because of the risk of inducing or aggravating cardiac arrhythmias. Tachyarrhythmias caused by myocardial sensitization may be treated with **propranolol** (p 373), 1–2 mg IV, or **esmolol** (p 338), 25–100 µg/kg/min IV.

3. Monitor for a minimum of 4–6 hours after significant exposure.

B. Specific drugs and antidotes. There is no specific antidote.

C. Decontamination (see p 41)

1. **Inhalation.** Remove the victim from exposure and administer supplemental oxygen, if available.

2. **Skin and eyes.** Remove contaminated clothing and wash exposed skin with soap and water. Irrigate exposed eyes with copious tepid water or saline.

3. **Ingestion** (see p 44)

a. **Prehospital.** Administer activated charcoal, if available. Do *not* induce emesis because of the danger of rapid absorption and abrupt onset of seizures or coma.

b. **Hospital.** Administer activated charcoal and a cathartic orally or by gastric tube. Consider gastric lavage; for small ingestions (< 30 mL), oral activated charcoal alone without gut emptying may be sufficient.

D. Enhanced elimination. These procedures are not effective or necessary.

VACOR (PNU)
Neal L. Benowitz, MD

ANTIDOTE   IPECAC   LAVAGE   CHARCOAL

Vacor rat killer (2% N-3-pyridylmethyl-N'-p-nitrophenylurea; PNU) is a unique rodenticide that causes irreversible insulin-dependent diabetes and autonomic nervous system injury. It was removed from general sale in the USA in 1979 but is still available in some homes and for use by licensed exterminators. The product was sold in 39-g packets of cornmeallike material containing 2% PNU.

I. **Mechanism of toxicity.** PNU is believed to antagonize the actions of nicotinamide and, in a manner similar to that of alloxan and streptozocin, injure pancreatic beta cells. The mechanisms of autonomic neuropathy and central nervous system effects are unknown. Adrenergic neurons acting on blood vessels but not the heart are affected. As a result, orthostatic hypotension associated with an intact reflex tachycardia is the usual picture.

II. **Toxic dose.** Acute toxicity has usually occurred after ingestion of one 39-g packet of Vacor (approximately 8 g of PNU). The smallest dose reported to cause toxicity was 390 mg.

III. **Clinical presentation.** Initial symptoms include nausea and vomiting. Occasionally, confusion, stupor, and coma occur after several hours. After a delay of several hours to days, irreversible autonomic neuropathy, peripheral neuropathy, and diabetes may occur.

    A. **Autonomic dysfunction.** Dizziness or syncope or both caused by severe orthostatic hypotension occur with an onset from 6 hours to 2 days following ingestion. Orthostatic hypotension is usually accompanied by intact reflex tachycardia. Other manifestations of autonomic neuropathy include dysphagia, recurrent vomiting, and constipation.

    B. **Insulin-dependent diabetes mellitus,** with polyuria, polydipsia, hyperglycemia, and ketoacidosis, occurs after a few days. Hypoglycemia, resulting from insulin release, occasionally precedes hyperglycemia.

    C. **Peripheral neuropathy** may cause paresthesias and muscle weakness.

IV. **Diagnosis.** Sudden onset of orthostatic hypotension or diabetes mellitus should suggest the possibility of Vacor ingestion. A careful investigation should be performed to determine what rat-killing chemicals may be present in the home.

    A. **Specific levels.** PNU levels are not available.

    B. **Other useful laboratory studies.** Electrolytes, glucose, BUN, creatinine.

V. **Treatment**

    A. **Emergency and supportive measures**

        1. Maintain the airway and assist ventilation if necessary (see p 4).

        2. Orthostatic hypotension usually responds to supine positioning and intravenous fluids. Chronic therapy includes a high-salt diet and fludrocortisone (0.1–1 mg/d).

        3. Treat diabetes in the usual manner with fluids and insulin.

    B. **Specific drugs and antidotes.** Immediately administer **nicotinamide** (see p 359). Although its efficacy in humans is not proved, nicotinamide can prevent PNU-induced diabetes in rats.

    C. **Decontamination** (see p 44)

        1. **Prehospital.** Administer activated charcoal, if available. Ipecac-induced emesis may be useful for initial treatment at the scene (eg, children at home) if it can be given within a few minutes of exposure.

        2. **Hospital.** Administer activated charcoal and a cathartic. For large ingestions (eg, more than 1 packet), consider gastric lavage and extra doses of charcoal (ie, to maintain 10:1 ratio of charcoal to PNU).

    D. **Enhanced elimination.** Forced diuresis, dialysis, and hemoperfusion are not effective. Repeat-dose charcoal treatment has not been studied.

VALPROIC ACID
Thomas E. Kearney, PharmD

ANTIDOTE   IPECAC   LAVAGE   CHARCOAL

Valproic acid (Depakene, Depakote [divalproex sodium]) is a structurally unique anticonvulsant and represents one of the newer agents marketed since 1978. It is used alone or in combination with other agents for the treatment of absence, partial complex, and generalized seizure disorders, and is a secondary agent for refractory status epilepticus.

I. **Mechanism of toxicity**

A. Valproic acid is a small-molecular-weight (144.21), branched-chain carboxylic acid (pKa = 4.8) that increases levels of the inhibitory neurotransmitter γ-aminobutyric acid (GABA). These properties may be responsible for its action as a general central nervous system (CNS) depressant, as well as disruption of amino acid and fatty acid metabolism and other metabolic pertubations observed in overdose.

B. **Pharmacokinetics**

1. Valproic acid is rapidly and completely absorbed from the gastrointestinal tract. There is a delay in the absorption with the preparation Depakote (divalproex sodium), because of its delayed-release formulation as well as the sequential process of intestinal conversion of divalproex to 2 molecules of valproic acid.

2. At therapeutic levels, valproic acid is highly protein-bound (80–95%) and primarily confined to the extracellular space with a small (0.13–0.22 L/kg) volume of distribution (Vd). In overdose, and at levels exceeding 90 μg/mL, saturation of protein-binding sites occurs, resulting in a greater circulating free fraction of valproic acid and a larger Vd.

3. Valproic acid is predominantly metabolized by the liver and may undergo some degree of enterohepatic recirculation. The elimination half-life is 5–20 hours (average 10.6 hours). In overdose, the half-life may be prolonged to as long as 30 hours. A level exceeding 1000 μg/mL may not drop into the therapeutic range for at least 3 days.

II. **Toxic dose.** The usual daily dose for adults is 1.2–1.5 g, to achieve therapeutic serum levels of 50–100 μg/mL, and the suggested maximum daily dose is 60 mg/kg. Acute ingestions exceeding 200 mg/kg are associated with high risk for significant CNS depression. The lowest published fatal dose is 15 g (750 mg/kg) in a 20-month-old, but adult patients have survived after ingestion of 75 g.

III. **Clinical presentation**

A. **Acute overdose**

1. Acute ingestion commonly causes gastrointestinal upset, variable CNS depression (confusion, disorientation, obtundation, coma with respiratory failure), and occasionally hypotension with tachycardia. The pupils may be miotic, and the presentation may mimic an opiate poisoning. Cardiorespiratory arrest has been associated with severe intoxication; and the morbidity and mortality from valproic acid poisoning seem to be related primarily to hypoxia.

2. Paradoxic seizures may occur in patients with a preexisting seizure disorder.

3. Transient rises of transaminase levels have been observed, without evidence of liver toxicity. Hyperammonemia with encephalopathy has been observed with therapeutic levels and in overdose. At very high serum levels (> 1000 μg/mL) after large ingestions, other metabolic and electrolyte abnormalities may be observed, including an increased anion gap acidosis, hypocalcemia, and hypernatremia.

4. Other complications or late sequelae (days after ingestion) associated with severe intoxication may include optic nerve atrophy, cerebral edema, noncardiogenic pulmonary edema, anuria, and pancreatitis (in one fatal case).

B. **Adverse effects of chronic valproic acid therapy** include hepatic failure (high-risk patients are less than 2 years of age, receiving multiple anticonvulsants, or have other long-term neurologic complications), red cell aplasia, thrombocytopenia, and neutropenia. These effects are not dose-related and are not seen after an acute overdose. Pancreatitis is usually considered a non–dose related effect. Alopecia has been associated with both acute and chronic valproic acid intoxication.

C. Valproic acid is a known human teratogen.

IV. **Diagnosis** is based on the history of exposure and typical findings of CNS depression and metabolic disturbances. The differential diagnosis is broad and includes most CNS depressants. Encephalopathy and hyperammonemia may mimic Reye's syndrome.

A. Specific levels. Obtain a stat serum valproic acid level. Serial valproic acid level determinations should be obtained, particularly after ingestion of divalproex-containing preparations (Depakote) owing to the potential for delayed absorption. Note that the enzyme-multiplied immunoassay technique (EMIT) assay for valproic acid may provide serum level results that are 50% higher than actual levels because of cross-reactivity of metabolites.

1. In general, serum levels exceeding 180 µg/mL are associated with coma, and levels greater than 1000 µg/mL are associated with coma with metabolic pertubations. However, there appears to be no or little correlation of serum levels with outcome; inconsistency with clinical effects probably results from several variables, including chronicity of usage with development of tolerance, alteration of protein binding, synergism with other sedative-hypnotics, presence of metabolic abnormalities, and hypoxia-related sequelae.

2. Death from acute valproic acid poisoning has been associated with peak levels ranging from 106–2728 µg/mL, and survival was reported in a patient with a peak level of 2120 µg/mL.

B. Other useful laboratory studies. Electrolytes, glucose, BUN, creatinine, calcium, ammonia, liver transaminases, bilirubin, prothrombin time (PT), amylase, serum osmolality and osmolar gap (see p 30; serum levels > 1500 µg/mL may increase the osmolar gap), arterial blood gases or oximetry, ECG monitoring. Valproic acid may cause a false-positive urine ketone determination.

V. Treatment

A. Emergency and supportive measures

1. Maintain the airway and assist ventilation if needed (see p 4). Administer supplemental oxygen.

2. Treat coma (p 18), hypotension (p 15), and seizures (p 22) if they occur. Corticosteroids, hyperventilation, barbiturates, and osmotic agents have been used anecdotally to treat cerebral edema.

3. Treat acidosis, hypocalcemia, or hypernatremia if they are severe and symptomatic.

4. Monitor patients for at least 6 hours after ingestion, and for up to 12 hours after ingestion of Depakote (divalproex sodium) because of the potential for delayed absorption.

B. Specific drugs and antidotes. There is no specific antidote. Naloxone (see p 355) has been reported to increase arousal, but inconsistently, with greatest success in patients with serum valproic acid levels of 185–190 µg/mL.

C. Decontamination (see p 44)

1. **Prehospital.** Administer activated charcoal, if available. Ipecac-induced emesis may be useful for initial treatment at the scene (eg, children at home) if it can be given within a few minutes of exposure. *Note:* Valproic acid may cause abrupt onset of CNS depression and paradoxic seizures in some patients.

2. **Hospital.** Administer activated charcoal and a cathartic. Consider gastric lavage for large ingestions. Moderately large ingestions (eg, > 5–10 g) theoretically require extra doses of activated charcoal to maintain the desired charcoal:drug ratio of 10:1. The charcoal is not given all at once, but in repeated 25- to 50-g quantities over the first 12–24 hours.

D. Enhanced elimination (see p 49). Although valproic acid is highly protein bound at therapeutic serum levels, saturation of protein-binding in overdose makes valproic acid favorably disposed to enhanced removal methods.

1. **Hemodialysis and hemoperfusion.** Hemodialysis may result in a four- to fivefold decrease in elimination half-life in overdose patients. Dialysis also corrects metabolic disturbances and removes valproic acid metabolites. Consider dialysis in patients with serum valproic acid levels exceeding 1500–2000 µg/mL, where otherwise 4–5 days may be required for levels to

drop to the therapeutic range, since these cases are associated with higher morbidity and mortality. Charcoal hemoperfusion has also been utilized with clearances similar to those observed with hemodialysis.

2. **Repeat-dose activated charcoal.** Theoretically, repeated doses of charcoal may enhance clearance by interruption of enterohepatic recirculation, but no data exist to confirm or quantify this benefit. Another benefit is enhanced gastrointestinal decontamination after large or massive ingestion, since single doses of charcoal are inadequate to adsorb all ingested drug. Also consider repeat-dose charcoal in comatose patients with moderately high serum levels (eg, > 200–1000 µg/mL), as long as the airway is adequately protected.

VASODILATORS
Olga F. Woo, PharmD

ANTIDOTE IPECAC LAVAGE CHARCOAL

A variety of vasodilators and alpha-receptor blockers are used in clinical medicine (see Table II–54). Alpha-adrenergic blocking agents (eg, phenoxybenzamine, phentolamine, tolazoline) have been used in clinical practice since the 1940s. The first selective α_1 inhibitor, prazosin, was introduced in the early 1970s; doxazosin, indoramin, terazosin, trimazosin, and urapidil are newer α_1-selective agents. Serious acute overdoses of these agents seldom occur. Nitroprusside (see p 231) and nitrates (see p 229) are discussed elsewhere.

I. **Mechanism of toxicity.** All these drugs dilate peripheral arterioles to lower blood pressure. A reflex sympathetic response results in tachycardia and occasionally cardiac arrhythmias. Prazosin and other newer α_1 specific agents are associated with little or no reflex tachycardia.

II. **Toxic dose.** The minimum toxic or lethal doses of these drugs have not been established. No fatalities have been reported except with indoramin overdose and excessive intravenous doses of phentolamine.

A. **Indoramin.** A 43-year-old woman died 6 hours after ingesting 250 mg.

B. **Prazosin.** A young man developed priapism 24 hours after an overdose of 150

TABLE II–54. PHARMACOKINETIC PROPERTIES OF SOME VASODILATORS

Drug	Volume of Distribution (L/kg)	Peak Absorption (h)	Elimination Half-Life (h)
Diazoxide	0.19–0.25	3–6	24
Doxazosin		2–3	22
Hydralazine	1.6	0.5–1	2–8
Indoramin	7.4	1–2	1–2[a]
Minoxidil	2.8–3.3	1	2.8–4.2
Phenoxybenzamine			24
Phentolamine			2–5
Prazosin	0.6–1.7	2–4	2–4
Terazosin		1–2	9–12
Urapidil			4.7

[a]6.6 to 32.8 in elderly patients

mg. A 19-year-old man became hypotensive after taking 200 mg and recovered within 36 hours. Two elderly men ingesting 40–120 mg were found comatose with Cheyne-Stokes breathing and recovered after 15–18 hours.

C. Pharmacokinetics. Most vasodilators are eliminated by hepatic metabolism (see Table II–54).

III. Clinical presentation. Acute overdose may cause headache, nausea, dizziness, weakness, syncope, orthostatic hypotension, warm flushed skin, and palpitations. Lethargy and ataxia may occur in children. Severe hypotension may result in cerebral and myocardial ischemia and acute renal failure.

IV. Diagnosis is based on a history of exposure and the presence of orthostatic hypotension, which may or may not be accompanied by reflex tachycardia.

A. Specific levels. Blood levels of these drugs are not routinely available or clinically useful.

B. Other useful laboratory studies. Electrolytes, glucose, BUN, creatinine, ECG and ECG monitoring.

V. Treatment

A. Emergency and supportive measures

1. Maintain the airway and assist ventilation if necessary (see p 4).
2. Hypotension usually responds to supine positioning and intravenous crystalloid fluids. Occasionally, pressor therapy is needed (p 15).

B. Specific drugs and antidotes. There is no specific antidote.

C. Decontamination (see p 44)

1. **Prehospital.** Administer activated charcoal, if available. Ipecac-induced emesis may be useful for initial treatment at the scene (eg, children at home) if it can be given within 30 minutes of exposure.
2. **Hospital.** Administer activated charcoal and a cathartic. Gastric emptying is not necessary if activated charcoal can be given promptly.

D. Enhanced elimination. There is no clinical experience with extracorporeal drug removal for these agents. Terazosin and doxazosin are long-acting and eliminated 60% in feces; thus, repeat-dose activated charcoal may enhance their elimination.

VITAMINS
Gerald Joe, PharmD

ANTIDOTE   IPECAC   LAVAGE   CHARCOAL

Acute toxicity is unlikely following ingestion of vitamin products that do not contain iron (when iron is present, see p 189). Vitamins A and D may cause toxicity but usually only after chronic use. The essential amino acid L-tryptophan is not a vitamin, but has been considered a dietary supplement and was widely used for treatment of depression, premenstrual symptoms, and insomnia until it was linked to the eosinophiliamyalgia syndrome and its sale was banned by the FDA.

I. Mechanism of toxicity

A. Vitamin A. The mechanism by which excessive amounts of vitamin A produce increased intracranial pressure is not known.

B. Vitamin D. Chronic ingestion of excessive amounts of vitamin D enhances calcium absorption and produces hypercalcemia.

C. Niacin. Histamine release results in cutaneous flushing and pruritus.

D. Pyridoxine. Chronic overdose may alter neuronal conduction, resulting in paresthesias and muscular incoordination.

E. Vitamin C. Chronic excessive use and large intravenous doses can produce increased levels of the metabolite oxalic acid. Urinary acidification promotes calcium oxalate crystal formation, which can result in nephropathy or acute renal failure.

F. Tryptophan. L-tryptophan can enhance brain serotonin levels, especially in patients taking monoamine oxidase (MAO) inhibitors (see p 22). The mechanism involved in causing eosinophilia-myalgia syndrome is unknown, but appears to be related to a contaminant associated with mass production of the amino acid by one Japanese producer.

II. Toxic dose

A. Vitamin A. Acute ingestion of more than 12,000 IU/kg is considered toxic. Chronic ingestion of more than 25,000 IU/d for 2–3 weeks may produce toxicity.

B. Vitamin D. Acute ingestion is highly unlikely to produce toxicity. Chronic ingestion in children of more than 5000 IU/d for several weeks (adults > 25,000 IU/d) may result in toxicity.

C. Niacin. Acute ingestion of more than 100 mg may cause dermal flushing reaction.

D. Pyridoxine. Chronic ingestion of 2–5 g/d for several months has resulted in neuropathy.

E. Vitamin C. Acute intravenous doses of more than 1.5 g and chronic ingestion of more than 4 g/d have produced nephropathy.

III. Clinical presentation. Most acute overdoses of multivitamins are associated with nausea, vomiting, and diarrhea.

A. Chronic **vitamin A** toxicity is characterized by dry, peeling skin and signs of increased intracranial pressure (headache, altered mental status, blurred vision). Bulging fontanelles have been described in infants. Liver injury may cause jaundice and ascites.

B. Chronic excessive use of **vitamin D** is associated with hypercalcemia, producing weakness, altered mental status, gastrointestinal upset, renal tubular injury, and occasionally cardiac arrhythmias.

C. Acute ingestion of **niacin** but not niacinamide (nicotinamide) may produce unpleasant cutaneous flushing and pruritus. Chronic excessive use has been associated with hepatitis.

D. Chronic excessive **pyridoxine** use may result in peripheral neuropathy.

E. Large doses of **B vitamins** may intensify the yellow color of urine, and **riboflavin** may produce yellow perspiration.

F. Vitamin C. Calcium oxalate crystals may cause acute renal failure or chronic nephropathy.

G. Tryptophan

1. Use of L-tryptophan by persons taking monoamine oxidase (MAO) inhibitors may cause myoclonus and hyperthermia ("serotonin syndrome," see p 21).

2. Chronic use of L-tryptophan has been associated with development of eosinophilia-myalgia syndrome, characterized by high eosinophil counts (> 1000/microL), severe generalized myalgias, and swelling and induration of the skin. Fever, polyneuropathy, and death have also been reported.

IV. Diagnosis of vitamin overdose is usually based on a history of ingestion. Cutaneous flushing and pruritus suggest a niacin reaction but may be caused by other histaminergic agents.

A. Specific levels. Serum vitamin A (retinol) or carotenoid assays may assist in the diagnosis of hypervitaminosis A. Other serum vitamin concentration measurements are not useful.

B. Other useful laboratory studies. CBC, electrolytes, glucose, BUN, calcium, creatinine, liver transaminases, urinalysis.

V. Treatment

A. Emergency and supportive measures

1. Treat fluid losses caused by gastroenteritis with intravenous crystalloid solutions (see p 15).

2. Treat vitamin A–induced elevated intracranial pressure and vitamin D–induced hypercalcemia if they occur.

3. Antihistamines may alleviate niacin–induced histamine release.

B. Specific drugs and antidotes. There is no specific antidote.

    C. Decontamination (see p 44). Usually, gut decontamination is unnecessary unless a toxic dose of vitamin A or D has been ingested, or if the product contains a toxic amount of iron (see p 189).

        1. Prehospital. Administer activated charcoal, if available. Ipecac-induced emesis may be useful for initial treatment at the scene (eg, children at home) if it can be given within 30 minutes of exposure.

        2. Hospital. Administer activated charcoal and a cathartic. Gastric emptying is not necessary if activated charcoal can be given promptly.

    D. Enhanced elimination. Forced diuresis, dialysis, and hemoperfusion are of no clinical benefit.

Section III. **Therapeutic Drugs and Antidotes**

Thomas E. Kearney, PharmD

INTRODUCTION

This section provides detailed descriptions of antidotes and other therapeutic agents used in the management of a poisoned patient. For each agent, a summary is provided of its pharmacologic effects, clinical indications, adverse effects and contraindications, usage in pregnancy, dosage, available formulations, and recommended minimum stocking levels for the hospital pharmacy. This information was obtained from a variety of resources, as noted in the bibliography.

I. **Use of antidotes in pregnancy.** It is always prudent to avoid or minimize drug exposure during pregnancy, and physicians are often reluctant to use an antidote for fear of potential fetal harm. This reluctance, however, must be tempered with a case-by-case risk/benefit analysis of use of the particular therapeutic agent. An acute drug overdose or poisoning in pregnancy may threaten the life of the mother as well as the fetus, and the antidote or therapeutic agent, despite unknown or questionable effects on the fetus, may have lifesaving benefit. The inherent toxicity and large body burden of the drug or toxic chemical involved in the poisoning may far exceed that of the indicated therapeutic agent or antidote.

With most agents discussed in this section, there is little or no information regarding their use in pregnant patients. The **Food and Drug Administration (FDA)** has established 5 categories of required labeling to indicate the potential for teratogenicity (see Table III–1). The distinction between categories depends mainly on the amount and reliability of animal and human data and the risk/benefit assessment for use of the agent. Note that the categorization may be based on anticipated chronic or repeated use and may not be relevant to a single or brief antidotal treatment.

II. **Hospital planning and stocking.** As hospitals prepare for reaccreditation by the Joint Commission on Accreditation of Healthcare Organizations (JCAHO), they need to be familiar with the specific requirements pertaining to toxicology information and resources listed in the "Emergency Services" and "Pharmaceutical Services" chapters of the *Accreditation Manual for Hospitals*.

A. **Reference materials.** The JCAHO recommends that current toxicologic reference materials and antidote information be readily available in the Emergency

TABLE III–1. FDA PREGNANCY CATEGORIES FOR TERATOGENIC EFFECTS

FDA Pregnancy Category	Definition
A	Adequate and well-controlled studies in pregnant women have failed to demonstrate a risk to the fetus in the first trimester, and there is no evidence of a risk in later pregnancy. The possibility of fetal harm appears remote.
B	Either (1) animal reproduction studies have failed to demonstrate any adverse effect (other than a decrease in fertility), but there are no adequate and well-controlled studies in pregnant women, or (2) animal studies have shown an adverse effect that was not confirmed by adequate and well-controlled studies in pregnant women. The possibility of fetal harm is probably remote.
C	Either (1) animal reproduction studies have shown an adverse effect on the fetus and there are no adequate and well-controlled human studies, or (2) there are no animal or human studies. The drug should be given only if the potential benefit outweighs the potential risk to the fetus.
D	There is positive evidence of human fetal risk based on adverse reaction data from investigational or marketing experience or human studies, but the potential risks may be acceptable in light of potential benefits (eg, use in a life-threatening situation for which safer drugs are ineffective or unavailalbe).
X	Studies in animals or humans have demonstrated fetal abnormalities, or there is positive evidence of fetal risk based on human experience, or both, and the risk of using the drug in a pregnant patient outweighs any possible benefit. The drug is contraindicated in women who are or who may become pregnant.

Reference: *Code of Federal Regulations*, title 21, section 201.57 (4/1/90).

Department, along with the telephone number of the regional poison control center (see p 53). In addition, up-to-date pharmaceutical reference materials should be available to pharmaceutical, medical, and nursing staffs.

B. Stocking levels. The pharmacy should maintain the medical staff–approved stock of antidotes and other emergency drugs. Many antidotes are used only infrequently, have a short shelf life, or are expensive. Optimal case management, however, requires having adequate supplies of antidotes readily available. Fortunately, only a minimal acquisition and maintenance cost is required to adequately stock many of these drugs.

1. The basis for our **suggested minimum stocking level** is a combination of factors to anticipate the highest total dose of a drug generally given during a 24-hour time period as quoted in the literature, the maximum manufacturer's recommended or tolerated daily dose, and estimation of these quantities for a 70-kg adult.

2. The possibility exists that larger quantities of a drug may be needed in unusual situations, particularly if multiple patients are treated simultaneously or for extended periods of time. Hospitals in close proximity to one another may wish to explore the practicality of sharing stocks, but should carefully consider the logistics of such arrangements (eg, transferring stocks after hours or on weekends).

ACETYLCYSTEINE
(N-ACETYLCYSTEINE, NAC)

Thomas E. Kearney, PharmD

I. Pharmacology. Acetylcysteine (N-acetylcysteine, NAC) is a mucolytic agent that acts as a sulfhydryl group donor, substituting for the liver's usual sulfhydryl donor glutathione. It rapidly binds (detoxifies) the highly reactive intermediates of metabolism. It is most effective in preventing acetaminophen-induced liver injury when given early in the course of intoxication (within 8–10 hours), but may also be of benefit in reducing the severity of liver injury even when given after 24 hours. It may be used empirically when the severity of ingestion is unknown or serum concentrations of the ingested drug are not immediately available.

II. Indications

A. Acetaminophen overdose.

B. Carbon tetrachloride, chloroform, mercury, or lead poisoning (unproved).

C. Pennyroyal oil (one case report). The mechanism of hepatic injury by pennyroyal oil is similar to that of acetaminophen, and empiric use of NAC seems justified for any significant pennyroyal oil ingestion.

III. Contraindications. Known hypersensitivity (rare).

IV. Adverse effects

A. Acetylcysteine typically causes nausea and vomiting when given **orally.** If the dose is vomited, it should be repeated. Use of a gastric tube, slower rate of administration, and a strong antiemetic agent (eg, metoclopramide, ondansetron) may be necessary.

B. Rapid **intravenous** administration can cause flushing, hypotension, and bronchospasm (anaphylactoid reaction). One death was reported in a small child rapidly receiving a large dose rapidly intravenously. Reactions can be minimized by giving each dose slowly over 45–60 minutes.

C. Use in pregnancy. There is no evidence for teratogenicity. Use of this drug to treat acetaminophen overdose is considered beneficial to both mother and developing fetus.

V. Drug or laboratory interactions. Activated charcoal adsorbs acetylcysteine and may interfere with its systemic absorption when both are given orally together; data suggest that peak acetylcysteine levels are decreased by about 30% and that the time to reach peak level may be delayed. However, these effects are not considered clinically important.

VI. Dosage and method of administration

A. Oral loading dose. Give 140 mg/kg of the 10% or 20% solution diluted to 5% in juice or soda.

B. Maintenance oral dose. 70 mg/kg every 4 hrs for 17 doses (FDA protocol) , or 6 doses if no evident hepatotoxicity and serum level has fallen to zero.

C. Intravenous administration is *not* approved in the USA. Contact a medical toxicologist or regional poison center (see p 53) for advice. A 48-hour investigational protocol showed safety and efficacy using the same doses and intervals as for oral administration. In the UK, the dosing regimen is 150 mg/kg in 200 mL of 5% dextrose in water (D5W) over 15 minutes, followed by 50 mg/kg in 500 mL of D5W over 4 hours, and then 100 mg/kg in 1000 mL of D5W over 16 hours.

D. Dosage during dialysis. Although acetylcysteine is removed during dialysis, no change in dosage is necessary.

VII. Formulations

A. The usual formulation is as a 10% (100 mg/mL) or 20% (200 mg/mL) solution, supplied as an inhaled mucolytic agent (Mucomyst). This form is available through most hospital pharmacies or respiratory therapy departments. This preparation is *not* approved for parenteral use. In rare circumstances when intravenous administration of this preparation is required, a 3% solution and a micropore filter should be used.

B. In the USA, the investigational intravenous formulation is available only at medical centers participating in an approved study.

C. Suggested minimum stocking level for treatment of a 70-kg adult for the first 24 hours: 20% solution, 7 vials (30 mL each).

ANTIVENIN, CROTALIDAE (RATTLESNAKE)

Thomas E. Kearney, PharmD

I. Pharmacology. To produce the antivenin, horses are hyperimmunized with the pooled venoms of *Crotalus adamanteus* (eastern diamondback rattlesnake), *Crotalus atrox* (western diamondback), *Crotalus durissus terrificus* (tropical rattlesnake, cascabel), and *Bothrops atrox* (fer-de-lance). The lyophilized protein product from pooled equine sera is a combination of several antibodies against venom constituents and also contains residual serum components. After intravenous administration, the antivenin is distributed widely throughout the body where it binds to venom.

II. Indications. Antivenin is used for treatment of significant envenomation by Crotalidae species (see **II**, p 285).

III. Contraindications. Known hypersensitivity to the antivenin or to horse serum is a relative contraindication; antivenin may still be indicated for severe envenomation despite allergic history.

IV. Adverse effects

A. Immediate hypersensitivity reactions (including life-threatening anaphylaxis) may occur, even in patients with no history of horse serum sensitivity and negative skin test results.

B. Mild flushing and wheezing often occur within the first 30 minutes of intravenous administration and often improve after slowing the rate of infusion.

C. Delayed hypersensitivity (serum sickness) occurs in over 75% of patients receiving more than 4 vials of antivenin and in virtually all patients who receive more than 12 vials. The onset is 5–14 days.

D. Use in pregnancy. There are no data on teratogenicity. Anaphylactic reaction resulting in shock or hypoxemia in the mother could conceivably adversely affect the fetus.

V. Drug or laboratory interactions. No known interactions.

VI. Dosage and method of administration. The initial dose is based on severity of symptoms, not on body weight (Table III–2). Children may require doses as large as or larger than those for adults. The end point of antivenin therapy is the rever-

TABLE III–2. INITIAL DOSE OF CROTALIDAE ANTIVENIN

Severity of Envenomation	Initial Dose (vials)
None or minimal	None
Mild (local pain and swelling)	5
Moderate (proximal progression of swelling, ecchymosis, mild systemic symptoms)	10
Severe (hypotension, rapidly progressive swelling and ecchymosis, coagulopathy	15

sal of systemic manifestations (eg, shock, coagulopathy, paresthesias) and the halting of progressive edema and pain. Antivenin may be effective up to 3 days or more following envenomation.

If envenomation by the Mojave rattlesnake *(Crotalus scutulatus scutulatus)* is suspected, especially if there is an increased serum CPK (creatine phosphokinase) level, administer 10 vials of antivenin even if there is minimal swelling or local pain.

A. Treat all patients in an intensive care setting.

B. Before skin test or antivenin administration, insert at least 1 and preferably 2 secure intravenous lines.

C. Perform skin test for horse serum sensitivity, using a 1:10 dilution of antivenin (some experts prefer this method) or the sample of horse serum provided in the antivenin kit (according to package instructions). Do **not** perform the skin test unless signs of envenomation are present and imminent antivenin therapy is anticipated. If the skin test is positive, reconsider the need for antivenin as opposed to supportive care, but do not abandon antivenin therapy if it is needed. Even if the skin test is negative, anaphylaxis may still occur unpredictably.

D. If antivenin is used in a patient with a positive skin test, pretreat with intravenous diphenhydramine (see p 331), 1 mg/kg slowly, and have ready at the bedside a preloaded syringe containing epinephrine (1:10,000 for intravenous use) in case of anaphylaxis. Dilute the antivenin 1:10 to 1:1000 before administration, and give each vial over 30–45 minutes, increasing the rate of infusion as tolerated.

E. Reconstitute the lyophilized product with the 10 mL of diluent provided and gently swirl for 10–30 minutes to solubilize the material. Avoid shaking, which destroys the immunoglobulins (indicated by foam formation). Further dilution with 50–200 mL of saline may facilitate solubilization.

F. Administer the diluted antivenin slowly (10–15 min/vial) by the intravenous route only.

VII. Formulations

A. Antivenin (Crotalidae) Polyvalent. Supplies can be located by a regional poison center (see Table I–41, p 53).

B. **Suggested minimum stocking level** to treat a 70-kg adult for the first 24 hours: 20 vials.

ANTIVENIN, *LATRODECTUS MACTANS* (BLACK WIDOW SPIDER)

Thomas E. Kearney, PharmD

I. Pharmacology. To produce the antivenin, horses are hyperimmunized with *Latrodectus mactans* (black widow spider) venom. The lyophilized protein product from pooled equine sera contains antibody specific to certain venom fractions, as well as residual serum proteins such as albumin and globulins. After intravenous administration, the antivenin distributes widely throughout the body where it binds to venom.

II. Indications

A. Severe hypertension or muscle cramping not alleviated by muscle relaxants, analgesics, or sedation, particularly in patients at the extremes of age (ie, younger than 1 year or older than 65 years).

 B. Black widow envenomation in **pregnancy** may cause abdominal muscle spasm severe enough to threaten spontaneous abortion or early onset of labor.

III. Contraindications. Known hypersensitivity to horse serum.

IV. Adverse effects

 A. Immediate hypersensitivity may occur, including life-threatening anaphylaxis.

 B. Delayed-onset serum sickness may occur after 10–14 days.

 C. Use in pregnancy. There are no data on teratogenicity. Anaphylactic reaction resulting in shock or hypoxemia in the mother could conceivably adversely affect the fetus.

V. Drug or laboratory interactions. No known interactions.

VI. Dosage and method of administration. Generally, one vial of antivenin is sufficient to treat black widow envenomation in adults or children.

 A. Treat all patients in an intensive care setting.

 B. Before skin test or antivenin administration, insert at least 1 and preferably 2 secure intravenous lines.

 C. Perform skin test for horse serum sensitivity, using a 1:10 dilution of antivenin (some experts prefer this method) or the sample of horse serum provided in the antivenin kit (according to package instructions). Do *not* perform the skin test unless signs of envenomation are present and imminent antivenin therapy is anticipated. If the skin test is positive, reconsider the need for antivenin as opposed to supportive care, but do not abandon antivenin therapy if it is needed. Even if the skin test is negative, anaphylaxis may still occur unpredictably.

 D. If antivenin is used in a patient with horse serum sensitivity, pretreat with intravenous diphenhydramine (see p 331), 1 mg/kg slowly, and have ready at the bedside a preloaded syringe containing epinephrine (1:10,000 for intravenous use) in case of anaphylaxis. Dilute the antivenin (1:10 to 1:1000) and give very slowly.

 E. Reconstitute the lyophilized product to 2.5 mL with the supplied diluent, using gentle swirling for 15–30 minutes to avoid shaking and destroying the immunoglobulins (indicated by the formation of foam).

 F. Dilute this solution to a total volume of 10–50 mL with normal saline.

 G. Administer the diluted antivenin slowly over 15–30 minutes.

VII. Formulations

 A. Lyophilized Antivenin *(L mactans),* 6000 units.

 B. Suggested minimum stocking level to treat a 70-kg adult for the first 24 hours: 1 vial.

ANTIVENIN, *MICRURUS FULVIUS* (CORAL SNAKE)

Thomas E. Kearney, PharmD

I. Pharmacology. To produce the antivenin, horses are hyperimmunized with venom from *Micrurus fulvius,* the eastern coral snake. The lyophilized protein preparation from pooled equine sera contains antibody to venom fractions as well as residual serum proteins. Administered intravenously, the antibody distributes widely throughout the body where it binds the target venom.

II. Indications

 A. Envenomation by the eastern coral snake *(M fulvius)* or the Texas coral snake *(M fulvius tenere)* (see p 285).

 B. *Not* effective for envenomation by the western, Arizona, or Sonora coral snake *(M euryxanthus).*

III. Contraindications. Known hypersensitivity to the antivenin or to horse serum is a relative contraindication; if a patient with significant envenomation needs the antivenin, it should be given with caution.

IV. Adverse effects

A. Immediate hypersensitivity, including life-threatening anaphylaxis, may occur even after a negative skin test for horse serum sensitivity.

B. Delayed hypersensitivity (serum sickness) may occur 1–3 weeks after antivenin administration, the severity depending on the total quantity of antivenin administered.

C. Use in pregnancy. There are no data on teratogenicity. Anaphylactic reaction resulting in shock or hypoxemia in the mother could conceivably adversely affect the fetus.

V. Drug or laboratory interactions. No known interactions.

VI. Dosage and method of administration. Generally, the recommended initial dose is 3–5 vials. The drug is most effective if given prior to the onset of signs or symptoms of envenomation. An additional 3–5 vials may be given, depending on the severity of neurological manifestations and not on body weight (children may require doses as large as or even larger than those for adults).

A. Treat all patients in an intensive care unit setting.

B. Before skin test or antivenin administration, insert at least 1 and preferably 2 secure intravenous lines.

C. Perform skin test for horse serum sensitivity, using a 1:10 dilution of antivenin (some experts prefer this method) or the sample of horse serum provided in the antivenin kit (according to package instructions). If the skin test is positive, reconsider the need for antivenin as opposed to supportive care, but do not abandon antivenin therapy if it is needed. Even if the skin test is negative, anaphylaxis may still occur unpredictably.

D. If antivenin is used in a patient with a positive skin test, pretreat with intravenous diphenhydramine (see p 331), 1 mg/kg slowly, and have ready at the bedside a preloaded syringe containing epinephrine (1:10,000 for intravenous use) in case of anaphylaxis. Dilute the antivenin (1:10 to 1:1000) and administer very slowly.

E. Reconstitute the lyophilized material with the 10 mL of the diluent supplied, gently swirling for 10–30 minutes. Avoid shaking the preparation because this may destroy the immunoglobulins (indicated by the formation of foam). Dilution with 50–200 mL of saline may aid solubilization.

F. Administer the antivenin intravenously over 15–30 minutes.

VII. Formulations

A. Antivenin *(M fulvius).*

B. Suggested minimum stocking level to treat a 70-kg adult for the first 24 hours: 5–10 vials.

APOMORPHINE

Thomas E. Kearney, PharmD

I. Pharmacology. Apomorphine is an alkaloid salt derived from morphine that has minimal analgesic properties but marked emetic efficacy. Vomiting is produced by direct stimulation of the medullary chemoreceptor trigger zone. Following subcutaneous administration, emesis occurs within an average time period of 5 minutes; oral administration is *not* recommended because of erratic absorption.

II. Indications. Apomorphine was previously used for induction of emesis in the acute management of oral poisoning, but it has been abandoned because of its potential for respiratory depression and its inconvenient formulation (soluble tablets for parenteral injection). The drug is not discussed further in this book, but it remains popular in veterinary practice.

ATROPINE

Thomas E. Kearney, PharmD

I. Pharmacology. Atropine is a parasympatholytic agent that competitively blocks the action of acetylcholine at muscarinic receptors. Desired therapeutic effects for treating poisoning include decreased secretions from salivary and other glands, decreased bronchorrhea and wheezing, decreased intestinal peristalsis, increased heart rate, and enhanced atrioventricular conduction.

II. Indications

A. Correction of bronchorrhea and excessive salivation associated with organophosphate and carbamate insecticide intoxication.

B. Acceleration of the rate of sinus node firing and atrioventricular nodal conduction velocity in the presence of drug-induced atrioventricular conduction impairment (eg, digitalis, beta blockers, calcium antagonists, organophosphate or carbamate insecticides, physostigmine).

C. Reversal of central and peripheral muscarinic symptoms in patients with intoxication by *Clitocybe* or *Inocybe* mushroom species.

III. Contraindications

A. Angle-closure glaucoma in which pupillary dilation may increase intraocular pressure.

B. Patients with hypertension, tachyarrhythmias, congestive heart failure, and coronary artery disease who might not tolerate a rapid heart rate.

C. Partial or complete obstructive uropathy.

D. Myasthenia gravis.

IV. Adverse effects

A. Some adverse effects include dry mouth, blurred vision, cycloplegia, mydriasis, urinary retention, tachycardia, aggravation of angina, and constipation. Duration of effects may be prolonged (several hours).

B. Doses less than 0.5 mg (in adults) and those administered by very slow intravenous push may result in paradoxic slowing of heart rate.

C. Use in pregnancy. FDA category C (indeterminate). It readily crosses the placenta. However, this does not preclude its acute, short-term use for a seriously symptomatic patient (see p 310).

V. Drug or laboratory interactions

A. Atropinization may occur more rapidly if atropine and pralidoxime are given concurrently to patients with organophosphate or carbamate insecticide poisoning.

B. Atropine has an additive effect with other antimuscarinic and antihistaminic compounds.

C. Slowing of gastrointestinal motility may delay absorption of orally ingested materials.

VI. Dosage and method of administration

A. Organophosphate or carbamate insecticide poisoning. For adults, give 1–5 mg IV; for children, give 0.05 mg/kg IV. Repeat every 5–10 minutes until satisfactory atropinization is achieved. The goal of therapy is drying of bronchial secretions (this end point may be reached prematurely if the patient is dehydrated) and reversal of wheezing and significant bradycardia. Recrudescence of symptoms may occur, and in severe poisonings several grams of atropine may be required and may be administered by constant intravenous infusion.

B. Drug-induced bradycardia. For adults, give 0.5–1 mg IV; for children, give 0.01–0.05 mg/kg up to a maximum dose of 0.5 mg IV. Repeat as needed. Note that 3 mg is a fully vagolytic dose in adults. If response is not achieved by 3 mg, the patient is unlikely to benefit from further treatment unless bradycardia is caused by excessive cholinergic effect (eg, carbamate or organophosphate overdose).

VII. Formulations

A. Parenteral. Atropine sulfate injection, 0.05-, 0.1-, 0.3-, 0.4-, 0.5-, 0.6-, 0.8-, 1-, and 1.2-mg/mL solutions. Use preservative-free formulations when massive doses are required.

B. Suggested minimum stocking level to treat a 70-kg adult for the first 24 hours: 1 g.

BAL (DIMERCAPROL)

Thomas E. Kearney, PharmD

I. **Pharmacology.** BAL (British antilewisite, Dimercaprol) is a dithiol chelating agent used in the treatment of poisoning by the heavy metals arsenic, mercury, lead, and gold. It is of no value for the treatment of poisoning by selenium, iron, or cadmium; in fact, it is contraindicated in these poisonings because the BAL-metal (mercaptide) complex may be more toxic than the metal alone. Adequate doses of BAL must be given to ensure an excess of free BAL. An insufficient concentration of BAL may allow dissociation of the BAL-metal complex. This chelate dissociates more rapidly in an acid urine; adequate renal function must exist to allow elimination of the mercaptide complex.

II. **Indications**

A. Arsenic poisoning (except arsine, for which BAL is ineffective).

B. Mercury poisoning (except monoalkyl mercury). BAL is most effective in preventing renal damage if administered within 2 hours after ingestion; it is not effective in reversing neurologic damage caused by chronic mercury poisoning.

C. Lead poisoning (except alkyl lead compounds). Calcium EDTA (p 335) and DMSA (p 332) are the preferred chelating agents, but BAL is commonly used as adjunctive therapy in patients with acute lead encephalopathy.

D. Possibly effective for poisoning caused by antimony, bismuth, chromium, copper, gold, nickel, tungsten, or zinc.

III. **Contraindications**

A. Heavy metal poisoning resulting from iron, cadmium, selenium, or uranium (BAL-metal complex is more toxic than the metal alone).

B. Poisoning caused by thallium, tellurium, or vanadium (BAL is ineffective).

C. Glucose-6-phosphate dehydrogenase (G6PD) deficiency. BAL may cause hemolysis; use only in life-threatening situations.

D. Hepatic impairment (except arsenic-induced jaundice).

E. Renal impairment. Avoid BAL or use only with extreme caution.

IV. **Adverse effects**

A. Local pain at injection site, sterile or pyogenic abscess formation.

B. Dose-related hypertension, with or without tachycardia. Onset 15–30 minutes, duration 2 hours. Use with caution in hypertensive patients.

C. Nephrotoxicity. Urine should be kept alkaline to protect renal function and to prevent dissociation of metal-BAL complex.

D. Nausea, vomiting, headache, lacrimation, rhinorrhea, salivation, urticaria, myalgias, paresthesias, dysuria, fever (particularly in children), central nervous system depression, seizures.

E. Thrombocytopenia and increased prothrombin time, which may limit intramuscular administration.

F. Despite its capacity to increase survival in acutely intoxicated animals, use of BAL is associated with redistribution of mercury and arsenic into the brain.

G. **Use in pregnancy.** BAL is embryotoxic in mice. Safety of BAL in human pregnancy is not established, although it has been used in a pregnant patient with Wilson's disease without apparent harm. It should be used in pregnancy only for life-threatening acute intoxication.

V. **Drug or laboratory interactions**

A. BAL forms toxic complexes with iron, cadmium, selenium, and uranium. Avoid concurrent iron replacement therapy.

B. BAL may abruptly terminate gold therapy—induced remission of rheumatoid arthritis.

C. BAL interferes with iodine accumulation by the thyroid.

VI. **Dosage and method of administration (adults and children)**

A. **Arsenic, mercury, and gold poisoning.** Give BAL, 3 mg/kg deep IM every 4–6 hours for 2 days, then every 12 hours for 7–10 days or until recovery. In

patients with severe arsenic or mercury poisoning, an initial dose of up to 5 mg/kg may be used.
   B. Lead poisoning (in conjunction with calcium EDTA therapy [see p 335]). For symptomatic acute encephalopathy or blood lead greater than 100 µg/dL, give BAL, 4–5 mg/kg deep IM every 4 hours for 3–5 days.
VII. Formulations
   A. Parenteral (for deep IM injection only, must **not** be given as IV). BAL in oil, 100 mg/mL, 3 mL ampules.
   B. Suggested minimum stocking level to treat a 70-kg adult for the first 24 hours: 1200 mg (4 ampules).

BENZTROPINE

Thomas E. Kearney, PharmD

   I. Pharmacology. Benztropine is an antimuscarinic agent with pharmacologic activity similar to that of atropine. The drug also exhibits antihistaminic properties. Benztropine is used for the treatment of parkinsonism and for the control of extrapyramidal side effects associated with neuroleptic use.
   II. Indications. Benztropine is an alternative in adults to diphenhydramine (the drug of choice for children) for the treatment of acute dystonic reactions associated with neuroleptics or metoclopramide.
   Note: It is not effective for tardive dyskinesia or neuroleptic malignant syndrome (see p 20).
   III. Contraindications
   A. Angle-closure glaucoma.
   B. Obstructive uropathy (prostatic hypertrophy).
   C. Myasthenia gravis.
   D. Not recommended for children under 3 years (use diphenhydramine; see p 20).
   IV. Adverse effects
   A. Adverse effects include sedation, blurred vision, tachycardia, urinary hesitancy or retention, and dry mouth. Adverse effects are minimal following single doses.
   B. Use in pregnancy. FDA category C (indeterminate). However, this does not preclude its acute, short-term use for a seriously symptomatic patient (see p 331).
   V. Drug or laboratory interactions
   A. Benztropine has additive effects with other drugs exhibiting antimuscarinic properties (eg, antihistamines, phenothiazines, cyclic antidepressants, disopyramide).
   B. Slowing of gastrointestinal motility may delay or inhibit absorption of certain drugs.
   VI. Dosage and method of administration
   A. Parenteral. Give 1–2 mg IV or IM (children > 3 years old, 0.02 mg/kg, 1 mg maximum).
   B. Oral. Give 1–2 mg PO every 12 hours (children > 3 years old, 0.02 mg/kg, 1 mg maximum) for 2–3 days to prevent recurrence of symptoms.
   VII. Formulations
   A. Parenteral. Benztropine mesylate (Cogentin), 1 mg/mL, 2-mL ampules.
   B. Oral. Benztropine mesylate (Cogentin), 0.5-, 1-, 2-mg tablets.
   C. Suggested minimum stocking level to treat a 70-kg adult for the first 24 hours: 6 mg (3 ampules, 2 mL each).

BICARBONATE, SODIUM

Thomas E. Kearney, PharmD

   I. Pharmacology
   A. Sodium bicarbonate is a buffering agent that reacts with hydrogen ions to cor-

rect acidemia and produce alkalemia. Urinary alkalinization from renally excreted bicarbonate ion enhances the renal elimination of certain acidic drugs (eg, salicylate, phenobarbital) and helps prevent renal tubular myoglobin deposition in patients with rhabdomyolysis. In addition, maintenance of a normal or high serum pH may prevent intracellular distribution of salicylate.

B. The sodium ion load and alkalemia produced by hypertonic sodium bicarbonate reverse sodium channel-dependent membrane-depressant ("quinidine-like") effects of several drugs (eg, cyclic antidepressants, type Ia and type Ic antiarrhythmic agents).

C. Sodium bicarbonate given orally or by gastric lavage forms an insoluble salt with iron and may help prevent absorption of ingested iron tablets (unproved).

II. Indications

A. Severe metabolic acidosis resulting from intoxication by methanol, ethylene glycol, or salicylates or from excessive lactic acid production (eg, resulting from status epilepticus or shock).

B. To produce urinary alkalinization, to enhance elimination of salicylate or phenobarbital, or to prevent renal deposition of myoglobin after severe rhabdomyolysis.

C. Cardiotoxicity (as evidenced by prolonged QRS and QT intervals) caused by cyclic antidepressants, type Ia or type Ic antiarrhythmics, and other membrane-depressant drugs.

D. Sodium bicarbonate has been used in lavage fluid to treat excessive iron ingestion (effectiveness unproved).

III. Contraindications. The following contraindications are relative.

A. Significant metabolic or respiratory alkalemia or hypernatremia.

B. Severe pulmonary edema.

IV. Adverse effects

A. Excessive alkalemia: impaired oxygen release from hemoglobin, hypocalcemic tetany, paradoxic intracellular acidosis (from elevated P_{CO2} concentrations), hypokalemia.

B. Hypernatremia, hyperosmolality.

C. Aggravation of congestive heart failure and pulmonary edema.

D. Extravasation leading to tissue inflammation and necrosis.

E. Use in pregnancy. FDA category C (indeterminate). However, this does not preclude its acute, short-term use for a seriously symptomatic patient (see p 310).

V. Drug or laboratory interactions. Do not mix with other parenteral drugs because of the possibility of drug inactivation or precipitation.

VI. Dosage and method of administration (adults and children)

A. Metabolic acidemia. Give 0.5–1 meq/kg IV bolus; repeat as needed to correct serum pH to at least 7.2. For salicylates, methanol, or ethylene glycol, raise the pH to at least 7.4–7.5.

B. Urinary alkalinization. Give 50–100 meq in 1 L of 5% dextrose in 0.25 normal saline at 2–3 mL/kg/h. Check urine pH frequently and adjust flow rate to maintain urine pH level at 6–7.

Note: Hypokalemia and fluid depletion prevent effective urinary alkalinization: add 20 meq of potassium to each liter, unless renal failure is present.

C. Cardiotoxic drug intoxication. Give 1–2 meq/kg IV bolus; repeat as needed to improve cardiotoxic manifestations and to maintain serum pH at 7.45–7.5. There is no evidence that constant infusions are as effective as boluses given as needed.

D. Gastric iron complexation. Make a 1–2% solution by diluting sodium bicarbonate with normal saline, and use 4–5 mL/kg as a gastric lavage solution.

VII. Formulations

A. Several products are available, ranging from 4.2% (0.5 meq/mL) to 8.4% (1 meq/mL) in volumes of 10–500 mL. The most commonly used formulation available in most emergency "crash carts" is 8.4% ("hypertonic") sodium bicarbonate, 1 meq/mL, in 50-mL ampules or prefilled syringes.

B. Suggested minimum stocking level to treat a 70-kg adult for the first 24 hours: 10 ampules or syringes (approximately 500 meq).

BOTULIN ANTITOXIN

Thomas E. Kearney, PharmD

I. Pharmacology. Botulin antitoxin contains concentrated equine-derived antibodies directed against the toxins produced by the various strains of *Clostridium botulinum* (A, B, and E). The trivalent form (A, B, E) provides the greatest degree of coverage and is preferred over the older bivalent (A, B) type. The antibodies bind and inactivate freely circulating botulin toxins but do **not** remove toxin that is already bound to nerve terminals. Because antitoxin will not reverse established paralysis once it occurs, it must be administered before paralysis sets in. Treatment within 24 hours of the onset of symptoms may shorten the course of intoxication and may prevent progression to total paralysis.

II. Indications. Botulin antitoxin is used to treat clinical botulism to prevent progression of neurologic manifestations. It is generally not recommended for treatment of infant botulism; however, clinical trials are underway in California with human-derived botulism immune globulin (BIG).

III. Contraindications. No absolute contraindications. Known hypersensitivity to botulin antitoxin or horse serum requires extreme caution if this product is given.

IV. Adverse effects
  A. Immediate hypersensitivity reactions (anaphylaxis) resulting from the equine source of antibodies.
  B. Delayed Arthus reaction (serum sickness) 1–2 weeks after antitoxin administration.
  C. Use in pregnancy. There are no data on teratogenicity. Anaphylactic reaction resulting in shock or hypoxemia in the mother could conceivably adversely affect the fetus.

V. Drug or laboratory interactions. No known interactions.

VI. Dosage and method of administration
  A. For established clinical botulism, give 1–2 vials IV every 4 hours for 4–5 doses (for suspected botulism, 1–2 vials are usually given empirically). Intramuscular administration is not recommended. Duration of therapy depends on clinical response, particularly any progression of muscular paralysis.
  B. Perform skin test prior to administration according to the package instructions. Should the patient have known sensitivity to horse serum or demonstrate a positive skin test, provide desensitization as indicated in the package insert. Even if the skin test is negative, anaphylaxis may still occur unpredictably. Pretreat the patient with diphenhydramine (see p 331), 1–2 mg/kg IV, and have epinephrine (see p 337) ready in case anaphylaxis occurs.

VII. Formulations
  A. Parenteral. Trivalent botulin antitoxin (7500 IU type A, 5500 IU type B, 8500 IU type E); available through the Centers for Disease Control (CDC), telephone (404) 639-3753. To obtain BIG for suspected infant botulism in the state of California, call (510) 540-2646.
  B. Suggested minimum stocking level. Not relevant—available only through federal (CDC) or state (California) government.

BRETYLIUM

Thomas E. Kearney, PharmD

I. Pharmacology. Bretylium is a quaternary ammonium compound that is an effective type III antifibrillatory drug and also suppresses ventricular ectopic activity. It increases the threshold for ventricular fibrillation and reduces the disparity in action potential duration between normal and ischemic tissue, which is believed to abolish boundary currents responsible for reentrant arrhythmias. Its pharmacologic actions are complex. Initially, norepinephrine is released from sympathetic neurons; this is followed by a block of further norepinephrine release. In addition, norepinephrine uptake is inhibited at adrenergic neurons. The result is a transient increase in heart rate, blood pressure, and cardiac output that may last from a few minutes to 1 hour. Subsequent adrenergic blockade produces vasodilation, which may result in hypotension.

II. Indications
- **A.** Prophylaxis and treatment of ventricular fibrillation. May be particularly effective in hypothermic patients.
- **B.** Ventricular tachycardia resistant to other antiarrhythmic agents. However, it has not been proved beneficial for drug- or chemical-induced ventricular dysrhythmias.

III. Contraindications
- **A.** Use with extreme caution in patients with intoxication by digitalis, chloral hydrate, or halogenated hydrocarbons, because the initial release of catecholamines may aggravate arrhythmias.
- **B.** Use with extreme caution in patients with arrhythmias caused by intoxication with cyclic antidepressants or type Ia or type Ic antiarrhythmic agents because of additive cardiac depression.
- **C.** Use with extreme caution in patients with severe pulmonary hypertension or aortic stenosis.
- **D.** Not recommended for children under 12 years old.

IV. Adverse effects
- **A.** Hypotension (both supine and orthostatic).
- **B.** Nausea and vomiting from rapid intravenous administration.
- **C.** Initial catecholamine release may cause transient hypertension and worsening of arrhythmias.
- **D. Use in pregnancy.** FDA category C (indeterminate). However, this does not preclude its acute, short-term use for a seriously symptomatic patient (see p 310).

V. Drug or laboratory interactions
- **A.** The pressor effect of sympathomimetic amines may be enhanced with initial catecholamine release.
- **B.** Cardiac-depressant effects may be additive with other antiarrhythmic drugs, particularly type Ia and type Ic drugs.

VI. Dosage and method of administration
- **A. For ventricular fibrillation,** give 5 mg/kg IV over 1 minute (in addition to cardiopulmonary resuscitation and defibrillation). If not effective, may repeat with 10 mg/kg.
- **B. For ventricular tachycardia,** give adults and children older than 12 years 5–10 mg/kg IV over 8–10 minutes or IM, repeated as necessary at 15-minute intervals to a maximum dose of 30 mg/kg; repeat every 6 hours as needed.
- **C. The continuous infusion rate** following the loading dose is 1–2 mg/min (children > 12 years old, 20–30 µg/kg/min).

VII. Formulations
- **A. Parenteral.** Bretylium tosylate (Bretylol, others), 50 mg/mL.
- **B. Suggested minimum stocking level** to treat a 70-kg adult for the first 24 hours: 6 vials, 10 mL each.

BROMOCRIPTINE

Thomas E. Kearney, PharmD

I. Pharmacology. Bromocriptine mesylate is a semisynthetic derivative of the ergopeptide group of ergot alkaloids with dopaminergic agonist effects. It also has minor α-adrenergic antagonist properties. The dopaminergic effects account for its inhibition of prolactin secretion and its beneficial effects in the treatment of parkinsonism, neuroleptic malignant syndrome (NMS; see p 20), and cocaine craving, as well as its adverse effect profile and drug interactions. A key limitation is the inability to administer bromocriptine by the parenteral route coupled with poor bioavailability (only about 6% of an oral dose is absorbed). In addition, the onset of therapeutic effects (eg, alleviation of muscle rigidity, hypertension, and hyperthermia) in the treatment of NMS may take several hours to days.

II. Indications

A. Treatment of NMS caused by neuroleptic drugs (eg, haloperidol, other antipsychotics) or levodopa withdrawal.

Note: If the patient has significant hyperthermia (eg, rectal or core temperature > 40 °C), bromocriptine should be considered secondary and adjunctive therapy to immediate measures such as neuromuscular paralysis and aggressive external cooling.

B. Bromocriptine has been used experimentally to alleviate craving for cocaine. **Caution:** There is one case report of a severe adverse reaction (hypertension, seizures, blindness) when bromocriptine was used in a cocaine abuser during the postpartum period.

C. Note: Bromocriptine is **not** considered appropriate first-line therapy for acute drug-induced extrapyramidal or parkinsonian symptoms (see p 24).

III. Contraindications

A. Uncontrolled hypertension or toxemia of pregnancy.

B. Known hypersensitivity to the drug.

C. A relative contraindication is a history of angina, myocardial infarction, stroke, vasospastic disorders (eg, Raynaud's disease), or bipolar affective disorder. In addition, there is no published experience in children.

IV. Adverse effects. Most adverse effects are dose-related and of minor clinical consequence; some are unpredictable.

A. The most common side effect is nausea. Epigastric pain, dyspepsia, and diarrhea also have been reported.

B. Hypotension (usually transient) and syncope may occur at the initiation of treatment, and hypertension may occur later. Other cardiovascular effects include dysrhythmias (with high doses), exacerbation of angina and vasospastic disorders such as Raynaud's disease, and intravascular thrombosis resulting in acute myocardial infarction (one case report).

C. Nervous system side effects vary considerably and include headache, drowsiness, fatigue, hallucinations, mania, psychosis, agitation, seizures, and cerebrovascular accident. Multiple interrelated risk factors include dose, concurrent drug therapy, and preexisting medical and psychiatric disorders.

D. Rare effects include pulmonary toxicity (infiltrates, pleural effusion and thickening) and myopia with long-term, high-dose treatment (months). There has been one case of retroperitoneal fibrosis.

E. Sulfite preservatives in some preparations may cause hypersensitivity reactions. SnapTabs tablets do not contain sulfites.

F. Use in pregnancy. No FDA category. This drug has been used therapeutically during the last trimester of pregnancy for treatment of a pituitary tumor. It has been shown to inhibit fetal prolactin secretion, and it may precipitate premature labor and inhibit lactation in the mother.

V. Drug or laboratory interactions

A. Bromocriptine may accentuate hypotension in patients receiving antihypertensive drugs.

B. Theoretically, this drug may have additive effects with other ergot alkaloids; and its potential to cause peripheral vasospasm may be exacerbated by propranolol.

C. Bromocriptine may reduce ethanol tolerance.

D. There has been one case report of apparent serotonin syndrome (see p 21) in a patient with Parkinson's disease receiving levodopa and carbidopa.

VI. Dosage and method of administration for NMS: in adults, administer 2.5–10 mg orally or by gastric tube 2–6 times daily. The pediatric dose is unknown. Use small, frequent dosing to minimize nausea.

A. A therapeutic response is usually achieved with total daily doses of 5–30 mg.

B. Continue treatment until rigidity and fever have completely resolved, then slowly taper dose. Several days of therapy may be required for complete reversal of NMS.

VII. Formulations

    A. Oral. Bromocriptine mesylate (Parlodel), 2.5- and 5-mg capsules and scored (SnapTabs) tablets.

    B. Suggested minimum stocking level to treat a 70-kg adult for the first 24 hours: 30 mg, or one 30-tablet (SnapTabs) package. SnapTabs tablets do not contain sulfite preservatives.

CALCIUM

Thomas E. Kearney, PharmD

  I. Pharmacology

    A. Calcium is a cation necessary for the normal functioning of a variety of enzymes and organ systems, including muscle and nervous tissue. Hypocalcemia, or a blockade of calcium's effects, may cause muscle cramps, tetany, and ventricular fibrillation. Antagonism of calcium-dependent channels results in hypotension, bradycardia, and atrioventricular block.

    B. Calcium ion rapidly binds to fluoride ion, abolishing its toxic effects.

    C. The neuromuscular effects of black widow spider venom can be antagonized to some degree by the administration of calcium, through a mechanism not fully understood.

    D. Calcium can reverse the negative inotropic effects of calcium antagonists; however, depressed automaticity and atrioventricular nodal conduction velocity and vasodilation may not respond to calcium administration.

    E. Calcium is directly antagonistic to the cardiotoxic effects of hyperkalemia.

  II. Indications

    A. Symptomatic hypocalcemia resulting from intoxication by fluoride, oxalate, or the intravenous anticoagulant citrate.

    B. Topical hydrofluoric acid exposure.

    C. Black widow spider envenomation with muscle cramping or rigidity.

    D. Calcium antagonist (eg, verapamil) overdose with hypotension.

    E. Severe hyperkalemia with cardiotoxic manifestations (except in patients with digitalis toxicity, see **III.B,** below).

  III. Contraindications

    A. Hypercalcemia.

    B. Digitalis intoxication (may aggravate digitalis-induced ventricular tachyarrhythmias).

    C. *Note:* Calcium *chloride* salt should ***not*** be used for intradermal or subcutaneous injection because it is too concentrated.

  IV. Adverse effects

    A. Tissue irritation, particularly with calcium chloride salt; extravasation may cause local cellulitis or necrosis.

    B. Hypercalcemia, especially in patients with diminished renal function.

    C. Hypotension, bradycardia, syncope, and cardiac arrhythmias caused by rapid intravenous administration.

    D. Constipation caused by orally administered calcium salts.

    E. Use in pregnancy. FDA category C (indeterminate). This does not preclude its acute, short-term use for a seriously symptomatic patient (see p 310).

  V. Drug or laboratory interactions

    A. Inotropic and arrhythmogenic effects of digitalis are potentiated by calcium.

    B. A precipitate will form with solutions containing soluble salts of carbonates, phosphates, or sulfates and with various antibiotics.

  VI. Dosage and method of administration

    A. Oral fluoride ingestion. Administer calcium-containing antacid (calcium carbonate) orally to complex fluoride ion.

    B. Symptomatic hypocalcemia, hyperkalemia, black widow spider envenomation, or calcium antagonist poisoning. Give 10% calcium gluconate, 10–

20 mL (children, 0.2–0.3 mL/kg), or 10% calcium chloride, 5–10 mL (children, 0.1–0.2 mL/kg), slowly IV. Repeat as needed.

Note: Calcium chloride contains nearly 3 times the milliequivalents of Ca^{2+} per milliliter of 10% solution compared with calcium gluconate.

- **C. Dermal hydrofluoric acid exposure.** For any exposure involving the hand or fingers, obtain immediate consultation from an experienced hand surgeon.
    - 1. For **topical** application of calcium gel, prepare gel by combining the proportion of 1 g of calcium gluconate or calcium chloride per 30 g (approximately 30 mL) of water-soluble base material (Surgilube, K-Y Jelly).
    - 2. For **subcutaneous** injection (when topical treatment fails to relieve pain), inject 5–10% calcium gluconate (***not*** chloride) SQ, 0.5 mL/cm^2 of affected skin, using a 27-gauge or smaller needle. May repeat 2–3 times at 1- to 2-hour intervals if pain is not relieved.
    - 3. For **intra-arterial** administration, infuse 20 mL of 10% calcium gluconate (***not*** chloride) diluted in 250 mL D_5W saline via the radial or brachial artery proximal to the injury over 3–4 hours.
    - 4. **Nebulized** inhalation and **ocular** administration of 2.5% calcium gluconate solutions are of unproved efficacy.

VII. Formulations
- **A. Oral.** Calcium carbonate; suspension, tablets, chewable tablets, 300–800 mg.
- **B. Parenteral.** Calcium gluconate 10%, 10 mL (1 g, contains 4.5 meq calcium); calcium chloride 10%, 10 mL (1 g, contains 13.6 meq).
- **C. Topical.** No commercial formulation is approved currently in the US.
- **D. Suggested minimum stocking level** to treat a 70-kg adult for the first 24 hours: 5–10 vials (1 g each) of calcium gluconate 10%.

CHARCOAL, ACTIVATED

Thomas E. Kearney, PharmD

- **I. Pharmacology.** Activated charcoal, by virtue of its large surface area, adsorbs many drugs and toxins. Small or highly ionic salts (eg, iron, lithium, cyanide) or small molecules (eg, alcohols) are poorly adsorbed. Repeated oral doses of activated charcoal can increase the rate of elimination of some drugs that have a small volume of distribution (Vd) and that undergo enterogastric or enterohepatic recirculation (eg, digitoxin) or diffuse into the gastrointestinal lumen from the intestinal circulation (eg, phenobarbital, theophylline). See also discussion in Section I, p 47.
- **II. Indications**
    - **A.** Activated charcoal is used orally after an ingestion to limit drug or toxin absorption. Although traditionally given after the stomach has been emptied by ipecac-induced emesis or gastric lavage, recent studies suggest that it may be used alone for most ingestions.
    - **B.** Repeated doses of activated charcoal may be indicated to enhance elimination of some drugs if (1) more rapid elimination will benefit the patient (and the benefits outweigh the risks of repeated doses; see **IV.C.** and **V.C,** below), and (2) more aggressive means of removal (eg, hemodialysis or hemoperfusion) are not immediately indicated or available (see p 49).
    - **C.** Repeated doses of activated charcoal may be useful when the quantity of drug or toxin ingested is greater than one-tenth of the usual charcoal dose (eg, an aspirin ingestion of more than 6–10 g) or when surface contact with the drug is hindered (eg, pharmacobezoars, wrapped or packaged drugs).
- **III. Contraindications**
    - **A.** Gastrointestinal ileus or obstruction may prevent the administration of more than 1–2 doses.
    - **B.** Acid or alkali ingestions, unless other drugs have also been ingested (charcoal makes endoscopic evaluation more difficult).
- **IV. Adverse effects**
    - **A.** Constipation (may be prevented by coadministration of a cathartic).

B. Distention of the stomach, with potential risk of aspiration.

C. Diarrhea, dehydration, and hypernatremia resulting from coadministered cathartics, especially with repeated doses of charcoal and cathartics, or even after a single large dose of a premixed, sorbitol-containing charcoal product.

D. Intestinal bezoar with obstruction.

E. Use in pregnancy. Activated charcoal is not systemically absorbed. Diarrhea resulting in shock or hypernatremia in the mother could conceivably adversely affect the fetus.

V. Drug or laboratory interactions

A. Activated charcoal may reduce, prevent, or delay the absorption of orally administered antidotes or other drugs (eg, nifedipine, acetylcysteine).

B. The adsorptive capacity of activated charcoal may be diminished by the concurrent ingestion of ice cream, milk, or sugar syrup; the clinical significance is unknown but is probably minor.

C. Repeated doses of charcoal may enhance the elimination of some necessary therapeutic drugs (eg, anticonvulsants).

VI. Dosage and method of administration

A. Initial dose. Activated charcoal, 1 g/kg orally or via gastric tube, is administered, or if the quantity of toxin ingested is known, 10 times the amount of ingested toxin by weight is given. For massive overdoses (eg, 60–100 g aspirin), this may need to be given in divided doses over 1–2 days.

B. Repeat-dose charcoal. Activated charcoal, 15–20 g (0.25–0.5 g/kg) every 4–6 hours is given orally or by gastric tube. Administer a small dose of cathartic with every second or third charcoal dose. Do **not** use cathartic with every activated charcoal dose.

End points for repeat-dose charcoal therapy include clinical improvement and declining serum drug level; the usual empiric duration is 24–48 hours.

VII. Formulations

A. There are a variety of formulations and a large number of brands of activated charcoal. It is available as a powder, a liquid aqueous suspension, and a liquid suspension in sorbitol or propylene glycol.

B. Suggested minimum stocking level to treat a 70-kg adult for the first 24 hours: 3 bottles containing 50 g of activated charcoal each. Preferred stock is the plain aqueous suspension.

CYANIDE ANTIDOTE KIT

See Nitrite (p 361) and Thiosulfate (p 376).

DANTROLENE

Thomas E. Kearney, PharmD

I. Pharmacology. Dantrolene relaxes skeletal muscle by inhibiting the release of calcium from the sarcoplasmic reticulum, thereby reducing actin-myosin contractile activity. Dantrolene can help control hyperthermia that results from excessive muscle hyperactivity, particularly when hyperthermia is caused by a defect within the muscle cell (eg, malignant hyperthermia). Dantrolene is not a substitute for other temperature-controlling measures (eg, sponging, fanning).

II. Indications

A. The primary indication for dantrolene is malignant hyperthermia (see p 20).

B. Dantrolene may be useful in treating hyperthermia and rhabdomyolysis caused by drug-induced muscular hyperactivity not controlled by usual cooling measures or neuromuscular paralysis.

C. Dantrolene is not likely to be effective for hyperthermia caused by conditions other than muscular hyperactivity, such as increased metabolic rate (eg, salicylate or dinitrophenol poisoning), impaired heat dissipation (eg, anticholinergic syndrome), or environmental exposure (heat stroke).

III. Contraindications. No absolute contraindications exist. Patients with muscular weakness or respiratory impairment must be observed closely for possible respiratory arrest.

IV. Adverse effects
   A. Muscle weakness, which may aggravate respiratory depression.
   B. Drowsiness, diarrhea.
   C. Hypersensitivity hepatitis, occasionally fatal, reported after chronic therapy.
   D. Use in pregnancy. FDA category C (indeterminate). This does not preclude its acute, short-term use for a seriously symptomatic patient (see p 310).
V. Drug or laboratory interactions
   A. Dantrolene may have additive central nervous system—depressant effects with sedative and hypnotic drugs.
   B. Each 20-mg vial of Dantrium contains 3 g of mannitol; this should be taken into consideration as it may have additive effects with any mannitol given to treat rhabdomyolysis.
VI. Dosage and method of administration (adults and children)
   A. Parenteral. Give 1–2 mg/kg rapidly IV; may be repeated as needed every 5–10 minutes, to a total dose of 10 mg/kg. Satisfactory response is usually achieved with 2–5 mg/kg.
   B. Oral. To prevent recurrence of hyperthermia, administer 1–2 mg/kg intravenously or orally (up to 100 mg maximum) 4 times a day for 2–3 days.
VII. Formulations
   A. Parenteral. Dantrolene sodium (Dantrium), 20 mg of lyophilized powder for reconstitution (after reconstitution, protect from light and use within 6 hours to ensure maximal activity). Each 20-mg vial contains 3 g of mannitol.
   B. Oral. Dantrolene sodium (Dantrium), 25-, 50-, 100-mg capsules.
   C. Suggested minimum stocking level to treat a 70-kg adult for the first 24 hours: 35 vials, 20 mg each.

DEFEROXAMINE

Thomas E. Kearney, PharmD

I. Pharmacology. Deferoxamine is a specific chelating agent for iron. It binds free iron and, to some extent, loosely bound iron (eg, from ferritin or hemosiderin). Iron bound to hemoglobin, transferrin, cytochrome enzymes, and all other sites is unaffected. The red iron-deferoxamine (ferrioxamine) complex is water-soluble and is excreted renally, where it imparts an orange-pink, or "vin rosé," color to the urine. One hundred milligrams of deferoxamine is capable of binding 8.5 mg of elemental iron.

II. Indications
   A. Deferoxamine is used to treat iron intoxication when the serum iron is greater than 450–500 μg/dL or when clinical signs of significant iron intoxication exist (eg, shock, acidosis, severe gastroenteritis, numerous radiopaque tablets visible in the gastrointestinal tract by x-ray).
   B. Deferoxamine is sometimes used as a "test dose" to determine the presence of free iron by observing for the characteristic "vin rosé" color in the urine; however, urine color change is not reliable.
III. Contraindications. No absolute contraindications to deferoxamine use in patients with serious iron poisoning. The drug should be used with caution in patients with known sensitivity to deferoxamine.
IV. Adverse effects
   A. Hypotension or an anaphylactoid-type reaction may occur from very rapid intravenous bolus administration; this may be avoided by limiting the rate of administration to 15 mg/kg/h.
   B. Local pain, induration, and sterile abscess formation may occur at intramuscular injection sites. Large intramuscular injections may also cause hypotension.
   C. The ferrioxamine complex may itself cause hypotension and may accumulate in patients with renal impairment; hemodialysis may be necessary to remove the ferrioxamine complex.

D. Deferoxamine, as a siderophore, promotes the growth of certain bacteria such as *Yersinia enterocolitica* and may predispose patients to *Yersinia* sepsis.

E. Infusions exceeding 24 hours have been associated with pulmonary complications (acute respiratory distress syndrome [ARDS]).

F. Use in pregnancy. FDA category C (indeterminate). Although it is a teratogen in animals, it has relatively poor placental transfer, and there is no evidence that short-term treatment is harmful in human pregnancy (see p 310). More importantly, failure to treat a serious acute iron intoxication may result in maternal and fetal morbidity or death.

V. Drug or laboratory interactions. Deferoxamine may interfere with determinations of serum iron (falsely low) and total iron-binding capacity (falsely high).

VI. Dosage and method of administration

A. The intravenous route is preferred in all cases. In children or adults, give at an infusion rate generally not to exceed 15 mg/kg/h (although rates up to 40–50 mg/kg/h have been given in patients with massive iron intoxication). The maximum cumulative daily dose should generally not exceed 6 g (up to 16 g have been tolerated). The end points of therapy include loss of "vin rosé"-colored urine; serum iron level less than 350 μg/dL; and resolution of clinical signs of intoxication.

B. Oral complexation is *not* recommended.

C. "Test dose" intramuscular injection is *not* recommended. If the patient is symptomatic, use the intravenous route. If the patient is not symptomatic but serious toxicity is expected to occur, intravenous access is essential (eg, for fluid boluses), and intravenous dosing provides more reliable administration.

VII. Formulations

A. Parenteral. Deferoxamine mesylate (Desferal), vials containing 500 mg of lyophilized powder.

B. Suggested minimum stocking level to treat a 70-kg adult for the first 24 hours: 12 vials.

DIAZEPAM

Thomas E. Kearney, PharmD

I. Pharmacology

A. Diazepam and other benzodiazepines potentiate inhibitory γ-aminobutyric acid (GABA) neuronal activity in the central nervous system. Pharmacologic effects include reduction of anxiety, suppression of seizure activity, central nervous system depression (possible respiratory arrest when given rapidly intravenously), and inhibition of spinal afferent pathways to produce skeletal muscle relaxation. In addition, diazepam has been reported to antagonize the cardiotoxic effect of chloroquine, although the mechanism is unknown.

B. Diazepam generally has little effect on the autonomic nervous system or cardiovascular system.

C. Diazepam is well absorbed orally but not intramuscularly. It is eliminated entirely by hepatic metabolism, with a serum half-life of approximately 40 hours. Active metabolites further extend the duration of effect.

II. Indications

A. Anxiety. Diazepam is used for the treatment of anxiety or agitation (eg, caused by sympathomimetic or hallucinogenic drug intoxication).

B. Convulsions. Diazepam is used for the treatment of acute seizure activity or status epilepticus resulting from idiopathic epilepsy or convulsant drug overdose. It is *not* effective for seizure prophylaxis or chronic treatment (see also Phenytoin [p 370], Phenobarbital [p 368], and Pentobarbital [p 367]).

C. Muscle relaxant. Diazepam is used for relaxation of excessive muscle rigidity and contractions (eg, caused by strychnine poisoning or black widow spider envenomation).

D. Chloroquine poisoning. Diazepam may antagonize cardiotoxicity.

E. Alcohol or sedative-hypnotic withdrawal. Diazepam is used to abate symptoms and signs of alcohol and hypnosedative withdrawal (eg, anxiety, tremor, seizures).

III. **Contraindications.** Do not use diazepam in patients with a known sensitivity to benzodiazepines.

IV. **Adverse effects**
   A. Central nervous system–depressant effects may interfere with evaluation of neurologic function.
   B. Excessive or rapid intravenous administration may cause respiratory arrest.
   C. The drug may precipitate or worsen heptic encephalopathy.
   D. **Use in pregnancy.** FDA category D. It readily crosses the placenta. However, this does not preclude its acute, short-term use for a seriously symptomatic patient (see p 310).

V. **Drug or laboratory interactions**
   A. Diazepam will potentiate central nervous system–depressant effects of opioids, ethanol, and other sedative-hypnotic and depressant drugs.
   B. **Flumazenil** (see p 340) will reverse the effects of diazepam and may trigger an acute abstinence syndrome in patients using diazepam chronically. Patients who have received flumazenil will have an unpredictable but reduced or absent response to diazepam.
   C. Diazepam may produce a false-positive glucose reaction with Clinistix and Diastix test strips.

VI. **Dosage and method of administration.** Do *not* give diazepam intramuscularly (absorbed erratically by this route). Rectal administration of 5–10 mg has been reported to be effective in children with status epilepticus when there is no intravenous access.
   A. **Anxiety or agitation.** Give 0.1–0.2 mg/kg IV initially (no faster than 5 mg/min in adults; administer over 3 min in children), depending on severity; may repeat every 1–4 hours as needed. Oral dose is 0.1–0.3 mg/kg.
   B. **Convulsions.** Give 0.1–0.2 mg/kg IV every 10–15 minutes (usual initial doses: adult, 5–10 mg; children > 5 years, 1–2 mg; children < 5 years, 0.2–0.5 mg), to a maximum total of 30 mg (adults) or 5 mg (young children) or 10 mg (older children). If convulsions persist, use an alternative anticonvulsant (see Phenytoin [p 370], Phenobarbital [p 368], or Pentobarbital [p 367]).
   C. **Muscle relaxation.** Give 0.1–0.2 mg/kg IV initially; may repeat every 1–4 hours as needed.
   D. **Chloroquine intoxication.** There is reported improvement of cardiotoxicity with high-dose administration of 1 mg/kg intravenously. *Caution:* This will likely cause apnea; the patient must be intubated, and ventilation must be controlled.
   E. **Alcohol withdrawal syndrome.** Administer 5–10 mg IV initially, then 5 mg every 10 minutes until patient is calm. Large doses may be required to sedate patients with severe withdrawal. Oral dose is 10–20 mg initially.

VII. **Formulations**
   A. **Parenteral.** Diazepam (Valium, others), 5 mg/mL solution, 2-mL prefilled syringe.
   B. **Oral.** Diazepam (Valium, others), 2-, 5-, and 10-mg tablets.
   C. **Suggested minimum stocking level** to treat a 70-kg adult for the first 24 hours: 200 mg.

DIAZOXIDE

Thomas E. Kearney, PharmD

   I. **Pharmacology**
   A. Diazoxide, a nondiuretic thiazide, is a direct arterial vasodilator formerly used to treat severe hypertension. Heart rate and cardiac output increase owing to a reflex response to decreased peripheral vascular resistance. The duration of the hypotensive effect ranges from 3 to 12 hours, although the elimination half-life is 20–40 hours.

B. Diazoxide is currently used in the treatment of oral hypoglycemic overdose because it increases serum glucose by inhibiting insulin secretion, diminishing peripheral glucose utilization, and enhancing hepatic glucose release.

II. Indications
A. Acute management of hypertensive crisis, although other newer antihypertensive agents generally are preferred (see Nifedipine [p 360], Phentolamine [p 369], Nitroprusside [p 362], and Labetalol [p 347]).
B. Oral hypoglycemic overdose, when serum glucose concentrations cannot be adequately maintained by intravenous 5% dextrose infusions.

III. Contraindications
A. Hypertension associated with aortic stenosis, aortic coarctation, hypertrophic cardiomyopathy, or arteriovenous shunt.
B. Known hypersensitivity to thiazides.

IV. Adverse effects
A. Hypotension or excessive blood pressure reduction must be avoided in patients with compromised cerebral or cardiac circulation.
B. Fluid retention from prolonged therapy may compromise patients with congestive heart failure.
C. Hyperglycemia may occur, particularly in patients with diabetes or hepatic dysfunction.
D. Use in pregnancy. FDA category C (indeterminate). This drug has caused skeletal, cardiac, and pancreatic abnormalities in animals, but no adequate human data exist. Use of this drug near term may cause hyperbilirubinemia and altered carbohydrate metabolism in the fetus or neonate, and intravenous administration during labor may cause cessation of uterine contractions. These cautions, however, do not necessarily preclude acute, short-term use of the drug for a seriously symptomatic patient (see p 310).

V. Drug or laboratory interactions
A. The hypotensive effect is potentiated by concomitant therapy with diuretics or β-adrenergic blockers.
B. Diazoxide displaces warfarin from protein-binding sites and may transiently potentiate its anticoagulant effects.

VI. Dosage and method of administration (adults and children)
A. For oral hypoglycemic-induced hypoglycemia
  1. Give 0.1–2 mg/kg/h infusion; initiate at lower infusion rate and titrate up as needed. Hypotension is minimized by keeping the patient supine and increasing the infusion rate slowly. Duration of therapy has ranged from 22 to 60 hours.
  2. An oral dosing regimen of 200 mg every 4 hours has also been used.
B. For hypertensive crisis, give 1–3 mg/kg IV (150 mg maximum) every 5–15 minutes as needed. *Note:* The use of a 300-mg rapid bolus is no longer recommended.

VII. Formulations
A. Parenteral. Diazoxide (Hyperstat), 15 mg/mL.
B. Oral. Diazoxide (Proglycem), 50-mg capsules, or 50-mg/mL oral suspension.
C. Suggested minimum stocking level to treat a 70-kg adult for the first 24 hours: parenteral, 2 vials (20 mL each); oral, 1 bottle (100 tablets) or 30 mL of suspension.

DIGOXIN-SPECIFIC ANTIBODIES

Thomas E. Kearney, PharmD

I. Pharmacology. Digoxin-specific antibodies are produced in immunized sheep and have a high binding affinity for digoxin and (to a lesser extent) digitoxin and other cardiac glycosides. The Fab fragments used to treat poisoning are derived by cleaving the whole antibodies. Once the digoxin-Fab complex is formed, the digoxin molecule is no longer pharmacologically active. The complex enters the circulation, is renally eliminated, and has a half-life of 16–20 hours. Reversal of signs of digitalis intoxication occurs within 30–60 minutes of administration, with complete reversal by 4 hours.

II. **Indications.** Digoxin-specific antibodies are used for life-threatening arrhythmias or hyperkalemia (> 5 meq/L) caused by cardiac glycoside intoxication (see p 124).

III. **Contraindications.** No contraindications are known. Caution is warranted in patients with known sensitivity to ovine (sheep) products; a skin test for hypersensitivity may be performed in such patients, using diluted reconstituted drug. There are no reports of hypersensitivity reactions in patients who have received the drug more than once.

IV. **Adverse effects**
   A. Monitor the patient for potential hypersensitivity reactions and serum sickness.
   B. In patients with renal insufficiency and impaired clearance of the digitalis-Fab complex, the complex may theoretically degrade, releasing active glycoside (this has not been reported).
   C. Removal of the inotropic effect of digitalis may exacerbate preexisting heart failure.
   D. With removal of digitalis effect, patients with preexisting atrial fibrillation may develop accelerated ventricular response.
   E. Removal of the digitalis effect may reactivate sodium-potassium ATPase and shift potassium into cells, causing a drop in the serum potassium level.
   F. **Use in pregnancy.** FDA category C (indeterminate). This does not preclude its acute, short-term use for a seriously symptomatic patient (see p 310).

V. **Drug or laboratory interactions**
   A. Digoxin-specific Fab fragments will bind other cardiac glycosides including digitoxin, ouabain, and (potentially) glycosides in oleander, lily of the Nile, and strophanthus.
   B. The digoxin-Fab complex cross-reacts with the antibody commonly utilized in quantitative immunoassay techniques. This results in falsely high serum concentrations of digoxin owing to measurement of the inactive Fab complex.

VI. **Dosage and method of administration.** Each vial (40 mg) of digoxin-immune Fab binds 0.6 mg of digoxin.
   A. Estimation of the dose of Fab is based on the body burden of digitalis. This may be calculated if the approximate amount ingested is known (Table III–3) or if the steady-state (postdistributional) serum drug concentration is known (Table III–4). (Steady-state serum drug concentration should be determined at least 12–16 hours after the last dose.)
   B. If the amount ingested or the postdistributional level is not known and the patient has life-threatening dysrhythmias, dosing may have to be empiric. Aver-

TABLE III–3. APPROXIMATE DIGOXIN-FAB DOSE IF AMOUNT INGESTED IS KNOWN

Tablets Ingested (0.25 mg)	Approximate Dose Absorbed (mg)	Recommended Dose	
		Fab (mg)	Vials
5	1	68	1.7
10	2	136	3.4
25	5	340	8.5
50	10	680	17
75	15	1000	25
100	20	1360	34
150	30	2000	50

TABLE III–4. APPROXIMATE DIGOXIN-FAB DOSE BASED ON SERUM CONCENTRATION AT STEADY STATE (AFTER EQUILIBRATION)

Digoxin: No. of digoxin-Fab vials $\cong \dfrac{\text{Serum digoxin (ng/mL)} \times \text{Body weight (kg)}}{100}$

Digitoxin No. of digoxin-Fab vials $\cong \dfrac{\text{Serum digitoxin (ng/mL)} \times \text{Body weight (kg)}}{1000}$

age dose requirements are 10 and 5 vials for acute and chronic digoxin intoxication, respectively.

C. Theoretically, Fab may be used to neutralize a *portion* of the digoxin body burden to reverse toxicity but maintain therapeutic benefits. The Fab dose can be estimated by subtracting the desired digoxin level from the measured postdistributional level before completing the calculation. Alternately, if the patient is hemodynamically stable, the drug can be given empirically, a vial at a time, titrating to clinical effect.

D. Reconstitute the drug according to package instructions, and administer intravenously over 30 minutes using a 0.22 micron filter. It may be given as a rapid bolus for immediately life-threatening arrhythmias.

VII. Formulations

    A. Parenteral. Digibind, 40 mg of lyophilized digoxin-specific Fab fragments per vial.

    B. Suggested minimum stocking level to treat a 70-kg adult for the first 24 hours: 20 vials.

DIPHENHYDRAMINE

Thomas E. Kearney, PharmD

    I. Pharmacology. Diphenhydramine is an antihistamine with anticholinergic, antitussive, antiemetic, and local anesthetic properties. The antihistaminic property affords relief from itching and minor irritation caused by plant-induced dermatitis and insect bites and, when used as pretreatment, provides partial protection against anaphylaxis caused by animal serum–derived antivenins or antitoxins. Drug-induced extrapyramidal symptoms respond to the anticholinergic effect of diphenhydramine. The effects of diphenhydramine are maximal 1 hour after intravenous injection and last up to 7 hours. The drug is eliminated by hepatic metabolism, with a serum half-life of 3–7 hours.

    II. Indications

        A. Relief of symptoms caused by excessive histamine effect (eg, ingestion of scombroid-contaminated fish or niacin, rapid intravenous administration of acetylcysteine).

        B. Pretreatment before administration of animal serum–derived antivenins or antitoxins, especially in patients with a history of hypersensitivity or with a positive skin test.

        C. Neuroleptic drug-induced extrapyramidal symptoms (and priapism, one case report).

        D. Pruritus caused by poison oak, poison ivy, or minor insect bites.

    III. Contraindications

        A. Angle-closure glaucoma.

        B. Prostatic hypertrophy with obstructive uropathy.

        C. Concurrent therapy with monoamine oxidase inhibitors.

    IV. Adverse effects

        A. Sedation, drowsiness, and ataxia may occur. Paradoxic excitation is possible in small children.

B. Excessive doses may cause flushing, tachycardia, blurred vision, delirium, toxic psychosis, urinary retention, and respiratory depression.

C. Some preparations may contain sulfite preservatives, which can cause allergic-type reactions in susceptible persons.

D. Use in pregnancy. FDA category B (see p 310). Fetal harm is extremely unlikely.

V. Drug or laboratory interactions

A. Additive sedative effect with opioids, ethanol, and other sedatives.

B. Additive anticholinergic effect with other antimuscarinic drugs.

VI. Dosage and method of administration

A. Pruritus. Give 25–50 mg orally every 6–8 hours (children, 5 mg/kg/d in divided doses), maximum adult daily dose 300 mg. The drug may also be applied topically, although systemic absorption and toxicity have been reported, especially when used on large areas with blistered or nonintact skin.

B. Pretreatment before antivenin administration. Give 50 mg (children, 0.5–1 mg/kg) IV; if possible, it should be given at least 15–20 minutes before antivenin use.

C. Drug-induced extrapyramidal symptoms. Give 50 mg (children, 0.5–1 mg/kg) IV or IM; if no response within 30–60 minutes, repeat dose to maximum 100 mg (adults). Provide oral maintenance therapy, 25–50 mg (children, 0.5–1 mg/kg) every 4–6 hours for 2–3 days to prevent recurrence.

VII. Formulations

A. Oral. Diphenhydramine hydrochloride (Benadryl, others), 25- and 50-mg tablets and capsules; elixir, 12.5 mg/5 mL.

B. Parenteral. Diphenhydramine hydrochloride (Benadryl, others), 10- and 50-mg/mL solutions.

C. Suggested minimum stocking level to treat a 70-kg adult for the first 24 hours: 5 vials (10 mg/mL, 10 mL each).

DMSA (SUCCIMER)

Michael J. Kosnett, MD, MPH

I. Pharmacology. DMSA (meso 2, 3-dimercaptosuccinic acid, succimer) is a chelating agent used in the treatment of intoxication from several heavy metals. A water-soluble analog of dimercaprol (BAL, see p 317), DMSA enhances the urinary excretion of lead and mercury. Its effect on elimination of the endogenous minerals calcium, iron, and magnesium is insignificant. Minor increases in zinc and copper excretion may occur. In an animal model, oral DMSA was not associated with increased gastrointestinal absorption of lead; the effect of oral DMSA on gastrointestinal absorption of mercury and arsenic is not known.

DMSA is rapidly but variably absorbed after oral administration, with peak levels occurring between 1 and 2 hours. The drug is eliminated primarily by the kidney, with peak urinary excretion of the parent drug and its metabolites after 2–4 hours.

II. Indications

A. DMSA is approved for treatment of intoxication by lead and mercury, where it is associated with increased urinary excretion of the metals and concurrent reversal of metal-induced enzyme inhibition. Oral DMSA is comparable to parenteral calcium EDTA (see p 335) in decreasing blood lead concentrations. Although DMSA treatment has been associated with subjective clinical improvement, controlled clinical trials demonstrating therapeutic efficacy have yet to be reported.

B. DMSA is protective against acute lethal effects of arsenic in animal models, and may have potential utility in human arsenic poisoning.

III. Contraindications. History of allergy to the drug.

IV. Adverse effects

A. Gastrointestinal disturbances including anorexia, nausea, vomiting, and diarrhea are the most common side effects, and occur in less than 10% of pa-

tients. There may be a mercaptanlike odor to the urine, which has no clinical significance.
  B. Mild, reversible increases in liver transaminases have been observed in 6–10% of patients.
  C. Rashes, some requiring discontinuation of treatment, have been reported in less than 5% of patients.
  D. Mild to moderate neutropenia has been noted occasionally.
  E. Minimal increases (less than 2-fold) in urinary excretion of zinc and copper have been observed, and have minor or no clinical significance.
  F. Use in pregnancy. FDA category C (indeterminate). DMSA has produced adverse fetal effects when administered to pregnant animals in amounts 1–2 orders of magnitude greater than recommended human doses; its effect on human pregnancy has not been determined (see p 310).
V. Drug or laboratory interactions. No known interactions. Concurrent administration with other chelating agents has not been adequately studied.
VI. Dosage and method of administration (adults and children)
  A. Lead poisoning. Availability in the USA is limited to an oral formulation (100-mg capsules) officially approved by the FDA for use in children with blood lead levels greater than 45 μg/dL. However, DMSA can also lower lead concentrations in adults.
    Note: Administration of DMSA should never be a substitute for removal from lead exposure. In adults, the federal OSHA Lead Standard requires removal from occupational lead exposure of any worker with a single blood lead concentration in excess of 60 μg/dL or an average of 3 successive values in excess of 50 μg/dL. **Prophylactic chelation,** defined as the *routine* use of chelation to prevent elevated blood lead concentrations or to lower blood lead levels below the standard in asymptomatic workers, *is not permitted.* Consult the local or state health department or OSHA (see Table IV–12, p 395) for more detailed information.
    1. Give 10 mg/kg (or 350 mg/m^2) orally every 8 hours for 5 days, then the same dose every 12 hours for 2 weeks.
    2. An additional course of treatment may be considered based on posttreatment blood lead levels and on the persistence or recurrence of symptoms. Although blood lead levels may decline by more than 50% during treatment, patients with high body lead burdens may experience rebound to within 20% of pretreatment levels as bone stores equilibrate with tissue levels. An interval of 2 or more weeks may be needed to assess the extent of posttreatment rebound.
    3. Experience with oral DMSA for severe lead intoxications (ie, lead encephalopathy) is very limited. In such cases, consideration should be given to parenteral therapy with calcium EDTA (see p 335).
  B. Mercury and arsenic poisoning
    1. Intoxication by inorganic mercury compounds and arsenic compounds may result in severe gastroenteritis and shock. In such circumstances, the capacity of the gut to absorb orally administered DMSA may be severely impaired, and use of an available parenteral agent such as BAL (see p 317) may be preferable.
    2. Give 10 mg/kg (or 350 mg/m^2) orally every 8 hours for 5 days, then the same dose every 12 hours for 2 weeks. The value of extending the duration of treatment in the presence of continuing symptoms or high levels of urinary metal excretion is undetermined.
VII. Formulations
  A. Oral. DMSA, meso 2, 3-dimercaptosuccinic acid, Succimer (Chemet), 100-mg capsules in bottles of 100.
  B. Parenteral. A parenteral form of DMSA (sodium 2, 3-dimercaptosuccinate), infused at a dose of 1–2 g per day, has been in use in the People's Republic of China, but is not available in the USA.

   C. Suggested minimum stocking level to treat a 70-kg adult for the first 24 hours: 20 capsules.

DOPAMINE

Neal L. Benowitz, MD

   I. Pharmacology. Dopamine is an endogenous catecholamine and the immediate metabolic precursor of norepinephrine. It stimulates α- and β-adrenergic receptors directly and indirectly. In addition, it acts on specific dopaminergic receptors. Its relative activity at these various receptors is dose-related. At low infusion rates (1–5 μg/kg/min), dopamine stimulates β_1 activity (increased heart rate and contractility) and increases renal and mesenteric blood flow through dopaminergic agonist activity. At high infusion rates (> 10–20 μg/kg/min), α-adrenergic stimulation predominates, resulting in increased peripheral vascular resistance. Dopamine is not effective orally. Following intravenous administration, its onset of action occurs within 5 minutes and the duration of effect is less than 10 minutes. The plasma half-life is about 2 minutes.

  II. Indications

    A. Dopamine is used to increase blood pressure, cardiac output, and urine flow in patients with shock who have not responded to intravenous fluid challenge, correction of hypothermia, or reversal of acidosis (see p 15).

    B. Low-dose infusion is most effective for hypotension caused by venodilation or reduced cardiac contractility; high-dose dopamine is indicated for shock resulting from decreased peripheral arterial resistance.

  III. Contraindications

    A. Uncorrected tachyarrhythmias or ventricular fibrillation, and uncorrected hypovolemia.

    B. High-dose infusion is relatively contraindicated in the presence of peripheral arterial occlusive disease with thrombosis or in patients with ergot poisoning (see p 158).

  IV. Adverse effects

    A. Severe hypertension, which may result in intracranial hemorrhage, pulmonary edema, or myocardial necrosis.

    B. Aggravation of tissue ischemia, resulting in gangrene (with high-dose infusion).

    C. Ventricular arrhythmias, especially in patients intoxicated by halogenated or aromatic hydrocarbon solvents or anesthetics.

    D. Tissue necrosis after extravasation (see p VI.A., below, for treatment of extravasation).

    E. Anaphylactoid reaction induced by sulfite preservatives in sensitive patients.

    F. Use in pregnancy. FDA category C (indeterminate). There may be a dose-related effect on uterine blood flow. This does not preclude its acute, short-term use for a seriously symptomatic patient (see p 310).

  V. Drug or laboratory interactions

    A. Enhanced pressor response may occur in the presence of cocaine and cyclic antidepressants owing to inhibition of neuronal reuptake.

    B. Enhanced pressor response may occur in patients taking monoamine oxidase inhibitors, owing to inhibition of neuronal metabolic degradation.

    C. Chloral hydrate and halogenated hydrocarbon anesthetics may enhance the arrhythmogenic effect of dopamine owing to sensitization of the myocardium to effects of catecholamines.

    D. Alpha- and beta-blocking agents antagonize the adrenergic effects of dopamine; haloperidol and other dopamine antagonists may antagonize the dopaminergic effects.

    E. There may be a reduced pressor response in patients with depleted neuronal stores of catecholamines (eg, chronic disulfiram or reserpine use, possibly acute cyclic antidepressant overdose).

VI. Dosage and method of administration (adults and children)

A. **Avoid extravasation.** ***Caution:*** The intravenous infusion must be free-flowing, and the infused vein should be observed frequently for signs of subcutaneous infiltration (pallor, coldness, induration). If extravasation occurs, immediately infiltrate the affected area with phentolamine (see p 369), 5–10 mg in 10–15 mL of normal saline (children, 0.1–0.2 mg/kg; maximum 10 mg total) via a fine (25- to 27-gauge) hypodermic needle; improvement is evidenced by hyperemia and return to normal temperature.

B. For **predominantly inotropic effects,** begin with 1 μg/kg/min and increase infusion rate as needed to 5–10 μg/kg/min.

C. For **predominantly vasopressor effect,** infuse 10–20 μg/kg/min and increase as needed. Doses above 50 μg/kg/min may result in severe peripheral vasoconstriction and gangrene.

VII. Formulations

A. Dopamine hydrochloride (Intropin, others), concentrate for admixture to intravenous solutions (40, 80, and 160 mg/mL in 5-mL vials) or premixed parenteral for injection (0.8, 1.6, and 3.2 mg/mL in 5% dextrose). All contain sodium bisulfite as a preservative.

B. **Suggested minimum stocking level** to treat a 70-kg adult for the first 24 hours: approximately 1800–2000 mg (2–3 vials, 160 mg/mL, 5 mL each).

EDTA, CALCIUM (CALCIUM DISODIUM EDTA, CALCIUM DISODIUM EDETATE, CALCIUM DISODIUM VERSENATE)

Michael J. Kosnett, MD, MPH

I. Pharmacology. Calcium EDTA has been used as a chelating agent to enhance elimination of certain toxic metals, principally lead. The elimination of endogenous metals, including zinc, manganese, iron, and copper, may also occur to a lesser extent. The plasma half-life of the drug is 20–60 minutes, and 50% of the injected dose is excreted in the urine within 1 hour. Increased urinary excretion of lead begins within 1 hour of EDTA administration, and is followed by a decrease in whole blood lead concentration over the course of treatment. Calcium EDTA mobilizes lead from soft tissues and from a fraction of the larger lead stores present in bone. In persons with high body lead burdens, cessation of EDTA chelation is often followed by an upward rebound in blood lead levels as bone stores equilibrate with lower soft tissue levels.

Note: Calcium EDTA should ***not*** be confused with sodium EDTA (edetate disodium), which is occasionally used to treat life-threatening severe hypercalcemia.

II. Indications

A. Calcium EDTA has been used to decrease blood lead concentrations and increase urinary lead excretion in individuals with symptomatic lead intoxication (see p 196) and in asymptomatic persons with high blood lead levels. Although clinical experience associates calcium EDTA chelation with relief of symptoms (particularly lead colic) and decreased mortality, controlled clinical trials demonstrating therapeutic efficacy are lacking, and treatment recommendations have been largely empiric.

B. Calcium EDTA may have possible utility in poisoning by zinc, manganese, and certain heavy radioisotopes.

III. Contraindications. Since calcium EDTA increases renal excretion of lead, anuria is a contraindication. Use reduced doses, with extreme caution, in patients with renal dysfunction, because accumulation of EDTA increases the risk of nephropathy.

IV. Adverse effects

A. Nephrotoxicity (eg, acute tubular necrosis, proteinuria, hematuria) may be minimized by adequate hydration, establishment of adequate urine flow, avoidance of excessive doses, and limitation of continuous administration to 5 days or less. Laboratory assessment of renal function should be performed daily during treatment for severe intoxication, and after the 2nd and 5th days in other cases.

B. In individuals with lead encephalopathy, rapid or high-volume infusions may exacerbate increased intracranial pressure. In such cases, the use of intramuscular injections or lower-volume, more concentrated intravenous infusions may be preferable.

C. Local pain may occur at intramuscular injection sites. Lidocaine (1 mL of 1% lidocaine for each mL of EDTA concentrate) may be added to intramuscular injections to decrease discomfort.

D. Inadvertent use of sodium EDTA (edetate disodium) may cause serious hypocalcemia.

E. Calcium EDTA may result in short-term zinc depletion, which has uncertain clinical significance.

F. **Use in pregnancy.** The safety of calcium EDTA in human pregnancy has not been established. Fetal malformations with high doses have been noted in animal studies.

V. **Drug or laboratory interactions.** Intravenous infusions may be incompatible with 10% dextrose solutions, amphotericin, or hydralazine.

VI. **Dosage and method of administration for lead poisoning (adults and children).** *Note:* Administration of EDTA should never be a substitute for removal from lead exposure. In adults, the federal OSHA Lead Standard requires removal from occupational lead exposure of any worker with a single blood lead concentration in excess of 60 μg/dL or an average of 3 successive values in excess of 50 μg/dL. *Prophylactic chelation,* defined as the *routine* use of chelation to prevent elevated blood lead concentrations or to lower blood lead levels below the standard in asymptomatic workers, *is not permitted.* Consult the local or state health department or OSHA (see Table VI–12, p 395) for more detailed information.

A. **Lead poisoning with encephalopathy, or blood lead levels greater than 100 μg/dL.** Administer calcium EDTA at a dose of 1500 mg/m^2/d (approximately 30 mg/kg) in 2–3 divided doses (every 8–12 hours) deep IM or as a continuous slow IV infusion (diluted to 2–4 mg/mL in 5% dextrose or normal saline). Treatment is usually continued for 5 days. Some clinicians advocate that treatment of patients with lead encephalopathy be initiated with a single dose of BAL (dimercaprol, see p 317), followed 4 hours later by the concomitant administration of BAL and calcium EDTA.

B. **Symptomatic lead poisoning without encephalopathy, and blood lead levels 50–100 μg/dL.** Administer calcium EDTA at a dose of 1000–1500 mg/m^2/d (approximately 20–30 mg/kg) in 2–3 divided doses deep IM or as a continuous IV infusion (diluted to 2–4 mg/mL) for 3–5 days.

C. An additional course of treatment may be considered based on posttreatment blood lead concentrations and the persistence or recurrence of symptoms. Treatment courses should be separated by a minimum of 2 days, and an interval of 2 or more weeks may be indicated to assess the extent of posttreatment rebound in blood lead levels.

D. Single-dose EDTA chelation lead mobilization tests have been advocated by some clinicians to evaluate body lead burden or to assess the need for a full course of treatment in patients with moderately elevated blood lead levels, but the value and necessity of these tests are controversial.

E. Oral EDTA therapy is *not* recommended for prevention or treatment of lead poisoning, because it may increase the absorption of lead from the gastrointestinal tract.

VII. **Formulations**

A. **Parenteral.** Calcium disodium edetate (Versenate), 200 mg/mL, 5-mL ampules. For intravenous infusion, dilute to 2–4 mg/mL in normal saline or 5% dextrose solution.

B. **Suggested minimum stocking level** to treat a 70-kg adult for the first 24 hours: 3 boxes (6 ampules per box, 18 g).

EPINEPHRINE

Neal L. Benowitz, MD

I. **Pharmacology.** Epinephrine is an endogenous catecholamine with α- and β-adrenergic agonist properties, used primarily in emergency situations to treat anaphylaxis or cardiac arrest. Beneficial effects include inhibition of histamine release from mast cells and basophils, bronchodilation, positive inotropic effects, and peripheral vasoconstriction.

Epinephrine is not active after oral administration. Subcutaneous injection produces effects within 5–10 minutes, with peak effects at 20 minutes. Intravenous or inhalational administration produces much more rapid onset. Epinephrine is rapidly inactivated in the body, with an elimination half-life of 2 minutes.

II. **Indications**
   A. Anaphylaxis and anaphylactoid reactions.
   B. Occasionally used for hypotension resulting from overdose by beta blockers, calcium antagonists, and other cardiac-depressant drugs.

III. **Contraindications**
   A. Uncorrected tachyarrhythmias or ventricular fibrillation, and uncorrected hypovolemia.
   B. Epinephrine is relatively contraindicated in patients with organic heart disease, peripheral arterial occlusive vascular disease with thrombosis, or ergot poisoning (see p 158).
   C. Narrow-angle glaucoma.

IV. **Adverse effects**
   A. Anxiety, restlessness, tremor, headache.
   B. Severe hypertension, which may result in intracranial hemorrhage, pulmonary edema, or myocardial necrosis or infarction.
   C. Use with caution in patients intoxicated by halogenated or aromatic hydrocarbon solvents and anesthetics, because these may sensitize the myocardium to the arrhythmogenic effects of epinephrine.
   D. Tissue necrosis after extravasation or intra-arterial injection.
   E. Aggravation of tissue ischemia, resulting in gangrene.
   F. Anaphylactoid reaction, which may occur owing to the bisulfite preservative in patients with sulfite hypersensitivity.
   G. Hypokalemia, hypophosphatemia, hyperglycemia, and leukocytosis may occur owing to β-adrenergic effects of epinephrine.
   H. **Use in pregnancy.** FDA category C (indeterminate). It is teratogenic in animals, crosses the placenta, can cause placental ischemia, and may suppress uterine contractions, but these effects do not preclude its acute, short-term use for a seriously symptomatic patient (see p 310).

V. **Drug or laboratory interactions**
   A. Enhanced arrhythmogenic effect occurs when epinephrine is given to patients with chloral hydrate overdose or anesthetized with cyclopropane or halogenated general anesthetics.
   B. Use in patients taking propranolol and other nonselective beta blockers may produce severe hypertension owing to blockade of β2-mediated vasodilation, resulting in unopposed α-mediated vasoconstriction.
   C. Cocaine and cyclic antidepressants may enhance stimulant effects owing to inhibition of neuronal epinephrine reuptake.
   D. Monoamine oxidase inhibitors may enhance pressor effects because of decreased neuronal epinephrine metabolism.
   E. Digitalis intoxication may enhance arrhythmogenicity of epinephrine.

VI. **Dosage and method of administration**
   A. **Avoid extravasation.** *Caution:* The intravenous infusion must be free-flowing, and the infused vein should be observed frequently for signs of subcutaneous infiltration (pallor, coldness, induration). If extravasation occurs, immediately infiltrate the affected area with phentolamine (see p 369), 5–10 mg in 10–15 mL of normal saline (children, 0.1–0.2 mg/kg; maximum 10 mg total) via

a fine (25- to 27-gauge) hypodermic needle; improvement is evidenced by hyperemia and return to normal temperature.

B. Mild to moderate allergic reaction. Give 0.3–0.5 mg SC or IM (children, 0.01 mg/kg of 1:1000 solution or 1:200 suspension; maximum 0.5 mg). May be repeated after 10–15 minutes if needed.

C. Severe anaphylaxis. Give 0.05–0.1 mg IV (0.5–1 mL of a 1:10,000 solution) every 5–10 minutes (children, 0.01 mg/kg; maximum 0.1 mg), or an intravenous infusion at 1–4 μg/min. If intravenous access is not available, the endotracheal route may be used; give 0.5 mg (5 mL of a 1:10,000 solution) down the endotracheal tube.

D. Hypotension. Infuse at 1 μg/min; titrate upward every 5 minutes as necessary.

VII. Formulations

   A. Parenteral. Epinephrine hydrochloride (Adrenalin, others), 0.01 mg/mL (1:100,000), 0.1 mg/mL (1:10,000), 0.5 mg/mL (1:2000), and 1 mg/mL (1:1000), in 1-, 2-, and 30-mL ampules, vials, and prefilled syringes. Most preparations contain sodium bisulfite or sodium metabisulfite as a preservative.

   B. Suggested minimum stocking level to treat a 70-kg adult for the first 24 hours: 10 mg (10 ampules, 1:1000, 1 mL, or equivalent).

ESMOLOL

Thomas E. Kearney, PharmD

  I. Pharmacology. Esmolol is a short-acting, intravenous, cardioselective β-adrenergic blocker with no intrinsic sympathomimetic or membrane-depressant activity. In usual therapeutic doses, it causes little or no bronchospasm in patients with asthma. Esmolol produces peak effects within 6–10 minutes of administration of an intravenous bolus. It is rapidly hydrolyzed by red blood cell esterases, with an elimination half-life of 9 minutes; therapeutic and adverse effects disappear within 30 minutes after the infusion is discontinued.

  II. Indications

   A. Rapid control of supraventricular and ventricular tachyarrhythmias and hypertension, especially if caused by excessive sympathomimetic activity (eg, stimulant drugs, hyperthyroid state).

   B. Reversal of hypotension and tachycardia caused by excessive β-adrenergic activity resulting from theophylline or caffeine overdose.

   C. Control of ventricular tachyarrhythmias caused by excessive myocardial catecholamine sensitivity (eg, chloral hydrate, chlorinated hydrocarbon solvents).

  III. Contraindications

   A. Contraindications include hypotension, bradycardia, or congestive heart failure secondary to intrinsic cardiac disease or cardiac-depressant effects of drugs and toxins (eg, cyclic antidepressants, barbiturates).

   B. Hypertension caused by α-adrenergic or generalized stimulant drugs, unless coadministered with a vasodilator (eg, nitroprusside, phentolamine).

  IV. Adverse effects

   A. Hypotension and bradycardia may occur, especially in patients with intrinsic cardiac disease or cardiac-depressant drug overdose.

   B. Bronchospasm may occur in patients with asthma or chronic bronchospasm, but it is less likely than with propranolol or other nonselective beta blockers and it is rapidly reversible after the infusion is discontinued.

   C. Esmolol may mask physiologic responses to hypoglycemia (tremor, tachycardia, glycogenolysis) and therefore should be used with caution in patients with diabetes.

   D. Use in pregnancy. FDA category C (indeterminate). This does not preclude its acute, short-term use for a seriously symptomatic patient (see p 310). High-dose infusion may contribute to placental ischemia.

  V. Drug or laboratory interactions

  A. Esmolol may transiently increase the serum digoxin level by 10–20%, but the clinical significance of this is unknown.
  B. Recovery from succinylcholine-induced neuromuscular blockade may be slightly delayed (5–10 minutes). Similarly, esmolol metabolism may be inhibited by anticholinesterase agents (eg, organophosphates).
  C. Esmolol is not compatible with sodium bicarbonate solutions.
VI. Dosage and method of administration
  A. Dilute before intravenous injection to a final concentration of 10 mg/mL, with 5% dextrose, lactated Ringer's injection, or saline solutions.
  B. Give as an intravenous infusion, starting at 50 µg/kg/min and increasing as needed up to 100 µg/kg/min. Steady state concentrations are reached approximately 30 minutes after each infusion adjustment. A loading dose of 500 µg/kg should be given if more rapid onset of clinical effects (5–10 minutes) is desired.
  C. Infusion rates greater than 200 µg/kg/min are likely to produce excessive hypotension.
VII. Formulations
  A. Parenteral. Esmolol hydrochloride (Brevibloc), 2.5 g in 10-mL ampules (250 mg/mL) and 100 mg in 10-mL vials (10 mg/mL).
  B. Suggested minimum stocking level to treat a 70-kg adult for the first 24 hours: 2 ampules (250 mg/mL, 10 mL) or 25 vials (10 mg/mL, 10 mL).

ETHANOL

Thomas E. Kearney, PharmD

  I. Pharmacology. Ethanol (ethyl alcohol) acts as a competitive substrate for the enzyme alcohol dehydrogenase, preventing the metabolic formation of toxic metabolites from methanol or ethylene glycol. Blood ethanol concentrations of 100 mg/dL effectively saturate alcohol dehydrogenase and prevent further methanol and ethylene glycol metabolism. Ethanol is well absorbed from the gastrointestinal tract when given orally, but the onset is more rapid and predictable when it is given intravenously. The elimination of ethanol is zero order; the average rate of decline is 15 mg/dL/h; however, this is highly variable and will be influenced by prior chronic use of alcohol, recruitment of alternate metabolic pathways, and concomitant hemodialysis (eg, to remove methanol or ethylene glycol).
 II. Indications. Methanol (methyl alcohol, see p 215) or **ethylene glycol** (see p 163) poisoning with a reliable history of ingestion but no available blood concentration measurements, with metabolic acidosis and an unexplained elevated osmolar gap see p 30, or with a serum concentration greater than 20 mg/dL.
III. Contraindications. Use of interacting drugs, which may cause disulfiram-type reaction (see **V.B.,** below).
IV. Adverse effects
  A. Nausea, vomiting, and gastritis may occur with oral administration.
  B. Inebriation, sedation, and hypoglycemia (particularly in children and malnourished adults) may occur. Ethanol may also exacerbate chronic pancreatitis.
  C. Intravenous use is sometimes associated with local phlebitis (especially with ethanol solutions > 10%). Hyponatremia may result from large doses of sodium-free intravenous solutions.
  D. Acute flushing, palpitations, and postural hypotension may occur in patients with atypical aldehyde dehydrogenase enzyme (up to 50–80% of Japanese, Chinese, and Korean individuals).
  E. Use in pregnancy. FDA category C (indeterminate). It crosses the placenta. Chronic overuse in pregnancy is associated with birth defects (fetal alcohol syndrome). The drug reduces uterine contractions and may slow or stop labor. However, these effects do not preclude its acute, short-term use for a seriously symptomatic patient (see p 310).
 V. Drug or laboratory interactions

A. Ethanol potentiates the effect of central nervous system—depressant drugs and hypoglycemic agents.

B. Disulfiram reaction (see p 155), including flushing, palpitations, and postural hypotension, may occur in patients taking disulfiram as well as a variety of other medications (eg, metronidazole, furazolidone, procarbazine, chlorpropamide, some cephalosporins, *Coprinus* mushrooms). In such cases, hemodialysis is the recommended alternative to ethanol treatment.

VI. Dosage and method of administration. Obtain serum ethanol levels after the loading dose and frequently during maintenance therapy to ensure a concentration of 100 mg/dL.

A. Ethanol may be given orally or intravenously. The desired serum concentration is 100 mg/dL (20 mmol/L); this can be achieved by giving approximately 750 mg/kg (Table III–5) as a loading dose, followed by a maintenance infusion of approximately 100–150 mg/kg/h (give a larger dose to chronic alcoholics).

B. Increase the infusion rate to 175–250 mg/kg/h (larger dose for chronic alcoholics) during hemodialysis to offset the increased rate of ethanol elimination. Alternately, ethanol may be added to the dialysate.

VII. Formulations

A. Oral. Pharmaceutical grade ethanol (96% USP).

Note: Commercial liquor may be used orally if pharmaceutical grade ethanol is not available; multiply the "proof" by 0.5 to obtain the percentage by volume, and then administer (100 mL per kg)/percentage.

B. Parenteral. Ethanol, 5% in 5% dextrose solution; 10% in 5% dextrose solution.

C. Suggested minimum stocking level to treat a 70-kg adult for the first 24 hours: 3 bottles (10% ethanol, 1 L each).

FLUMAZENIL

Thomas E. Kearney, PharmD

I. Pharmacology. Flumazenil (Romazicon) is a highly selective competitive inhibitor of central nervous system benzodiazepine receptors. It has no demonstrable benzodiazepine agonist activity and no significant toxicity even in high doses. It has no effect on alcohol or opioid receptors. Flumazenil is most effective parenterally (high first-pass effect with oral). After intravenous administration, the onset of benzodiazepine reversal occurs within 1–2 minutes, peaks at 6–10 minutes, and lasts for 1–5 hours, depending on the dose of flumazenil and the degree of preex-

TABLE III–5. ETHANOL DOSING (ADULTS AND CHILDREN)

	Intravenous[c]		
Dose	5%	10%	50% Oral
Loading[a]	15 mL/kg	7.5 mL/kg	1.5 mL/kg
Maintenance[b]	2–4 mL/kg/h	1–2 mL/kg/h	0.2–0.4 mL/kg/h
Maintenance during hemodialysis[b]	4–7 mL/kg/h	2–3.5 mL/kg/h	0.4–0.7 mL/kg/h

[a]If the patient's serum ethanol level is greater than 0, reduce the loading dose in a proportional manner. Multiply the calculated loading dose by the following factor:

$$\frac{100 - [\text{patient's serum ethanol in mg/dL}]}{100}$$

[b]Doses may vary depending on the individual. Chronic alcoholics have a higher rate of ethanol elimination, and maintenance doses should be adjusted to maintain an ethanol level of approximately 100 mg/dL.
[c]Infuse intravenous loading dose over 20–30 minutes or longer.

isting benzodiazepine effect. It is eliminated by hepatic metabolism with a serum half-life of approximately 1 hour.

II. Indications
A. Rapid reversal of benzodiazepine overdose–induced coma and respiratory depression, both as a diagnostic aid and potential substitute for endotracheal intubation.
B. Postoperative reversal of benzodiazepine sedation for surgical procedures and as an adjunct in weaning patients from ventilators.

III. Contraindications
A. Known hypersensitivity to flumazenil or benzodiazepines.
B. Suspected serious cyclic antidepressant overdose.
C. The patient has been given a benzodiazepine for control of a potentially life-threatening condition (eg, status epilepticus or increased intracranial pressure).

IV. Adverse effects
A. Anxiety, agitation, headache, dizziness, nausea, vomiting, tremor, and transient facial flushing.
B. Rapid reversal of benzodiazepine effect in patients with benzodiazepine addiction or high tolerance may result in acute withdrawal state, including hyperexcitability, tachycardia, and seizures (rarely reported).
C. Seizures or arrhythmias may be precipitated in patients with serious cyclic antidepressant overdose.
D. Flumazenil has precipitated arrhythmias in a patient with mixed benzodiazepine and chloral hydrate overdose.
E. Use in pregnancy. FDA category C (indeterminate). This does not preclude its acute, short-term use for a seriously symptomatic patient (see p 310).

V. Drug or laboratory interactions. No known interactions. Flumazenil does not appear to alter kinetics of benzodiazepines or other drugs.

VI. Dosage and method of administration
A. Benzodiazepine overdose. Titrate the dosage until desired response is achieved.
   1. Administer 0.2 mg IV over 30 seconds (pediatric dose not established; start with 0.01 mg/kg). If no response, give 0.3 mg. If no response, give 0.5 mg, and repeat every 30 seconds if needed to a total maximum dose of 3 mg (1 mg in children).
   2. Because effects last only 1–5 hours, continue to monitor patient closely for resedation. If multiple repeated doses are needed, consider a continuous infusion (0.2–1 mg/h).
B. Reversal of conscious sedation or anesthetic doses of benzodiazepine. A dose of 0.2 mg given intravenously is usually sufficient and may be repeated, titrating up to 1 mg.

VII. Formulations
A. Parenteral. Flumazenil (Romazicon), 0.1 mg/mL, 5-mL and 10-mL vials.
B. Suggested minimum stocking level to treat a 70-kg adult for the first 24 hours: 10 vials (0.1 mg/mL, 10 mL).

FOLIC ACID

Kathryn H. Keller, PharmD

I. Pharmacology. Folic acid is a B-complex vitamin that is essential for protein synthesis and erythropoiesis. In addition, the administration of folate to patients with methanol (and possibly ethylene glycol) poisoning may enhance the elimination of the toxic metabolite formic acid.
Note: Folic acid requires metabolic activation and is not effective for treatment of poisoning by dihydrofolate reductase inhibitors (eg, methotrexate, trimethoprim). Leucovorin (see p 348) is the proper agent in these situations.

II. Indications

    A. Adjunctive treatment for methanol poisoning.

    B. May be administered in ethylene glycol poisoning.

III. Contraindications. No known contraindications.

IV. Adverse effects

    A. Rare allergic reactions have been reported following intravenous administration.

    B. Use in pregnancy. Folic acid is a recommended supplement.

  V. Drug or laboratory interactions. This agent may increase metabolism of phenytoin.

 VI. Dosage and method of administration. The dose required for methanol or ethylene glycol poisoning is not established, although 50 mg IV (children, 1 mg/kg) every 4 hours for 6 doses has been recommended.

VII. Formulations

    A. Parenteral. Sodium folate (Folvite), 5 mg/mL and 10 mg/mL, 10-mL vials.

    B. Suggested minimum stocking level to treat a 70-kg adult for the first 24 hours: 6 vials (5 mg/mL, 1 mL each).

GLUCAGON

Thomas E. Kearney, PharmD

  I. Pharmacology. Glucagon is a polypeptide hormone that stimulates the formation of adenyl cyclase, which in turn increases the intracellular concentration of cyclic adenosine monophosphate (cAMP). This results in enhanced glycogenolysis and elevated serum glucose concentration; vascular smooth muscle relaxation; and positive inotropic, chronotropic, and dromotropic effects. These effects occur independently of β-adrenergic stimulation. Glucagon is destroyed in the gastrointestinal tract and must be given parenterally. After intravenous administration, effects are seen within 1–2 minutes and persist for 10–20 minutes. The serum half-life is about 3–10 minutes.

 II. Indications

    A. Hypotension, bradycardia, or conduction impairment caused by β-adrenergic blocker intoxication (see p 99).

    B. Possibly effective for severe cardiac depression caused by intoxication with calcium antagonists, quinidine, or other type Ia and type Ic antiarrhythmic drugs.

    C. Because of the benign side effect profile of glucagon, consider its early empiric use in any patient with myocardial depression (bradycardia, hypotension, low cardiac output) who does not respond rapidly to usual measures.

III. Contraindications. Known hypersensitivity to the drug (rare), or pheochromocytoma.

IV. Adverse effects

    A. Hyperglycemia.

    B. Nausea and vomiting.

    C. Use in pregnancy. FDA category B. Fetal harm is extremely unlikely (see p 310).

 V. Drug or laboratory interactions. Concurrent administration of epinephrine potentiates and prolongs the hyperglycemic and cardiovascular effects of glucagon.

 VI. Dosage and method of administration. Give 5–10 mg IV, followed by 1–5 mg/h infusion (children, 0.15 mg/kg IV, followed by 0.05–0.1 mg/kg/h). For very large doses, consider using sterile water or saline to reconstitute, rather than the phenol-containing diluent provided with the drug.

VII. Formulations

    A. Parenteral. Glucagon for injection, 1 unit (approximately 1 mg, with 1 mL diluent), 10 units (approximately 10 mg, with 10 mL diluent). Diluent contains phenol 0.2%.

    B. Suggested minimum stocking level to treat a 70-kg adult for the first 24 hours: 100 mg (10 vials, 10 units each).

GLUCOSE

Thomas E. Kearney, PharmD

  I. Pharmacology. Glucose is an essential carbohydrate used as a substrate for energy production within the body. Although many organs use fatty acids as an alternative energy source, the brain is totally dependent on glucose as its major energy source; thus, hypoglycemia may rapidly cause serious brain injury.

 II. Indications
  A. Hypoglycemia.
  B. Empiric therapy for patients with stupor, coma, or seizures who may have unsuspected hypoglycemia.

III. Contraindications. No absolute contraindications for empiric treatment of comatose patients with possible hypoglycemia. However, hyperglycemia and (possibly) recent ischemic brain injury may be aggravated by excessive glucose administration.

IV. Adverse effects
  A. Hyperglycemia and serum hyperosmolarity.
  B. Local phlebitis and cellulitis following extravasation (occurs with concentrations > 10%) from the intravenous injection site.
  C. Administration of a large glucose load may precipitate acute Wernicke-Korsakoff syndrome in thiamine-depleted patients. For this reason, thiamine (see p 19) is routinely given along with glucose to alcoholic or malnourished patients.
  D. Administration of large volumes of sodium-free dextrose solutions may contribute to hyponatremia.
  E. Use in pregnancy. FDA category C (indeterminate). This does not preclude its acute, short-term use for a seriously symptomatic patient (see p 310).

 V. Drug or laboratory interactions. No known interactions.

VI. Dosage and method of administration
  A. As empiric therapy for coma, give 50–100 mL of 50% dextrose via a secure intravenous line (children, 2–4 mL/kg of 25% dextrose; do *not* use 50% dextrose in children).
  B. Persistent hypoglycemia (eg, resulting from poisoning by hypoglycemic agent) may require repeated boluses of 25% (for children) or 50% dextrose and infusion of 5–10% dextrose, titrated as needed. Consider use of diazoxide (see p 328) in such situations.

VII. Formulations
  A. Parenteral. Dextrose injection, 50%, 50-mL prefilled injector; 25% dextrose, 10 mL; various solutions of 5–10% dextrose, some in combination with saline or other crystalloids.
  B. Suggested minimum stocking level to treat a 70-kg adult for the first 24 hours: 4 prefilled injectors (50% and 25%), 4 bottles or bags (5% and 10%, 1 L each).

HALOPERIDOL

Thomas E. Kearney, PharmD

  I. Pharmacology. Haloperidol is a butyrophenone neuroleptic drug useful for the management of acutely agitated psychotic patients. It has strong central antidopaminergic activity and weak anticholinergic effects. Haloperidol is well absorbed from the gastrointestinal tract and by the intramuscular route. Peak pharmacologic effects occur within 30–40 minutes of an intramuscular injection. The drug is metabolized and excreted slowly in the urine and feces. Although the serum half-life is 12–24 hours, the drug is detectable in the serum and urine for up to several weeks after a single dose.

 II. Indications. Haloperidol is used for the management of acute agitated functional psychosis or extreme agitation induced by stimulants or hallucinogenic drugs, especially when drug-induced agitation has not responded to diazepam (see p 327) or midazolam (see p 353).

III. Contraindications
A. Severe central nervous system depression in the absence of airway and ventilatory control.

B. Severe parkinsonism.

C. Known hypersensitivity to haloperidol.

IV. Adverse effects
A. Haloperidol produces less sedation and less hypotension than chlorpromazine but is associated with a higher incidence of extrapyramidal side effects.

B. Rigidity, diaphoresis, and hyperpyrexia may be a manifestation of **neuroleptic malignant syndrome** (see p 20) induced by haloperidol and other neuroleptic agents.

C. Haloperidol lowers the seizure threshold and should be used with caution in patients with known seizure disorder or who have ingested a convulsant drug.

D. Some oral haloperidol tablets contain tartrazine dye, which may precipitate allergic reactions in susceptible patients.

E. Use in pregnancy. This drug is teratogenic and fetotoxic in animals, and it crosses the placenta. Its safety in human pregnancy has not been established.

V. Drug or laboratory interactions
A. Haloperidol potentiates central nervous system—depressant effects of opioids, antidepressants, phenothiazines, ethanol, barbiturates, and other sedatives.

B. Combined therapy with lithium may increase the risk of neuroleptic malignant syndrome (see p 20).

VI. Dosage and method of administration
A. Oral. Give 2–5 mg of haloperidol orally; may repeat once if necessary; usual daily dose is 3–5 mg 2–3 times daily (children > 3 years old, 0.05–0.15 mg/kg/d or 0.5 mg in 2–3 divided doses).

B. Parenteral. Give 2–5 mg of haloperidol IM; may repeat once after 20–30 minutes and hourly if necessary (children > 3 years old, same as orally). Haloperidol is not approved for intravenous use in the USA, but that route has been widely used and is reportedly safe (except the decanoate salt formulation).

VII. Formulations
A. Oral. Haloperidol (Haldol), 0.5-, 1-, 2-, 5-, 10-, and 20-mg tablets.

B. Parenteral. Haloperidol (Haldol), 2 mg/mL and 5 mg/mL, 10-mL vials.

C. Suggested minimum stocking level to treat a 70-kg adult for the first 24 hours: 2 vials (5 mg/mL, 10 mL each).

HYDROXOCOBALAMIN

Kathryn H. Keller, PharmD

I. Pharmacology. Hydroxocobalamin and cyanocobalamin are synthetic forms of vitamin B_{12} used for the treatment of pernicious anemia. When administered to patients with cyanide poisoning, hydroxocobalamin exchanges its hydroxyl group with free cyanide in the plasma to produce the nontoxic cyanocobalamin.

II. Indications
A. Acute cyanide poisoning (concentrated formulation for this use has orphan drug status in USA). This drug may be synergistic with sodium thiosulfate (see p 376).

B. Prophylaxis against cyanide poisoning during nitroprusside infusion.

III. Contraindications. Do not use in patients with a known hypersensitivity to the drug.

IV. Adverse effects
A. Urine, sweat, tears, and other secretions become brownish-red after hydroxocobalamin administration.

B. Nausea, vomiting, hypertension, and mild muscle twitching or spasms.

C. Allergic reactions have been reported.

D. Use in pregnancy. No assigned FDA category; no reported experience with use during pregnancy is available. This does not preclude its acute, short-term use for a seriously symptomatic patient (see p 310), and it may be preferable to nitrite administration for cyanide poisoning.

V. Drug or laboratory interactions. Coloration of the serum sample may interfere with some general laboratory tests (AST, bilirubin, creatinine, magnesium).

VI. Dosage and method of administration. *Note:* In the USA, the only readily available formulation of hydroxocobalamin contains 1 mg/mL, which is impractical for acute cyanide poisoning because of the preparation time and the large volume (up to 4 g) that would need to be administered.

    A. Acute cyanide poisoning. Administer hydroxocobalamin intravenously in a dose equivalent to 50 times the amount of the cyanide exposure. If the amount of cyanide exposure is unknown, the recommended empiric dose is 4 g (or 50 mg/kg).

    B. Prophylaxis during nitroprusside infusion. Administer 25 mg/h by intravenous infusion.

VII. Formulations

    A. Parenteral (USA). Hydroxocobalamin, 1 mg/mL for intramuscular use, 10- and 30-mL vials.

    B. A preparation of 4 g of hydroxocobalamin in combination with 8 g of sodium thiosulfate is used in France for intravenous administration. This preparation has been granted orphan drug status by the FDA. Contact the National Information Center for Orphan Drugs and Rare Diseases in Washington, DC (1-800-456-3505 or 1-202-565-4167), for information on supplies and status.

    C. Suggested minimum stocking level to treat a 70-kg adult for the first 24 hours: for nitroprusside prophylaxis, 500 mg; for acute cyanide poisoning, orphan drug status means the drug is not commercially available for stocking.

IPECAC SYRUP

Thomas E. Kearney, PharmD

I. Pharmacology. Ipecac syrup is a mixture of plant-derived alkaloids, principally emetine and cephaeline, that produce emesis by direct irritation of the stomach and by stimulation of the central chemoreceptor trigger zone. Vomiting occurs in 90% of patients, usually within 20–30 minutes. Depending on the time after ingestion of the toxin, ipecac-induced emesis removes 30–50% of the stomach contents.

II. Indications. For a more complete discussion of gastric decontamination, see p 44.

    A. Early, on-scene management of oral poisonings, immediately following ingestion, in the home or at industrial on-site health care facilities without access to activated charcoal or the capacity to perform gastric lavage.

    B. In health care facilities, its use is generally limited to recent ingestions involving substances poorly adsorbed by activated charcoal (eg, iron, lithium, potassium, sodium) or sustained-release or enteric-coated tablets.

III. Contraindications

    A. Comatose or obtunded mental state.

    B. Ingestion of a caustic or corrosive substance or sharp object.

    C. Ingestion of most petroleum distillates or hydrocarbons (see p 178).

    D. Ingestion of a drug or toxin likely to result in abrupt onset of seizures or coma (eg, cyclic antidepressants, strychnine, camphor, nicotine, cocaine, amphetamines, isoniazid).

    E. Severe hypertension.

    F. Patient at high risk for hemorrhagic diathesis (eg, coagulopathy, esophageal varices).

IV. Adverse effects

    A. Persistent gastrointestinal upset following emesis may significantly delay administration of activated charcoal or other oral antidotes, or food or fluids, for up to several hours.

B. Severe and repeated vomiting may cause Mallory-Weiss tear, pneumomediastinum, hemorrhagic gastritis, or intracranial hemorrhage.

C. Vomiting may stimulate vagal reflex, resulting in bradycardia or atrioventricular block.

D. Drowsiness occurs in about 20% and diarrhea in 25% of children.

E. Single ingestions of therapeutic doses of ipecac syrup are not toxic (the former fluid extract was more potent), and failure to induce vomiting does not require removal of the ipecac. However, **chronic repeated ingestion** of ipecac (eg, in bulemics) may result in accumulation of cardiotoxic alkaloids and may lead to fatal cardiomyopathy and arrhythmias.

F. Use in pregnancy. FDA category C (indeterminate). There is minimal systemic absorption, but it may induce uterine contractions in late pregnancy.

V. Drug or laboratory interactions

A. Ipecac syrup potentiates nausea and vomiting associated with the ingestion of other gastric irritants.

B. Ipecac syrup is adsorbed in vitro by activated charcoal; however, ipecac still produces vomiting when given concurrently with charcoal.

C. Ipecac syrup contains 1.5–2% ethanol, which may cause an adverse reaction in patients taking disulfiram (see p 155) or other agents that have disulfiramlike effects (eg, metronidazole, *Coprinus* mushrooms).

VI. Dosage and method of administration

A. Children 6–12 months old. Give 5–10 mL.
   Note: Not recommended for non–health care facility use in this age group.

B. Children 1–12 years old. Give 15 mL.

C. Adults and children over 12 years old. Give 30 mL.

D. Follow ipecac administration with 4–8 oz of water or clear liquid (not essential for emetic effect). If emesis does not occur within 30 minutes, repeat the dose of ipecac and fluid.

VII. Formulations

A. Ipecac syrup, 30 mL.

B. Suggested minimum stocking level to treat a 70-kg adult for the first 24 hours: 2 bottles, 30 mL each.

ISOPROTERENOL

Thomas E. Kearney, PharmD

I. Pharmacology. Isoproterenol is a catecholaminelike drug that stimulates β-adrenergic receptors (β$_1$ and β$_2$). Pharmacologic properties include positive inotropic and chronotropic cardiac effects, peripheral vasodilation, and bronchodilation. Isoproterenol is not absorbed orally and shows variable and erratic absorption from sublingual and rectal sites. The effects of the drug are rapidly terminated by tissue uptake and metabolism; effects persist only a few minutes after intravenous injection.

II. Indications

A. Severe bradycardia or conduction block resulting in hemodynamically significant hypotension.
   Note: After beta-blocker overdose, even exceedingly high doses of isoproterenol may not overcome the pharmacologic blockade of β-receptors, and glucagon (see p 342) is the preferred agent.

B. Use isoproterenol to increase heart rate and normalize conduction to abolish polymorphous ventricular tachycardia (torsades de pointes) associated with QT interval prolongation (see p 14).

III. Contraindications

A. Do not use isoproterenol for ventricular fibrillation or ventricular tachycardia (other than torsades de pointes).

B. Use with extreme caution in the presence of halogenated or aromatic hydrocarbon solvents or anesthetics, or chloral hydrate.

IV. Adverse effects
A. Increased myocardial oxygen demand may result in angina pectoris or acute myocardial infarction.
B. Peripheral β_2-mediated vasodilation may worsen hypotension.
C. The drug may precipitate ventricular arrhythmias.
D. Sulfite preservative in some parenteral preparations may cause hypersensitivity reactions.
E. Hypokalemia may occur secondary to β-adrenergic–mediated intracellular potassium shift.
F. Use in pregnancy. FDA category C (indeterminate). This does not preclude its acute, short-term use for a seriously symptomatic patient (see p 310). However, it may cause fetal ischemia and also can reduce or stop uterine contractions.

V. Drug or laboratory interactions
A. Additive β-adrenergic stimulation occurs in the presence of other sympathomimetic drugs, theophylline, or glucagon.
B. Administration in the presence of cyclopropane, halogenated anesthetics, or other halogenated or aromatic hydrocarbons may enhance risk of ventricular arrhythmias because of sensitization of the myocardium to the arrhythmogenic effects of catecholamines.
C. Digitalis-intoxicated patients are more prone to develop ventricular arrhythmias when isoproterenol is administered.
D. Beta blockers may interfere with the action of isoproterenol by competitive blockade at β-adrenergic receptors.

VI. Dosage and method of administration
A. For intravenous infusion, use a solution containing 2–4 µg/mL, and begin with 0.5–1 µg/min infusion (children, 0.1 µg/kg/min) and increase as needed for desired effect or as tolerated (by monitoring for arrhythmias). The usual upper dosage is 20 µg/min (1.5 µg/kg/min in children), but as high as 200 µg/min has been given in adults with propranolol overdose.
B. If a dilute solution is not available, make a solution of 1:50,000 (20 µg/mL) by diluting 1 mL of the 1:5000 solution to a volume of 10 mL with normal saline.

VII. Formulations
A. Parenteral. Isoproterenol hydrochloride (Isuprel), 0.02 mg/mL (1:50,000) or 0.2 mg/mL (1:5000), which contains sodium bisulfite or sodium metabisulfite as a preservative.
B. Suggested minimum stocking level to treat a 70-kg adult for the first 24 hours: 10 ampules.

LABETALOL

Thomas E. Kearney, PharmD

I. Pharmacology. Labetalol is a mixed α- and β-adrenergic antagonist; after intravenous administration, the nonselective β-antagonist properties are approximately 7 times greater than the α_1-antagonist activity. Hemodynamic effects generally include a decrease in heart rate, blood pressure, and systemic vascular resistance. Atrioventricular conduction velocity may be decreased. After intravenous injection, hypotensive effects are maximal within 10–15 minutes and persist about 2–4 hours. The drug is eliminated by hepatic metabolism and has a half-life of 5–6 hours.

II. Indications. Labetalol may be used to treat hypertension and tachycardia associated with stimulant drug overdose (eg, cocaine, amphetamines).
Note: Hypertension with bradycardia suggests excessive α-mediated vasoconstriction (see p 18, 253); in this case, a pure alpha blocker such as phentolamine (see p 369) is preferable, because the reversal of β_2-mediated vasodilation may worsen hypertension.

III. Contraindications
A. Asthma.

B. Congestive heart failure.

C. Atrioventricular block.

IV. Adverse effects

A. Paradoxic hypertension may result when labetalol is used in the presence of stimulant intoxicants possessing strong mixed α- and β-adrenergic agonist properties (eg, cocaine, amphetamines) owing to the relatively weak α-antagonist properties of labetalol compared with its beta-blocking ability. (This has been reported with propranolol but not with labetalol.)

B. Orthostatic hypotension and negative inotropic effects may occur.

C. Dyspnea and bronchospasm may result, particularly in asthmatics.

D. Nausea, abdominal pain, diarrhea, and lethargy have been reported.

E. Use in pregnancy. FDA category C (indeterminate). This does not preclude its acute, short-term use for a seriously symptomatic patient (see p 310).

V. Drug or laboratory interactions

A. Additive blood pressure lowering with other antihypertensive agents, halothane, or nitroglycerin.

B. Cimetidine increases oral bioavailability of labetalol.

C. Labetalol is incompatible with 5% sodium bicarbonate injection (forms a precipitate).

D. Labetalol may cause false-positive elevation of urinary catecholamine levels.

VI. Dosage and method of administration

A. Adult. Give 20 mg slow IV bolus initially; may repeat with 40- to 80-mg doses at 10-minute intervals until blood pressure is controlled or a cumulative dose of 300 mg is achieved (most patients will respond to total doses of 50–200 mg). Alternatively, administer a constant infusion of 2 mg/min until blood pressure is controlled or a 300-mg cumulative dose is reached. After this, give oral labetalol starting at 100 mg twice daily.

B. Children older than 12 years. Initial 0.25 mg/kg dose is given intravenously over 2 minutes.

VII. Formulations

A. Parenteral. Labetalol hydrochloride (Normodyne, Trandate), 5 mg/mL, 40-mL vials.

B. Oral. Labetalol hydrochloride (Normodyne, Trandate), 100-, 200-, 300-mg tablets.

C. Suggested minimum stocking level to treat a 70-kg adult for the first 24 hours: 2 vials (5 mg/mL, 40 mL each).

LEUCOVORIN CALCIUM

Kathryn H. Keller, PharmD

I. Pharmacology. Leucovorin (folinic acid, citrovorum factor) is a metabolically functional form of folic acid. Unlike folic acid, leucovorin does not require reduction by dihydrofolate reductase, and therefore it can participate directly in the one-carbon transfer reactions necessary for purine biosynthesis and cellular DNA and RNA production. In animal models of methanol intoxication, both leucovorin and folic acid reduce morbidity and mortality by catalyzing the oxidation of the highly toxic metabolite, formic acid, to nontoxic products.

II. Indications

A. Folic acid antagonists (eg, methotrexate, trimethoprim, pyrimethamine). *Note:* Leucovorin treatment is essential because cells are incapable of utilizing folic acid owing to inhibition of dihydrofolate reductase.

B. Methanol poisoning. Leucovorin is an alternative to folic acid.

III. Contraindications. No known contraindications.

IV. Adverse effects

A. Allergic reactions as a result of prior sensitization have been reported.

B. Hypercalcemia from the calcium salt may occur (limit infusion rate to 16 mL/min).

TABLE III–6. LEUCOVORIN DOSE DETERMINATION

Methotrexate Concentration (10^{-6} mol/L)	Hours After Methotrexate Exposure	Leucovorin Dose (Adults and Children)
0.1–1	24	10–15 mg/m² q6h for 12 doses
1–5	24	50 mg/m² q6h until serum level is < 1 × 10^{-7} mol/L
5–10[a]	24	100 mg/m² q6h until serum level is < 1 × 10^{-7} mol/L

Reference: Methotrexate Management, in Rumack, B H et al (eds); *Poisindex.* Denver, 1989.
[a]If serum creatinine increases by 50% in the first 24 hours after methotrexate, increase the dose frequency to every 3 hours until the methotrexate level is less than 5 × 10^{-6} mol/L.

    C. Use in pregnancy. FDA category C (indeterminate). This does not preclude its acute, short-term use for a seriously symptomatic patient (see p 310).
  V. Drug or laboratory interactions. Leucovorin antagonizes the antifolate effect of methotrexate.
 VI. Dosage and method of administration
    A. Methotrexate poisoning. *Note:* Efficacy depends on early administration; the drug should be given within 1 hour of poisoning if possible. Administer intravenously a dose equal to or greater than the dose of methotrexate. If the dose is large but unknown, administer 75 mg (children, 10 mg/m²/dose) and then 12 mg every 6 hours for 4 doses. Serum methotrexate levels can be used to guide leucovorin therapy (Table III–6). Do not use oral therapy.
    B. Other folic acid antagonists. Administer 5–15 mg/d IM, IV, or orally for 5–7 days.
    C. Methanol poisoning. For adults and children, give 1 mg/kg (up to 50–70 mg) IV every 4 hours for 1–2 doses. Oral folic acid is given thereafter at the same dosage every 4–6 hours until resolution of symptoms and adequate elimination of methanol from the body (usually 2 days). Although leucovorin could be used safely for the entire course of treatment, its cost does not justify such prolonged use in place of folic acid.
VII. Formulations
    A. Parenteral. Leucovorin calcium (Wellcovorin, others), 3- and 10-mg/mL vials; and 50, 100, 350 mg for reconstitution (use sterile water rather than diluent provided, which contains benzyl alcohol).
    B. Oral. Leucovorin calcium (Wellcovorin, others), 5-, 10-, 15-, 25-mg tablets.
    C. Suggested minimum stocking level to treat a 70-kg adult for the first 24 hours: 2 100-mg vials or 1 350-mg vial.

LIDOCAINE

Thomas E. Kearney, PharmD

 I. Pharmacology
    A. Lidocaine is a local anesthetic and a type Ib antiarrhythmic agent. It inhibits fast sodium channels, depresses automaticity within the His-Purkinje system and the ventricles, and prolongs the effective refractory period and action potential duration. Conduction within ischemic myocardial areas is depressed, abolishing reentrant circuits. Unlike quinidine and related drugs, lidocaine exerts minimal effect on the automaticity of the sinoatrial node and on conduction through the atrioventricular node and does not decrease myocardial contractility or blood pressure in usual doses.
    B. The oral bioavailability of lidocaine is poor owing to extensive first-pass hepatic metabolism. After intravenous administration of a single dose, the onset of action is within 60–90 seconds and the duration of effect is 10–20 minutes. The elimination half-life of lidocaine is approximately 1.5–2 hours; active me-

tabolites have elimination half-lives of 2–10 hours. Drug accumulation may occur in patients with congestive heart failure or liver or renal disease.

II. **Indications.** Lidocaine is used for the control of ventricular arrhythmias arising from poisoning by a variety of cardioactive drugs and toxins (eg, digoxin, cyclic antidepressants, stimulants, theophylline). Patients with atrial arrhythmias do not usually respond to this drug.

III. **Contraindications**

   A. The presence of nodal or ventricular rhythms in the setting of third-degree atrioventricular or intraventricular block. These are usually reflex escape rhythms that may provide lifesaving cardiac output, and abolishing them may result in asystole.

   B. Hypersensitivity to lidocaine or other amide-type local anesthetics (rare).

IV. **Adverse effects**

   A. Excessive doses produce dizziness, confusion, agitation, and seizures.

   B. Conduction defects, bradycardia, and hypotension may occur with extremely high serum concentrations or in patients with underlying conduction disease.

   C. **Use in pregnancy.** FDA category B. Fetal harm is extremely unlikely (see p 310).

V. **Drug or laboratory interactions**

   A. Cimetidine and propranolol may decrease the hepatic clearance of lidocaine.

   B. Lidocaine may produce additive effects with other local anesthetics. In severe cocaine intoxication, lidocaine theoretically may cause additive neuronal depression.

VI. **Dosage and method of administration (adults and children).** Administer 1 mg/kg IV bolus over 1 minute, followed by infusion of 1–4 mg/min (20–50 µg/kg/min) to maintain serum concentrations of 1.5–5 mg/L. If significant ectopy persists after the initial bolus, a repeat dose of 0.5 mg/kg IV can be given if needed at 10-minute intervals (to maximum 300 mg or 3 mg/kg total dose). In patients with congestive heart failure or liver disease, use half the recommended dose.

VII. **Formulations**

   A. **Parenteral.** Lidocaine hydrochloride (Xylocaine, others), 50-mg (5-mL) and 100-mg (5-mL) prefilled syringes without preservatives; 1- and 2-g single use vials or additive syringes for preparing intravenous infusions.

   B. **Suggested minimum stocking level** to treat a 70-kg adult for the first 24 hours: 10 prefilled 100-mg syringes, 6 1-g vials for infusions.

METHOCARBAMOL

Thomas E. Kearney, PharmD

   I. **Pharmacology.** Methocarbamol is a centrally acting muscle relaxant. It does not directly relax skeletal muscle, and it does not depress neuromuscular transmission or muscle excitability; muscle relaxation is probably related to its sedative effects. After intravenous administration, the onset of action is nearly immediate. Elimination occurs by hepatic metabolism, with a serum half-life of 0.9–2.2 hours.

  II. **Indications**

   A. Control of painful muscle spasm caused by black widow spider envenomation (see p 288). Methocarbamol should be used as an adjunct to other medications (eg, calcium, diazepam) that are considered more effective.

   B. Management of muscle spasm caused by mild tetanus (see p 293) or strychnine (see p 290) poisoning.

 III. **Contraindications**

   A. Known hypersensitivity to the drug.

   B. History of epilepsy (intravenous methocarbamol may precipitate seizures).

 IV. **Adverse effects**

   A. Dizziness, drowsiness, nausea, flushing, and metallic taste may occur.

   B. Extravasation from intravenous site may cause phlebitis and sloughing. Do not administer subcutaneously.

    C. Hypotension, bradycardia, and syncope have occurred after intramuscular or intravenous administration. (Keep patient in a recumbent position for 10–15 minutes after injection.)

    D. Urticaria and anaphylactic reactions have been reported.

    E. Use in pregnancy. There is no reported experience, and no FDA category has been assigned.

V. Drug or laboratory interactions

    A. Lidocaine produces additive sedation with alcohol and other central nervous system depressants.

    B. Lidocaine may cause false-positive urine 5-HIAA and VMA results.

    C. The urine may turn brown, black, or blue after it stands.

VI. Dosage and method of administration

    A. Parenteral

        1. Administer 1 g (children, 15 mg/kg) IV over 5 minutes, followed by 0.5 g in 250 mL of 5% dextrose (children, 10 mg/kg in 5 mL of 5% dextrose) over 4 hours. Repeat every 6 hours to a maximum of 3 g daily.

        2. For tetanus, higher doses are usually recommended. Give 1–2 g IV initially, no faster than 300 mg/min; if needed, use a continuous infusion up to a total of 3 g.

        3. The usual intramuscular dose is 500 mg every 8 hours for adults and 10 mg/kg every 8 hours for children. Do not give subcutaneously.

    B. Oral. Switch to oral administration as soon as tolerated. Give 0.5–1 g (children, 10–15 mg/kg) orally or by gastric tube every 6 hours. The maximum dose is 1.5 g every 6 hours; for tetanus, the maximum adult dose is 24 g/d.

VII. Formulations

    A. Parenteral. Methocarbamol (Robaxin), 100 mg/mL.

    B. Oral. Methocarbamol (Robaxin, others), 500-, 750-mg tablets.

    C. Suggested minimum stocking level to treat a 70-kg adult for the first 24 hours: 24 vials (100 mg/mL, 10 mL each).

METHYLENE BLUE

Kathryn H. Keller, PharmD

    I. Pharmacology. Methylene blue is a thiazine dye that reverses drug-induced methemoglobinemia by increasing the conversion of methemoglobin to hemoglobin. This requires the presence of adequate amounts of the enzymes methemoglobin reductase and glucose-6-phosphate dehydrogenase (G6PD). The onset is rapid, with a maximum effect within 30 minutes. Methylene blue is excreted in the urine and bile, which turn blue or green.

    II. Indications. Methylene blue is used to treat methemoglobinemia (see p 217) in which the patient has symptoms or signs of hypoxemia (eg, dyspnea, confusion, chest pain) or has a methemoglobin level greater than 30%. **Note:** Methylene blue is not effective for sulfhemoglobinemia.

    III. Contraindications

        A. Glucose-6-phosphate dehydrogenase (G6PD) deficiency; treatment with methylene blue is ineffective and may cause hemolysis.

        B. Severe renal failure.

        C. Known hypersensitivity to methylene blue.

        D. Methemoglobin reductase deficiency.

        E. Reversal of nitrite-induced methemoglobinemia for treatment of cyanide poisoning.

    IV. Adverse effects

        A. Gastrointestinal upset, headache, and dizziness may occur.

        B. Excessive doses of methylene blue (> 7 mg/kg) can actually cause methemoglobinemia by directly oxidizing hemoglobin. Doses greater than 15 mg/kg are associated with hemolysis, particularly in neonates.

        C. Long-term administration may result in marked anemia.

        D. Extravasation may result in local tissue necrosis.

E. **Use in pregnancy.** There is no reported experience, and no FDA category has been assigned. This does not preclude its acute, short-term use for a seriously symptomatic patient (see p 310).

V. **Drug or laboratory interactions**
   A. No known drug interactions, but the intravenous preparation should not be mixed with other drugs.
   B. False-positive methemoglobin levels of about 15% are produced by dosages of 2 mL/kg of methylene blue.

VI. **Dosage and method of administration (adults and children)**
   A. Administer 1–2 mg/kg (0.1–0.2 mL/kg of 1% solution) IV slowly over 5 minutes. May be repeated in 30–60 minutes.
   B. If no response after 2 doses, do not repeat dosing; consider G6PD deficiency or methemoglobin reductase deficiency.
   C. Patients with continued production of methemoglobin from a long-acting oxidant stress (eg, dapsone) may require repeated dosing every 6–8 hours for 2–3 days.

VII. **Formulations**
   A. **Parenteral.** Methylene blue injection 1% (10 mg/mL).
   B. **Suggested minimum stocking level** to treat a 70-kg adult for the first 24 hours: 5 ampules (10 mg/mL, 10 mL each).

METOCLOPRAMIDE

Thomas E. Kearney, PharmD

I. **Pharmacology.** Metoclopramide, a dopamine antagonist, is an antiemetic that acts at the chemoreceptor trigger zone and may also increase gastrointestinal motility and facilitate gastric emptying. The onset of effect is 1–3 minutes after intravenous administration, and therapeutic effects persist for 1–2 hours after a single dose. The drug is excreted primarily by the kidney. The initial and terminal elimination half-lives are 5 minutes and 2.5–5 hours, respectively.

II. **Indications**
   A. Metoclopramide is used to prevent and control persistent nausea and vomiting, particularly when the ability to administer activated charcoal (eg, treatment of theophylline poisoning) or other oral antidotal therapy (eg, acetylcysteine for acetaminophen poisoning) is compromised.
   B. Theoretical (unproved) use to stimulate bowel activity in patients with ileus who require repeat-dose activated charcoal or whole bowel irrigation.

III. **Contraindications**
   A. Pheochromocytoma (metoclopramide may cause hypertensive crisis).
   B. Obstruction or perforation of the gastrointestinal tract.
   C. Known hypersensitivity to the drug; possible cross-sensitivity with procainamide.

IV. **Adverse effects**
   A. Sedation, restlessness, fatigue, and diarrhea may occur.
   B. Extrapyramidal reactions may result, particularly with high-dose treatment. Pediatric patients appear to be more susceptible. These reactions may be prevented by pretreatment with diphenhydramine.
   C. The drug may increase the frequency and severity of seizures in patients with seizure disorders.
   D. Parenteral formulations that contain sulfite preservatives may precipitate bronchoconstriction in susceptible individuals.
   E. **Use in pregnancy.** FDA category B. Fetal harm is extremely unlikely (see p 310).

V. **Drug or laboratory interactions**
   A. Additive sedation occurs in the presence of other central nervous system depressants.
   B. Risk of extrapyramidal reactions may be increased in the presence of other dopamine antagonist agents (eg, haloperidol, phenothiazines).

    C. Hypotensive reactions may occur when the drug is administered with anesthetics having hypotensive properties.

    D. The drug may enhance the absorption of ingested drugs by promoting gastric emptying.

    E. Anticholinergic agents may inhibit bowel motility effects.

VI. Dosage and method of administration

    A. Low dose. Give 10–20 mg IM or slowly IV (children, 0.1 mg/kg); this is reportedly effective for mild nausea.

    B. High dose. For adults and children, give 1–2 mg/kg IV infusion over 15 minutes in 50 mL dextrose or saline. May be repeated twice at 2- to 3-hour intervals. Pretreatment with 50 mg (children, 1 mg/kg) of diphenhydramine (see p 331) helps to prevent extrapyramidal reactions.

        1. Metoclopramide is most effective if given prior to emesis or 30 minutes before administration of nausea-inducing drug (eg, acetylcysteine).

        2. If no response to initial dose, may give additional 2 mg/kg at 3 hourly intervals up to maximum 12 mg/kg total dose.

VII. Formulations

    A. Parenteral. Metoclopramide hydrochloride (Reglan), 5 mg/mL; 2-, 10-, 30-, 50-, and 100-mL vials.

    B. Suggested minimum stocking level to treat a 70-kg adult for the first 24 hours: 1000 mg (4 vials, 50 mL each, or equivalent).

MIDAZOLAM

Thomas E. Kearney, PharmD

  I. Pharmacology. Midazolam is an ultrashort-acting and potent parenteral benzodiazepine used for the acute management of agitation and anxiety. Intravenous injection causes rapid sedation owing to high transient brain levels. Unlike diazepam, midazolam is well absorbed by subcutaneous and intramuscular routes. The serum half-life is 2–4 hours, but because central nervous system effects are determined by the rate of redistribution from the brain, the usual duration of sedation is only 30 minutes to 2 hours after a single dose. However, sedation may persist for 10 hours or longer after a prolonged infusion (see **VI.C.,** below).

 II. Indications

    A. Acute anxiety or agitation secondary to hallucinogenic or stimulant drug intoxication, psychosis, or metabolic encephalopathy.

    B. Sedation and amnesia during neuromuscular paralysis for endotracheal intubation.

    C. Status epilepticus (may be given intramuscularly if intravenous access for other anticonvulsants such as diazepam is not established).

III. Contraindications. No absolute contraindications. Midazolam must be used with caution in patients with compromised respiratory status, especially if the equipment and experienced personnel to manage respiratory arrest are not available.

IV. Adverse effects

    A. Respiratory arrest and hypotension may result, especially if the drug is given rapidly or in excessive doses or to elderly patients or those already intoxicated by other depressant drugs.

    B. Use in pregnancy. FDA category D (possible fetal risk). It readily crosses the placenta. This does not necessarily preclude its acute, short-term use for a seriously symptomatic patient (see p 310).

 V. Drug or laboratory interactions

    A. Additive depressant effects with other sedative-hypnotic agents, ethanol, or opiates.

    B. Central nervous system–depressant effects inhibited or reversed by flumazenil (see p 340).

VI. Dosage and method of administration

    A. Agitation or excessive muscle hyperactivity. Give 0.05 mg/kg IV over 20–30 seconds, or 0.1 mg/kg IM; may repeat every 20–30 minutes as needed.

Caution: There have been several reports of respiratory arrest and hypotension after rapid intravenous administration of midazolam, especially when given in combination with intravenous opioids.

B. Status epilepticus with no intravenous access. Give 0.1–0.2 mg/kg IM, may repeat after 5–10 minutes.

C. Continuous IV infusion or prolonged repeated dosing is *not* recommended because such use nullifies the short duration of effect from tissue redistribution, resulting in prolonged sedation or coma. Midazolam is also very expensive compared with other intermediate or long-acting agents (eg, diazepam).

VII. Formulations

    A. Parenteral. Midazolam (Versed), 1- and 5-mg/mL solutions; 1-, 2-, 5-, and 10-mL vials.

    B. Suggested minimum stocking level to treat a 70-kg adult for the first 24 hours: 2 vials (5 mg/mL, 5 mL each) or equivalent.

MORPHINE

Thomas E. Kearney, PharmD

    I. Pharmacology. Morphine is the principal alkaloid of opium and is a potent analgesic and sedative agent. In addition, it decreases venous tone and systemic vascular resistance, resulting in reduced preload and afterload. Morphine is variably absorbed from the gastrointestinal tract and is usually used parenterally. After intravenous injection, peak analgesia is attained within 20 minutes and usually lasts 3–5 hours. Morphine is eliminated by hepatic metabolism, with a serum half-life of about 3 hours; however, the clearance of morphine is slowed and duration of effect is prolonged in patients with renal failure.

  II. Indications

    A. Severe pain associated with black widow spider envenomation, rattlesnake envenomation, or other bites or stings.

    B. Pain caused by corrosive injury to the eyes, skin, or gastrointestinal tract.

    C. Pulmonary edema resulting from congestive heart failure. Chemical-induced noncardiogenic pulmonary edema is *not* an indication for morphine therapy.

  III. Contraindications

    A. Known hypersensitivity to morphine.

    B. Respiratory or central nervous system depression with impending respiratory failure, unless the patient is intubated or equipment and trained personnel are standing by to intervene if necessary.

    C. Suspected head injury. Morphine may obscure or cause exaggerated central nervous system depression.

  IV. Adverse effects

    A. Respiratory and central nervous system depression may result in respiratory arrest. Depressant effects may be prolonged in patients with liver disease and chronic renal failure.

    B. Hypotension may occur owing to decreased systemic vascular resistance and venous tone.

    C. Nausea, vomiting, and constipation may occur.

    D. Bradycardia, wheezing, flushing, pruritus, urticaria, and other histaminelike effects may occur.

    E. Use in pregnancy. FDA category C (indeterminate). This does not preclude its acute, short-term use for a seriously symptomatic patient (see p 310).

  V. Drug or laboratory interactions

    A. Additive depressant effects with other opioid agonists, ethanol and other sedative-hypnotic agents, tranquilizers, and antidepressants.

    B. Morphine is physically incompatible with solutions containing a variety of drugs, including aminophylline, phenytoin, phenobarbital, and sodium bicarbonate.

  VI. Dosage and method of administration

    A. Morphine may be injected subcutaneously, intramuscularly, or intravenously.

The oral and rectal routes produce erratic absorption and are not recommended for use in acutely ill patients.

B. The usual initial dose is 5–10 mg IV or 10–15 mg SC or IM, with maintenance analgesic doses of 5–20 mg every 4 hours. The pediatric dose is 0.1–0.2 mg/kg every 4 hours.

VII. Formulations

A. Parenteral. Morphine sulfate for injection; variety of available concentrations from 0.5 to 25 mg/mL.

B. Suggested minimum stocking level to treat a 70-kg adult for the first 24 hours: 150 mg.

NALOXONE

Thomas E. Kearney, PharmD

I. Pharmacology. Naloxone is a pure opioid antagonist that competitively blocks mu, kappa, and sigma opiate receptors within the central nervous system. Naloxone has no opioid agonist properties and can be given safely in large doses without producing respiratory or central nervous system depression. Naloxone is not effective orally but may be given subcutaneously, intramuscularly, intravenously, or even endotracheally. After intravenous administration, opioid antagonism occurs within 1–2 minutes and persists for approximately 1–4 hours. The plasma half-life is about 60 minutes.

II. Indications

A. Reversal of acute opioid intoxication manifested by coma, respiratory depression, or hypotension.

B. Empiric therapy for stupor or coma suspected to be caused by opioid overdose.

C. Anecdotal reports suggest that high-dose naloxone may partially reverse the central nervous system and respiratory depression associated with clonidine (see p 137), ethanol (see p 160), benzodiazepine (see p 97), or valproic acid (see p 302) overdoses, although these effects are inconsistent.

III. Contraindications. Do not use in patients with a known hypersensitivity to naloxone.

IV. Adverse effects

A. Use in opiate-dependent patients may precipitate acute withdrawal syndrome.

B. Pulmonary edema or ventricular fibrillation has occasionally occurred shortly after naloxone administration in opioid-intoxicated patients.

C. Agitation, hypertension, and ventricular irritability may occur following opioid antagonism when stimulant drugs are also present. Such reactions have been associated with postanesthetic use of naloxone when catecholamines and large fluid volumes have been administered.

D. There has been one case report of hypertension following naloxone administration in a patient with clonidine overdose.

E. Use in pregnancy. FDA category B (see p 310). In an opioid-dependent mother, acute naloxone-induced withdrawal may precipitate labor.

V. Drug or laboratory interactions. Naloxone antagonizes the analgesic effect of opioids.

VI. Dosage and method of administration. Avoid intramuscular route; absorption is erratic and incomplete. Do not give orally.

A. Suspected opioid-induced coma

1. Administer 0.4–2 mg IV; may repeat at 2- to 3-minute intervals until desired response achieved. Titrate carefully in opioid-dependent patients. The dose for children is the same as for adults.

2. The total dose required to reverse the effects of the opioid is highly variable and is dependent on the concentration and receptor affinity of the opioid. Some drugs (eg, propoxyphene) do not respond to usual doses of naloxone. However, if no response is achieved by a total dose of 10–15 mg, the diagnosis of opioid overdose should be questioned.

3. *Caution:* Resedation can occur when the naloxone wears off in 1–2 hours. Repeated doses of naloxone may be required to maintain reversal of the effects of opioids with prolonged elimination half-lives (eg, methadone) or sustained-release formulations or ingested packets or vials.

B. Infusion. Give 0.4–0.8 mg/h in 5% dextrose, titrated to clinical effect. Another method is to estimate two-thirds of the initial dose needed to awaken the patient and give this amount each hour.

VII. Formulations

A. Parenteral. Naloxone hydrochloride (Narcan), 0.02, 0.4, or 1 mg/mL; 1-, 2-, or 10-mL syringes, ampules, or vials.

B. Suggested minimum stocking level to treat a 70-kg adult for the first 24 hours: 30 mg (3 vials, 1 mg/mL, 10 mL each, or equivalent).

NALTREXONE

Thomas E. Kearney, PharmD

I. Pharmacology. Naltrexone, like naloxone, is a competitive antagonist for all opioid receptors (mu, kappa, delta). It is 2–9 times more potent than naloxone, and is effective when given orally, despite a high first-pass effect. One active metabolite, 6-β-naltrexol, has opiate antagonist effects while another, noroxymorphine, can cause opiate agonist effects including miosis in some patients. The degree and duration of naltrexone-induced opioid antagonism depends on the dose, but ranges from 24–72 hours.

II. Indications

A. Naltrexone is used to prevent recidivism in patients detoxified from opioid abuse, coupled with a comprehensive drug abuse treatment program including counseling and behavior modification.

B. Naltrexone has been used, along with clonidine, to detoxify methadone-dependent patients.

C. It is *not* used for acute reversal of opioid intoxication (see Naloxone [p 355]).

III. Contraindications

A. Active liver disease or hepatic insufficiency.

B. Patients receiving opioids or with known opioid dependence.

IV. Adverse effects

A. Dose-dependent hepatocellular injury when used in high doses for several weeks.

B. Use in opiate-dependent patients may precipitate acute withdrawal syndrome (see **V.A.,** below).

C. Most other reported effects are minor or inconsequential. Those with an incidence greater than 10% include nausea, vomiting, abdominal pain, headache, irritability, dizziness, anxiety, and chills.

D. Use in pregnancy. FDA category C (indeterminate) (see p 310). It is embryocidal in animals. In an opioid-dependent mother, acute withdrawal may precipitate labor.

V. Drug or laboratory interactions

A. Naltrexone may precipitate a severe and prolonged withdrawal syndrome in patients who are opioid-dependent. Symptoms include nausea, abdominal cramps, vomiting, hallucinations, fever, chills, hypersecretions, anxiety, and mydriasis, and may begin within 5 minutes and last up to 48 hours. Wait at least 7–10 days after discontinuing opioids before starting naltrexone (longer periods may be advisable after use of long-acting agents such as methadone). To ensure an adequate drug holiday period, administer a "naloxone challenge" dose (see **VI.A.1.,** below). Also consider coadministration of clonidine to alleviate potential opioid withdrawal symptoms (see **VI.B.,** below).

B. Naltrexone will nullify the therapeutic effects of opioids. Administration of this drug should be stopped at least 48–72 hours before planned surgical procedures or other situations requiring opioid analgesia.

C. The drug may augment lethargy and drowsiness after initial doses in patients receiving phenothiazines.

VI. Dosage and method of administration

A. Stepwise approach for maintenance of opioid sobriety

1. **Naloxone challenge** prior to initiating naltrexone therapy. Administer naloxone subcutaneously (0.8 mg) or intravenously (start with 0.2 mg, wait 30 seconds; if no withdrawal symptoms, administer additional 0.6 mg). Observe for 20–40 minutes. If no withdrawal symptoms occur, administer additional 1.2 mg to confirm the absence of opioid dependence. If withdrawal symptoms occur, rechallenge after waiting 24 hours.

2. **Initiation of naltrexone**
   a. Administer 25 mg orally, and observe for 1 hour. If no withdrawal symptoms, then give another 25 mg; or
   b. Give 5–12.5 mg orally, observe for 1 hour, then give repeated incremental doses to a total of 50 mg.

3. **Maintenance dosing.** The usual dose is 50 mg orally daily for the period of treatment (usually 6 months). Compliance may be enhanced by increasing the dose and interval (eg, 100 mg every other day or 150 mg every 3rd day).

B. Naltrexone-clonidine regimen for opioid detoxification of the methadone-dependent patient.

1. Initiate therapy with clonidine (0.005 mg/kg) and titrate upward as necessary (highest mean daily dose 2.3 mg).

2. On the second day, give naltrexone, 1 mg orally, and repeat by increasing increments of 1–2 mg every 4 hours for the next 2 days. After the third day, clonidine may be used only as needed to reduce opioid withdrawal symptoms. Naltrexone can be gradually increased to 50 mg daily.

VII. Formulations

A. Oral. Naltrexone hydrochloride (Trexan), 50-mg tablets (scored).

B. Suggested minimum stocking level to treat a 70-kg adult for the first 24 hours: 1 bottle (50 tablets).

NEUROMUSCULAR BLOCKERS

Thomas E. Kearney, PharmD

I. Pharmacology

A. Neuromuscular-blocking agents produce skeletal muscle paralysis by inhibiting the action of acetylcholine at the neuromuscular junction. **Depolarizing agents** (eg, succinylcholine; Table III–7) depolarize the motor end plate and block recovery; transient muscle fasciculations occur with the initial depolarization. **Nondepolarizing agents** (eg, pancuronium, vecuronium) competitively block the action of acetylcholine at the motor end plate; therefore, no initial muscle fasciculations occur. They also block acetylcholine at sympathetic ganglia, which may result in hypotension.

TABLE III–7. COMPARISON OF NEUROMUSCULAR-BLOCKING AGENTS

Drug	Type	Onset	Duration
Succinylcholine	Depolarizing	30–60 s	2–3 min, dissipates over 10 min
Pancuronium	Nondepolarizing	2–3 min	Dose-dependent; at 0.06 mg/kg, duration of effect is 35–45 min
Vecuronium[a]	Nondepolarizing	1–2 min	Dose-dependent; average, 25–40 min
Atracurium[a]	Nondepolarizing	3–5 min	Dose-dependent; average, 20–45 min
Mivacurium	Nondepolarizing	1–8 min	Dose-dependent; average, 15–20 min

[a]These agents have minimal cardiovascular effects compared with other nondepolarizing agents.

B. The neuromuscular blockers produce complete muscle paralysis with no depression of central nervous system function. Thus, patients who are conscious will remain awake but unable to move and patients with status epilepticus may continue to have central nervous system seizure activity despite flaccid paralysis.

C. Succinylcholine produces the most rapid onset of effects, with total paralysis within 30–60 seconds after intravenous administration. It is rapidly hydrolyzed by plasma cholinesterases, and its effects dissipate in 10–20 minutes. Pancuronium produces paralysis within 2–3 minutes, and its effects subside after about 45 minutes. Vecuronium produces paralysis within about 1 minute, with recovery after about 15–20 minutes.

II. Indications

A. Neuromuscular blockers are used to abolish excessive muscular activity, rigidity, or peripheral seizure activity when continued hyperactivity may produce or aggravate rhabdomyolysis and hyperthermia. Examples of such situations include the following.

Note: The preferred agent for these conditions is pancuronium.

1. Drug overdoses involving stimulants (eg, amphetamines, cocaine, phencyclidine, monoamine oxidase inhibitors) or strychnine.

2. Tetanus.

3. Hyperthermia associated with muscle rigidity or hyperactivity (eg, status epilepticus, neuroleptic malignant syndrome [see p 20], or serotonin syndrome [see p 21]).

Note: Neuromuscular blockers are not effective for malignant hyperthermia (see p 20); in fact, inability to induce paralysis with these agents should suggest the diagnosis of malignant hyperthermia.

B. Neuromuscular blockers provide prompt flaccid paralysis to facilitate orotracheal intubation. The preferred agents for this purpose are succinylcholine and vecuronium.

III. Contraindications

A. Unpreparedness or inability to intubate the trachea and ventilate the patient after total paralysis ensues. Proper equipment and trained personnel must be assembled before the drug is given.

B. Known history of malignant hyperthermia. Succinylcholine use is associated with malignant hyperthermia in susceptible patients (incidence approximately 1 in 50,000).

IV. Adverse effects

A. Complete paralysis results in respiratory depression and apnea.

B. Succinylcholine can stimulate vagal nerves, resulting in sinus bradycardia and atrioventricular block. Children are particularly sensitive to vagotonic effects.

C. Muscle fasciculations may cause increased intraocular and intragastric pressure (the latter of which may result in emesis and aspiration of gastric contents). Rhabdomyolysis and myoglobinuria may be observed, especially in children.

D. Succinylcholine may produce hyperkalemia in patients with myopathy, recent severe burns, or spinal cord injury (this risk is maximal a few months after the injury).

E. Clinically significant histamine release with bronchospasm may occur, especially with succinylcholine.

F. Neuromuscular blockade is potentiated by hypokalemia and hypocalcemia (nondepolarizing agents) and by hypermagnesemia (depolarizing and nondepolarizing agents).

G. Prolonged effects may occur after succinylcholine use in patients with genetic deficiency of plasma cholinesterase.

H. Prolonged effects may occur in patients with neuromuscular disease (eg, myasthenia gravis, Eaton-Lambert syndrome).

I. **Use in pregnancy.** FDA category C (indeterminate). This does not preclude their acute, short-term use for a seriously ill patient (see p 310).

V. Drug or laboratory interactions

   A. Actions of the nondepolarizing agents are potentiated by ether, methoxyflurane, and enflurane and are inhibited or reversed by anticholinesterase agents (eg, neostigmine, physostigmine, carbamate and organophosphate insecticides).

   B. Organophosphate (see p 240) or carbamate (see p 118) insecticide intoxication may potentiate or prolong the effect of succinylcholine.

   C. Numerous drugs may potentiate neuromuscular blockade. These include calcium antagonists, aminoglycoside antibiotics, propranolol, membrane-stabilizing drugs (eg, quinidine), magnesium, lithium, and thiazide diuretics.

   D. Anticonvulsants (carbamazepine, phenytoin) and theophylline may delay the onset and shorten the duration of action of some nondepolarizing agents.

VI. Dosage and method of administration

   A. Succinylcholine

   1. Give 0.6 mg/kg IV (infants, 2 mg/kg; children, 1 mg/kg) over 10–20 seconds; may repeat as needed.

   2. To prevent fasciculations, administer a small dose of a nondepolarizing agent (eg, pancuronium, 0.01 mg/kg) 2–3 minutes prior to the succinylcholine.

   3. Pretreat children with atropine (0.005–0.01 mg/kg) to prevent bradycardia or atrioventricular block.

   B. Pancuronium. Give 0.06–0.1 mg/kg IV push, then 0.01–0.02 mg/kg every 20–40 minutes as needed.

   C. Vecuronium. For children older than 1 year and adults, give 0.08–0.1 mg/kg IV push, then 0.01–0.02 mg/kg every 10–20 minutes as needed.

VII. Formulations

   A. Succinylcholine chloride (Anectine, others), 20, 50, 100 mg/mL; 5-, 10-mL vials and ampules. **Suggested minimum stocking level** to treat a 70-kg adult for the first 24 hours: 2 vials of each concentration.

   B. Pancuronium bromide (Pavulon), 1, 2 mg/mL; 2-, 5-, and 10-mL vials and ampules. **Suggested minimum stocking level** to treat a 70-kg adult for the first 24 hours: 8 vials (2 mg/mL, 5 mL each).

   C. Vecuronium bromide (Norcuron), 10 mg of lyophilized powder for reconstitution. **Suggested minimum stocking level** to treat a 70-kg adult for the first 24 hours: 3 vials.

NICOTINAMIDE (NIACINAMIDE)

Thomas E. Kearney, PharmD

   I. Pharmacology. Nicotinamide (niacinamide, vitamin B_3), one of the B vitamins, is required for the functioning of the coenzymes nicotinamide adenine dinucleotide (NAD) and nicotinamide adenine dinucleotide phosphate (NADP). NAD and NADP are responsible for energy transfer reactions. Niacin deficiency, which results in pellagra, can be corrected with nicotinamide.

   II. Indications. Nicotinamide is used to prevent the neurologic and endocrinologic toxicity associated with the ingestion of Vacor (PNU), a rodenticide that is believed to act by antagonizing nicotinamide (see p 301). Best results are achieved when nicotinamide therapy is instituted within 3 hours of ingestion. It may also be effective for treatment of Vacor analogs such as alloxan and streptozocin.

   III. Contraindications. No known contraindications.

   IV. Adverse effects

   A. Headache, dizziness.

   B. Hyperglycemia.

   C. Hepatotoxicity (reported after chronic use with daily dose > 3 g).

   D. Use in pregnancy. No assigned FDA category. This does not preclude its acute, short-term use for a seriously symptomatic patient (see p 310).

   V. Drug or laboratory interactions. No known interactions.

   VI. Dosage and method of administration (adults and children). *Note:* The parenteral preparation is no longer available in the US. The oral form may be substituted, but is of unknown efficacy.

    1. Give 500 mg IV initially, followed by 100–200 mg IV every 4 hours for 48 hours. Then give 100 mg orally 3–5 times daily for 2 weeks. If clinical deterioration from the Vacor progresses during initial therapy with nicotinamide, change dosing interval to every 2 hours. The maximum suggested daily dose is 3 g.

    2. *Note:* Nicotinic acid (niacin) is ***not*** a substitute for nicotinamide in the treatment of Vacor ingestions.

VII. Formulations

    A. Parenteral. Niacinamide, 100 mg/mL (not available in the US).

    B. Oral. Niacinamide, 50-, 100-, 125-, 250-, 500-mg tablets. **Suggested minimum stocking level** to treat a 70-kg adult for the first 24 hours: 3 g.

NIFEDIPINE

Thomas E. Kearney, PharmD

  I. Pharmacology. Nifedipine is a calcium antagonist that inhibits the influx of calcium ions through calcium channels. It acts primarily by dilating systemic and coronary arteries. Unlike some other calcium antagonists (eg, verapamil, diltiazem), nifedipine has minimal effects on cardiac conduction and contractility. Nifedipine is administered orally. The rapid onset of effect (15–30 minutes) following sublingual administration of the capsule contents appears to be caused by swallowing of the liquid rather than actual buccal absorption. The drug is metabolized by the liver and has a serum half-life of 2–5 hours.

  II. Indications

    A. Hypertension following overdose with vasoconstrictive substances such as phenylpropanolamine, cocaine, amphetamines, phencyclidine, or other stimulants. However, for rapid and titratable effect in patients with severe hypertension, a parenteral vasodilator such as phentolamine (see p 369) or nitroprusside (see p 362) is preferred.

    B. Adjunctive use as a vasodilator for treatment of arterial spasm (ie, ergot poisoning).

  III. Contraindications

    A. Known hypersensitivity to the drug.

    B. Volume depletion (relative contraindication).

  IV. Adverse effects. The main disadvantage of nifedipine is that it is administered orally, with less titratability than other agents and the potential to "overshoot" the desired drop in blood pressure.

    A. Hypotension may result, especially in volume-depleted patients.

    B. Tachycardia, headache, and flushing may occur.

    C. Cerebral perfusion may be compromised if blood pressure is lowered too rapidly in a patient with intracranial hypertension resulting from stroke or hypertensive encephalopathy.

    D. Use with extreme caution in patients with obstructive cardiomyopathy or aortic stenosis; increased gradient across the aortic valve may cause pulmonary edema and hypotension.

    E. Use in pregnancy. FDA category C (indeterminate). However, this does not preclude its acute, short-term use for a seriously symptomatic patient (see p 310).

  V. Drug or laboratory interactions. Nifedipine has an additive blood pressure–lowering effect when given with other antihypertensives or beta blockers.

  VI. Dosage and method of administration. The usual dose is a 10-mg capsule—punctured, chewed, and contents swallowed (do not use extended-release formulations). It may be repeated as needed. Most hypertensive patients respond to 10–20 mg. For childhood hypertensive emergencies, give 0.25–0.5 mg/kg/dose.

  VII. Formulations

    A. Oral. Nifedipine (Procardia, Adalat), 10- and 20-mg fluid-filled capsules.

B. Suggested minimum stocking level to treat a 70-kg adult for the first 24 hours: 1 bottle (10 mg, 100 capsules).

NITRITE, SODIUM AND AMYL

Kathryn H. Keller, PharmD

I. Pharmacology. Sodium nitrite injectable solution and amyl nitrite crushable ampules for inhalation are components of the cyanide antidote kit. The value of nitrites as an antidote to cyanide poisoning is 2-fold: they oxidize hemoglobin to methemoglobin, which binds free cyanide, and they may enhance endothelial cyanide detoxification by producing vasodilation. Inhalation of an ampule of amyl nitrite produces a methemoglobin level of about 5%. Intravenous administration of a single dose of sodium nitrite is anticipated to produce a methemoglobin level of about 20–30%.

II. Indications

A. Symptomatic cyanide poisoning (see p 145). Nitrites are not usually used for empiric treatment unless cyanide is very strongly suspected, and they are not recommended for smoke inhalation victims.

B. Possibly effective for hydrogen sulfide poisoning, if given within 30 minutes of exposure (see p 182).

III. Contraindications

A. Significant preexisting methemoglobinemia (> 40%).

B. Severe hypotension is a relative contraindication, as it may be worsened by nitrites.

C. Administration to patients with concurrent carbon monoxide poisoning is a relative contraindication; generation of methemoglobin may further compromise oxygen transport to the tissues.

IV. Adverse effects

A. Headache, facial flushing, dizziness, nausea, vomiting, tachycardia, and sweating may occur. These side effects may be masked by the symptoms of cyanide poisoning.

B. Rapid intravenous administration may result in hypotension.

C. Excessive and potentially fatal methemoglobinemia may result.

D. Use in pregnancy. No assigned FDA category. These agents may compromise blood flow and oxygen delivery to the fetus, and they may induce fetal methemoglobinemia. However, this does not preclude their acute, short-term use for a seriously symptomatic patient (see p 310).

V. Drug or laboratory interactions

A. Hypotension may be exacerbated by the concurrent presence of alcohol or other vasodilators, or any antihypertensive agent.

B. Methylene blue should not be administered to a cyanide-poisoned patient, because it may reverse nitrite-induced methemoglobinemia and result in release of free cyanide ion. However, it may be considered when severe and life-threatening excessive methemoglobinemia (eg, > 70%) is present.

C. Binding of methemoglobin to cyanide (cyanomethemoglobin) may lower the measured free methemoglobin level.

VI. Dosage and method of administration

A. Amyl nitrite crushable ampules. Crush 1–2 ampules in gauze, cloth, or sponge and place under the nose of the victim, who should inhale deeply for 30 seconds. Rest for 30 seconds, then repeat. Each ampule lasts about 2–3 minutes. If the victim is receiving respiratory support, place the ampules in the face mask or port access to the endotracheal tube. Stop ampule use when administering IV sodium nitrite.

B. Sodium nitrite parenteral

1. Adults. Administer 300 mg of sodium nitrite (10 mL of 3% solution) IV over 3–5 minutes.

2. Children. Give 0.15–0.33 mL/kg to a maximum of 10 mL. Pediatric dosing should be based on the hemoglobin concentration, if known (see Table

III–8). If anemia is suspected or hypotension is present, start with the lower dose, dilute in 50–100 mL of saline, and give over at least 5 minutes.

3. Oxidation of hemoglobin to methemoglobin occurs within 30 minutes. If no response to treatment occurs within 30 minutes, an additional half-sized dose of intravenous sodium nitrite may be given.

VII. Formulations
   A. Amyl nitrite. A component of the Lilly Cyanide Antidote kit, 0.3 mL in crushable ampules, 12 per kit. The drug may also be acquired separately in aspirols. ***Note:*** The ampules have a shelf life of only 1 year, and may disappear because of the potential for abuse (as "poppers").
   B. Sodium nitrite parenteral. A component of the Lilly Cyanide Antidote kit, 300 mg in 10 mL of sterile water (3%), 2 ampules per kit.
   C. Suggested minimum stocking level to treat a 70-kg adult for the first 24 hours: 2 Lilly Cyanide Antidote kits, or equivalent (one kit should be kept in the Emergency Department).

NITROPRUSSIDE

Thomas E. Kearney, PharmD

   I. Pharmacology. Nitroprusside is an ultrashort-acting and titratable parenteral hypotensive agent that acts by directly relaxing vascular smooth muscle. Both arterial and venous dilation occur; the effect is more marked in patients with hypertension. A small increase in heart rate may be observed in hypertensive patients. Intravenous administration produces nearly immediate onset of action, with a duration of effect of 1–10 minutes. Nitroprusside is rapidly metabolized, with a serum half-life of about 1–2 minutes. Cyanide is produced during metabolism and is converted to the less toxic thiocyanate. Thiocyanate has a half-life of 2–3 days, and accumulates in patients with renal insufficiency.

   II. Indications
   A. Rapid control of severe hypertension (eg, in patients with stimulant intoxication or monoamine oxidase inhibitor toxicity).
   B. Arterial vasodilation in patients with ergot-induced peripheral arterial spasm.

   III. Contraindications
   A. Compensatory hypertension, eg, in patients with intracranial hemorrhage or mass lesion, or in patients with coarctation of the aorta.
   B. Use with caution in patients with hepatic insufficiency, because cyanide metabolism may be impaired.

   IV. Adverse effects
   A. Nausea, vomiting, headache, and sweating may be caused by excessively rapid lowering of the blood pressure.

TABLE III–8. PEDIATRIC DOSING OF SODIUM NITRITE BASED ON HEMOGLOBIN CONCENTRATION

Hemoglobin (g/dL)	Initial Dose (mg/kg)	Initial Dose of 3% Sodium Nitrite (mL/kg)
7	5.8	0.19
8	6.6	0.22
9	7.5	0.25
10	8.3	0.27
11	9.1	0.3
12	10	0.33
13	10.8	0.36
14	11.6	0.39

B. **Cyanide toxicity,** manifested by altered mental status and metabolic acidosis, may occur with rapid high-dose infusion (> 10–15 µg/kg/min) for periods of 1 hour or longer. Continuous intravenous infusion of hydroxocobalamin, 25 mg/h (see p 344), or thiosulfate (see p 376) has been used to limit cyanide toxicity. If severe cyanide toxicity occurs, discontinue the nitroprusside infusion and give antidotal doses of thiosulfate and sodium nitrite (see p 361).

C. **Thiocyanate intoxication,** manifested by disorientation, delirium, muscle twitching, and psychosis, may occur with prolonged high-dose infusions (usually > 3 µg/kg/min for 48 hours or longer), particularly in patients with renal insufficiency (may occur at rates as low as 1 µg/kg/min). Thiocyanate production is also enhanced by coadministration of sodium thiosulfate. Monitor thiocyanate levels if the nitroprusside infusion lasts more than 1–2 days; toxicity is associated with thiocyanate levels of 50 mg/L or greater.

D. Rebound hypertension may be observed after sudden discontinuance.

E. **Use in pregnancy.** FDA category C (indeterminate; see p 310). It may cross the placenta, and it may affect uterine blood flow; however, it has been used successfully in pregnant women.

V. **Drug or laboratory interactions.** Hypotensive effect is potentiated by other antihypertensive agents and inhalational anesthetics.

VI. **Dosage and method of administration**

A. Use only in an emergency or intensive care setting with the capability of frequent or continuous blood pressure monitoring.

B. Dissolve 50 mg of sodium nitroprusside in 3 mL of 5% dextrose; then dilute this solution in 250, 500, or 1000 mL of 5% dextrose to achieve a concentration of 200, 100, or 50 µg/mL, respectively. Protect the solution from light to avoid photodegradation (as evidenced by a color change) by covering the bottle and tubing with paper or aluminum foil.

C. Start with an intravenous infusion rate of 0.3 µg/kg/min using a controlled infusion device, and titrate to desired effect. The average dose is 3 µg/kg/min in children and adults (range, 0.5–10 µg/kg/min). The maximum rate should not exceed 10 µg/kg/min to avoid risk of acute cyanide toxicity. If there is no response after 10 minutes at the maximum rate, discontinue the infusion and use an alternate vasodilator (eg, phentolamine, see p 369).

VII. **Formulations**

A. **Parenteral.** Nitroprusside sodium (Nipride, others), 50 mg of lyophilized powder for reconstitution.

B. **Suggested minimum stocking level** to treat a 70-kg adult for the first 24 hours: 24 vials.

NOREPINEPHRINE

Neal L. Benowitz, MD

I. **Pharmacology.** Norepinephrine is an endogenous catecholamine that stimulates mainly α-adrenergic receptors. It is used primarily as a vasopressor to increase systemic vascular resistance and venous return to the heart. Norepinephrine is also a weak β_1-adrenergic receptor agonist, and it may increase heart rate and cardiac contractility in patients with shock.

Norepinephrine is not effective orally and is erratically absorbed after subcutaneous injection. After intravenous administration, the onset of action is nearly immediate, and the duration of effect is 1–2 minutes after the infusion is discontinued.

II. **Indications.** Norepinephrine is used to increase blood pressure and cardiac output in patients with shock caused by venodilation or low systemic vascular resistance, or both. Hypovolemia, depressed myocardial contractility, hypothermia, and electrolyte imbalance should be corrected first or concurrently.

III. **Contraindications**

A. Uncorrected hypovolemia.

B. Norepinephrine is relatively contraindicated in patients with organic heart disease, peripheral arterial occlusive vascular disease with thrombosis, or in those with ergot poisoning (see p 158).

IV. Adverse effects
  A. Severe hypertension, which may result in intracranial hemorrhage, pulmonary edema, or myocardial necrosis.
  B. Aggravation of tissue ischemia, resulting in gangrene.
  C. Tissue necrosis after extravasation.
  D. Anxiety, restlessness, tremor, and headache.
  E. Anaphylaxis induced by sulfite preservatives in sensitive patients. Use with extreme caution in patients with known hypersensitivity to sulfite preservatives.
  F. Use with caution in patients intoxicated by chloral hydrate or halogenated or aromatic hydrocarbon solvents or anesthetics.
  G. Use in pregnancy. This drug crosses the placenta, and it can cause placental ischemia and reduce uterine contractions.

V. Drug or laboratory interactions
  A. Enhanced pressor response may occur in the presence of cocaine and cyclic antidepressants owing to inhibition of neuronal reuptake.
  B. Enhanced pressor response may occur in patients taking monoamine oxidase inhibitors owing to inhibition of neuronal metabolic degradation.
  C. Alpha- and beta-blocking agents may antagonize the adrenergic effects of norepinephrine.
  D. Anticholinergic drugs may block reflex bradycardia, which normally occurs in response to norepinephrine-induced hypertension, enhancing the hypertensive response.
  E. Chloral hydrate overdose, and cyclopropane and halogenated or aromatic hydrocarbon solvents and anesthetics, may enhance myocardial sensitivity to arrhythmogenic effects of norepinephrine.

VI. Dosage and method of administration
  A. Avoid extravasation. *Caution:* The intravenous infusion must be free-flowing, and the infused vein should be observed frequently for signs of infiltration (pallor, coldness, induration). If extravasation occurs, immediately infiltrate the affected area with phentolamine (see p 361), 5–10 mg in 10–15 mL of normal saline (children, 0.1–0.2 mg/kg; maximum 10 mg) via a fine (25- to 27-gauge) hypodermic needle; improvement is evidenced by hyperemia and return to normal temperature.
  B. Intravenous infusion. Begin at 4–8 μg/min (children, 1–2 μg/min or 0.1 μg/kg/min) and increase as needed every 5–10 minutes.

VII. Formulations. Norepinephrine bitartrate is rapidly oxidized on exposure to air; it must be kept in its airtight ampule until immediately before use. If the solution appears brown or contains a precipitate, do not use it. The stock solution must be diluted in 5% dextrose or 5% dextrose-saline for infusion; usually, a 4-mg ampule is added to 1 L of fluid to provide 4 μg/mL of solution.
  A. Parenteral. Norepinephrine bitartrate (Levophed), 1 mg/mL, 4-mL ampule. Contains sodium bisulfite as a preservative.
  B. Suggested minimum stocking level to treat a 70-kg adult for the first 24 hours: 5 ampules.

OXYGEN

Thomas E. Kearney, PharmD

  I. Pharmacology. Oxygen is a necessary oxidant to drive biochemical reactions. Room air contains 21% oxygen.
  II. Indications
  A. Supplemental oxygen is indicated when normal oxygenation is impaired because of pulmonary injury, which may result from aspiration (chemical pneumonitis) or inhalation of toxic gases. The P_{O2} should be maintained at 70–80 mm Hg if possible.

B. Supplemental oxygen is usually given empirically to patients with altered mental status or suspected hypoxemia.

C. Oxygen (100%) is indicated for carbon monoxide poisoning to increase the conversion of carboxyhemoglobin and carboxymyoglobin to hemoglobin and myoglobin and to increase oxygen saturation of the plasma and subsequent delivery to tissues. It may also be of benefit in patients poisoned by inhibitors of cellular respiration, such as cyanide or hydrogen sulfide.

D. Hyperbaric oxygen (100% oxygen delivered to the patient in a pressurized chamber at 2–3 atm) is advocated by some clinicians in patients with carbon monoxide poisoning (see p 121) for rapid reversal of carbon monoxide binding to hemoglobin, intracellular myoglobin, and possibly cytochrome oxidase, and for its potentially beneficial effects on cerebral edema and postischemic cellular damage. It has also been advocated for treatment of poisoning by carbon tetrachloride, cyanide, hydrogen sulfide, and for severe methemoglobinemia, but the experimental and clinical evidence is scanty.

III. Contraindications

A. In **paraquat** poisoning, oxygen may contribute to lung injury. In fact, slightly *hypoxic* environments (10–12% oxygen) have been advocated to reduce the risk of pulmonary fibrosis from paraquat.

B. Relative contraindications to hyperbaric oxygen therapy include a history of recent middle ear or thoracic surgery, untreated pneumonthorax, seizure disorder, or severe sinusitis.

IV. Adverse effects. *Caution:* Oxygen is extremely flammable.

A. Prolonged, high concentrations of oxygen are associated with pulmonary alveolar tissue damage. In general, the FI_{O2} should not be maintained at greater than 80% for more than 24 hours.

B. Oxygen therapy may increase the risk of retrolental fibroplasia in neonates.

C. Administration of high oxygen concentrations to patients with severe chronic obstructive pulmonary disease and chronic carbon dioxide retention who are dependent on hypoxemia to provide a drive to breathe may result in respiratory arrest.

D. Use in pregnancy. No known adverse effects.

V. Drug or laboratory interactions

A. May potentiate pulmonary toxicity associated with paraquat poisoning.

B. May potentiate toxicity via enhanced generation of free radicals with some chemotherapeutic agents (eg, bleomycin, adriamycin, daunorubicin).

VI. Dosage and method of administration

A. Supplemental oxygen. Provide supplemental oxygen to maintain a P_{O2} of approximately 70–80 mm Hg. If a P_{O2} greater than 50 mm Hg cannot be maintained with an FI_{O2} of at least 60%, consider positive end-expiratory pressure or continuous positive airway pressure.

B. Carbon monoxide poisoning. Provide 100% oxygen by tight-fitting face mask with a good seal, or endotracheal tube, and oxygen reservoir. Consider hyperbaric oxygen if the patient does not respond rapidly or is pregnant (see p 121) and is stable enough for transport to a hyperbaric facility.

VII. Formulations

A. Nasal cannula. See Table III–9.

TABLE III–9. AMOUNT OF OXYGEN PROVIDED BY NASAL CANNULA

Flow Rate (L/min)	Approximate Inspired Oxygen Concentration (%)
1	24
2	28
5	40

    B. Ventimask. Provides variable inspired oxygen concentrations from 24 to 40%.
    C. Nonrebreathing reservoir mask. Provides 60–90% inspired oxygen concentrations.
    D. Hyperbaric oxygen. One hundred percent oxygen can be delivered at a pressure of 2–3 atm.

PENICILLAMINE

Thomas E. Kearney, PharmD

  I. Pharmacology. Penicillamine is a derivative of penicillin that has no antimicrobial activity but effectively chelates some heavy metals such as lead, mercury, and copper. It has been used as adjunctive therapy following initial treatment with calcium EDTA (see p 335) or BAL (dimercaprol; see p 317). Penicillamine is well absorbed orally, and the penicillamine-metal complex is eliminated in the urine. No parenteral form is available.

  II. Indications
    A. Penicillamine may be used to treat heavy metal poisoning caused by lead (penicillamine may be used alone for minor intoxications or as adjunctive therapy after calcium EDTA or BAL in moderate to severe intoxications), mercury (after initial BAL therapy), copper, and possibly gold.
    B. For lead or mercury poisoning, oral DMSA (see p 332) is preferable, as it may result in greater metal excretion with fewer adverse effects.

  III. Contraindications
    A. Penicillin allergy is a contraindication.
    B. Renal insufficiency is a relative contraindication because the complex is eliminated only through the urine.
    C. Concomitant administration with other hematopoietic-depressant drugs (eg, gold salts, immunosuppressants, antimalarial agents, phenylbutazone) is not recommended.

  IV. Adverse effects
    A. Hypersensitivity reactions: rash, pruritus, drug fever, hematuria, and proteinuria.
    B. Leukopenia, thrombocytopenia, hemolytic anemia, agranulocytosis.
    C. Hepatitis, pancreatitis.
    D. Anorexia, nausea, vomiting, epigastric pain, impairment of taste.
    E. The requirement for pyridoxine is increased, and patient may require daily supplementation.
    F. Use in pregnancy. Birth defects have been associated with its use during pregnancy. No assigned FDA category (see p 310).

  V. Drug or laboratory interactions. Penicillamine may potentiate hematopoietic-depressant effects of drugs such as gold salts, immunosuppressants, antimalarial agents, and phenylbutazone.

  VI. Dosage and method of administration
    A. Penicillamine should be taken on an empty stomach, at least 1 hour before meals and at bedtime.
    B. The usual dose is 25–35 mg/kg/d, administered in 3–4 divided doses. Initiating treatment at 25% of this dose and gradually increasing to the full dose over 2–3 weeks may minimize adverse reactions.
    C. Weekly measurement of urinary and blood concentrations of the intoxicating metal is indicated to assess the need for continued therapy. Treatment for as long as 3 months has been tolerated.

  VII. Formulations. *Note:* Although the chemical derivative *N*-acetylpenicillamine may demonstrate better central nervous system and peripheral nerve penetration, it is not currently available in the USA.
    A. Oral. Penicillamine (Cuprimine, Depen), 125-, 250-mg capsules, 250-mg tablets.

B. **Suggested minimum stocking level** to treat a 70-kg adult for the first 24 hours: 1500 mg.

PENTOBARBITAL

Thomas E. Kearney, PharmD

I. **Pharmacology.** Pentobarbital is a short-acting barbiturate with anticonvulsant as well as sedative-hypnotic properties. It is used as a third-line drug in the treatment of status epilepticus. It may also reduce intracranial pressure in patients with cerebral edema. Following intravenous administration of a single dose, the onset of effect occurs within about 1 minute and lasts about 15 minutes. Pentobarbital demonstrates a biphasic elimination pattern; the half-life of the initial phase is 4 hours, and the terminal phase half-life is 35–50 hours. Effects are prolonged after termination of a continuous infusion.

II. **Indications**
   A. Pentobarbital is used for the management of status epilepticus that is unresponsive to conventional anticonvulsant therapy (eg, diazepam, phenytoin, phenobarbital). If the use of pentobarbital for seizure control is considered, consultation with a neurologist is recommended.
   B. It is used to manage elevated intracranial pressure, in conjunction with other agents.
   C. It may be used therapeutically or diagnostically for patients with suspected alcohol or sedative-hypnotic drug withdrawal syndrome.

III. **Contraindications**
   A. Known sensitivity to the drug.
   B. Manifest or latent porphyria.

IV. **Adverse effects**
   A. Central nervous system depression, coma, and respiratory arrest may occur, especially with rapid bolus or excessive doses.
   B. Hypotension may result, especially with rapid intravenous infusion.
   C. Laryngospasm and bronchospasm have been reported after rapid intravenous injection, although the mechanism is unknown.
   D. **Use in pregnancy.** FDA category D (possible fetal risk). Pentobarbital readily crosses the placenta, and chronic use may cause hemorrhagic disease of the newborn (owing to vitamin K deficiency) or neonatal dependency and withdrawal syndrome. However, these potential effects do not preclude its acute, short-term use for a seriously symptomatic patient (see p 310).

V. **Drug or laboratory interactions**
   A. Pentobarbital has additive central nervous system and respiratory depression effects with other barbiturates, as well as sedative and opioid drugs.
   B. Hepatic enzyme induction is generally not encountered with acute pentobarbital overdose, although it may occur within 24–48 hours.
   C. Clearance may be enhanced by hemoperfusion, requiring supplemental doses during the procedure.

VI. **Dosage and method of administration**
   A. **Intermittent intravenous bolus.** Give 100 mg IV slowly over at least 2 minutes; may repeat as needed at 2-minute intervals, to a maximum dose of 300–500 mg (children, 1 mg/kg IV, repeated as needed to a maximum of 5–6 mg/kg).
   B. **Continuous intravenous infusion.** Administer a loading dose of 5–6 mg/kg IV over 1 hour (not to exceed 50 mg/min; children, 1 mg/kg/min), followed by maintenance infusion of 0.5–3 mg/kg/h titrated to the desired effect. Electroencephalographic achievement of burst suppression usually occurs with serum pentobarbital concentration of 25–40 μg/mL.
   C. **Oral.** The oral regimen for treatment of barbiturate or other sedative drug withdrawal syndrome is administration of 200 mg orally, repeated every hour until signs of mild intoxication appear (eg, slurred speech, drowsiness, nystagmus).

Most patients respond to 600 mg or less. Repeat the total initial dose every 6 hours as needed. Phenobarbital is an alternative (see below).

VII. Formulations

    A. Parenteral. Pentobarbital sodium (Nembutal, others), 50 mg/mL, in 1- and 2-mL tubes and vials, and 20- and 50-mL vials.

    B. Oral. 50- and 100-mg capsules and suppositories. Also available as an elixir.

    C. Suggested minimum stocking level to treat a 70-kg adult for the first 24 hours: 2 vials, 50 mL each, or equivalent.

PHENOBARBITAL

Thomas E. Kearney, PharmD

  I. Pharmacology. Phenobarbital is a barbiturate commonly used as an anticonvulsant. Because of the delay in onset of the therapeutic effect of phenobarbital, diazepam (see p 327) is usually the initial agent for parenteral anticonvulsant therapy. After an oral dose of phenobarbital, peak brain concentrations are achieved within 10–15 hours. Onset of effect following intravenous administration is usually within 5 minutes, although peak effects may take up to 30 minutes. Therapeutic plasma levels are 15–35 mg/mL. The drug is eliminated by metabolism and renal excretion, and the elimination half-life is 48–100 hours.

  II. Indications

    A. Control of tonic-clonic seizures and status epilepticus, generally as a second- or third-line agent after diazepam or phenytoin have been tried.

     Note: For treatment of drug-induced seizures, especially seizures caused by theophylline, phenobarbital is often tried before phenytoin.

    B. Management of withdrawal from ethanol and other sedative-hypnotic drugs.

  III. Contraindications

    A. Known sensitivity to barbiturates.

    B. Manifest or latent porphyria.

  IV. Adverse effects

    A. Central nervous system depression, coma, and respiratory arrest may result, especially with rapid bolus or excessive doses.

    B. Hypotension may result from rapid intravenous administration. This can be prevented by limiting the rate of administration to less than 50 mg/min (children, 1 mg/kg/min).

    C. Use in pregnancy. FDA category D (possible fetal risk). It readily crosses the placenta, and chronic use may cause hemorrhagic disease of the newborn (owing to vitamin K deficiency) or neonatal dependency and withdrawal syndrome. However, these potential effects do not preclude its acute, short-term use for a seriously symptomatic patient (see p 310).

  V. Drug or laboratory interactions

    A. Phenobarbital has additive central nervous system and respiratory depression effects with other sedative drugs.

    B. Hepatic enzyme induction with chronic use, although this is *not* encountered with acute phenobarbital dosing.

    C. Extracorporeal removal techniques (eg, hemodialysis, hemoperfusion, and repeat-dose activated charcoal; see p 49) may enhance the clearance of phenobarbital, possibly requiring supplemental dosing to maintain therapeutic levels.

  VI. Dosage and method of administration

    A. Parenteral. Administer slowly intravenously (rate < 50 mg/min; children, < 1 mg/kg/min) until seizures are controlled or the loading dose of 10–15 mg/kg is achieved (children have required as much as 30 mg/kg in the first 24 hours to treat status epilepticus). Slow the infusion rate if hypotension develops. Intermittent infusions of 2 mg/kg every 5–15 minutes may diminish the risk of respiratory depression or hypotension.

     1. If intravenous access is not immediately available, phenobarbital may be given intramuscularly; the initial dose in adults and children is 3–5 mg/kg IM.

2. It may also be given by the intraosseous route.

B. Oral. For treatment of barbiturate or sedative drug withdrawal, give 60–120 mg orally and repeat every hour until signs of mild intoxication appear (eg, slurred speech, drowsiness, nystagmus).

VII. Formulations

A. Parenteral. Phenobarbital sodium (Luminal, others), 30, 60, 65, 130 mg/mL in tubex syringes, vials, and ampules.

B. Oral. 8-, 15-, 30-, 60-, 65-, 100-mg tablets; also elixir.

C. Suggested minimum stocking level to treat a 70-kg adult for the first 24 hours: 16 ampules (130 mg each) or equivalent.

PHENTOLAMINE

Thomas E. Kearney, PharmD

I. Pharmacology. Phentolamine is a competitive presynaptic and postsynaptic α-adrenergic receptor blocker that produces peripheral vasodilation. By acting on both venous and arterial vessels, it decreases total peripheral resistance and venous return. It may also stimulate β-adrenergic receptors, causing cardiac stimulation. Phentolamine has a rapid onset of action (usually 2 minutes) and short duration of effect (approximately 15–20 minutes).

II. Indications

A. Hypertensive crisis associated with phenylpropanolamine or stimulant drug overdose (eg, amphetamines, cocaine, ephedrine).

B. Hypertensive crisis resulting from interaction between monoamine oxidase inhibitors and tyramine or other sympathomimetic amines.

C. Hypertensive crisis associated with sudden withdrawal of sympatholytic antihypertensive drugs (eg, clonidine).

D. Extravasation of vasoconstrictive agents (eg, epinephrine, norepinephrine, dopamine).

III. Contraindications. Use with extreme caution in patients with intracranial hemorrhage or ischemic stroke; excessive lowering of blood pressure may aggravate brain injury.

IV. Adverse effects

A. Hypotension and tachycardia may occur from excessive doses.

B. Anginal chest pain and cardiac arrhythmias may occur.

C. Slow intravenous infusion (< 0.3 mg/min) may result in transient increased blood pressure caused by stimulation of β-adrenergic receptors.

D. Use in pregnancy. No assigned FDA category. However, this does not preclude its acute, short-term use for a seriously symptomatic patient (see p 310).

V. Drug or laboratory interactions. Additive or synergistic effects may occur with other antihypertensive agents, especially other α-adrenergic antagonists (eg, prazosin, terazosin, yohimbine).

VI. Dosage and method of administration

A. Parenteral. Give 1–5 mg IV (children, 0.02–0.1 mg/kg) as a bolus; may repeat at 5- to 10-minute intervals (or constant infusion of 0.1–2 mg/min) as needed to lower blood pressure to a desired level (usually < 100 mm Hg diastolic in adults, 80 mm Hg diastolic in children, but may vary depending on the clinical situation).

B. Catecholamine extravasation. Infiltrate 5–10 mg in 10–15 mL of normal saline (children, 0.1–0.2 mg/kg; maximum 10 mg) into affected area with a fine (25- to 27-gauge) hypodermic needle; improvement is evidenced by hyperemia and return to normal temperature.

VII. Formulations

A. Parenteral. Phentolamine mesylate (Regitine), 5 mg in 1-mL vials.

B. Suggested minimum stocking level to treat a 70-kg adult for the first 24 hours: 20 vials.

PHENYTOIN

Kathryn H. Keller, PharmD

I. **Pharmacology.** The neuronal membrane-stabilizing actions of phenytoin make this a popular drug for sustained control of acute and chronic seizure disorders and a useful drug for certain cardiac arrhythmias. Because of the relatively slow onset of anticonvulsant action, phenytoin is usually administered after diazepam. At serum concentrations considered therapeutic for seizure control, phenytoin acts similarly to lidocaine to reduce ventricular premature depolarizations and suppress ventricular tachycardia. After intravenous administration, peak therapeutic effects are attained within 1 hour. The therapeutic serum concentration for seizure control is 10–20 mg/L. Elimination is nonlinear, with an apparent half-life averaging 22 hours.

II. **Indications**

   A. Control of generalized tonic-clonic seizures or status epilepticus.

   B. Control of cardiac arrhythmias, particularly those associated with digitalis intoxication.

III. **Contraindications.** Known hypersensitivity to phenytoin or other hydantoins.

IV. **Adverse effects**

   A. Rapid intravenous administration (> 50 mg/min in adults or 1 mg/kg/min in children) may produce hypotension, atrioventricular block, and cardiovascular collapse, probably owing to the propylene glycol diluent.

   B. Extravasation may result in local tissue necrosis and sloughing.

   C. Drowsiness, ataxia, nystagmus, and nausea may occur.

   D. **Use in pregnancy.** No assigned FDA category. Congenital malformations (fetal hydantoin syndrome) and hemorrhagic disease of the newborn have occurred with chronic use. However, this does not preclude its acute, short-term use for a seriously symptomatic patient (see p 310).

V. **Drug or laboratory interactions**

   A. The various drug interactions associated with chronic phenytoin dosing (ie, accelerated metabolism of other drugs) are not applicable to its acute emergency use.

   B. Extracorporeal removal methods (eg, hemoperfusion, repeat-dose activated charcoal) will enhance phenytoin clearance. Supplemental dosing may be required during such procedures to maintain therapeutic levels.

VI. **Dosage and method of administration**

   A. **Parenteral.** Administer a loading dose of 15–20 mg/kg IV slowly at a rate not to exceed 50 mg/min (or 1 mg/kg/min in children). It may be diluted in 50–150 mL of normal saline with use of in-line filter. Phenytoin has been administered via the intraosseous route in children. Do **not** administer by the intramuscular route.

   B. **Maintenance dose.** Give 5 mg/kg/d as a single oral dose of capsules or twice daily for other dosage forms and in children. Monitor serum phenytoin levels.

VII. **Formulations**

   A. **Parenteral.** Phenytoin sodium (Dilantin, others), 50 mg/mL, 2- and 5-mL ampules and vials.

   B. **Oral.** Phenytoin sodium (Dilantin, others), 30- and 100-mg capsules.

   C. **Suggested minimum stocking level** to treat a 70-kg adult for the first 24 hours: 6 vials (50 mg/mL, 5 mL each) or equivalent.

PHYSOSTIGMINE

Thomas E. Kearney, PharmD

I. **Pharmacology.** Physostigmine is a reversible inhibitor of acetylcholinesterase, the enzyme that degrades acetylcholine. Physostigmine increases concentrations of acetylcholine, causing stimulation of both muscarinic and nicotinic receptors. The tertiary amine structure of physostigmine allows it to penetrate the blood-brain barrier and exert central cholinergic effects as well. Owing to cholinergic stimulation of the brain stem's reticular activating system, it has nonspecific analeptic (arousal) effects. After parenteral administration, the onset of action is within 3–8 minutes and the duration of effect is usually 30–60 minutes. The elimination half-life is 15–40 minutes.

II. Indications

A. Physostigmine is used for the management of severe anticholinergic syndrome (agitated delirium, urinary retention, severe sinus tachycardia, hyperthermia with absent sweating). Its overall utility is limited, because most patients with anticholinergic poisoning can be managed supportively.

B. Physostigmine is sometimes used diagnostically to differentiate functional psychosis from anticholinergic delirium.

III. Contraindications

A. Physostigmine should *not* be used as an antidote for cyclic antidepressant overdose because it may worsen cardiac conduction disturbances, cause bradyarrhythmias or asystole, and aggravate or precipitate seizures.

B. Do not use physostigmine with concurrent use of depolarizing neuromuscular blockers (eg, succinylcholine, decamethonium).

IV. Adverse effects

A. Bradycardia, heart block, asystole.

B. Seizures (particularly with rapid administration or excessive dose).

C. Nausea, vomiting, diarrhea.

D. Bronchorrhea, bronchospasm.

E. Fasciculations, muscle weakness.

F. Use in pregnancy. No assigned FDA category (see p 310). Transient weakness has been noted in neonates whose mothers were treated with physostigmine for myasthenia gravis.

V. Drug or laboratory interactions

A. Physostigmine may potentiate depolarizing neuromuscular-blocking agents (eg, succinylcholine, decamethonium) and cholinesterase inhibitors (eg, organophosphate and carbamate insecticides).

B. It may have additive depressant effects on cardiac conduction in patients with cyclic antidepressant overdose.

C. Through its nonspecific analeptic effects, it may induce arousal in patients with benzodiazepine or sedative-hypnotic intoxication.

VI. Dosage and method of administration.
Parenteral: 0.5–2 mg slow IV push (children, 0.02 mg/kg) while using a cardiac monitor; may repeat as needed every 20–30 minutes. Atropine (see p 315) should be kept nearby to reverse excessive muscarinic stimulation. Do *not* administer intramuscularly or as a continuous IV infusion.

VII. Formulations

A. Parenteral. Physostigmine salicylate (Antilirium), 1 mg/mL in 1-mL syringes and 2-mL vials.

B. Suggested minimum stocking level to treat a 70-kg adult for the first 24 hours: 10 ampules (2 mL each).

PRALIDOXIME (2-PAM)

Thomas E. Kearney, PharmD

I. Pharmacology. Pralidoxime (2-PAM) reverses organophosphate poisoning by reactivating phosphorylated cholinesterase enzyme and protecting the enzyme from further inhibition. The clinical effect of pralidoxime is most apparent at nicotinic receptors, with reversal of skeletal muscle weakness and muscle fasciculations. Its impact on muscarinic symptoms (salivation, sweating, bradycardia, bronchorrhea) is less pronounced than that of the antimuscarinic agent atropine (see p 315).

A. 2-PAM is most effective when given before the enzyme has been irreversibly bound ("aged") by the organophosphate (the rate of aging varies with each organophosphate: for most compounds, it occurs within 24 hours, but for some chemical warfare agents, it may occur in several minutes). However, late therapy with 2-PAM is appropriate, especially in patients poisoned by fat-soluble compounds (eg, fenthion, demeton) that can be released from tissue stores over days, causing continuous or recurrent intoxication.

    B. Inadequate dosing of 2-PAM may be linked to the "intermediate syndrome," which is characterized by prolonged muscle weakness.

    C. Peak plasma concentrations are reached within 5–15 minutes after intravenous administration. Pralidoxime is eliminated by renal excretion and hepatic metabolism, with a half-life of 0.8–2.7 hours.

II. Indications

    A. Pralidoxime is used to treat poisoning caused by organophosphate cholinesterase inhibitor insecticides. Because of its low toxicity, its possible ineffectiveness if treatment is delayed until after the cholinesterase enzyme has aged, its ability to reverse nicotinic as well as muscarinic effects, and its ability to reduce atropine requirements, it should be used early and empirically for suspected organophosphate poisoning.

    B. Pralidoxime is not required in carbamate poisoning because cholinesterase inhibition is transient and spontaneously resolves. Moreover, there is one animal study demonstrating enhanced Sevin (carbaryl) toxicity with 2-PAM. However, it is still recommended for empiric treatment of symptomatic patients with mixed or unknown cholinesterase inhibitor poisoning.

III. Contraindications

    A. Use in patients with myasthenia gravis may precipitate a myasthenic crisis.

    B. Use with caution and in reduced doses in patients with renal impairment.

IV. Adverse effects

    A. Nausea, headache, dizziness, diplopia, and hyperventilation may occur.

    B. Rapid intravenous administration may result in tachycardia, laryngospasm, muscle rigidity, and transient neuromuscular blockade.

    C. Use in pregnancy. FDA category C (indeterminate). This does not preclude its acute, short-term use for a seriously symptomatic patient (see p 310).

V. Drug or laboratory interactions.
Symptoms of atropinization may occur more quickly when atropine and pralidoxime are administered concurrently.

VI. Dosage and method of administration.
The intravenous route is preferred. Intramuscular or subcutaneous injection is possible when the intravenous route is not immediately available.

    A. Initial dose. Give 1–2 g (children, 20–40 mg/kg) IV over 5–10 minutes (rate not to exceed 200 mg/min in adults or 4 mg/kg/min in children), or give as a continuous intravenous infusion in 100 mL of saline (1–2 mL/kg) over 15–30 minutes. Repeat the dose if muscle weakness or fasciculations are not relieved. Several grams may be required in some cases.

    B. Maintenance infusion. Because of the short half-life of 2-PAM and the longer duration of many organophosphate compounds, toxicity frequently recurs, requiring repeated doses.

        1. Discrete intermittent boluses, which were recommended previously, may result in wide fluctuation in serum levels and erratic clinical effects. Therefore, after the initial dose it is preferable to give 2-PAM as a continuous intravenous infusion in a 1% solution (1 g in 100 mL saline) at a rate of 200–500 mg/h (children 5–10 mg/kg/h) and titrate to desired clinical response.

        2. Despite earlier recommendations that 2-PAM should be given only for 24 hours, therapy may need to be continued for several days, particularly when long-acting, lipid-soluble organophosphates are involved. Gradually reduce the dose and carefully observe the patient for signs of recurrent muscle weakness or other signs of toxicity.

        3. *Note:* 2-PAM may accumulate in patients with renal insufficiency.

VII. Formulations

    A. Parenteral. Pralidoxime chloride (Protopam), 1 g with 20 mL sterile water.

    B. Suggested minimum stocking level to treat a 70-kg adult for the first 24 hours: 12 vials.

PROPRANOLOL

Thomas E. Kearney, PharmD

I. **Pharmacology.** Propranolol is a nonselective β-adrenergic blocker that acts on β_1-receptors in the myocardium and β_2-receptors in the lung, vascular smooth muscle, and kidney. Within the myocardium, propranolol depresses heart rate, conduction velocity, myocardial contractility, and automaticity. Although propranolol is effective orally, for toxicologic emergencies it is usually administered by the intravenous route. After intravenous injection, the onset of action is nearly immediate and the duration of effect is 10 minutes to 2 hours, depending on the cumulative dose. The drug is eliminated by hepatic metabolism, with a half-life of about 2–3 hours.

II. **Indications**

A. To control excessive sinus tachycardia or ventricular arrhythmias caused by catecholamine excess (eg, theophylline, caffeine), sympathomimetic drug intoxication (eg, amphetamines, pseudoephedrine, cocaine), or excessive myocardial sensitivity (eg, chloral hydrate, freons, chlorinated and other hydrocarbons).

B. To control hypertension in patients with excessive β_1-mediated increase in heart rate and contractility; use in conjunction with a vasodilator (eg, phentolamine; see p 369) in patients with mixed α- and β-adrenergic hyperstimulation.

C. To raise the diastolic blood pressure in patients with hypotension caused by excessive β_2-mediated vasodilation (eg, theophylline, metaproterenol).

D. May ameliorate or reduce β-adrenergic–mediated electrolyte and other metabolic abnormalities (eg, hypokalemia, hyperglycemia, lactic acidosis).

III. **Contraindications**

A. Use with extreme caution in patients with asthma, congestive heart failure, sinus node dysfunction, or other cardiac conduction disease and in those receiving calcium antagonists and other cardiac-depressant drugs.

B. Do not use as single therapy for hypertension resulting from sympathomimetic overdose. Propranolol produces peripheral vascular beta-blockade, which may abolish β_2-mediated vasodilation and allow unopposed α-mediated vasoconstriction, resulting in paradoxic worsening of hypertension.

IV. **Adverse effects**

A. Bradycardia, sinus and atrioventricular block.

B. Hypotension, congestive heart failure.

C. Bronchospasm in patients with asthma or bronchospastic chronic obstructive pulmonary disease.

Note: Propranolol has been used successfully in asthmatic patients overdosed on theophylline or β_2 agonists without precipitating bronchospasm.

D. **Use in pregnancy.** FDA category C (indeterminate). It may cross the placenta; and neonates delivered within 3 days of administration of this drug may have persistent β-adrenergic blockade. However, this does not preclude its acute, short-term use for a seriously symptomatic patient (see p 310).

V. **Drug or laboratory interactions**

A. Propranolol may allow unopposed α-adrenergic stimulation in patients with mixed adrenergic stimulation (eg, epinephrine surge in patients with acute hypoglycemia, pheochromocytoma, or cocaine or amphetamine intoxication), resulting in severe hypertension or end-organ ischemia.

B. Propranolol has an additive hypotensive effect with other antihypertensive agents.

C. This drug may potentiate competitive neuromuscular blockers (see p 357).

D. The drug has additive depressant effects on cardiac conduction and contractility when given with calcium antagonists.

E. Cimetidine reduces hepatic clearance of propranolol.

F. Propranolol may worsen vasoconstriction caused by ergot alkaloids.

VI. **Dosage and method of administration**

A. **Parenteral.** Give 0.5–3 mg IV (children, 0.01–0.02 mg/kg IV; maximum 1 mg/dose) while monitoring heart rate and blood pressure; dose may be repeated as needed after 5–10 minutes. The dose required for complete β-receptor blockade is about 0.2 mg/kg.

B. Oral. Oral dosing may be initiated after the patient is stabilized; the dosage range is about 1–5 mg/kg/d in 3–4 divided doses for both children and adults.

VII. Formulations

A. Parenteral. Propranolol hydrochloride (Inderal), 1 mg/mL in 1-mL ampules and prefilled syringes.

B. Oral. Propranolol hydrochloride (Inderal, others), 60-, 80-, 120-, 160-mg capsules; 10-, 20-, 40-, 60-, 80-, 90-mg tablets.

C. Suggested minimum stocking level to treat a 70-kg adult for the first 24 hours: 10 ampules or syringes.

PROTAMINE

Thomas E. Kearney, PharmD

I. Pharmacology. Protamine is a cationic protein that rapidly binds to and inactivates heparin. The onset of action after intravenous administration is nearly immediate (30–60 s).

II. Indications

A. Protamine is used for the reversal of the anticoagulant effect of heparin when an excessively large dose has been inadvertently administered. Protamine is generally not needed for treatment of bleeding during standard heparin therapy because discontinuance of the heparin infusion is generally sufficient.

B. Protamine may be used for reversal of regional anticoagulation in the hemodialysis circuit in cases in which anticoagulation of the patient would be contraindicated (ie, active gastrointestinal or central nervous system bleeding).

III. Contraindications

A. Do not give protamine to patients with known sensitivity to the drug. Diabetic patients who have used protamine insulin may be at the greatest risk for hypersensitivity reactions.

B. Protamine reconstituted with benzyl alcohol should not be used in neonates because of suspected toxicity from the alcohol.

IV. Adverse effects

A. Rapid intravenous administration is associated with hypotension, bradycardia, and anaphylactoid reactions. Have epinephrine (see p 337) and diphenhydramine (see p 331) ready.

B. Rebound effect owing to heparin may occur within 8 hours of protamine administration.

C. Use in pregnancy. FDA category C (indeterminate). Maternal hypersensitivity reaction or hypotension could result in placental ischemia. However, this does not preclude its acute, short-term use for a seriously symptomatic patient (see p 310).

V. Drug or laboratory interactions. No known drug interactions, other than the reversal of the effect of heparin.

VI. Dosage and method of administration

A. Administer protamine by slow intravenous injection, over at least 1–3 minutes, not to exceed 50 mg in a 10-minute period.

B. The dose of protamine depends on the total dose and time since administration of heparin.

1. Immediately after heparin administration, give 1–1.5 mg of protamine for each 100 units of heparin.

2. At 30–60 minutes after heparin administration, give only 0.5–0.75 mg of protamine for each 100 units of heparin.

3. Two hours or more after heparin administration, give only 0.25–0.375 mg of protamine for each 100 units of heparin.

4. If heparin was administered by constant infusion, give 25–50 mg of protamine.

VII. Formulations

A. Parenteral. Protamine sulfate, 50 mg in 5-mL ampules or 250 mg in 25-mL vials.

B. Suggested minimum stocking level to treat a 70-kg adult for the first 24 hours: 4 ampules or 1 vial.

PYRIDOXINE (VITAMIN B$_6$)

Thomas E. Kearney, PharmD

I. Pharmacology. Pyridoxine (vitamin B$_6$) is a water-soluble B-complex vitamin that acts as a cofactor in many enzymatic reactions. Overdose involving isoniazid or other monomethylhydrazines (eg, gyromitrin mushrooms) may cause seizures by interfering with pyridoxine utilization in the brain, and pyridoxine given in high doses can rapidly control these seizures. It can also correct the lactic acidosis secondary to isoniazid-induced impaired lactate metabolism. In ethylene glycol intoxication, pyridoxine theoretically may enhance metabolic conversion of the toxic metabolite, glyoxylic acid, to the nontoxic product, glycine. Pyridoxine is well absorbed orally but is usually given intravenously for urgent uses. The biologic half-life is about 15–20 days.

II. Indications

A. Acute management of seizures caused by intoxication with isoniazid (see p 192), *Gyromitra* mushrooms (see p 223), or possibly cycloserine. Pyridoxine may act synergistically with diazepam (see p 327).

B. Adjunct to therapy for ethylene glycol intoxication.

III. Contraindications. No known contraindications.

IV. Adverse effects

A. Usually no adverse effects are noted from acute dosing of pyridoxine.

B. Chronic excessive doses may result in peripheral neuropathy.

C. Use in pregnancy. FDA category A (see p 310). However, chronic excessive use in pregnancy has resulted in pyridoxine withdrawal seizures in neonates.

V. Drug or laboratory interactions. No adverse interactions are associated with acute dosing.

VI. Dosage and method of administration

A. Isoniazid poisoning. Give 1 g of pyridoxine intravenously for each gram of isoniazid known to have been ingested (as much as 52 grams have been administered and tolerated). Dilute in 50 mL dextrose or saline and give over 5 minutes. If ingested amount is unknown, administer 4–5 g IV empirically and repeat as needed.

B. Monomethylhydrazine poisoning. Give 25 mg/kg IV; may repeat as necessary.

C. Ethylene glycol poisoning. Give 50 mg IV or IM every 6 hours until intoxication is resolved.

D. Cycloserine poisoning. A dosage of 300 mg/d has been recommended.

VII. Formulations

A. Parenteral. Pyridoxine hydrochloride (Beesix, Hexa-Betalin), 100 mg/mL (10% solution) in 10- and 30-mL vials.

B. Suggested minimum stocking level to treat a 70-kg adult for the first 24 hours: 20 g (20 vials, 10 mL each, or equivalent).

THIAMINE (VITAMIN B$_1$)

Thomas E. Kearney, PharmD

I. Pharmacology. Thiamine (vitamin B$_1$) is a water-soluble vitamin that acts as an essential cofactor for various pathways of carbohydrate metabolism. Thiamine also acts as a cofactor in the metabolism of glyoxylic acid (produced in ethylene glycol intoxication). Thiamine deficiency may result in beriberi and Wernicke–

Korsakoff syndrome. Thiamine is rapidly absorbed after oral, intramuscular, or intravenous administration.

II. **Indications**

    A. Empiric therapy to prevent and treat Wernicke–Korsakoff syndrome in alcoholic or malnourished patients. Thiamine should be given concurrently with glucose in such patients.

    B. Adjunctive treatment in patients poisoned with ethylene glycol to possibly enhance the detoxification of glyoxylic acid.

III. **Contraindications.** Use caution in patients with known sensitivity to thiamine.

IV. **Adverse effects**

    A. Anaphylactoid reactions, vasodilation, hypotension, weakness, and angioedema following rapid intravenous injection.

    B. Acute pulmonary edema in patients with beriberi owing to sudden increase in vascular resistance.

    C. Use in pregnancy. FDA category A (see p 310).

V. **Drug or laboratory interactions.** Theoretically, thiamine may enhance the effect of neuromuscular blockers, although the clinical significance is unclear.

VI. **Dosage and method of administration.** Parenteral: 100 mg (children, 50 mg) slow IV (over 5 minutes) or IM; repeat every 6 hours. Doses as high as 1 gram over the first 12 hours have been given to patients with acute Wernicke–Korsakoff syndrome.

VII. **Formulations**

    A. Parenteral. Thiamine hydrochloride (Betalin, others), 100 and 200 mg/mL, in 1-, 2-, 10- and 30-mL ampules, vials, and prefilled syringes.

    B. Suggested minimum stocking level to treat a 70-kg adult for the first 24 hours: 1 g (one 10-mL vial or equivalent).

THIOSULFATE, SODIUM

Susan Kim, PharmD

    I. **Pharmacology.** Sodium thiosulfate is a sulfur donor that promotes the conversion of cyanide to less toxic thiocyanate by the sulfur transferase enzyme rhodanese. Unlike nitrites, thiosulfate is essentially nontoxic and may be given empirically in suspected cyanide poisoning.

II. **Indications**

    A. May be given alone or in combination with nitrites (see p 361) in patients with acute cyanide poisoning.

    B. Empiric treatment of possible cyanide poisoning associated with smoke inhalation.

    C. Prophylaxis during nitroprusside infusions (see p 362).

    D. Extravasation of mechlorethamine (use topically).

    E. Bromate salt ingestion (unproved).

III. **Contraindications.** No known contraindications.

IV. **Adverse effects**

    A. May produce burning sensation during infusion.

    B. Use in pregnancy. FDA category C (indeterminate). This does not preclude its acute, short-term use for a seriously symptomatic patient (see p 310).

V. **Drug or laboratory interactions.** No known interactions.

VI. **Dosage and method of administration.** Parenteral: Administer 12.5 g (50 mL of 25% solution) IV at 2.5–5 mL/min. The pediatric dose is 400 mg/kg (1.6 mL/kg of 25% solution) up to 50 mL. Half the initial dose may be given after 30–60 minutes if needed.

VII. **Formulations**

    A. Parenteral. As a component of the Lilly Cyanide Antidote kit: thiosulfate sodium, 25% solution, 50 mL. Also available separately in vials and ampules containing 2.5 g/10 mL or 1 g/10 mL.

    B. Suggested minimum stocking level to treat a 70-kg adult for the first 24 hours: 2 Lilly Cyanide Antidote kits (one should be kept in the Emergency Department).

VITAMIN K₁ (PHYTONADIONE)

Thomas E. Kearney, PharmD

I. **Pharmacology.** Vitamin K_1 is an essential cofactor in the hepatic synthesis of coagulation factors II, VII, IX, X, and prothrombin. In adequate doses, vitamin K_1 reverses the inhibitory effects of coumarin and indanedione derivatives on the synthesis of these factors. *Note:* Vitamin K_3 (menadione) is *not* effective in reversing excessive anticoagulation caused by these agents. After parenteral vitamin K_1 administration, there is a 6- to 8-hour delay before vitamin K–dependent coagulation factors begin to achieve significant levels, and peak effects are not seen until 1–2 days after initiation of therapy. The duration of effect is 5–10 days. The response to vitamin K_1 is variable; it is influenced by the potency of the ingested anticoagulant and the patient's hepatic biosynthetic capability. Fresh-frozen plasma or whole blood is indicated for immediate control of serious hemorrhage.

II. **Indications**
   A. Excessive anticoagulation caused by coumarin and indanedione derivatives, as evidenced by elevated prothrombin time. It is *not* indicated for empiric treatment of anticoagulant ingestion, as most cases do not require treatment.
   B. Vitamin K deficiency (eg, malnutrition, malabsorption, hemorrhagic disease of the newborn) with coagulopathy.
   C. Hypoprothrombinemia resulting from salicylate intoxication.

III. **Contraindications.** Do not use in patients with known hypersensitivity.

IV. **Adverse effects**
   A. Anaphylactoid reactions have been reported after intravenous administration. Intravenous use should be restricted to true emergencies; the patient must be closely monitored in an intensive care setting.
   B. Intramuscular administration in anticoagulated patients may cause large, painful hematomas. This can be avoided by using oral or subcutaneous routes.
   C. Patients receiving anticoagulants for medical reasons (eg, deep vein thrombosis, prosthetic heart valves) may experience untoward effects from complete reversal of their anticoagulation status. Preferably, such patients should receive small quantities of fresh frozen plasma or extremely small titrated doses (0.5–1 mg) until the prothrombin time is in the desired therapeutic range (eg, 1.5–2 times normal). Anticoagulation with heparin may be indicated until the desired prothrombin time is achieved.
   D. **Use in pregnancy.** FDA category C (indeterminate). It crosses the placenta readily. However, this does not preclude its acute, short-term use for a seriously symptomatic patient (see p 310).

V. **Drug or laboratory interactions.** Empiric use after an acute anticoagulant overdose will delay (for up to several days) the onset of elevation of prothrombin time, which may give a false impression of insignificant ingestion in a case of serious "superwarfarin" overdose (see p 143).

VI. **Dosage and method of administration**
   A. **Oral** administration may be considered for maintenance therapy after initial parenteral treatment of symptomatic "superwarfarin" poisonings. The usual oral dose of vitamin K_1 (*not* menadione, vitamin K_3) is 10–25 mg/d in adults and 5–10 mg/d in children. Recheck the prothrombin time after 48 hours, and increase the dose as needed. Daily doses of 50–200 mg have been required in some cases. Therapy may be required for several weeks or even months.
   B. **Subcutaneous** administration is the preferred route. The adult dose is 5–10 mg, and that for children is 1–5 mg; may be repeated in 6–8 hours. Switch to oral therapy as soon as possible.
   C. **Intravenous** administration is rarely used, and only when hemorrhage is pres-

ent or imminent (in such cases, consider fresh-frozen plasma for rapid replacement of coagulation factors). The usual dose is 10–50 mg (0.6 mg/kg in children under 12 years), depending on the severity of anticoagulation, diluted in preservative-free dextrose or sodium chloride solution. Give slowly at a rate not to exceed 1 mg/min or 5% of the total dose per minute, whichever is slower.

VII. Formulations
  A. Parenteral. Phytonadione (AquaMEPHYTON, Konakion) 2 and 10 mg/mL, in 0.5-, 1-, 2.5-, and 5-mL ampules.
  B. Oral. Phytonadione (Mephyton), 5-mg tablets.
  C. Suggested minimum stocking level to treat a 70-kg adult for the first 24 hours: 100 mg (2 5-mL ampules, 10 mg/mL each, or equivalent).

REFERENCES

Gilman AG et al (editors): *Goodman & Gilman's The Pharmacological Basis of Therapeutics*, 8th ed. Macmillan, 1990.

Kastrup EK et al (editors): *Drug Facts & Comparisons 1993*. Lippincott, 1993.

Martindale W (editor): *The Extra Pharmacopoeia*, 28th ed. Rittenhouse, 1982.

McEnvoy GK (editor): *American Hospital Formulary Service Drug Information 1993*. American Society of Hospital Pharmacists, 1993.

US Pharmacopoeial Convention: *Drug Information for the Health Care Provider*. USPC, 1992.

Section IV. Environmental and Occupational Toxicology

EMERGENCY MEDICAL RESPONSE
TO HAZARDOUS MATERIALS INCIDENTS

Kent R. Olson, MD, and Frank J. Mycroft, PhD

With the constant threat of accidental incidents involving hazardous materials, local emergency response providers must be prepared to handle victims who may be contaminated with chemical substances. Many local jurisdictions have developed **Hazardous Materials (HazMat) teams,** usually comprised of fire and paramedical personnel who are trained to identify hazardous situations quickly and to take the lead in organizing a response. Health care providers such as ambulance personnel, nurses, physicians, and local hospital officials should participate in emergency response planning and drills with their local HazMat team before a chemical disaster occurs.

I. **General considerations.** The most important elements of successful medical management of a hazardous materials incident are as follows:
   A. Use extreme caution when dealing with unknown or unstable conditions.
   B. Rapidly assess the potential acute hazard of the substances involved.
   C. Determine the potential for secondary contamination of downstream personnel and facilities.
   D. Perform any needed decontamination on scene *before* victim transport, if possible.
II. **Organization of the incident.** Most incidents are operated under the control of the **Incident Commander,** usually the senior fire chief or police or coast guard officer. The first priorities will be to secure the area, establish a command post, create hazard zones, and appoint a health and safety officer.
   A. **Hazard zones** (Fig IV–1) are determined by the nature of the spilled substance and wind and geographic conditions. In general, the command post and support area will be upwind and upgrade from the spill, with sufficient distance to allow rapid escape if conditions change.
      1. The **"hot" area** is the most dangerous and may require carefully selected personal protective gear as well as vigorous decontamination when leaving the area.
      2. Basic decontamination, if indicated, should be carried out in the **"contamination reduction" area.**
      3. Patients in the hot and contamination reduction areas will generally receive only rudimentary first aid such as cervical spine stabilization and placement on a backboard. Additional first aid or more sophisticated medical treatment will generally be provided in the **"support" area** after the victim has undergone basic decontamination.
   B. **Health and safety officer.** A predesignated member of the HazMat team should be placed in charge of health and safety. This person will determine the nature and degree of any hazard, the need for specialized personal protective gear, and the decontamination requirements; the officer will also monitor entry into and exit from the spill site.
III. **Assessment of hazard potential.** Be prepared to recognize dangerous situations and to respond appropriately. The potential for toxic or other injury depends on the identities of the chemicals involved, their toxicities, their chemical and physical properties, the conditions of exposure, and the circumstances surrounding their release. Be aware that a substance's reactivity, flammability, explosivity, or corrosivity may be a source of greater hazard than its systemic toxicity.
   A. **Identify the substances involved.** Make inquiries and look for labels, warning placards, or shipping papers.
      1. The **National Fire Protection Association (NFPA)** has developed a labeling system for describing chemical hazards that is widely used (Fig IV–2).
      2. The **US Department of Transportation (DOT)** has developed a system of warning placards for vehicles carrying hazardous materials. The DOT placards usually bear a 4-digit substance identification code and also a single-digit hazard classification code (Fig IV–3). Identification of the substance

FIGURE IV–1. Control zones at a hazardous materials incident site.

from the 4-digit code can be provided by the regional poison control center, CHEMTREC, or the DOT manual (see **B,** below).

3. **Shipping papers,** which may include Material Safety Data Sheets (MSDSs), are usually carried by the driver or pilot or may be found in the cab of the truck.

B. Obtain acute toxicity information. Determine the acute health effects and obtain advice on general hazards, decontamination procedures, and medical management of victims. Resources include:

1. **Regional poison control centers** (see Table I–41, p 53). The regional poison control center can provide information on immediate health effects, the need for decontamination or specialized protective gear, and specific treatment including the use of antidotes. The regional center can also provide consultation with a medical toxicologist.

2. **CHEMTREC** ([800] 424-9300). Operated by the Chemical Manufacturers' Association, this 24-hour hotline can provide information on the identity and

NATIONAL FIRE PROTECTION ASSOCIATION
IDENTIFICATION OF THE FIRE HAZARDS OF MATERIALS

NFPA 704
HAZARD SIGNAL SYSTEM

Flammability (Red)

4 – Highly flammable and volatile
3 – Highly flammable
2 – Flammable
1 – Low flammability
0 – Does not burn

Health Hazard (Blue)

4 – Extremely hazardous
3 – Moderately hazardous
2 – Hazardous
1 – Slightly hazardous
0 – No health hazard

Reactivity (Yellow)

4 – Highly explosive, detonates readily
3 – Explosive, less readily detonated
2 – Violently reactive but does not detonate
1 – Not violently reactive
0 – Normally stable

Other Hazards

☢ – Radioactive

OX – Oxidizer

〰 – Water-reactive

FIGURE IV–2. National Fire Protection Association (NFPA) identification of the hazards of materials. (Reproduced, with permission, from *Fire Protection Guide on Hazardous Materials,* 9th ed. National Fire Protection Association, 1986.)

hazardous properties of chemicals and, when appropriate, can put the caller in touch with industry representatives and medical toxicologists.

   3. **Table IV–13** (p 396) and specific chemicals covered in Section II of this manual.
   4. A variety of texts, journals, and computerized information systems are available but are of uneven scope or depth. See the reference list at the end of this section (p 387).
C. **Recognize dangerous environments.** In general, environments likely to expose the rescuer to the same conditions that caused grave injury to the victim are not safe for unprotected entry. **These situations require trained and properly equipped rescue personnel.** Examples include the following:
   1. Any indoor environment where the victim was rendered unconscious or otherwise disabled.
   2. Environments causing acute onset of symptoms in rescuers such as chest tightness, shortness of breath, eye or throat irritation, coughing, dizziness, headache, nausea, or incoordination.
   3. Confined spaces such as large tanks or crawl spaces: their poor ventilation and small size can result in extremely high levels of airborne contaminants. In addition, such spaces permit only a slow or strenuous exit, which may become physically impossible for an intoxicated individual.
   4. Spills involving substances with poor warning properties or high vapor pressures (see p 399–400), especially when they occur in an indoor or enclosed environment. Substances with poor warning properties can cause serious injury without any warning signs of exposure such as smell or eye irritation. High vapor pressures increase the likelihood that dangerous air concentrations may be present. Also note that gases or vapors with a density greater than air may concentrate in low-lying areas.

Identification of Health Hazard Color Code: BLUE		Identification of Flammability Color Code: RED		Identification of Reactivity (Stability) Color Code: YELLOW	
Signal	Type of Possible Injury	Signal	Susceptibility of Materials to Burning	Signal	Susceptibility to Release of Energy
4	Materials which on very short exposure could cause death or major residual injury even though prompt medical treatment were given.	4	Materials which will rapidly or completely vaporize at atmospheric pressure and normal ambient temperature, or which are readily dispersed in air and which will burn readily.	4	Materials which in themselves are readily capable of detonation or of explosive decomposition or reaction at normal temperatures and pressures.
3	Materials which on short exposure could cause serious temporary or residual injury even though prompt medical treatment were given.	3	Liquids and solids that can be ignited under almost all ambient temperature conditions.	3	Materials which in themselves are capable of detonation or explosive reaction but require a strong initiating source or which must be heated under confinement before initiation or which react explosively with water.
2	Materials which on intense or continued exposure could cause temporary incapacitation or possible residual injury unless prompt medical treatment is given.	2	Materials that must be moderately heated or exposed to relatively high ambient temperatures before ignition can occur.	2	Materials which in themselves are normally unstable and readily undergo violent chemical change but do not detonate. Also materials which may react violently with water or which may form potentially explosive mixtures with water.
1	Materials which on exposure would cause irritation but only minor residual injury even if no treatment is given.	1	Materials that must be preheated before ignition can occur.	1	Materials which in themselves are normally stable, but which can become unstable at elevated temperatures and pressures or which may react with water with some release of energy but not violently.
0	Materials which on exposure under fire conditions would offer no hazard beyond that of ordinary combustible material.	0	Materials that will not burn.	0	Materials which in themselves are normally stable, even under fire exposure conditions, and which are not reactive with water.

FIGURE IV-2. National Fire Protection Association (NFPA) identification of the hazards of materials. (Continued)

EXAMPLE OF PLACARD AND PANEL WITH ID NUMBER

The Identification Number (ID No.) may be displayed on placards or on orange panels on tanks. Check the sides of the transport vehicle if the ID number is not displayed on the ends of the vehicle.

ID NUMBER ➔ **1090**

This panel must not be confused with the Maryland Petroleum Transporters' orange-colored marker which contains abbreviated words and a four-digit registration number.

FIGURE IV–3. Example of US Department of Transportation (DOT) vehicle warning placard and panel with DOT identification number.

- **D. Determine the potential for secondary contamination.** Although the threat of secondary contamination of emergency response personnel, equipment, and downstream facilities *may* be significant, it varies widely depending on the chemical, its concentration, and whether basic decontamination has already been performed. Not all toxic substances carry a risk of downstream contamination even though they may be extremely hazardous to rescuers in the hot zone. Exposures involving inhalation only and no external contamination do not pose a risk of secondary contamination.
    1. Examples of substances with **no significant risk** for secondary contamination of personnel outside the hot zone are **gases,** such as carbon monoxide, arsine, and chlorine, and **vapors,** such as those of xylene, toluene, or perchloroethylene.
    2. Examples of substances with **significant potential** for secondary contamination and requiring aggressive decontamination and protection of downstream personnel include potent organophosphate insecticides, oily nitro compounds, and highly radioactive compounds such as plutonium.
    3. In many cases involving substances with a high potential for secondary contamination, this risk can be minimized by removal of grossly contaminated clothing and thorough washing in the contamination reduction corridor, including soap or shampoo wash. Following these measures, only rarely will the downstream medical team face significant persistent personal threat to their health from an exposed victim.
- **IV. Personal protective equipment.** Personal protective equipment includes chemical-resistant clothing and gloves and respiratory protective gear. The use of such equipment should be supervised by experts in industrial hygiene or others with appropriate training and experience. Equipment that is incorrectly selected, improperly fitted, poorly maintained, or inappropriately used may provide a false sense of security and may fail, resulting in serious injury.
    - **A. Protective clothing** may be as simple as a disposable apron or as sophisticated as a fully encapsulated chemically resistant suit. However, no chemically resistant clothing is completely impervious to all chemicals over the full range of exposure conditions. Each suit is rated for its resistance to specific chemicals, and many are also rated for chemical breakthrough time.
    - **B. Protective respiratory gear** may be a simple paper mask, a cartridge filter respirator, or a positive-pressure air-supplied respirator. Respirators must be properly fitted for each user.
        1. **A paper mask** provides partial protection against gross quantities of airborne dust particles but does not prevent exposure to gases, vapors, or fumes.

    2. Cartridge filter respirators filter certain chemical gases and vapors out of the ambient air. They are used only when the toxic substance is known to be adsorbed by the filter, the airborne concentration is low, and there is adequate oxygen in the ambient air.

    3. Air-supplied respirators provide an independent source of clean air. They may be fully self-contained units or masks supplied by a long hose. Self-contained breathing apparatus (SCBA) has a limited duration of air supply, from 5 to 30 minutes. Users must be fitted for their specific gear.

V. Victim management. Victim management includes rapid stabilization and removal from the hot zone, initial decontamination, delivery to emergency medical services personnel at the clean zone perimeter, and medical assessment and treatment in the support area. Usually only the HazMat team or other fire department personnel with appropriate training and protective gear will be responsible for rescue from the hot zone, where skin and respiratory protection may be critical. Emergency medical personnel without specific training and appropriate equipment must not enter the hot zone unless it is determined to be safe by the incident commander or safety officer.

A. Stabilization in the hot zone. If there is suspicion of trauma, the patient should be placed on a backboard and a cervical collar applied if appropriate. Gross contamination may be brushed off the patient. No further medical intervention can be expected from rescuers who are wearing bulky suits, masks, and heavy gloves. Therefore, every effort should be made to get the seriously ill patient out of this area as quickly as possible. Victims who are ambulatory should be directed to walk to the contamination reduction area.

B. Initial decontamination. Gross decontamination may take place in the hot zone (eg, brushing off chemical powder, removing soaked clothing), but most decontamination occurs in the contamination reduction corridor before the victim is transferred to waiting emergency medical personnel in the support area. Do not delay critical treatment while decontaminating the victim unless the nature of the contaminant makes such treatment too dangerous. Consult a regional poison control center (see Table I–41, p 53) for specific advice on decontamination. See also Section I, p 41.

    1. Pull or cut off contaminated clothing and flush exposed skin, hair, or eyes with copious plain water from a high-volume low-pressure fire hose. For oily substances, additional washing with soap or shampoo may be required. Ambulatory, cooperative victims may be able to perform their own decontamination.

    2. For eye exposures, remove contact lenses if present, and irrigate using plain water or, if available, normal saline dribbled from an intravenous bag. Continue irrigation until symptoms resolve or, if the contaminant is an acid or base, until the pH of the conjunctival sac is near normal (6–8).

    3. Double-bag and save all removed clothing and jewelry.

    4. Collect run-off water if possible, but generally rapid flushing of exposed skin or eyes should not be delayed because of environmental concerns.

    5. For ingestions, if the material is a suspected corrosive substance or the patient is experiencing painful swallowing or has oral burns, give the patient a glass of water to drink. If available, administer activated charcoal (see p 47); even though this may obscure the view during later endoscopy, it may prevent absorption of systemic toxins.

    6. In the majority of incidents, basic victim decontamination as outlined above will substantially reduce or eliminate the potential for secondary contamination of downstream personnel or equipment. Procedures for cleaning equipment and people are contaminant-specific and depend on the risk of chemical persistence as well as toxicity.

C. Treatment in the support area. Once the patient is decontaminated (if required) and released into the support area, basic medical assessment and treatment by emergency medical providers may begin. In the majority of incidents, once the victim has been removed from the hot zone and is stripped and flushed, there is little or no risk of secondary contamination of these providers and sophisticated protective gear is not necessary. Simple surgical latex gloves and a plain apron or disposable outer clothing are generally sufficient.

1. Maintain a patent airway and assist breathing if necessary (see p 4). Administer supplemental oxygen.
2. Provide supportive care for shock (p 15), arrhythmias (p 10–14), coma (p 18), or seizures (p 22).
3. Treat with specific antidotes if appropriate and available.
4. Further skin, hair, or eye washing may be necessary. If the victim ingested a toxic substance, give activated charcoal (p 47).
5. Take notes on the probable or suspected level of exposure for each victim, the initial symptoms and signs, and treatment provided. For chemicals with delayed toxic effects, this could be lifesaving.

VI. Ambulance transport and hospital treatment. For skin or inhalation exposures, no special precautions should be required if adequate decontamination has been carried out in the field prior to transport.

A. Patients who have ingested toxic substances may vomit en route; carry a large plastic bag-lined basin and extra towels to soak up and immediately isolate spillage. Vomitus may contain the original toxic material or even toxic gases created by action of stomach acid on the substance (eg, hydrogen cyanide from ingested cyanide salts). When performing gastric lavage in the emergency department, isolate gastric washings (eg, using closed wall suction container system).

B. For those unpredictable situations in which **a contaminated victim arrives at the hospital before decontamination,** it is important to have a strategy ready that will minimize exposure to hospital personnel:

1. Ask the local HazMat team to set up a contamination reduction area outside the hospital emergency department entrance.
2. Prepare in advance a hose with 85 °F water, soap, and an old gurney for rapid decontamination *outside* the emergency department entrance. Have a child's inflatable pool or other container ready to collect water runoff, if possible.
3. Do not bring patients soaked with volatile liquids into the emergency department until they have been stripped and flushed outside.
4. For incidents involving radioactive materials or other highly contaminating substances that are not volatile, utilize the hospital's radiation accident protocol, which will generally include:
   a. Restricted access zones.
   b. Isolation of ventilation ducts leading out of the treatment room to prevent spreading the contamination throughout the hospital.
   c. Paper covering for floors, using absorbent materials if liquids are involved.
   d. Protective clothing for hospital staff (gloves, paper masks, shoe covers, caps, and gowns).
   e. Double-bagging and saving all contaminated clothing and equipment.
   f. Instituting monitoring to detect the extent and persistence of contamination (ie, a Geiger counter for radiation incidents).
   g. Contacting appropriate local, state, and federal offices to notify them of the incident and to obtain advice on laboratory testing and decontamination of equipment.

VII. Summary. The emergency medical response to a hazardous materials incident requires prior training and planning to protect the health of response personnel and victims.

A. Response plans and training should be flexible. The hazard and the required actions vary greatly with the circumstances at the scene and the chemicals involved.

B. First responders should be able to:
1. Recognize potentially hazardous situations.

2. Take steps to protect themselves from injury.
3. Obtain accurate information about the identity and toxicity of each chemical substance involved.
4. Use appropriate protective gear.
5. Perform victim decontamination before transport to a hospital.
6. Provide appropriate first-aid and advanced supportive measures as needed.
7. Coordinate their actions with other responding agencies such as the HazMat team, police and fire departments, and regional poison control centers.

REFERENCES

ATSDR: *Medical Management Guidelines for Acute Chemical Exposures, Final Draft.* US Department of Health & Human Services, US Government Printing Office, 1992.

Borak J, Callan M, Abbott W: *Hazardous Materials Exposure: Emergency Response and Patient Care.* Brady, 1991.

Bronstein AC, Currance PL: *Emergency Care for Hazardous Materials Exposure.* Mosby, 1988.

California Emergency Medical Services Authority: *Hazardous Materials Medical Management Protocols,* 2nd ed. California State Emergency Medical Services Authority, Sacramento, 1989.

Emergency Response Guidebook. US Department of Transportation, 1992.

Fire Protection Guide on Hazardous Materials, 9th ed. National Fire Protection Association, 1986.

NIOSH Pocket Guide to Chemical Hazards. US Department of Health and Human Services, US Government Printing Office, 1990.

OSHA: Hazardous waste operations and emergency response: Interim final rule. 29 CFR Part 1910. *Fed Reg* 1986;**51**:45654.

Stutz DR, Ulin S: *Hazardous Materials Injuries: A Handbook for Prehospital Care,* 3rd ed. Bradford Communications, 1992.

Sullivan JB, Krieger GR: *Hazardous Materials Toxicology: Clinical Principles of Environmental Health.* Williams & Wilkins, 1992.

INITIAL EVALUATION OF THE PATIENT WITH OCCUPATIONAL CHEMICAL EXPOSURES

Charles E. Becker, MD, and Kent R. Olson, MD

I. General considerations
   A. The patient with an occupational chemical exposure may come to the physician with a chronic work-related medical condition or with an acute illness requiring urgent medical attention. It is important to always maintain a high index of suspicion about occupational illness in any patient who is working.
   1. Chronic illness may not be correctly associated with work if there is no easily recognized temporal relationship between the work schedule and the disease. In addition, for illnesses with a long latency period between exposure and disease (eg, cancer), the connection may not be made unless one asks about prior occupations.
   2. Occupational exposure may masquerade as an exacerbation of a chronic disease (eg, worsening angina caused by exposure to carbon monoxide).
   3. Acute illnesses may not be recognized as work-related if there is a delay of more than a few hours before onset of symptoms or if there is no history of a dramatic incident at the workplace such as an explosion, fire, or major spill.
   B. This chapter outlines the initial evaluation of the patient with an occupational chemical exposure. This material is designed for the emergency department or urgent care center physician rather than the practitioner who is providing continuing health care or workplace medical surveillance programs. For a more detailed discussion of occupational illness, refer to one of the several textbooks of occupational medicine listed in the references (p 395).
II. Urgent evaluation of the patient
   A. Stabilize the patient
   1. If the patient is acutely ill, refer immediately to Section I (p 4) of this hand-

TABLE IV–1. SELECTED OCCUPATIONS AND SPECIFIC EXPOSURES

Occupation or Industry	Exposures (Syndrome)
Bakers	Flour, fungi, grain dust (asthma)
Battery manufacturing or repair	Lead, cadmium
Butchers	Vinyl plastic fumes (asthma)
Cement workers	Potassium chromate, dichromate (asthma)
Coal miners	Dust, silica (lung disease)
Dentists	Mercury, waste anesthetic gases
Dry cleaners	Solvents (liver, skin, and neurologic disease [neuropathy])
Electronics workers	Toluene diisocyanate (asthma); solvent exposure, hydrofluoric acid (skin burns).
Electroplating	Cyanide, chromium, nickel
Explosives manufacturing	Nitrates (headache and rebound vasoconstriction)
Farm workers	Pesticides; infectious agents; NO_2, pentachlorophenol, H_2S
Fire fighters	Carcinogens, smoke products (eg, CO, CN, nitrogen dioxide)
Foundry workers	Silica (lung disease), resins (asthma)
Fumigators	Methyl bromide (encephalopathy, neuropathy), sulfuryl fluoride (pulmonary edema), organophosphates and carbamates
Hospital workers	Infectious agents, radiation, cleansers, ethylene oxide
Insulation industry	Formaldehyde, asbestos, fiberglass
Insulators	Asbestos, fiberglass
Jackhammer operators	Vibration (vascular disease)
Meat packing or weighing	Polyvinylchloride or papain (asthma), infectious agents (Q fever)
Miners	Dust (lung disease)
Office workers	Poorly designed workplace (joint and eye problems)
Painters	Solvents, lead, isocyanates
Pathology technicians	Fluorocarbons (palpitations), formaldehyde, phenol
Petroleum industry	Benzene (leukemia), NH_3 and H_2S, polycyclic aromatic hydrocarbons
Pottery industry	Silica, lead
Poultry workers	Infectious agents (psittacosis), dusts (asthma)
Radiator repairmen	Lead
Rubber manufacturing	Ethylenediamine (asthma)
Seamen	Asbestos
Sewer workers	H_2S, methane
Shoe repairmen	Benzene (leukemia), benzidine (bladder cancer)
Sterilizer operators	Ethylene oxide (polyneuropathy)
Vintners	Arsenic (cancer and dermatitis)
Welders	Metal and polymer fume fever, ultraviolet radiation (skin and corneal burns), lead
Woodworkers	N-Hexane (neuropathy), other solvents, dust (asthma), wood preservatives

book for step-by-step guidance on management of common complications of poisoning. In general, establish a patent airway, assist ventilation if needed, give supplemental oxygen, and monitor the vital signs and electrocardiogram.

   2. If the patient has not been decontaminated at the scene, determine whether the patient poses a risk of secondary contamination to the emergency department, office personnel, or facility. Simple removal of clothing and showering or flushing with copious amounts of water is satisfactory for most chemical exposures (see Section I, p 41, and Section IV, p 385). Bag and save any contaminated clothing for possible chemical identification.

B. Obtain history of the incident

   1. From the victim or a coworker. The patient may be unable to provide accurate details about the incident. Determine whether the patient was accompanied by a coworker who can provide information about the specific incident and the work environment. Find out what activity the patient was involved in when the illness occurred. Find out whether there was a loss of consciousness, seizures, or other signs or symptoms, some of which may have resolved by the time medical attention was available. Ask about treatment already provided at the scene (eg, skin or eye irrigation, oxygen administration).

   2. Chemical identification. Ask the patient or coworker to identify the chemicals involved in the incident. Often they may have only a vague idea of the chemicals used or may refer to them by common or slang terms (ie, "solvent" or "dopant"), so it is important to determine the proper names of specific chemicals the worker may have been exposed to (see **3,** below). In addition, check Table IV–1 for a list of possible exposures associated with several common occupations.

   3. Work environment. Obtain a description of the work environment and the specific chemicals used. Was the room excessively hot or poorly ventilated? Was the patient working in an enclosed space or tank? These situations can cause heat exhaustion or hypoxia, which may masquerade as chemical intoxication.

   4. Protective gear. Was the patient using protective gear? If the patient smelled an odor or experienced eye or throat irritation, this may suggest protective suit failure, improper fitting, or use of the wrong equipment. Also, be aware that fully encapsulated suits may not allow for proper ventilation or sweating, resulting in hypoxia or heat exhaustion.

   5. Work practices. Ask whether there have been recent changes in work practices or manufacturing processes. Has the patient recently changed specific job duties? Has a new chemical been introduced?

   6. Other medical problems. Consider preexisting medical conditions that may mimic or aggravate chemical intoxication, such as alcoholism, coronary artery disease, or chronic obstructive pulmonary disease.

C. Obtain useful information from the worksite

   1. Worksite contacts. The following persons at the worksite may have access to useful information: the work supervisor, the health and safety officer, the industrial hygienist, an on-site nurse or physician, a union health and safety representative, a company personnel representative. **Note:** It is important to enlist the agreement of the exposed employee before contacting the worksite, as worker concerns about job security often complicate management of occupational exposures.

   2. Chemical identification. Obtain the Material Safety Data Sheets for information on chemical products used at the patient's workstation. If there is a Department of Transportation (DOT) identification placard (see Fig IV–3, p 384) on the container, check the DOT guidebook to identify the chemical and then locate it in Table IV–13 or in Section II.

   3. Air measurements. If an accidental overexposure has occurred, ask whether an industrial hygienist has measured air concentrations of the in-

TABLE IV–2. SELECTED OCCUPATIONAL SKIN DISORDERS

Disorders	Selected Causes
Contact dermatitis	
Irritant	Fibrous glass, corrosives, soaps
Allergic	Nickel, chromates
Chemical burns	Corrosive acids and alkali, phenols, hydrofluoric acid, phosphorus
Acne	Oils, fats, tars
Chloracne	Dibenzofurans, PCB dioxin
Pigmentary changes	Aniline, arsenic, phenols
Cancer	Ultraviolet radiation, arsenic
Hair loss	Thallium, arsenic, radiation

volved chemicals during or shortly after the incident. These measurements can be compared with recommended workplace exposure limits (Table IV–13). Generally, air levels at or below the permissible exposure limit (PEL) or threshold limit value (TLV) are not likely to be responsible for serious acute illness (unless, perhaps, skin exposure or ingestion has occurred).

4. **Baseline health data.** Obtain information from the patient's company medical file on any previous baseline physical examination and laboratory testing (eg, cholinesterase levels, blood lead levels, pulmonary function tests, chest radiographs) that could be compared with current data.

D. **Perform physical examination and laboratory testing**

1. **Organ system evaluation.** In addition to the routine examination, emphasis should be placed on organ systems most likely to be affected by specific chemicals and those that yield the most clues to occupational exposures or illness. For acute illness, the most common sites affected are the central nervous system and the cardiorespiratory system. Tables IV–2 through IV–11 describe considerations for several organ systems affected by occupational exposures.

a. **Skin.** The skin is the organ most commonly exposed to occupational toxins. Many chemicals are irritating to the skin, and some are sensitizers, capable of producing chronic allergic skin disorders. Solvents generally cause skin defatting, resulting in loss of the protective stratum corneum barrier and allowing enhanced penetration by toxic chemicals. Alkali, acids, and other corrosive materials cause chemical burns. Other chemicals may cause acne, chloracne, depigmentation, cancer, or hair loss (Table IV–2). Skin exposure may also result in systemic absorption and toxicity (see Table IV–13).

b. **Eyes, ears, nose, and throat.** Many chemicals that are highly water-soluble rapidly dissolve in the moist mucous membranes of the eyes,

TABLE IV–3. OCCUPATIONAL EXPOSURE OF THE EYES, EARS, NOSE, AND THROAT

Warning Properties	Selected Examples
None	Carbon monoxide, diethylamine
Weak	Ethylene oxide, nitrogen oxides
Strong	Acetone, ammonia, chlorine

TABLE IV–4. SELECTED OCCUPATIONAL PULMONARY EXPOSURES

Lung Diseases	Selected Causes
Acute and subacute	
Irritation, bronchitis, pulmonary edema	Sulfur dioxide, methyl isocyanate, chlorine, nitrogen oxides, ammonia, phosgene, formaldehyde, many others
Induction of asthma	Isocyanates, wood pulp dust, nickel
Extrinsic alveolitis	Woodworking, farming
Metal fume fever	Zinc oxides (welding galvanized steel)
Chronic (with latency before effect)	
Interstitial	Asbestosis, silicosis, coal dust
Granulomatous	Berylium
Cancer	Asbestos, arsenic, bischloromethyl ether, cigarette smoke, chromates

nose, and throat, providing excellent warning properties of local irritation. Others may have distinctive odors, although this may be unreliable because of concurrent upper respiratory infection or olfactory fatigue (Table IV–3).

c. **Lungs.** Along with the skin, the lungs are a very common route of chemical exposure. With highly water-soluble or irritating gases, early warning properties usually prevent prolonged exposure and symptoms are most severe early after exposure. On the other hand, with less soluble gases symptoms may be delayed 6–24 hours. Several lung exposures have long latency periods before overt disease appears, such as asbestosis and other pneumoconioses (Table IV–4).

d. **Musculoskeletal system.** Injuries to the musculoskeletal system are the most common type of reported on-the-job injuries. Many types of work involving repetitive motion may cause acute tendinitis and, with cumulative trauma, may result in chronic pain syndromes. Consider that a chemical exposure (eg, solvent or pesticide causing dizziness, incoordination,

TABLE IV–5. SELECTED OCCUPATIONAL MUSCULOSKELETAL DISORDERS

Disorders	Selected Causes
Local injuries	
Low back pain	Heavy labor, lifting
Reynaud's syndrome	Vibration, cold
Carpal tunnel syndrome	Vibration, assemblers, packers
Degenerative arthritis	Housekeeping, heavy labor
Systemic illnesses	
Scleroderma	Some organic solvents
Gout	Lead
Osteosclerosis	Fluoride
Aseptic necrosis	Scuba divers
Osteonecrosis	Phosphorus
Osteosarcoma	Radium

TABLE IV–6. SELECTED OCCUPATIONAL NEUROLOGIC DISORDERS

Disorders	Selected Causes
CNS tumors	Vinyl chloride, petroleum products
Parkinsonism	Manganese, carbon monoxide, carbon disulfide, MPTP
Headache	Carbon monoxide, nitrites, solvents
Acute encephalopathy	Carbon monoxide, solvents, lead, carbon disulfide, methyl bromide
Peripheral neuropathy	Lead, arsenic, mercury, thallium, *n*-hexane, methyl butyl ketone, methyl bromide, acrylamide, triorthocresyl phosphate

   or syncope) may enhance the risk of an accident resulting in traumatic injury (Table IV–5).
  e. Nervous system. The central and peripheral nervous systems are frequently involved in acute and chronic occupational chemical exposures. Ask about paresthesias, dysesthesias, local weakness, fatigue, disturbed sleep patterns, or headache (Table IV–6).
   f. Gastrointestinal system. Symptoms are often nonspecific. Gastroenteritis may be confused with viral or food-borne illness. Colic and constipation should suggest lead exposure. Many toxins can cause subtle or severe hepatic damage. Be sure to elicit a history of alcohol use or dependency, which may aggravate workplace chemical hepatitis (Table IV–7).
  g. Cardiovascular system. Workplace chemical exposures may cause acute myocardial abnormalities (eg, cardiac ischemia or arrhythmias) or may affect vascular tone. Hydrocarbon solvents as a group, and in particular halogenated hydrocarbons, may sensitize the myocardium to arrhythmogenic effects of epinephrine. Chronic exposures may be associated with a higher risk of coronary disease (Table IV–8).
  h. Hematopoietic system. The hematopoietic system can be affected by acute and chronic workplace chemical exposures. Exposures in the distant past may have a long latency period before causing cancer (eg, benzene; Table IV–9).
  i. Renal system. Many occupational chemical exposures produce acute or chronic kidney dysfunction and bladder abnormalities. Up to 60–70% of kidney function may be lost before the decrease is clinically apparent (Table IV–10).
  j. Endocrine system. Table IV–11 shows selected disorders of the endocrine and reproductive systems caused by occupational chemical exposures.
 2. General laboratory panel. In general, the following empiric tests are recommended for most patients with an occupational chemical exposure.
  a. CBC (complete blood count).

TABLE IV–7. SELECTED OCCUPATIONAL GASTROINTESTINAL DISORDERS

Disorders	Selected Causes
Nausea and vomiting	Organophosphates and carbamates, epoxy resins, copper fumes, solvents
Diarrhea	Organophosphates and carbamates, arsenic, thallium, phosphorus
Jaundice	Hemolysis (eg, arsine), hepatitis (carbon tetrachloride, nitrobenzene, hydrazine, phosphorus, dioxin)

TABLE IV–8. SELECTED OCCUPATIONAL CARDIOVASCULAR DISORDERS

Disorders	Selected Causes
Coronary artery disease	Carbon disulfide, carbon monoxide
Arrhythmias	Halogenated hydrocarbons, barium
Hypertension	Lead
Cor pulmonale	Fibrogenic restrictive lung disease
Angina pectoris	Carbon monoxide, methylene chloride
Hypotension	Nitrites, nitroglycerin

    b. BUN (blood urea nitrogen) and creatinine.
    c. Glucose and electrolytes.
    d. Liver enzymes.
    e. Urinalysis.
  3. Specific laboratory tests. If the exposure agent is known, order specific tests as recommended in Section II. In general, focus attention on the organ systems affected. For example, a chest radiograph and assessment of oxygenation (arterial blood gases or pulse oximetry), and possibly pulmonary function tests, would be appropriate after symptomatic exposure to a pulmonary irritant gas.
  4. Baseline tests. Check to see whether baseline tests are available in the patient's company file to compare with current data.
  5. Consultation. A regional poison center (see p 53), medical toxicologist, or occupational medicine specialist may be able to assist in the selection and interpretation of laboratory tests.

III. Treatment and disposition
  A. Treatment
    1. Treatment recommendations are provided in Sections I and II for common complications of poisoning and for many specific chemicals and other toxic agents.
    2. Other sources of information on treatment of acute occupational poisoning are listed in the references.
  B. Disposition
    1. Remember that many chemicals may cause delayed-onset effects (for example, pulmonary edema may occur several hours after exposure to nitrogen dioxide). In such cases, prolonged observation in the emergency department or in the hospital may be necessary.
    2. Be sure that a method is established to notify the patient of laboratory test

TABLE IV–9. SELECTED OCCUPATIONAL HEMATOPOIETIC DISORDERS

Disorders	Selected Causes
Hemolysis	Arsine, naphthalene, stibine
Methemoglobinemia	Nitrites, aniline, oxidizers
Bone marrow suppression	Arsenic, radiation, benzene
Porphyria	Hexachlorobenzene, lead
Neutropenia	Chlorinated hydrocarbons
Anemia	Lead

TABLE IV–10. SELECTED OCCUPATIONAL RENAL DISORDERS

Disorders	Selected Causes
Acute tubular necrosis	Glycols, inorganic mercury, arsine
Chronic renal failure	Lead, cadmium, radiation
Bladder cancers	Benzidine, β-naphthylamine

    results, to explain abnormal findings, and to provide treatment when appro-
    priate.
  3. Patients should be referred to a qualified occupational medicine specialist
    for follow-up. An occupational medicine physician may already be available
    at the worksite or may be found through a local medical school or govern-
    ment agency.
C. Mandated reporting
  1. There are a variety of specific legal requirements for reporting of occupa-
    tional exposures to state and federal agencies. In some cases, specific lab-
    oratory testing and workplace exclusion are mandated by law (for example,
    for lead exposure).
  2. If you are not already familiar with local, state, or federal reporting require-
    ments, contact the local health officer or environmental health officer or a
    regional Occupational Safety and Health Administration (OSHA) office.
    Table IV–12 (see p 395) lists regional federal OSHA offices and their tele-
    phone numbers. *Note:* Some states have their own programs (eg, Cal-
    OSHA in California). Obtain referral from regional OSHA office.
  3. Be certain to ensure strict confidentiality of all patient information other than
    that required by law to be reported.
  4. Check to determine whether other workers have been affected. Some may
    have stayed at work or may have gone to other treatment facilities. If a po-
    tentially life-threatening hazard still exists at the worksite, then workers may
    need to be evacuated and immediate reporting to local officials is manda-
    tory.
  5. Determine whether there has been potential contamination of the environ-
    ment in the neighborhood of the workplace, which might necessitate evacu-
    ation of local residents. Once again, reporting of the incident to local officials
    is essential.
IV. Summary: Characteristics of occupational exposures
  A. There may be a delay in onset of symptoms.
  B. The exposure may be difficult to identify and quantify.
  C. Other workers may be exposed.
  D. Potential for contamination of health care providers and the environment
    should be determined.
  E. Expert consultation may be available through local agencies and federal OSHA
    offices.
  F. There may be special reporting requirements mandated by law.

TABLE IV–11. SELECTED OCCUPATIONAL ENDOCRINE AND REPRODUCTIVE DISORDERS

Disorders	Selected Causes
Thyroiditis	Polychlorinated biphenyls
Aspermia	Dibromochloropropane
Miscarriage	Lead, nitrous oxide

TABLE IV–12. REGIONAL OFFICES OF THE OCCUPATIONAL SAFETY AND HEALTH ADMINISTRATION (OSHA)

Region	Regional Office and Phone Number	States Served
I	Boston (617) 565–7164	Connecticut, Maine, Massachusetts, New Hampshire, Vermont
II	New York City (212) 337–2325	New York, New Jersey
III	Philadelphia (215) 596–1201	Delaware, District of Columbia, Maryland, Pennsylvania, Virginia, West Virginia
IV	Atlanta (404) 347–3573	Alabama, Florida, Georgia, Kentucky, Mississippi, North Carolina, South Carolina, Tennessee
V	Chicago (312) 353–2220	Illinois, Indiana, Michigan, Minnesota, Ohio, Wisconsin
VI	Dallas (214) 767–4731	Arkansas, Louisiana, New Mexico, Oklahoma, Texas
VII	Kansas City (816) 426–5861	Iowa, Kansas, Missouri, Nebraska
VIII	Denver (303) 844–3061	Colorado, Montana, North Dakota, South Dakota, Utah, Wyoming
IX	San Francisco (415) 995–5672	Arizona, California, Hawaii, Nevada, South Pacific Islands
X	Seattle (206) 442–5930	Alaska, Idaho, Oregon, Washington

REFERENCES

Hathaway G et al (editors): *Proctor and Hughes' Chemical Hazards of the Workplace,* 3rd ed. Lippincott, 1991.

LaDou J (editor): *Occupational Medicine.* Appleton & Lange, 1990.

National Institute of Occupational Safety and Health: *Recommendations for Occupational Safety and Health Standards 1988.* US Department of Health & Human Services/Centers for Disease Control, 1988.

Rom WN (editor): *Environmental and Occupational Medicine,* 2nd ed. Little, Brown, 1992.

THE TOXIC HAZARDS OF INDUSTRIAL AND OCCUPATIONAL CHEMICALS

Frank J. Mycroft, PhD, and Patricia Hess Hiatt, BS

Table IV–13 provides basic information on the toxicity of many of the most commonly encountered and toxicologically significant industrial chemicals. The table is intended to expedite the recognition of potentially hazardous exposure situations and therefore provides information such as vapor pressures, warning properties, physical appearance, occupational exposure standards and guidelines, and hazard classification codes, which may also be useful in the assessment of an exposure situation. Table IV–13 is divided into 3 sections: **health hazards, exposure guidelines,** and **comments.** To use the table correctly, it is important to understand the scope and limitations of the information it provides.

The chemicals included in Table IV–13 were selected according to the following criteria: (1) toxic potential; (2) prevalence of use; (3) public health concern; and (4) availability of adequate toxicologic, regulatory, and physical/chemical properties information. Several governmental and industrial lists of "hazardous chemicals" were used. A number of chemicals for which no toxicologic information could be found, for which there are no regulatory standards, or that have very limited use were omitted. Chemicals that were of specific interest, those with existing exposure recommendations, and those of high use (even if of low toxicity) were included.

 I. Health hazards information. The health hazards section focuses primarily on the basic hazards associated with inhalation of or skin exposures to chemicals that might occur in a workplace. It is based almost entirely on the occupational health literature. Most of our understanding of the potential effects of chemicals on human health derive from occupational exposures, which are typically many times greater than environmental exposures. Moreover, the information in Table IV–13 unavoidably emphasizes *acute* health effects. Much more is known about the acute effects of chemicals on human health than about their chronic effects. The rapid onset of symptoms following exposure makes the causal association more readily apparent for acute health effects.

A. The table is *not* a comprehensive source of the toxicology and medical information needed to manage a severely symptomatic or poisoned patient. Medical management information and advice for specific poisonings are found in Section I (see pulmonary problems, pp 2–9, and pulmonary and skin decontamination, pp 41–44) and Section II (see caustics and corrosives, p 126; gases, p 176; and hydrocarbons, p 178).

Hydrocarbons, broadly defined as chemicals containing carbon and hydrogen, make up the majority of substances in Table IV–13. Hydrocarbons have a wide range of chemical structures, and, not surprisingly, a variety of toxic effects. There are a few common features of hydrocarbon exposure, and the reader is directed to Section II, p 178, for general diagnosis and treatment. Some common features include:

1. Skin. A dermatitis caused by defatting or removal of oils in the skin is common, especially with prolonged contact. Some agents can cause frank burns.

2. Arrhythmias. Many hydrocarbons, most notably fluorinated, chlorinated, and aromatic compounds, can sensitize the heart to arrhythmogenic effects of epinephrine, resulting in premature ventricular contractions (PVCs), ventricular tachycardia, or fibrillation. This effect occasionally can be caused by even simple aliphatic compounds such as butane.

    a. Because arrhythmias may not occur immediately, cardiac monitoring for 24 hours is recommended for all victims who have had significant hydrocarbon exposure (eg, syncope, coma, arrhythmias).

    b. Ventricular arrhythmias are preferably treated with a β-adrenergic blocker (eg, esmolol, propranolol) rather than lidocaine (see p 15).

3. Pulmonary aspiration of most hydrocarbons, especially those with relatively high volatility and low viscosity (eg, gasoline, kerosene, naphtha) can cause a severe chemical pneumonitis.

B. To broaden the scope of the table, the findings of human and animal studies relating to the carcinogenic or reproductive toxicity of a chemical are included when available. The International Agency for Research on Cancer (IARC) is the foremost authority in evaluating the carcinogenic potential of chemical agents for humans. The overall IARC evaluations are provided, when available, in the health hazards section of the table. The IARC evaluations are based primarily upon human and animal data:

1. IARC 1 substances are considered human carcinogens; generally there is sufficient epidemiologic information to support a causal association between exposure and human cancer.

2. IARC 2 compounds are suspected of being carcinogenic to humans based upon a combination of animal and human data. Group 2 is subdivided into two parts.

    a. IARC 2A indicates that a chemical is *probably* carcinogenic to humans. Most often there is limited evidence of carcinogenicity in humans combined with sufficient evidence of carcinogenicity in animals.

    b. IARC 2B indicates that a chemical is *possibly* carcinogenic to humans. This category may be used when there is limited evidence from epidemiologic studies and less than sufficient evidence for carcinogenicity in animals. It also may be used when there is inadequate evidence of carcinogenicity in humans and sufficient evidence in animals.

3. IARC 3 substances cannot be classified in regard to their carcinogenic potential for humans because of inadequate data.

4. If a chemical is described in the table as carcinogenic but an IARC category is not given, this indicates that although IARC has not classified the chemical, other sources (eg, US Environmental Protection Agency, California Department of Health Services Hazard Evaluation Service and Information System) consider it carcinogenic.

C. Problems in assessing health hazards. The nature and magnitude of the health hazards associated with occupational or environmental exposures to any chemical depend on its intrinsic toxicity and the conditions of exposure.

1. Characterization of these hazards is often difficult. Important considerations include the potency of the agent, the route of exposure, the level and temporal pattern of exposure, genetic susceptibility, overall health status, and lifestyle factors that may alter individual sensitivities (eg, alcohol consumption may cause "degreaser's flush" in workers exposed to trichloroethylene). Despite their value in estimating the likelihood and potential severity of an effect, quantitative measurements of the level of exposure are not often available.

2. Hazard characterizations cannot address undiscovered or unappreciated health effects. The limited information available on the health effects of most chemicals makes this a major concern. For example, of the more than 5 million compounds known to science, only about 100,000 have any listing in the *Registry of the Toxic Effects of Chemical Substances* published by the National Institute for Occupational Safety and Health (NIOSH). Of these 100,000 substances, less than 5,000 have any toxicity studies relating to their potential tumorigenic or reproductive effects in animals or humans. Because of these gaps, the absence of information does not imply the absence of hazard.

3. The predictive value of animal findings for humans is sometimes uncertain. For many effects, however, there is considerable concordance between test animals and humans.

4. The developmental toxicity information presented here is not a sufficient basis on which to make clinical judgments as to whether a given exposure might adversely affect a pregnancy. For most chemicals that are known to have adverse effects on fetal development in test animals, there are insufficient epidemiologic data in humans. The predictive value of these animal findings for humans, who are typically exposed to levels much lower than those used in animal tests, is thought to be poor. In general, so little is known about the effects of substances on fetal development that it is prudent to conservatively manage all chemical exposures. The information here is presented solely to identify those compounds for which available data further indicate the need to control exposures.

II. Exposure guidelines and National Fire Protection Association rankings

A. Threshold limit values (TLVs) are workplace exposure guidelines established by the American Conference of Governmental Industrial Hygienists (ACGIH), a professional society. Although the ACGIH has no regulatory authority, its recommendations are highly regarded and widely followed by the occupational health community.

The toxicologic basis for each TLV varies. A TLV may be set on the basis of such diverse effects as respiratory sensitization, sensory irritation, narcosis, or asphyxia. Therefore, the TLV is not a relative index of toxicity. Because the degree of health hazard is a continuous function of exposure, TLVs are not fine lines separating safe from dangerous levels of exposure. The *Documentation of the Threshold Limit Values,* which is published by the ACGIH and describes in detail the rationale for each value, should be consulted for specific information on the toxicologic significance of a particular TLV.

Common units for a TLV are **ppm** (parts of chemical per million parts of air) and **mg/m³** (milligrams of chemical per cubic meter of air). At standard temperature and pressure, **TLV values in ppm can be converted to their equivalent concentrations in mg/m³** by multiplying the TLV in ppm by the molecular weight (MW) in mg of the chemical and dividing the result by 22.4 (1 mol of gas displaces 22.4 L of air at standard temperature and pressure):

$$mg/m^3 = \frac{ppm \times MW}{22.4}$$

1. The **threshold limit value time-weighted average (TLV-TWA)** refers to airborne contaminants and is the time-weighted average concentration for a normal 8-hour workday and 40-hour workweek to which nearly all workers may be repeatedly exposed, day after day, without adverse effect. Unless otherwise indicated, the values listed under the ACGIH TLV heading are the TLV-TWA values. Because TLV-TWAs are often set to protect against worker discomfort, nonspecific minor health complaints such as eye or throat irritation, cough, headache, or nausea may indicate overexposure.
2. The **threshold limit value ceiling (TLV-C)** is the airborne concentration that should not be exceeded during any part of a working exposure. Ceiling guidelines are often set for rapidly acting agents for which an 8-hour time-weighted average exposure limit would be inappropriate. TLV-Cs are listed under the ACGIH TLV heading and are noted by a **"(C)."**
3. Compounds for which **skin contact** is a significant route of exposure are designated with an **"S."** This could refer to potential corrosive effects or systemic toxicity owing to skin absorption.
4. The ACGIH classifies some substances as being *confirmed* **(A1)** or *suspected* **(A2) human carcinogens.** These designations are also provided in the table.
5. The TLVs are heavily based on workplace exposures and conditions occurring within the USA. Their application, which requires training in industrial hygiene, is therefore limited to similar exposures and conditions.
B. **OSHA regulations** are standards for exposure to airborne contaminants set and enforced by the Occupational Safety and Health Administration (OSHA), an agency of the federal government.
1. The **permissible exposure limit (PEL)** set by federal OSHA is closely analogous to the ACGIH TLV-TWA. In fact, when OSHA was established in 1971, it formally adopted the 1969 ACGIH TLVs for nearly all of its PELs. In 1988, OSHA updated the majority of its PELs by adopting the 1986 TLVs. These revised PELs were printed in the 1990 edition of this manual. However, in early 1993, the 1988 PEL revisions were voided as a result of legal challenges, and the earlier values were restored. Because these restored values cannot be reliably assumed to protect worker health, and because the values may change again as a result of further administrative or legislative action, the PELs are not printed in this edition.
2. Substances that are specifically **regulated as carcinogens** by OSHA are indicated by **"OSHA CA"** under the ACGIH TLV heading. For these carcinogens, additional regulations apply. The notation **"NIOSH CA"** in the TLV column identifies those chemicals that the National Institute for Occupational Safety and Health recommends be treated as potential human carcinogens.
3. Some states operate their own occupational health and safety programs in cooperation with OSHA. In these states, stricter standards may apply.
C. **Immediately dangerous to life or health (IDLH)** represents "a maximum concentration from which one could escape within 30 minutes without any escape-impairing symptoms or any irreversible health effects." The IDLH values were jointly set by OSHA and NIOSH for the purpose of respirator selection.

Emergency Response Planning Guidelines (ERPGs) have been developed by the American Industrial Hygiene Association (AIHA) for 35 specific substances. The values are generally based upon limited human experience as well as available animal data and should be considered estimates. Although these values are printed in the IDLH column, they have different meanings:

1. **ERPG-1** is "the maximum air concentration below which it is believed nearly all individuals could be exposed for up to 1 hour without experiencing other than mild transient adverse health effects or perceiving a clearly defined objectionable odor."

2. **ERPG-2** is "the maximum air concentration below which it is believed that nearly all individuals could be exposed for up to 1 hour without experiencing or developing irreversible or other serious health effects or symptoms which could impair their abilities to take protective action."

3. **ERPG-3** is "the maximum air concentration below which it is believed that nearly all individuals could be exposed for up to 1 hour without experiencing or developing life-threatening health effects."

4. The ERPGs were developed for purposes of emergency planning and response. They are not exposure guidelines and do not incorporate the safety factors normally used in establishing acceptable exposure limits. Use of the ERPGs for periods longer than one hour is not safe.

D. **National Fire Protection Association (NFPA) codes** are part of the system created by the NFPA for identifying and ranking the potential fire hazards of materials. The system has 3 principal categories of hazard: **health (H), flammability (F),** and **reactivity (R).** Within each category, hazards are ranked from four (4), indicating a severe hazard, to zero (0), indicating no special hazard. The NFPA rankings for each substance are listed under their appropriate headings. The criteria for rankings within each category are found in Fig IV–2, p 383.

1. The NFPA health hazard category is based on both the intrinsic toxicity of a chemical and the toxicities of its combustion or breakdown products. The overall ranking is determined by the greater source of health hazard under fire or other emergency conditions. The common hazards from the ordinary combustion of materials are not considered in these rankings.

2. This system is intended to provide basic information to fire-fighting and emergency response personnel. Its application to specific situations requires skill. Conditions at the scene, such as the amount of material involved and its rate of release, wind conditions, and the proximity to various populations and their health status, are as important as the intrinsic properties of a chemical in determining the magnitude of hazard.

III. **Comments section.** The comments column of Table IV–13 provides supplementary information on the physical and chemical properties of substances that would be helpful in assessing their health hazards. Information such as physical state and appearance, vapor pressures, warning properties, and potential breakdown products is included.

A. Information on **physical state and appearance** of a compound may help in its identification and indicate whether dusts, mists, vapors, or gases are likely means of airborne exposure. ***Note:*** For many products, especially pesticides, appearance and some hazardous properties may vary with the formulation.

B. The **vapor pressure** of a substance determines its potential maximum air concentration and influences the degree of inhalation exposure or airborne contamination. Vapor pressures fluctuate greatly with temperature.

1. Substances with high vapor pressures tend to volatilize more quickly and can reach higher maximum air concentrations than substances with low vapor pressures. Some substances have such low vapor pressures that airborne contamination is a threat only if they are finely dispersed in a dust or mist.

2. Substances with a **saturated air concentration** below their TLVs do not pose a significant vapor inhalation hazard. Vapor pressures can be roughly converted to a saturated air concentration expressed in ppm by multiplying by a factor of 1300. This is equivalent to dividing by 760 mm Hg and then

multiplying the result by 1 million to adjust for the original units of parts per million (a pressure of 1 equals 760 mm Hg):

$$ppm = \frac{\text{Vapor pressure (mm Hg)}}{760} \times 10^6$$

C. **Warning properties,** such as odor and sensory irritation, can be valuable indicators of exposure. However, because of olfactory fatigue and individual differences in odor thresholds, the sense of smell is often unreliable for many compounds. There is no correlation between the quality of an odor and its toxicity. Pleasant-smelling compounds are not necessarily less toxic than foul-smelling ones.
   1. The warning property assessments found in the table are based on OSHA evaluations. For the purpose of this manual, chemicals described as having *good* warning properties can be detected at levels below the TLV by smell or irritation by most individuals. Chemicals described as having *adequate* warning properties can be detected at air levels near the TLV. Chemicals described as having *poor* warning properties can be detected only at levels significantly above the TLV or not at all.
   2. Reported values for odor threshold in the literature vary greatly for many chemicals and are uncertain. These differences make assessments of warning qualities difficult.
D. **Thermal breakdown products.** Under fire conditions, many organic substances will break down to other toxic substances. The amounts, kinds, and distribution of breakdown products vary with the fire conditions and are not easily modeled. Information on the likely thermal decomposition products is included because of their importance in the assessment of health hazards under fire conditions.
   1. In general, incomplete combustion of *any* organic material will produce some carbon monoxide (see p 121).
   2. The partial combustion of compounds containing sulfur, nitrogen, or phosphorus atoms will also release their oxides (see p 292, 230, 176).
   3. Compounds with chlorine atoms will release some hydrogen chloride or chlorine (see p 130) when exposed to high heat or fire; some chlorinated compounds may also generate phosgene (see p 256).
   4. Compounds containing the fluorine atom are similarly likely to break down to yield some hydrogen fluoride (see p 180) and fluorine.
   5. Some compounds (eg, polyurethane) that contain an unsaturated carbon-nitrogen bond will release cyanide (see p 145) during their decomposition.
   6. Polychlorinated aromatic compounds may yield polychlorinated dibenzo-dioxins and polychlorinated dibenzofurans (see p 154) when heated.
   7. In addition, smoke from a chemical fire is likely to contain large amounts of the volatilized original chemical and still other poorly characterized partial breakdown products.
   8. The thermal breakdown product information found in Table IV–13 is derived primarily from data found in the literature and the general considerations described immediately above. Aside from the NFPA codes, Table IV–13 does not otherwise cover the chemical reactivities or compatibilities of substances.
IV. **Summary.** Table IV–13 provides basic information that describes the potential health hazards associated with exposure to several hundred chemicals. The table is not a comprehensive listing of all the possible health hazards for each chemical. The information compiled here comes from a wide variety of respected sources (see references below) and focuses on the more likely or commonly reported health effects. Publications from the National Institute for Occupational Safety and Health, the Occupational Safety and Health Administration, the American Conference of Governmental Industrial Hygienists, the Hazard Evaluation System and

Information Service of the State of California, and the National Fire Protection Association; major textbooks in the fields of toxicology and occupational health; and major review articles were the primary sources of the information found here. Refer to the original sources for more complete information.

Table IV–13 is intended primarily to guide users in the quick qualitative assessment of common toxic hazards. Its application to specific situations requires skill. Because of the many data gaps in the toxicologic literature, exposures should generally be managed conservatively. Contact a regional poison control center (see Table I–41, p 53) or medical toxicologist for expert assistance in managing specific emergency exposures.

REFERENCES

Air contaminants: Permissible exposure limits. *Fed Reg* 1989;**54**:2332.

Barlow SM, Sullivan FM (editors): *Reproductive Hazards of Industrial Chemicals.* Academic Press, 1982.

Emergency Response Planning Committee: *Emergency Response Planning Guidelines.* American Industrial Hygiene Association, 1992.

Fire Protection Guide on Hazardous Materials, 9th ed. National Fire Protection Association, 1986.

Hathaway G et al: *Proctor and Hughes' Chemical Hazards of the Workplace,* 3rd ed. Lippincott, 1991.

Hayes WJ Jr: *Pesticides Studied in Man.* Williams & Wilkins, 1982.

IARC Monographs on the Evaluation of the Carcinogenic Risk of Chemicals to Humans. 54 vols. World Health Organization, 1972–1992.

Morgan DP: *Recognition and Management of Pesticide Poisonings,* 4th ed. US Environmental Protection Agency, 1989.

National Toxicology Program: *Sixth Annual Report on Carcinogens.* US Department of Health & Human Services, 1991.

NIOSH: *Occupational Diseases: A Guide to Their Recognition.* US Department of Health & Human Services, 1977.

NIOSH: Recommendations for occupational safety and health standards. *MMWR* 1988;**37(Suppl 7)**.

NIOSH/OSHA: *Occupational Health Guidelines for Chemical Hazards.* DHHS (NIOSH) Publication No. 81-123. US Department of Health & Human Services, 1981.

NIOSH/OSHA: *Pocket Guide to Chemical Hazards.* NIOSH Publication No. 78-210. US Department of Health & Human Services, 1985.

Rumack BH (editor): *TOMES.* Vol 16. Micromedex, 1993.

Schardein JL: *Chemically Induced Birth Defects.* Marcel Dekker, 1985.

Schardein JL, Schwetz BA, Kenel MF: Species sensitivities and prediction of teratogenic potential. *Environ Health Perspect* 1985;**61**:55.

Threshold Limit Values and Biological Exposure Indices, 6th ed. American Council of Governmental Industrial Hygienists, 1991.

TABLE IV–13. HEALTH HAZARD SUMMARIES FOR INDUSTRIAL AND OCCUPATIONAL CHEMICALS

Abbreviations and designations used in this table are defined as follows:

IARC = International Agency for Research on Cancer overall classification (see p 396): 1 = known human carcinogen; 2A = probable human carcinogen; 2B = possible human carcinogen; 3 = inadequate data available.

TLV = American Conference of Governmental Industrial Hygienists (ACGIH) threshold limit value time weighted average (TLV-TWA) air concentration (see p 397):
A1 = ACGIH-confirmed human carcinogen; A2 = ACGIH-suspected human carcinogen; A3 = ACGIH animal carcinogen; A4 = considered by ACGIH as not classifiable (inadequate data); A5 = not suspected as human carcinogen by ACGIH.

ppm = Parts of chemical per million parts of air.
mg/m³ = Milligrams of chemical per cubic meter of air.
mppcf = Million particles of dust per cubic foot of air.
(C) = Ceiling air concentration (TLV-C) that should not be exceeded at any time.
S = Skin absorption can be significant route of exposure.

NIOSH CA = Judged by National Institute for Occupational Safety and Health to be a known or suspected human carcinogen (see p 398).

OSHA CA = Regulated by the Occupational Safety and Health Administration as an occupational carcinogen (see p 398).

IDLH = Immediately dangerous to life or health air concentration (see p 398).
ERPG = Emergency Response Planning Guidelines air concentration values for a one-hour period of exposure (see p 398–399).

NFPA Codes = National Fire Protection Association hazard classification codes (see p 383 and p 399): 0 (no hazard) <—> 4 (severe hazard)
H = Health hazard
F = Fire hazard
R = Reactivity hazard
Ox = Oxidizing agent
W = Water-reactive substance

Health Hazard Summaries	ACGIH TLV	IDLH	NFPA Codes H F R	Comments
Acetaldehyde (CAS: 75-07-0): Corrosive; severe burns to eyes and skin may occur. Vapors strongly irritating to eyes and respiratory tract; evidence for adverse effects on fetal development in animals. A carcinogen in test animals (IARC 2B).	100 ppm [proposed: 25 ppm (C), A3]	10,000 ppm	2 4 2	Colorless liquid. Fruity odor and irritation are both adequate warning properties. Vapor pressure is 750 mm Hg at 20 °C (68 °F). Highly flammable.
Acetic acid (vinegar acid [CAS: 64-19-7]): Concentrated solutions are corrosive; severe burns to eyes and skin may occur. Vapors strongly irritating to eyes and respiratory tract.	10 ppm	1000 ppm	2 2 1	Colorless liquid. Pungent, vinegarlike odor and irritation both occur near the TLV and are adequate warning properties. Vapor pressure is 11 mm Hg at 20 °C (68 °F). Flammable.

Substance	TLV	Air concentration	H	F	R	Special	Comments
Acetic anhydride (CAS: 108-24-7): Corrosive; severe burns to eyes and skin may result. Dermal sensitization has been reported. Vapors highly irritating to eyes and respiratory tract.	5 ppm (C) [proposed: 5 ppm]	1000 ppm	2	2	1	W	Colorless liquid. Odor and irritation both occur below the TLV and are good warning properties. Vapor pressure is 4 mm Hg at 20 °C (68 °F). Flammable. Evolves heat upon contact with water.
Acetone (dimethyl ketone, 2-propanone [CAS: 67-64-1]): Vapors mildly irritating to eyes and respiratory tract. A CNS depressant at high levels. Eye irritation and headache are common symptoms of moderate overexposure.	750 ppm	20,000 ppm	1	3	0		Colorless liquid with a sharp, aromatic odor. Eye irritation is an adequate warning property. Vapor pressure is 266 mm Hg at 25 °C (77 °F). Highly flammable.
Acetonitrile (methyl cyanide, cyanomethane, ethanenitrile [CAS: 75-05-8]): Vapors mildly irritating to eyes and respiratory tract. Inhibits several metabolic enzyme systems. Dermal absorption occurs. Metabolized to cyanide (see p 145); fatalities have resulted. Symptoms include headache, nausea, vomiting, weakness, and stupor. Limited evidence for adverse effects on fetal development in test animals given large doses.	40 ppm	4000 ppm	2	3	0		Colorless liquid. Etherlike odor, detectable at the TLV, is an adequate warning property. Vapor pressure is 73 mm Hg at 20 °C (68 °F). Flammable. Thermal breakdown products include oxides of nitrogen and cyanide. May be found in products for removing sculptured nails.
Acetophenone (phenyl methyl ketone, [CAS: 98-86-2]): Direct contact mildly irritating to eyes and skin. A CNS depressant at high levels.	[proposed: 10 ppm]						
Acetylene tetrabromide (tetrabromoethane [CAS: 79-27-6]): Direct contact is irritating to eyes and skin. Vapors irritating to eyes and respiratory tract. Dermal absorption occurs. Highly hepatotoxic; liver injury can result from low-level exposures.	1 ppm	10 ppm	3	0	1		Viscous, pale yellow liquid. Pungent, chloroformlike odor. Vapor pressure is less than 0.1 mm Hg at 20 °C (68 °F). Not combustible. Thermal breakdown products include hydrogen bromide and carbonyl bromide.
Acrolein (acryaldehyde, 2-propenal [CAS: 107-02-8]): Highly corrosive; severe burns to eyes or skin may result. Vapors extremely irritating to eyes, skin, and respiratory tract; pulmonary edema has been reported. Permanent pulmonary function changes may result.	0.1 ppm	5 ppm ERPG-1:0.1 ppm ERPG-2: 0.5 ppm ERPG-3: 3 ppm	3	3	2		Colorless to yellow liquid. An unpleasant odor. Eye irritation occurs at low levels and provides a good warning property. Formed in the pyrolysis of many substances. Vapor pressure is 214 mm Hg at 20 °C (68 °F). Highly flammable.

(C) = ceiling air concentration (TLV-C); S = skin absorption can be significant; A1 = ACGIH-confirmed human carcinogen; A2 = ACGIH-suspected human carcinogen; NFPA Hazard Codes: H = health, F = fire, R = reactivity, Ox = oxidizer, W = water-reactive, 0 (none) <—> 4 (severe). ERPG = Emergency Response Planning Guideline. See p 402 for explanation of definitions.

continued

TABLE IV–13. HEALTH HAZARD SUMMARIES FOR INDUSTRIAL AND OCCUPATIONAL CHEMICALS (Continued)

Health Hazard Summaries	ACGIH TLV	IDLH	NFPA Codes H		Comments
Acrylamide (propenamide, acrylic amide [CAS: 79-06-1]): Concentrated solutions are slightly irritating. Well absorbed by all routes. A potent neurotoxin causing peripheral neuropathy. Contact dermatitis also reported. Testicular toxicity in test animals. A carcinogen in test animals (IARC 2B).	0.03 mg/m³ S, A2				Colorless solid. Vapor pressure is 0.007 mm Hg at 20 °C (68 °F). Not flammable. Decomposes around 80 °C (176 °F). Breakdown products include oxides of nitrogen. Monomer used in the synthesis of polyacrylamide plastics.
Acrylic acid (propenoic acid [CAS: 79-10-7]): Corrosive; severe burns may result. Vapors highly irritating to eyes, skin, and respiratory tract. Limited evidence of adverse effects on fetal development at high doses in test animals. Based on structural analogies, compounds containing the acrylate moiety may be carcinogens.	2 ppm, S	ERPG-1: 2 ppm ERPG-2: 50 ppm ERPG-3: 750 ppm	3	2	Colorless liquid with characteristic acrid odor. Vapor pressure is 31 mm Hg at 25 °C (77 °F). Flammable. Inhibitor added to prevent explosive self-polymerization.
Acrylonitrile (cyanoethylene, vinyl cyanide, propenenitrile [CAS: 107-13-1]): Direct contact can be strongly irritating to eyes and skin. Well absorbed by all routes. A CNS depressant at high levels. Metabolized to cyanide (see p 145). Moderate acute overexposure will produce headache, weakness, nausea, and vomiting. Evidence of adverse effects on fetal development at high doses in animals. A carcinogen in test animals with limited epidemiologic evidence for carcinogenicity in humans (IARC 2A).	2 ppm, S, A2 OSHA CA NIOSH CA	500 ppm	4	2	Colorless liquid with a mild odor. Vapor pressure is 83 mm Hg at 20 °C (68 °F). Flammable. Polymerizes rapidly. Thermal decomposition products include hydrogen cyanide and oxides of nitrogen. Used in the manufacture of ABS and SAN resins.
Aldicarb (CAS: 116-06-3): A potent, carbamate-type cholinesterase inhibitor (see p 118). Well absorbed dermally.					Absorption by fruits has caused human poisonings.
Aldrin (CAS: 309-00-2): Chlorinated insecticide (see p 129). Minor skin irritant. Convulsant. Hepatotoxin. Well absorbed dermally. Limited evidence for carcinogenicity in test animals (IARC 3).	0.25 mg/m³, S NIOSH CA	100 mg/m³	3 1 0 (solutions) 2 0 0 (dry)		Tan to dark brown solid. A mild chemical odor. Vapor pressure is 0.000006 mm Hg at 20 °C (68 °F). Not flammable but breaks down, yielding hydrogen chloride gas. Most uses have been banned in US.

Allyl alcohol (2-propen-1-ol [CAS: 107-18-6]): Strongly irritating to eyes and skin; severe burns may result. Vapors highly irritating to eyes and respiratory tract. Systemic poisoning can result from dermal exposures. May cause liver and kidney injury.

2 ppm, S — 150 ppm — — — Colorless liquid. Mustardlike odor and irritation occur near the TLV and serve as good warning properties. Vapor pressure is 17 mm Hg at 20 °C (68 °F). Flammable. Used in chemical synthesis and as a pesticide.

Allyl chloride (3-chloro-1-propene [CAS: 107-05-1]): Highly irritating to eyes and skin. Vapors highly irritating to eyes and respiratory tract. Well absorbed by the skin, producing both superficial and penetrating irritation and pain. Causes liver and kidney injury in test animals. Chronic exposures have been associated with reports of mild neuropathy.

1 ppm — 300 ppm ERPG-1: 3 ppm ERPG-2: 40 ppm ERPG-3: 300 ppm — 3 3 1 Colorless, yellow, or purple liquid. Pungent, disagreeable odor and irritation occur only at levels far above the TLV, so exposure is accompanied by poor warning. Vapor pressure is 295 mm Hg at 20 °C (68 °F). Highly flammable. Breakdown products include hydrogen chloride and phosgene.

Allyl glycidyl ether (AGE [CAS: 106-92-3]): Highly irritating to eyes and skin; severe burns may result. Vapors irritating to eyes and respiratory tract. Sensitization dermatitis has been reported. Hematopoietic and testicular toxicity occurs in test animals at modest doses. Well absorbed through the skin.

5 ppm — 270 ppm — — — — Colorless liquid. Unpleasant odor. Vapor pressure is 2 mm Hg at 20 °C (68 °F). Flammable.

Allyl propyl disulfide (onion oil [CAS: 2179-59-1]): Mucous membrane irritant and lacrimator.

2 ppm — — — — — — Liquid with a pungent, irritating odor. A synthetic flavorant and food additive. Thermal breakdown products include sulfur oxide fumes.

α-Alumina (aluminum oxide [CAS: 1344-28-1]): Nuisance dust and physical irritant.

10 mg/m³

(C) = ceiling air concentration (TLV-C); S = skin absorption can be significant; A1 = ACGIH-confirmed human carcinogen; A2 = ACGIH-suspected human carcinogen; NFPA Hazard Codes: H = health, F = fire, R = reactivity, Ox = oxidizer, W = water-reactive, 0 (none) <—> 4 (severe). ERPG = Emergency Response Planning Guideline. See p 402 for explanation of definitions.

continued

TABLE IV–13. HEALTH HAZARD SUMMARIES FOR INDUSTRIAL AND OCCUPATIONAL CHEMICALS (Continued)

Health Hazard Summaries	ACGIH TLV	IDLH	NFPA Codes H F R	Comments
Aluminum metal (CAS: 7429-90-5): Dusts can cause mild eye and respiratory tract irritation. Long-term inhalation of large amounts of fine aluminum powders or fumes from aluminum ore (bauxite) has been associated with reports of pulmonary fibrosis (Shaver's disease). Acute exposures in aluminum refining ("pot room") has been associated with asthmalike responses. Industrial processes used to produce aluminum have been associated with an increased incidence of cancer in workers.	10 mg/m³ (metal and oxide) 5 mg/m³ (pyrophoric powders, welding fumes) 2 mg/m³ (soluble salts, alkyls NOC)		0 1 1	Oxidizes readily. Fine powders and flakes are flammable and explosive when mixed with air. Reacts with acids and caustic solutions to produce flammable hydrogen gas.
Aluminum phosphide (CAS: 20859-73-8): Effects caused by phosphine gas that is produced on contact with moisture. Severe respiratory tract irritant.				
4-Aminodiphenyl (p-aminobiphenyl, p-phenylaniline [CAS: 92-67-1]): Potent bladder carcinogen in humans (IARC 1). Causes methemoglobinemia (see p 217).	S, A1 OSHA CA NIOSH CA			Colorless crystals.
2-Aminopyridine (CAS: 504-29-0): Mild irritant. Potent CNS convulsant. Very well absorbed by inhalation and skin contact. Signs and symptoms include headache, dizziness, nausea, elevated blood pressure, and convulsions.	0.5 ppm	5 ppm		Colorless solid with a distinctive odor and a very low vapor pressure at 20 °C (68 °F). Combustible.
Amitrole (3-amino-1,2,4-triazole [CAS: 61-82-5]): Mild irritant. Well absorbed by inhalation and skin contact. Shows antithyroid activity in test animals. Evidence of adverse effects on fetal development in test animals at high doses. A carcinogen in test animals (IARC 2B).	0.2 mg/m³			Crystalline solid. Appearance and some hazardous properties vary with the formulation.

Toxicity	TLV		NFPA (H F R)	Comments
Ammonia (CAS: 7664-41-7): Corrosive; severe burns to eyes and skin result. Vapors highly irritating to eyes and respiratory tract; pulmonary edema has been reported. Severe responses are associated with anhydrous ammonia or with concentrated ammonia solutions (see p 64).	25 ppm	500 ppm ERPG-1: 26 ppm ERPG-2: 200 ppm ERPG-3: 1000 ppm	3 1 0 (liquid) 2 1 0 (gas)	Colorless gas or aqueous solution. Pungent odor and irritation are good warning properties. Flammable. Breakdown products include oxides of nitrogen. Although widely used in industry, concentrated forms are most frequently encountered in agriculture and from its use as a refrigerant.
n-Amyl acetate (CAS: 628-63-7): Defats the skin, producing a dermatitis. Vapors mildly irritating to eyes and respiratory tract. A CNS depressant at very high levels. Reversible liver and kidney injury may occur at very high exposures.	100 ppm	4000 ppm	1 3 0	Colorless liquid. Its bananalike odor detectable below the TLV is a good warning property. Vapor pressure is 4 mm Hg at 20 °C (68 °F). Flammable.
sec-Amyl acetate (α-methylbutyl acetate [CAS: 628-38-0]): Defats the skin, producing a dermatitis. Vapors irritating to eyes and respiratory tract. A CNS depressant at very high levels. Reversible liver and kidney injury may occur at high-level exposures.	125 ppm	9000 ppm	1 3 0	Colorless liquid. A fruity odor occurs below the TLV and is a good warning property. Vapor pressure is 7 mm Hg at 20 °C (68 °F). Flammable.
Aniline (aminobenzene, phenylamine [CAS: 62-53-3]): Mildly irritating to eyes upon direct contact, with corneal injury possible. Potent inducer of methemoglobinemia (see p 217). Well absorbed via inhalation and dermal routes. Limited evidence of carcinogenicity in test animals (IARC 3).	2 ppm, S	100 ppm	3 2 0	Colorless to brown viscous liquid. Distinctive amine odor and mild eye irritation occur well below the TLV and are good warning properties. Vapor pressure is 0.6 mm Hg at 20 °C (68 °F). Combustible. Breakdown products include oxides of nitrogen.
o-Anisidine (o-methoxyaniline [CAS: 29191-52-4]): Mild skin sensitzer causing dermatitis. Causes methemoglobinemia (see p 217). Well absorbed through skin. Headaches and vertigo are signs of exposure. Possible liver and kidney injury. A carcinogen in test animals (IARC 2B).	0.1 ppm, S	50 mg/m³	2 1 0	Colorless, red, or yellow liquid with the fishy odor of amines. Vapor pressure is less than 0.1 mm Hg at 20 °C (68 °F). Combustible. Primarily used in the dyestuffs industry.

(C)₁ = ceiling air concentration (TLV-C); S = skin absorption can be significant; A1 = ACGIH-confirmed human carcinogen; A2 = ACGIH-suspected human carcinogen; NFPA Hazard Codes: H = health, F = fire, R = reactivity, Ox = oxidizer, W = water-reactive, 0 (none) <——> 4 (severe). ERPG = Emergency Response Planning Guideline. See p 402 for explanation of definitions.

continued

TABLE IV–13. HEALTH HAZARD SUMMARIES FOR INDUSTRIAL AND OCCUPATIONAL CHEMICALS (Continued)

Health Hazard Summaries	ACGIH TLV	IDLH	NFPA Codes H F R	Comments
Antimony and salts (antimony trichloride, antimony trioxide, antimony pentachloride [CAS: 7440-36-0]): Dusts and fumes irritating to eyes, skin, and respiratory tract. Toxicity through contamination with silica or arsenic may occur. Antimony trioxide is carcinogenic in test animals with limited evidence for carcinogenicity among antimony trioxide production in workers (IARC 2B). See also p 80.	0.5 mg/m³ (as Sb)	80 mg/m³		The metal is silver-white and has a very low vapor pressure. Some chloride salts release HCl upon contact with air.
ANTU (α-naphthylthiourea [CAS: 86-88-4]): Well absorbed by skin contact and inhalation. Pulmonary edema and liver injury may result from ingestion. Repeated exposures can injure the thyroid and adrenals, producing hypothyroidism. Possible slight contamination with a 2-naphthylamine, a human bladder carcinogen.	0.3 mg/m³	100 mg/m³		Colorless to gray solid powder. Odorless. A rodenticide. Breakdown products include oxides of nitrogen and sulfur dioxide.
Arsenic (CAS: 7440-38-2) Irritating to eyes and skin; hyperpigmentation, hyperkeratoses, and skin cancers have been described. A general cellular poison. May cause bone marrow suppression, peripheral neuropathy, and gastrointestinal, liver, and cardiac injury. Some arsenic compounds have adverse effects on fetal development in test animals. Exposure linked to skin, respiratory tract, and liver cancer in workers (IARC 1). See also p 87.	0.2 mg/m³ (as As) [proposed: 0.1 mg/m³ (as As) A1] OSHA CA NIOSH CA			Elemental forms vary in appearance. Crystals are gray. Amorphous forms may be yellow or black. Vapor pressure is very low—about 1 mm Hg at 372 °C (701 °F).
Arsine (CAS: 7784-42-1): Extremely toxic hemolytic agent. Symptoms include abdominal pain, jaundice, hemoglobinuria, and renal failure. Low-level chronic exposures reported to cause anemia. See also p 89.	0.05 ppm NIOSH CA	6 ppm		Colorless gas with an unpleasant garliclike odor. Flammable. Breakdown products include arsenic trioxide and arsenic fumes. Used in the semiconductor industry.
Asbestos (chrysotile, amosite, crocidolite, tremolite, anthophyllite): Effects of exposure include asbestosis (fibrosis of the lung). lung cancer, mesothelioma, and possible digestive tract cancer (IARC 1). Signs of toxicity are usually delayed at least 15–30 years. See also p 90.	[proposed: 0.2 fibers/cm³, A1] OSHA CA NIOSH CA			Fibrous materials. Not combustible. TLVs vary with type: amosite, 0.5 fibers/cm³, A1; chrysotile, 2 fibers/cm³, A1; crocidolite, 0.2 fibers/cm³, A1; other forms, 2 fibers/cm³, A1.

continued

Substance	ACGIH TLV	ERPG	NFPA Codes (H F R)	Comments
Asphalt fumes (CAS: 8052-42-4): Vapors and fumes irritating to eyes, skin, and respiratory tract. Skin contact can produce hyperpigmentation, dermatitis, or photosensitization. Some constituents are carcinogenic in test animals.	5 mg/m³			Smoke with an acrid odor. Asphalt is a complex mixture of parrafinic, aromatic, and heterocyclic hydrocarbons formed by the evaporation of lighter hydrocarbons from petroleum and the partial oxidation of the residue.
Atrazine (CAS: 1912-24-9): A triazine herbicide. Minor skin and eye irritant.	5 mg/m³			
Azinphos-methyl (Guthion [CAS: 86-50-0]): Low-potency organophosphate anticholinesterase insecticide (see p 240). Requires metabolic activation.	0.2 mg/m³, S			Brown waxy solid with a negligible vapor pressure. Not combustible. Breakdown products include sulfur dioxide, oxides of nitrogen, and phosphoric acid.
Barium and soluble compounds (CAS: 7440-39-3): Powders irritating to eyes, skin, and respiratory tract. Although not typical of workplace exposures, ingestion of soluble barium salts (as opposed to the insoluble medical compounds used in radiography) are associated with muscle paralysis. See also p 95.	0.5 mg/m³ (as Ba)			Most soluble barium compounds (eg. barium chloride, barium carbonate) are odorless white solids. Elemental barium spontaneously ignites on contact with air and reacts with water to form flammable hydrogen gas.
Benomyl (methyl 1-(butylcarbamoyl)-2-benzimidazolecarbamate, Benlate [CAS: 17804-35-2]): A carbamate cholinesterase inhibitor (see p 118). Mildly irritating to eyes and skin. Of low systemic toxicity in test animals by all routes. Evidence of adverse effects on fetal development in test animals.		0.8 ppm		
Benzene (CAS: 71-43-2): Vapors mildly irritating to eyes and respiratory tract. Well absorbed by all routes. A CNS depressant at high levels. Symptoms include headache, nausea, tremors, cardiac arrhythmias, and coma. Chronic exposure may result in hematopoietic system depression, aplastic anemia, and leukemia (IARC 1). See also p 96.	10 ppm, A2, S [proposed: 0.1 ppm, A1, S] OSHA CA NIOSH CA	3000 ppm	2 3 0	Colorless liquid. Aromatic hydrocarbon odor. Vapor pressure is 75 mm Hg at 20 °C (68 °F). Flammable.
Benzidine (p-diaminodiphenyl [CAS: 92-87-5]): Extremely well absorbed by inhalation and through skin. Caused bladder cancer in exposed workers (IARC 1).	S, A1 OSHA CA NIOSH CA			White or reddish solid crystals. Breakdown products include oxides of nitrogen. Found in dye-stuffs, rubber industry, and analytical laboratories.

(C) = ceiling air concentration (TLV-C); S = skin absorption can be significant; A1 = ACGIH-confirmed human carcinogen; A2 = ACGIH-suspected human carcinogen; NFPA Hazard Codes: H = health, F = fire, R = reactivity, Ox = oxidizer, W = water-reactive. 0 (none) <—> 4 (severe). ERPG = Emergency Response Planning Guideline. See p 402 for explanation of definitions.

TABLE IV–13. HEALTH HAZARD SUMMARIES FOR INDUSTRIAL AND OCCUPATIONAL CHEMICALS (Continued)

Health Hazard Summaries	ACGIH TLV	IDLH	NFPA Codes H F R	Comments
Benzoyl peroxide (CAS: 94-36-0): Dusts cause skin, eye, and respiratory tract irritation. A skin sensitizer.	5 mg/m³	7000 mg/m³	1 4 4 Ox	White granules or crystalline solids with a very faint odor. Vapor pressure is negligible at 20 °C (68 °F). Strong oxidizer, reacting with combustible materials. Decomposes at 75 °C (167 °F). Unstable and explosive at high temperatures.
Benzyl chloride (α-chlorotoluene, [chloro-methyl]benzene [CAS: 100-44-7]): Highly irritating to skin and eyes. A potent lacrimator. Vapors highly irritating to respiratory tract. Symptoms include weakness, headache, and irritability. May injure liver. Limited evidence for carcinogenicity and adverse effects on fetal development in test animals.	1 ppm	10 ppm	2 2 1	Colorless liquid with a pungent odor. Vapor pressure is 0.9 mm Hg at 20 °C (68 °F). Combustible. Breakdown products include phosgene and hydrogen chloride.
Beryllium (CAS: 7440-41-7): Very high acute exposure to dusts and fumes cause eye, skin, and respiratory tract irritation. However, more importantly, chronic low-level exposures to beryllium oxide dusts can produce interstitial lung disease called berylliosis, which is a sarcoid-like condition that can have extrapulmonary manifestations. A carcinogen in test animals. There is limited evidence of carcinogenicity in humans (IARC 2B).	0.002 mg/m³, A2 NIOSH CA		4 1 0	Silver-white metal or dusts. Reacts with some acids to produce flammable hydrogen gas.
Biphenyl (diphenyl [CAS: 92-52-4]): Fumes mildly irritating to eyes. Chronic overexposures can cause bronchitis and liver injury. Peripheral neuropathy and CNS injury have also been reported.	0.2 ppm	300 mg/m³	2 1 0	White crystals. Unusual but pleasant odor. Combustible.
Borates (anhydrous sodium tetraborate, borax [CAS: 1303-96-4]): Contact with dusts is highly irritating to eyes, skin, and respiratory tract. Contact with tissue moisture may cause thermal burns because hydration of borates generates heat. See also p 106.	1 mg/m³ (anhydrous and pentahydrate) 5 mg/m³ (decahydrate)			White or light gray solid crystals. Odorless.

Chemical	TLV	NFPA Codes	Comments
Boron oxide (boric anhydride, boric oxide [CAS: 1303-86-2]): Contact with moisture generates boric acid (see p 106). Direct eye or skin contact with dusts is irritating. Occupational inhalation exposure has caused sore throat and cough. Evidence for adverse effects on the testes in test animals.	10 mg/m³		Colorless glassy granules, flakes, or powder. Odorless. Not combustible.
Boron tribromide (CAS: 10294-33-4): Corrosive; decomposed by tissue moisture to hydrogen bromide (see p 110) and boric acid (see p 106). Severe skin and eye burns may result from direct contact. Vapors highly irritating to eyes and respiratory tract.	1 ppm (C)		Colorless fuming liquid. Reacts with water, forming hydrogen bromide and boric acid. Vapor pressure is 40 mm Hg at 14 °C (57 °F).
Boron trifluoride (CAS: 7637-07-2): Corrosive; decomposed by tissue moisture to hydrogen fluoride (see p 180) and boric acid (see p 106). Severe skin and eye burns may result. Vapors highly irritating to eyes, skin, and respiratory tract.	1 ppm (C)	3 0 1	Colorless gas. Dense white irritating fumes produced on contact with moist air. These fumes contain boric acid and hydrogen fluoride.
Brodifacoum (CAS: 56073-10-1): Long-acting anticoagulant causing hemmorhage. Blocks vitamin K 1-2,3 epoxide reductase to inhibit Vitamin K-dependent clotting factor synthesis. See also p 143.			
Bromine (CAS: 7726-95-6): Corrosive; severe skin and eye burns may result. Vapors highly irritating to eyes and respiratory tract; pulmonary edema may result. Measleslike eruptions may appear on the skin several hours after a severe exposure. See also p 163.	0.1 ppm ERPG-1: 0.2 ppm ERPG-2: 1 ppm ERPG-3: 5 ppm	4 0 0 Ox	Heavy red-brown fuming liquid. Odor and irritation thresholds are below the TLV and are adequate warning properties. Vapor pressure is 175 mm Hg at 20 °C (68 °F). Not combustible.
Bromine pentafluoride (CAS: 7789-30-2): Corrosive; severe skin and eye burns may result. Vapors extremely irritating to eyes and respiratory tract. Chronic overexposures caused severe liver and kidney injury in test animals. See also p 126.	0.1 ppm	4 0 3 W, Ox	Pale yellow liquid. Pungent odor. Not combustible. Highly reactive, igniting most organic materials and corroding many metals. Highly reactive with acids. Breakdown products include bromine and fluorine.

(C) = ceiling air concentration (TLV-C); S = skin absorption can be significant; A1 = ACGIH-confirmed human carcinogen; A2 = ACGIH-suspected human carcinogen; NFPA Hazard Codes: H = health, F = fire, R = reactivity, Ox = oxidizer, W = water-reactive, 0 (none) <—> 4 (severe). ERPG = Emergency Response Planning Guideline. See p 402 for explanation of definitions.

continued

TABLE IV–13. HEALTH HAZARD SUMMARIES FOR INDUSTRIAL AND OCCUPATIONAL CHEMICALS (Continued)

Health Hazard Summaries	ACGIH TLV	IDLH	NFPA Codes H			Comments
Bromoform (tribromomethane [CAS: 75-25-2]): Vapors highly irritating to eyes and respiratory tract. Well absorbed by inhalation and skin contact. CNS depressant. Liver and kidney injury may occur. Two preliminary tests indicate that it may be an animal carcinogen.	0.5 ppm, S					Colorless to yellow liquid. Chloroformlike odor and irritation are adequate warning properties. Vapor pressure is 5 mm Hg at 20 °C (68 °F). Not combustible. Thermal breakdown products include hydrogen bromide and bromine.
1,3-Butadiene [CAS: 106-99-0]: Vapors mildly irritating. A CNS depressant at very high levels. Evidence of adverse effects on reproductive organs and fetal development in test animals. A very potent carcinogen in test animals; limited evidence of carcinogenicity in exposed workers (IARC 2B).	10 ppm, A2 NIOSH CA	20,000 ppm ERPG-1: 10 ppm ERPG-2: 50 ppm ERPG-3: 5000 ppm	2	4	2	Colorless gas. Mild aromatic odor is a good warning property. Readily polymerizes. Inhibitor added to prevent peroxide formation. Used in the formation of styrene-butadiene and ABS plastics.
2-Butoxyethanol (ethylene glycol monobutyl ether, butyl Cellosolve [CAS: 111-76-2]): Liquid very irritating to eyes and slightly irritating to skin. Vapors irritating to eyes and respiratory tract. A hemolytic agent in test animals. Mild CNS depressant. Liver and kidney toxicity in test animals. Well absorbed dermally. Reproductive toxicity much less than certain other glycol ethers such as ethylene glycol monomethyl ether. See also p 163.	25 ppm, S	700 ppm				Colorless liquid with a mild etherlike odor. Irritation occurs below the TLV and is a good warning property. Vapor pressure is 0.6 mm Hg at 20 °C (68 °F). Flammable.
n-Butyl acetate (CAS: 123-86-4]): Vapors irritating to eyes and respiratory tract. A CNS depressant at high levels. Limited evidence for adverse effects on fetal development in test animals.	150 ppm [proposed: 20 ppm]	10,000 ppm	1	3	0	Colorless liquid. Fruity odor is a good warning property. Vapor pressure is 10 mm Hg at 20 °C (68 °F). Flammable.
sec-Butyl acetate (2-butanol acetate [CAS: 105-46-4]): Vapors irritating to eyes and respiratory tract. A CNS depressant at high levels.	200 ppm	10,000 ppm	1	3	0	
tert-Butyl acetate (tert-butyl ester of acetic acid [CAS: 540-88-5]): Vapors irritating to eyes and respiratory tract. A CNS depressant at high levels.	200 ppm	10,000 ppm				

n-Butyl acrylate (CAS: 141-32-2): Highly irritating to skin and eyes; corneal necrosis may result. Vapors highly irritating to eyes and respiratory tract. Based on structural analogies, compounds containing the acrylate moiety may be carcinogens (IARC 3).

10 ppm		2 2 2	Colorless liquid. Vapor pressure is 3.2 mm Hg at 20 °C (68 °F). Flammable. Contains inhibitor to prevent polymerization.

n-Butyl alcohol (CAS: 71-36-3): Irritating upon direct contact. Vapors mildly irritating to eyes and respiratory tract. A CNS depressant at very high levels. Chronic occupational overexposures associated with hearing loss and vestibular impairment.

50 ppm (C), S	8000 ppm	1 3 0	Colorless liquid. Strong odor and irritation occur below the TLV and are both good warning properties. Flammable.

sec-Butyl alcohol (CAS: 78-92-2): Vapors mildly irritating to eyes and respiratory tract. A CNS depressant at high levels.

100 ppm	10,000 ppm	1 3 0	Colorless liquid. Pleasant odor occurs well below the TLV and is an adequate warning property. Vapor pressure is 13 mm Hg at 20 °C (68 °F). Flammable.

tert-Butyl alcohol (CAS: 75-65-0): Vapors mildly irritating to eyes and respiratory tract. A CNS depressant at high levels.

100 ppm	8000 ppm	1 3 0	Colorless liquid. Camphorlike odor and irritation occur slightly below the TLV and are good warning properties. Vapor pressure is 31 mm Hg at 20 °C (68 °F). Flammable.

Butylamine (CAS: 109-73-9): Caustic alkali. Liquid highly irritating to eyes and skin upon direct contact; severe burns may result. Vapors highly irritating to eyes and respiratory tract. May cause histamine release.

5 ppm (C), S	2000 ppm	2 3 0	Colorless liquid. Ammonia or fishlike odor occurs below the TLV and is an adequate warning property. Vapor pressure is about 82 mm Hg at 20 °C (68 °F). Flammable.

tert-Butyl chromate (CAS: 1189-85-1): Liquid highly irritating to eyes and skin; severe burns may result. Vapors or mists irritating to eyes and respiratory tract. A liver and kidney toxin. By analogy to other Cr(VI) compounds, a possible carcinogen. See also p 135.

0.1 mg/m³ (C), S (as CrO₃) NIOSH CA	30 mg/m³		Liquid. Reacts with moisture.

(C) = ceiling air concentration (TLV-C); S = skin absorption can be significant; A1 = ACGIH-confirmed human carcinogen; A2 = ACGIH-suspected human carcinogen; NFPA Hazard Codes: H = health, F = fire, R = reactivity, Ox = oxidizer, W = water-reactive, 0 (none) <—> 4 (severe). ERPG = Emergency Response Planning Guideline. See p 402 for explanation of definitions.

continued

TABLE IV–13. HEALTH HAZARD SUMMARIES FOR INDUSTRIAL AND OCCUPATIONAL CHEMICALS (Continued)

Health Hazard Summaries	ACGIH TLV	IDLH	NFPA Codes H			Comments
n-Butyl glycidyl ether (BGE, glycidylbutylether, 1,2-epoxy-3-butoxy propane [CAS: 2426-08-6]): Liquid irritating to eyes and skin. Vapors irritating to the respiratory tract. A CNS depressant. Causes sensitization dermatitis upon repeated exposures. Testicular atrophy and hematopoietic injury at modest doses in test animals.	25 ppm	3500 ppm				Colorless liquid. Vapor pressure is 3 mm Hg at 20 °C (68 °F).
n-Butyl lactate (CAS: 138-22-7): Vapors irritating to eyes and respiratory tract. Workers have complained of sleepiness, headache, coughing, nausea, and vomiting.	5 ppm		1	2	0	Colorless liquid. Vapor pressure is 0.4 mm Hg at 20 °C (68 °F). Combustible.
n-Butyl mercaptan (butanethiol [CAS: 109-79-5]): Vapors mildly irritating to eyes and respiratory tract. Pulmonary edema occurred at high exposure levels in test animals. A CNS depressant at very high levels. Limited evidence for adverse effects on fetal development in test animals at high doses.	0.5 ppm	2500 ppm	2	3	0	Colorless liquid. Strong, offensive garliclike odor. Vapor pressure is 35 mm Hg at 20 °C (68 °F). Flammable.
o-sec-Butylphenol (CAS: 89-72-5): Irritating to skin upon direct, prolonged contact; burns have resulted. Vapors mildly irritating to eyes and respiratory tract.	5 ppm, S					A liquid.
p-tert-Butyltoluene (CAS: 98-51-1): Mild skin irritant upon direct contact. Defatting agent causing dermatitis. Vapors irritating to eyes and respiratory tract. A CNS depressant. Limited evidence of adverse effects on fetal development in test animals at high doses.	10 ppm [proposed: 1 ppm]	1000 ppm				Colorless liquid. Gasolinelike odor and irritation occur below the TLV and are both good warning properties. Vapor pressure is less than 1 mm Hg at 20 °C (68 °F). Combustible.

Substance / Toxicology	TLV / Air concentration	Other	NFPA (H F R)	Comments
Cadmium and compounds: Acute fumes and dust exposures can injure the respiratory tract; pulmonary edema can occur. Chronic exposures associated primarily with kidney injury and lung injury. Adverse effects on the testes and on fetal development in test animals. Cadmium and some of its compounds are carcinogenic in test animals. Limited direct evidence for carcinogenicity in humans (IARC 2A). See also p 111.	0.05 mg/m³ (as Cd), A2 [proposed: 0.01 mg/m³ (total dust), 0.002 mg/m³ (respirable dust), A2] NIOSH CA	50 mg/m³ (dust); 9 mg/m³ (fume)		Compounds vary in color. Give off fumes when heated or burned. Generally poor warning properties. Metal has a vapor pressure of about 1 mm Hg at 394 °C (741 °F) and reacts with acids to produce flammable hydrogen gas.
Calcium cyanamide (calcium carbimide, lime nitrogen [CAS: 156-62-7]): Dusts highly irritating to eyes, skin, and respiratory tract. Causes sensitization dermatitis. Systemic symptoms include nausea, fatigue, headache, chest pain, and shivering. A disulfiramlike interaction with alcohol (see p 155), "cyanamide flush," may occur in exposed workers.	0.5 mg/m³			Gray crystalline material. Reacts with water, generating ammonia and flammable acetylene.
Calcium hydroxide (hydrated lime, caustic lime [CAS: 1305-62-0]): Corrosive (see p 126); severe eye and skin burns may result. Dusts moderately irritating to eyes and respiratory tract.	5 mg/m³			White, deliquescent crystalline powder. Odorless.
Calcium oxide (lime, quicklime, burnt lime [CAS: 1305-78-8]): Corrosive (see p 126). Exothermic reactions with moisture. Highly irritating to eyes and skin upon direct contact. Dusts highly irritating to skin, eyes, and respiratory tract.	2 mg/m³	250 mg/m³	1 0 1	White or gray solid powder. Odorless. Hydration generates heat.
Camphor, synthetic (CAS: 76-22-2): Irritating to eyes and skin upon direct contact. Vapors irritating to eyes and nose; may cause loss of sense of smell. A convulsant at doses typical of overdose ingestion, rather than industrial exposure. See also p 115.	2 ppm	200 mg/m³	0 2 0	Colorless glassy solid. Sharp, obnoxious, aromatic odor near the TLV is an adequate warning property. Vapor pressure is 0.18 mm Hg at 20 °C (68 °F). Combustible.
Caprolactam (CAS: 105-60-2): Highly irritating to eyes and skin upon direct contact. Vapors, dusts, and fumes highly irritating to eyes and respiratory tract. Convulsant activity in test animals.	1 mg/m³ (dust); 5 ppm (vapor)			White solid crystals. Unpleasant odor. Vapor pressure is 6 mm Hg at 120 °C (248 °F). Thermal breakdown products include oxides of nitrogen.

(C) = ceiling air concentration (TLV-C); S = skin absorption can be significant; A1 = ACGIH-confirmed human carcinogen; A2 = ACGIH-suspected human carcinogen; NFPA Hazard Codes: H = health, F = fire, R = reactivity, Ox = oxidizer, W = water-reactive, 0 (none) <—> 4 (severe). ERPG = Emergency Response Planning Guideline. See p 402 for explanation of definitions.

continued

TABLE IV–13. HEALTH HAZARD SUMMARIES FOR INDUSTRIAL AND OCCUPATIONAL CHEMICALS (Continued)

Health Hazard Summaries	ACGIH TLV	IDLH	NFPA Codes H	Comments
Captafol (Difolatan [CAS: 2425-06-1]): Dusts irritating to eyes, skin, and respiratory tract. A skin and respiratory tract sensitizer. May cause photoallergic dermatitis. Evidence for carcinogenicity in animal tests (IARC 2A).	0.1 mg/m³, S			White solid crystals. Distinctive, pungent odor. Fungicide. Thermal breakdown products include hydrogen chloride and oxides of nitrogen or sulfur.
Carbaryl (1-naphthyl N-methylcarbamate, Sevin [CAS: 63-25-2]): A carbamate-type cholinesterase inhibitor (see p 118). Evidence of adverse effects on fetal development in test animals at high doses.	5 mg/m³	600 mg/m³		Colorless, white, or gray solid. Odorless. Vapor pressure is 0.005 mm Hg at 20 °C (68 °F). Breakdown products include oxides of nitrogen and methylamine.
Carbofuran (2,3-dihydro-2,2'-dimethyl-7-benzofuranylmethylcarbamate, Furadan [CAS: 1563-66-2]): A carbamate-type cholinesterase inhibitor (see p 118). Not well absorbed by skin contact.	0.1 mg/m³			White solid crystals. Odorless. Vapor pressure is 0.00005 mm Hg at 33 °C (91 °F). Thermal breakdown products include oxides of nitrogen.
Carbon disulfide (CAS: 75-15-0): Vapors mildly irritating to eyes and respiratory tract. A CNS depressant causing coma at high concentrations. Well absorbed by all routes. Acute symptoms include headache, dizziness, nervousness, and fatigue. Neuropathies, parkinsonianlike syndromes, and psychosis may occur. A liver and kidney toxin. An atherogenic agent causing stroke and heart disease. Adversely affects male and female reproductive systems in test animals and humans. Evidence for adverse effects on fetal development in test animals.	10 ppm, S	500 ppm ERPG-1: 1 ppm ERPG-2: 50 ppm ERPG-3: 500 ppm	2 3 0	Colorless to pale yellow liquid. Disagreeable odor occurs below the TLV and is a good warning property. Vapor pressure is 300 mm Hg at 20 °C (68 °F). Highly flammable. Major use in viscose rayon manufacture but is also used in chemical synthesis and as an industrial solvent.
Carbon monoxide (CAS: 630-08-0): Binds to hemoglobin, forming carboxyhemoglobin and causing cellular hypoxia. Persons with heart disease are more susceptible. Signs and symptoms include headache, dizziness, coma, and convulsions. Permanent CNS impairment and adverse effects on fetal development may occur after severe poisoning. See also p 121.	25 ppm	1500 ppm	2 4 0	Colorless, odorless gas. No warning properties. Important sources of exposure include indoor use of internal combustion engines, structural fires, and faulty space heaters.

Carbon tetrabromide (tetrabromomethane [CAS: 558-13-4]): Highly irritating to eyes upon direct contact. Vapors highly irritating to eyes and respiratory tract. The liver and kidneys are also likely target organs.

0.1 ppm

White to yellow-brown solid. Vapor pressure is 40 mm Hg at 96 °C (204 °F). Nonflammable; thermal breakdown products may include hydrogen bromide and bromine.

Carbon tetrachloride (tetrachloromethane [CAS: 56-23-5]): Mildly irritating upon direct contact. A CNS depressant. May cause cardiac arrhythmias. Highly toxic to kidney and liver. Alcohol abuse increases risk of liver toxicity. A carcinogen in test animals (IARC 2B). See also p 123.

5 ppm, S, A2 [proposed: 5 ppm, S, A3] NIOSH CA

300 ppm 3 0 0

Colorless. Etherlike odor is a poor warning property. Vapor pressure is 91 mm Hg at 20 °C (68 °F). Not combustible. Breakdown products include hydrogen chloride, chlorine gas, and phosgene.

Carbonyl fluoride (COF$_2$ [CAS: 353-50-4]): Extremely irritating to eyes and respiratory tract; pulmonary edema may result. Toxicity results from its hydrolysis to hydrofluoric acid (see p 180).

2 ppm

Colorless, odorless gas. Decomposes upon contact with water to produce hydrofluoric acid.

Catechol (1,2-benzenediol [CAS: 120-80-9]): Highly irritating upon direct contact; severe eye and deep skin burns result. Well absorbed by skin. Systemic toxicity similar to that of phenol (see p 249); however, catechol may be more likely to cause convulsions and hypertension. At high doses, renal and liver injury may occur.

5 ppm, S

Colorless solid crystals.

Cesium hydroxide (cesium hydrate [CAS: 21351-79-1]): Corrosive (see p 126). Highly irritating upon direct contact; severe burns may result. Dusts are irritating to eyes and respiratory tract.

2 mg/m^3

Colorless or yellow crystals that absorb moisture. Negligible vapor pressure.

Chlordane [CAS: 57-74-9]: Irritating to skin. A CNS convulsant. Skin absorption is rapid and has caused convulsions and death. Hepatotoxic. Evidence of carcinogenicity in test animals (IARC 2B). See also p 129.

0.5 mg/m^3, S

500 mg/m^3

Viscous amber liquid. Formulations vary in appearance. A chlorinelike odor. Vapor pressure is 0.00001 mm Hg at 20 °C (68 °F). Not combustible. Thermal breakdown products include hydrogen chloride, phosgene, and chlorine gas. EPA banned this insecticide in 1976.

(C) = ceiling air concentration (TLV-C); S = skin absorption can be significant; A1 = ACGIH-confirmed human carcinogen; A2 = ACGIH-suspected human carcinogen; NFPA Hazard Codes: H = health, F = fire, R = reactivity, Ox = oxidizer, W = water-reactive, 0 (none) <—> 4 (severe). ERPG = Emergency Response Planning Guideline. See p 402 for explanation of definitions.

continued

TABLE IV–13. HEALTH HAZARD SUMMARIES FOR INDUSTRIAL AND OCCUPATIONAL CHEMICALS (Continued)

Health Hazard Summaries	ACGIH TLV	IDLH	NFPA Codes H F R	Comments
Chlorinated camphene (toxaphene [CAS: 8001-35-2]): Moderately irritating upon direct contact. A CNS convulsant. Acute symptoms include nausea, confusion, tremors, and convulsions. Well absorbed by skin. Potential liver and kidney injury. See also p 129.	0.5 mg/m³, S	200 mg/m³		Waxy amber-colored solid. Formulations vary in appearance. Turpentinelike odor. Vapor pressure is about 0.3 mm Hg at 20 °C (68 °F).
Chlorinated diphenyl oxide (CAS: 55720-99-5): Chloracne may result from even small exposures. A hepatotoxin in chronically exposed test animals. Signs and symptoms include gastrointestinal upset, jaundice, and fatigue.	0.5 mg/m³	5 mg/m³		Waxy solid or liquid. Vapor pressure is 0.00006 mm Hg at 20 °C (68 °F).
Chlorine (CAS: 7782-50-5): Extremely irritating to eyes, skin, and respiratory tract; severe burns and pulmonary edema may occur. Symptoms include lacrimation, sore throat, headache, coughing, and wheezing. High concentrations may cause rapid tissue swelling and airway obstruction through laryngeal edema. See also p 130.	0.5 ppm	30 ppm ERPG-1: 1 ppm ERPG-2: 3 ppm ERPG-3: 20 ppm	3 0 0 Ox	Amber liquid or greenish-yellow gas. Irritating odor and irritation occur near the TLV and are both good warning properties. Can be formed when acid cleaners are mixed with hypochlorite bleach cleaners.
Chlorine dioxide (chlorine peroxide [CAS: 10049-04-4]): Extremely irritating to eyes and respiratory tract. Symptoms and signs are those of chlorine gas above (see p 130).	0.1 ppm	10 ppm	3 0 3 W	Yellow-green or orange gas or liquid. Sharp odor at the TLV is a good warning property. Reacts with water to produce perchloric acid. Decomposes explosively in sunlight, with heat, or with shock to produce chlorine gas. Bleaching agent widely used in paper industry.
Chlorine trifluoride (chlorine fluoride [CAS: 7790-91-2]): Upon contact with moist tissues, hydrolyzes to chlorine (see p 180), hydrogen fluoride (see p 180), and chlorine dioxide. Extremely irritating to eyes, skin, and respiratory tract; severe burns or delayed pulmonary edema could result.	0.1 ppm (C)	20 ppm	4 0 3 W	Greenish-yellow or colorless liquid or gas, or white solid. Possesses a suffocating, sweet odor. Not combustible. Water-reactive, yielding hydrogen fluoride and chlorine gas. Used as incendiary and rocket fuel additive.

	TLV	ERPG	H	F	R	Comments
Chloroacetaldehyde (CAS: 107-20-0): Extremely corrosive upon direct contact; severe burns will result. Vapors extremely irritating to eyes, skin, and respiratory tract.	1 ppm (C)	250 ppm				Colorless liquid with a pungent, irritating odor. Vapor pressure is 100 mm Hg at 20 °C (68 °F). Combustible. Readily polymerizes. Thermal breakdown products include phosgene and hydrogen chloride.
α-Chloroacetophenone (tear gas, chemical Mace [CAS: 532-27-4]): Extremely irritating to mucous membranes and respiratory tract. With extremely high inhalational exposures, lower respiratory injury is possible. A potent skin sensitizer. See also p 176.	0.05 ppm	100 mg/m³	2	1	0	Sharp, irritating odor and irritation occur near the TLV and are adequate warning properties. Vapor pressure is 0.012 mm Hg at 20 °C (68 °F). Mace is a common crowd control agent.
Chlorobenzene (monochlorobenzene [CAS: 108-90-7]): Irritating; skin burns may result from prolonged contact. Vapors irritating to eyes and respiratory tract. A CNS depressant. May cause methemoglobinemia (see p 217). Prolonged exposure to high levels has caused lung, liver, and kidney injury in test animals.	10 ppm	2400 ppm	2	3	0	Colorless liquid. Aromatic odor occurs below the TLV and is a good warning property. Vapor pressure is 8.8 mm Hg at 20 °C (68 °F). Flammable. Thermal breakdown products include hydrogen chloride and phosgene.
o-Chlorobenzylidenemalononitrile (tear gas, OCBM, CS [CAS: 2698-41-1]): Highly irritating on direct contact; severe burns may result. Aerosols and vapors very irritating to mucous membranes and upper respiratory tract. With extremely high inhalational exposures, lower respiratory injury is possible. Potent skin sensitizer. Symptoms include headache, nausea and vomiting, severe eye and nose irritation, excess salivation, and coughing. See also p 176.	0.05 ppm (C), S	2 mg/m³				White solid crystals. Pepperlike odor. Vapor pressure is much less than 1 mm Hg at 20 °C (68 °F). CS is a common crowd control agent.
Chlorobromomethane (bromochloromethane, Halon 1011 [CAS: 74-97-5]): Irritating upon direct contact. Vapors mildly irritating to eyes and respiratory tract. A CNS depressant. Disorientation, nausea, headache, seizures, and coma have been reported at high exposure. Chronic high doses caused liver and kidney injury in test animals.	200 ppm	5000 ppm				Colorless to pale yellow liquid. Sweet, pleasant odor detectable far below the TLV. Vapor pressure is 117 mm Hg at 20 °C (68 °F). Thermal breakdown products include hydrogen chloride, hydrogen bromide, and phosgene.

(C) = ceiling air concentration (TLV-C); S = skin absorption can be significant; A1 = ACGIH-confirmed human carcinogen; A2 = ACGIH-suspected human carcinogen; NFPA Hazard Codes: H = health, F = fire, R = reactivity, Ox = oxidizer, W = water-reactive, 0 (none) <—> 4 (severe). ERPG = Emergency Response Planning Guideline. See p 402 for explanation of definitions.

continued

TABLE IV–13. HEALTH HAZARD SUMMARIES FOR INDUSTRIAL AND OCCUPATIONAL CHEMICALS (Continued)

Health Hazard Summaries	ACGIH TLV	IDLH	NFPA Codes H F R	Comments
Chlorodifluoromethane (Freon 22 [CAS: 75-45-6]): Irritating upon direct contact. Vapors mildly irritating to eyes and respiratory tract. A CNS depressant. High-level exposure may cause arrhythmias. There is evidence at high doses for adverse effects on fetal development in test animals. See also p 175.	1000 ppm			Colorless, almost odorless gas. Nonflammable. Thermal breakdown products may include hydrogen fluoride.
Chloroform (trichloromethane [CAS: 67-66-3]): Mildly irritating upon direct contact; dermatitis may result from prolonged exposure. Vapors slightly irritating to eyes and respiratory tract. A CNS depressant. High levels (15,000–20,000 ppm) can cause coma and cardiac arrhythmias. Can produce liver and kidney damage. Limited evidence of adverse effects on fetal development in test animals. A carcinogen in test animals (IARC 2B). See also p 132.	10 ppm, A2 NIOSH CA	1000 ppm	2 0 0	Colorless liquid. Pleasant, sweet odor. Not combustible. Vapor pressure is 160 mm Hg at 20 °C (68 °F). Breakdown products include hydrogen chloride, phosgene, and chlorine gas.
bis(Chloromethyl) ether (BCME [CAS: 542-88-1]): A human and animal carcinogen (IARC 1).	0.001 ppm, A1 OSHA CA NIOSH CA			Colorless liquid with a suffocating odor. Vapor pressure is 100 mm Hg at 20 °C (68 °F). Used in the manufacture of ion-exchange resins.
Chloromethyl methyl ether (CMME, methyl chloromethyl ether [CAS: 107-30-2]): Vapors irritating to eyes and respiratory tract. Workers show increased risk of lung cancer, possibly owing to contamination of CMME with 1–7% BCME. (See above)	A2 OSHA CA NIOSH CA			Combustible. Breakdown products include oxides of nitrogen and hydrogen chloride. Used in the manufacture of ion-exchange resins.
1-Chloro-1-nitropropane (CAS: 600-25-9): Based on animal studies, vapors highly irritating to eyes and respiratory tract and may cause pulmonary edema. High levels may cause injury to cardiac muscle, liver, and kidney.	2 ppm	2000 ppm	— 2 3	Colorless liquid. Unpleasant odor and tearing occur near the TLV and are good warning properties. Vapor pressure is 5.8 mm Hg at 20 °C (68 °F).

Agent	Exposure Limits	H	F	R	Comments
Chloropentafluoroethane (fluorocarbon 115 [CAS: 76-15-3]): Irritating upon direct contact. Vapors mildly irritating to eyes and respiratory tract. Produces coma and cardiac arrhythmias, but only at very high levels in test animals. See also p 175.	1000 ppm				Colorless, odorless gas. Thermal breakdown products include hydrogen fluoride and hydrogen chloride.
Chloropicrin (trichloronitromethane) [CAS: 76-06-2]): Extremely irritating upon direct contact; severe burns may result. Vapors extremely irritating to eyes, skin, and respiratory tract; delayed pulmonary edema has been reported. Kidney and liver injuries have been observed in test animals.	0.1 ppm ERPG-2: 0.2 ppm ERPG-3: 3 ppm	4	0	3	Colorless, oily liquid. Sharp, penetrating odor and tearing occur near the TLV and are good warning properties. Vapor pressure is 20 mm Hg at 20 °C (68 °F). Breakdown products include oxides of nitrogen, phosgene, nitrosyl chloride, and chlorine gas. Used in fumigants.
β-Chloroprene (2-chloro-1,3-butadiene [CAS: 126-99-8]): Irritating upon direct contact. Vapors irritating to eyes and respiratory tract. A CNS depressant at high levels. Liver and kidneys are major target organs. Limited evidence for adverse effects on fetal development and male reproduction in test animals. Equivocal evidence of carcinogenicity in test animals (IARC 3).	10 ppm, S NIOSH CA	2	3	0	Colorless liquid with an etherlike odor. Vapor pressure is 179 mm Hg at 20 °C (68 °F). Highly flammable. Breakdown products include hydrogen chloride. Used in making neoprene.
o-Chlorotoluene (2-chloro-1-methylbenzene [CAS: 95-49-8]): In test animals, direct contact produced skin and eye irritation; high vapor exposures resulted in tremors, convulsions, and coma. By analogy to toluene and chlorinated compounds, may cause cardiac arrhythmias. See p 298.	50 ppm	2	2	0	Colorless liquid. Vapor pressure is 10 mm Hg at 43 °C (109 °F). Flammable.
Chlorpyrifos (Dursban, O,O-diethyl-O-(3,5,6-trichloro-2-pyridinyl [CAS: 2921-88-2]): An organophosphate-type cholinesterase inhibitor (see p 240).	0.2 mg/m³, S				White solid crystals. Vapor pressure is 0.00002 mm Hg at 25 °C (77 °F).
Chromic acid and chromates (chromium trioxide, sodium dichromate, potassium chromate): Highly irritating upon direct contact; severe eye and skin ulceration (chrome ulcers) may result. Dusts and mists highly irritating to eyes and respiratory tract. Skin and respiratory sensitization (asthma) may occur. Chromium trioxide is a teratogen in test animals. Certain hexavalent chromium compounds are carcinogenic in test animals and humans (IARC 1). See also p 135.	0.5 mg/m³ (CrII and III compounds) 0.05 mg/m³ (CrVI compounds), A1				Soluble chromate compounds are water-reactive.

(C) = ceiling air concentration (TLV-C); S = skin absorption can be significant; A1 = ACGIH-confirmed human carcinogen; A2 = ACGIH-suspected human carcinogen; NFPA Hazard Codes: H = health, F = fire, R = reactivity, Ox = oxidizer, W = water-reactive, 0 (none) <—> 4 (severe). ERPG = Emergency Response Planning Guideline. See p 402 for explanation of definitions.

continued

TABLE IV–13. HEALTH HAZARD SUMMARIES FOR INDUSTRIAL AND OCCUPATIONAL CHEMICALS (Continued)

Health Hazard Summaries	ACGIH TLV	IDLH	NFPA Codes H	Comments
Chromium metal and insoluble chromium salts: Irritating upon direct contact with skin and eyes; dermatitis may result. Ferrochrome alloys possibly associated with pneumoconiotic changes. See also p 135.	0.5 mg/m³ (metal, as Cr) 0.05 mg/m³ (CrVI compounds, as Cr), A1			Chromium metal, silver luster; copper chromite, greenish-blue solid. Odorless.
Chromyl chloride (CAS: 14977-61-8): Hydrolyzes upon contact with moisture to produce chromic trioxide, HCl, chromic trichloride, and chlorine. Highly irritating upon direct contact; severe burns may result. Mists and vapors highly irritating to eyes and respiratory tract. Certain hexavalent chromium VI compounds are carcinogenic in test animals and humans. See also p 135.	0.025 ppm NIOSH CA		3 0 1	Dark red fuming liquid. Water-reactive, yielding hydrogen chloride, chlorine gas, chromic acid, and chromic chloride.
Coal tar pitch volatiles (particulate polycyclic aromatic hydrocarbons [CAS: 65996-93-2]): Irritating upon direct contact. Contact dermatitis, acne, hypermelanosis, and photosensitization may occur. Fumes irritating to eyes and respiratory tract. A carcinogen in test animals and humans, p 178.	0.2 mg/m³, A1 NIOSH CA	700 mg/m³		A complex mixture composed of a high percentage of polycyclic aromatic hydrocarbons. A smoky odor. Combustible. Creosote is an important source of exposure.
Cobalt and compounds: Irritating upon direct contact; dermatitis and skin sensitization may occur. Fumes and dusts irritate the respiratory tract; chronic interstitial pneumonitis and respiratory tract sensitization reported. Cardiotoxicity associated with ingestion, but has not been well-documented with occupational exposures.	0.05 mg/m³ (metal dust and fume, as Co) [proposed: 0.02 mg/m³ (elemental and inorganic compounds, as Co), A3]	20 mg/m³		Elemental cobalt is a black or gray, odorless solid with a negligible vapor pressure. "Hard metal" used in specialty grinding and cutting is a tungsten carbide-cobalt amalgam.

Cobalt hydrocarbonyl (CAS: 16842-03-8): In animal testing, overexposure produces symptoms similar to those of nickel carbonyl and iron pentacarbonyl. Effects include headache, nausea, vomiting, dizziness, fever, and pulmonary edema. — 0.1 mg/m^3 (as Co) — Flammable gas.

Copper fumes, dusts, and salts: Irritation upon direct contact varies with the compound. The salts are more irritating and can cause corneal ulceration. Allergic contact dermatitis is rare. Dusts and mists irritating to the respiratory tract; nasal ulceration has been described. A syndrome like metal fume fever (see p 142) can result from overexposure to fumes or fine dusts. — 1 mg/m^3 (dusts and mists) / 0.2 mg/m^3 (copper fume) — Salts vary in color. Generally odorless.

Cotton dust: Chronic exposure causes a respiratory syndrome called byssinosis. Symptoms include cough and wheezing, typically appearing on the first day of the workweek and continuing for a few days or all week, although they may subside within an hour after leaving work. Can lead to irreversible obstructive airway disease. — 0.2 mg/m^3 — 500 mg/m^3 — Cotton textile manufacture is the principal source of exposure.

Creosote (coal tar creosote [CAS: 8001-58-9]): A primary irritant, photosensitizer, and corrosive. Direct eye contact can cause severe keratitis and corneal scarring. Prolonged skin contact can cause chemical acne, pigmentation changes, and severe penetrating burns. Exposure to the fumes or vapors causes irritation of mucous membranes and the respiratory tract. Systemic toxicity results from phenolic and cresolic constituents. Liver and kidney injury may occur with heavy exposure. A carcinogen in test animals. Some evidence for carcinogenicity in humans (IARC 2A). See also phenol, p 249. — NIOSH CA — 2 2 0 — Oily, dark liquid. Appearance and some hazardous properties vary with the formulation. Sharp, penetrating smoky odor. Combustible. Creosote is produced by the fractional distillation of coal tar. See entry on coal tar pitch volatiles.

(C) = ceiling air concentration (TLV-C); S = skin absorption can be significant; A1 = ACGIH-confirmed human carcinogen; A2 = ACGIH-suspected human carcinogen; NFPA Hazard Codes: H = health, F = fire, R = reactivity, Ox = oxidizer, W = water-reactive, 0 (none) <—> 4 (severe). ERPG = Emergency Response Planning Guideline. See p 402 for explanation of definitions.

continued

TABLE IV–13. HEALTH HAZARD SUMMARIES FOR INDUSTRIAL AND OCCUPATIONAL CHEMICALS (Continued)

Health Hazard Summaries	ACGIH TLV	IDLH	NFPA Codes H	Comments
Cresol (methylphenol, cresylic acid, hydroxymethylbenzene [CAS: 1319-77-3]): Corrosive. Skin and eye contact can cause severe burns. Exposure may be prolonged owing to local anesthetic action on skin. Well absorbed by all routes. Dermal absorption is a major route of systemic poisoning. Induces methemoglobinemia (see p 217). CNS depressant. Symptoms include headache, nausea and vomiting, tinnitus, dizziness, weakness, and confusion. Severe lung, liver and kidney injury may occur. See also phenol, p 249.	5 ppm, S	250 ppm	3 2 0 (ortho) 3 1 0 (meta, para)	Colorless, yellow, or pink liquid with a phenolic odor. Vapor pressure is 0.2 mm Hg at 20 °C (68 °F). Combustible.
Crotonaldehyde (2-butenal [CAS: 4170-30-3]): Highly irritating upon direct contact; severe burns may result. Vapors highly irritating to eyes and respiratory tract; delayed pulmonary edema may occur. Evidence for carcinogenicity in test animals.	2 ppm	400 mg/m³ ERPG-1: 2 ppm ERPG-2: 10 ppm ERPG-3: 50 ppm	3 3 2	Colorless to straw-colored liquid. Pungent, irritating odor occurs below the TLV and is an adequate warning property. A warning agent added to fuel gases. Vapor pressure is 30 mm Hg at 20 °C (68 °F). Flammable. Polymerizes when heated.
Crufomate (4-tert-butyl-2-chlorophenyl N-methyl O-methylphosphoramidate [CAS: 299-86-5]): An organophosphate cholinesterase inhibitor (see p 240).	5 mg/m³			Crystals or yellow oil. Pungent odor. Flammable.
Cumene (isopropylbenzene [CAS: 98-82-8]): Mildly irritating upon direct contact. A CNS depressant at moderate levels. Well absorbed through skin.	50 ppm, S	8000 ppm	2 3 0	Colorless liquid. Sharp, aromatic odor below the TLV is a good warning property. Vapor pressure is 8 mm Hg at 20 °C (68 °F). Flammable.
Cyanamide (carbodiimide [CAS: 420-04-2]): Causes transient vaso-motor flushing. Highly irritating and caustic to eyes and skin. Has a disulfiramlike interaction with alcohol, producing flushing, headache, and dyspnea (see p 155).	2 mg/m³		4 1 3	Combustible. Thermal breakdown products include oxides of nitrogen.

Chemical	TLV		H	F	R	Comments
Cyanide salts (sodium cyanide, potassium cyanide): Potent and rapidly fatal metabolic asphyxiants that inhibit cytochrome oxidase and stop cellular respiration. Well absorbed through skin; caustic action can promote dermal absorption. See also p 145.	5 mg/m³ (as cyanide), S	50 mg/m³ (as cyanide)				Solids. Mild, almondlike odor. In presence of moisture or acids, hydrogen cyanide may be released. Odor is a poor indicator of exposure to hydrogen cyanide. May be generated in fires from the pyrolysis of such products as polyurethane and polyacrylonitrile.
Cyanogen (dicyan, oxalonitrile) [CAS: 460-19-5]): Hydrolyzes to release hydrogen cyanide and cyanic acid. Toxicity similar to that of hydrogen cyanide (see p 145). Vapors irritating to eyes and respiratory tract.	10 ppm		4	4	2	Colorless gas. Pungent, almondlike odor. Breaks down on contact with water to yield hydrogen cyanide and cyanate. Flammable.
Cyanogen chloride (CAS: 506-77-4): Vapors extremely irritating to eyes and respiratory tract; pulmonary edema may result. Cyanide interferes with cellular respiration (see p 145).	0.3 ppm (C)					Colorless liquid or gas with a pungent odor. Thermal breakdown products include hydrogen cyanide and hydrogen chloride. Formed by a reaction with hypochlorite in the treatment of cyanide-containing waste water.
Cyclohexane (CAS: 110-82-7): Mildly irritating upon direct contact. Vapors irritating to eyes and respiratory tract. A CNS depressant at high levels. Chronically exposed test animals developed liver and kidney injury.	300 ppm	10,000 ppm	1	3	0	Colorless liquid with a sweet, chloroformlike odor. Vapor pressure is 95 mm Hg at 20 °C (68 °F). Highly flammable.
Cyclohexanol (CAS: 108-93-0): Irritating upon direct contact. Vapors irritating to eyes and respiratory tract. Well absorbed by skin. A CNS depressant at high levels. Based on animal tests, it may injure the liver and kidneys at high doses.	50 ppm, S	3500 ppm	1	2	0	Colorless viscous liquid. Mild camphorlike odor. Irritation occurs near the TLV and is a good warning property. Vapor pressure is 1 mm Hg at 20 °C (68 °F). Combustible.
Cyclohexanone (CAS: 108-94-1): Irritating upon direct contact. Vapors irritate the eyes and respiratory tract. A CNS depressant at very high levels. Chronic, moderate doses caused slight liver injury in test animals.	25 ppm, S	5000 ppm	1	2	0	Clear to pale yellow liquid with peppermintlike odor. Vapor pressure is 2 mm Hg at 20 °C (68 °F). Flammable.
Cyclohexene (1,2,3,4-tetrahydrobenzene [CAS: 110-83-8]): By structural analogy to cyclohexane, may cause respiratory tract irritation. A CNS depressant.	300 ppm	10,000 ppm	1	3	0	Colorless liquid with a sweet odor. Vapor pressure is 67 mm Hg at 20 °C (68 °F). Flammable. Readily forms peroxides and polymerizes.

(C) = ceiling air concentration (TLV-C); S = skin absorption can be significant; A1 = ACGIH-confirmed human carcinogen; A2 = ACGIH-suspected human carcinogen; NFPA Hazard Codes: H = health, F = fire, R = reactivity, Ox = oxidizer, W = water-reactive, 0 (none) <—> 4 (severe). ERPG = Emergency Response Planning Guideline. See p 402 for explanation of definitions.

continued

TABLE IV–13. HEALTH HAZARD SUMMARIES FOR INDUSTRIAL AND OCCUPATIONAL CHEMICALS (Continued)

Health Hazard Summaries	ACGIH TLV	IDLH	NFPA Codes H F R	Comments
Cyclohexylamine (aminocyclohexane [CAS: 108-91-8]): Corrosive and highly irritating upon direct contact. Vapors highly irritating to eyes and respiratory tract. Pharmacologically active, possessing sympathomimetic activity. Weak methemoglobin–forming activity (see p 217). Very limited evidence for adverse effects on reproduction in test animals. Animal studies suggest brain, liver, and kidneys are target organs.	10 ppm		2 3 0	Liquid with an obnoxious, fishy odor. Flammable.
Cyclonite (RDX, trinitrotrimethylenetriamine [CAS: 121-82-4]): Dermal and inhalation exposures affect the CNS with symptoms of confusion, headache, nausea, vomiting, convulsions, and coma. Does not have nitratelike toxicity.	1.5 mg/m³, S			Crystalline solid. Vapor pressure is negligible at 20 °C (68 °F). Thermal breakdown products include oxides of nitrogen. Explosive.
Cyclopentadiene [CAS: 542-92-7]): Mildly irritating upon direct contact. Vapors irritating to eyes and respiratory tract. A CNS depressant at high levels. Animal studies suggest some potential for kidney and liver injury at high doses.	75 ppm	2000 ppm		Colorless liquid. Sweet, turpentinelike odor. Irritation occurs near the TLV and is a good warning property. Vapor pressure is high at 20 °C (68 °F). Flammable.
Cyclopentane (CAS: 287-92-3): Mildly irritating to eyes and respiratory tract. A CNS depressant at very high levels. Solvent mixtures containing cyclopentane have caused peripheral neuropathy although this may have been related to n-hexane in combination.	600 ppm		1 3 0	Colorless liquid with a faint hydrocarbon odor. Vapor pressure is about 400 mm Hg at 31 °C (88 °F). Flammable.
DDT (dichlorodiphenyltrichloroethane [CAS: 50-29-3]): Dusts irritating to eyes. Ingestion may cause tremor and convulsions. Chronic low-level exposure results in bioaccumulation. A carcinogen in test animals (IARC 2B). See also p 129.	1 mg/m³ NIOSH CA			Colorless, white, or yellow solid crystals with a faint aromatic odor. Vapor pressure is 0.0000002 mm Hg at 20 °C (68 °F). Combustible. Banned for use in US in 1973.

Substance	(C) / TLV	ERPG / air conc.	H	F	R	Comments
Decaborane (CAS: 17702-41-9): A potent CNS toxin. Symptoms include headache, dizziness, nausea, loss of coordination, and fatigue. Symptoms may be delayed in onset for 1–2 days; convulsions occur in more severe poisonings. Systemic poisonings can result from dermal absorption. Animal studies suggest a potential for liver and kidney injury.	0.05 ppm, S	20 ppm	3	2	1	Colorless solid crystals with a pungent odor. Vapor pressure is 0.05 mm Hg at 25 °C (77 °F). Combustible. Reacts with water to produce flammable hydrogen gas. Used as a rocket fuel additive and as a rubber vulcanization agent.
Demeton (Systox, mercaptophos) [CAS: 8065-48-3]: An organophosphate-type cholinesterase inhibitor (see p 240).	0.01 ppm, S	20 mg/m³				A sulfurlike odor. A very low vapor pressure at 20 °C (68 °F). Thermal breakdown products include oxides of sulfur.
Diacetone alcohol (4-hydroxy-4-methyl-2-pentanone [CAS: 123-42-2]: Irritating upon direct contact. Vapors very irritating to eyes and respiratory tract. A CNS depressant at high levels. Possibly some hemolytic activity.	50 ppm	2100 ppm	1	2	0	Colorless liquid with an agreeable odor. Vapor pressure is 0.8 mm Hg at 20 °C (68 °F). Flammable.
Diazinon (*O,O*-diethyl *O*-2-isopropyl-4-methyl-6-pyrimidinylthiophosphate [CAS: 333-41-5]): An organophosphate-type cholinesterase inhibitor (see p 240). Well absorbed dermally. Limited evidence for adverse effects on male reproduction and fetal development in test animals at high doses.	0.1 mg/m³, S					Commercial grades are yellow to brown liquids with a faint odor. Vapor pressure is 0.00014 mm Hg at 20 °C (68 °F). Thermal breakdown products include oxides of nitrogen and sulfur.
Diazomethane (azimethylene, diazirine [CAS: 334-88-3]): Extremely irritating to eyes and respiratory tract; pulmonary edema has been reported. Immediate symptoms include cough, chest pain, and respiratory distress. A potent methylating agent and respiratory sensitizer.	0.2 ppm	10 ppm				Yellow gas with a musty odor. Air mixtures and compressed liquids can be explosive when heated or shocked.
Diborane (boron hydride [CAS: 19287-45-7]): Extremely irritating to the respiratory tract; pulmonary edema may result. Repeated exposures have been associated with headache, fatigue, and dizziness; muscle weakness or tremors; and chills or fever. Animal studies suggest the liver and kidney are also target organs.	0.1 ppm	40 ppm	3	4	3 W	Colorless gas. Obnoxious, nauseatingly sweet odor. Highly flammable. Water-reactive; ignites spontaneously with moist air at room temperatures. A strong reducing agent. Breakdown products include boron oxide fumes. Used in microelectronics industry.

(C) = ceiling air concentration (TLV-C); S = skin absorption can be significant; A1 = ACGIH-confirmed human carcinogen; A2 = ACGIH-suspected human carcinogen; NFPA Hazard Codes: H = health, F = fire, R = reactivity, Ox = oxidizer, W = water-reactive, 0 (none) <—> 4 (severe). ERPG = Emergency Response Planning Guideline. See p 402 for explanation of definitions.

continued

TABLE IV–13. HEALTH HAZARD SUMMARIES FOR INDUSTRIAL AND OCCUPATIONAL CHEMICALS (Continued)

Health Hazard Summaries	ACGIH TLV	IDLH	NFPA Codes H			Comments
1,2-Dibromo-3-chloropropane (DBCP [CAS: 96-12-8]): Irritant of eyes and respiratory tract. Has caused sterility (aspermia, oligospermia) in overexposed men. Well absorbed by skin contact and inhalation. A carcinogen in test animals (IARC 2B).	OSHA CA NIOSH CA					Brown liquid with a pungent odor. Combustible. Thermal breakdown products include hydrogen bromide and hydrogen chloride.
1,2-Dibromo-2,2-dichloroethyl dimethyl phosphate (Naled, Dibrom [CAS: 300-76-5]): An organophosphate anticholinesterase agent (see p 240). Highly irritating upon contact; eye injury is likely. Well absorbed dermally; localized muscular twitching results within minutes of contact.	3 mg/m³, S					Has a pungent odor. Vapor pressure is 0.002 mm Hg at 20 °C (68 °F). Not combustible. Thermal breakdown products include hydrogen bromide, hydrogen chloride, and phosphoric acid.
Dibutyl phosphate (di-*n*-butyl phosphate [CAS: 107-66-4]): A moderately strong acid likely to be irritating upon direct contact. Vapors and mists are irritating to the respiratory tract and have been associated with headache at low levels.	1 ppm	125 ppm				Colorless to brown liquid. Odorless. Vapor pressure is much less than 1 mm Hg at 20 °C (68 °F). Decomposes at 100 °C (212 °F) to produce phosphoric acid fumes.
Dibutyl phthalate (CAS: 84-74-2): Mildly irritating upon direct contact. Ingestion has produced nausea, dizziness, photophobia, and lacrimation but no permanent effects. Adverse effects on fetal development and male reproduction in test animals at very high doses.	5 mg/m³	9300 mg/m³	0	1	0	Colorless, oily liquid with a faint aromatic odor. Vapor pressure is less than 0.01 mm Hg at 20 °C (68 °F). Combustible.
1,2-Dichloroacetylene (CAS: 7572-29-4): Vapors extremely irritating to eyes and respiratory tract; pulmonary edema may result. CNS toxicity includes nausea and vomiting, headache, involvement of trigeminal nerve and facial muscles, and outbreaks of facial herpes. Limited evidence for carcinogenicity in test animals.	0.1 ppm (C)					Colorless liquid.

Substance	TLV-C	Air conc.	H	F	R	Comments
o-Dichlorobenzene (1,2-dichlorobenzene [CAS: 95-50-1]): Irritating upon direct contact; skin blisters and hyperpigmentation may result from prolonged contact. Vapor also irritating to eyes and respiratory tract. Highly hepatotoxic in test animals. Evidence for adverse effects on male reproduction in test animals.	25 ppm	1700 ppm	2	2	0	Colorless to pale yellow liquid. Aromatic odor and eye irritation occur well below the TLV and are adequate warning properties. Thermal breakdown products include hydrogen chloride and chlorine gas.
p-Dichlorobenzene (1,4-dichlorobenzene [CAS: 106-46-7]): Irritating upon direct contact with the solid. Vapors irritating to eyes and respiratory tract. Systemic effects include headache, nausea, vomiting, and liver injury. The *ortho* isomer is more toxic to the liver. A carcinogen in test animals (IARC 2B). See also p 226.	75 ppm [proposed: 10 ppm, A3]	1000 ppm	2	2	0	Colorless or white solid. Mothball odor and irritation occur near the TLV and are adequate warning properties. Vapor pressure is 0.4 mm Hg at 20 °C (68 °F). Combustible. Thermal breakdown products include hydrogen chloride. Used as a moth repellant.
3,3′-Dichlorobenzidine (CAS: 91-94-1): Well absorbed by the dermal route. Animal studies suggest that severe eye injury and respiratory tract irritation may occur. A potent carcinogen in test animals (IARC 2B).	S, A2 OSHA CA NIOSH CA					Crystalline needles with a faint odor.
Dichlorodifluoromethane (Freon 12, fluorocarbon 12 [CAS: 75-71-8]): Mild eye and respiratory tract irritant. Extremely high exposures (eg, 100,000 ppm) can cause coma and cardiac arrhythmias. See also p 175.	1000 ppm	50,000 ppm				Colorless gas. Etherlike odor is a poor warning property. Vapor pressure is 5.7 mm Hg at 20 °C (68 °F). Not combustible. Decomposes slowly on contact with water or heat to produce hydrogen chloride, hydrogen fluoride, and phosgene.
1,3-Dichloro-5,5-dimethylhydantoin (Halane, Dactin [CAS: 118-52-5]): Releases hypochlorous acid and chlorine gas (see p 130) on contact with moisture. Direct contact with the dust or concentrated solutions irritating to eyes, skin, and respiratory tract.	0.2 mg/m³	5 mg/m³	2	3	0	White solid with a chlorinelike odor. Odor and eye irritation occur below the TLV and are adequate warning properties. Not combustible. Thermal breakdown products include hydrogen chloride, phosgene, oxides of nitrogen, and chlorine gas.
1,1-Dichloroethane (ethylidene chloride [CAS: 75-34-3]): Mild eye and skin irritant. Vapors irritating to the respiratory tract. A CNS depressant at high levels. By analogy with its 1,2-isomer, may cause arrhythmias. Animal studies suggest some potential for kidney and liver injury.	100 ppm	4000 ppm	2	3	0	Colorless, oily liquid. Chloroformlike odor occurs at the TLV. Vapor pressure is 182 mm Hg at 20 °C (68 °F). Flammable. Thermal breakdown products include vinyl chloride, hydrogen chloride, and phosgene.

(C) = ceiling air concentration (TLV-C); S = skin absorption can be significant; A1 = ACGIH-confirmed human carcinogen; A2 = ACGIH-suspected human carcinogen; NFPA Hazard Codes: H = health, F = fire, R = reactivity, Ox = oxidizer, W = water-reactive, 0 (none) <—> 4 (severe). ERPG = Emergency Response Planning Guideline. See p 402 for explanation of definitions.

continued

TABLE IV–13. HEALTH HAZARD SUMMARIES FOR INDUSTRIAL AND OCCUPATIONAL CHEMICALS (Continued)

Health Hazard Summaries	ACGIH TLV	IDLH	NFPA Codes H F R			Comments
1,2-Dichloroethane (ethylene dichloride [CAS: 107-06-2]): Irritating upon prolonged contact; burns may occur. Well absorbed dermally. Vapors irritating to eyes and respiratory tract. A CNS depressant at high levels. May cause cardiac arrhythmias. Severe liver and kidney injury has been reported. A carcinogen in test animals (IARC 2B).	10 ppm NIOSH CA	1000 ppm	2	3	0	Flammable. Thermal breakdown products include hydrogen chloride and phosgene.
1,1-Dichloroethylene (vinylidine chloride [CAS: 75-35-4]): Irritating upon direct contact. Vapors very irritating to eyes and respiratory tract. A CNS depressant. May cause cardiac arrhythmias. In test animals, damages the liver and kidneys. Limited evidence of carcinogenicity in test animals (IARC 3).	5 ppm NIOSH CA		2	4	2	Colorless liquid. Sweet, etherlike or chloroformlike odor occurs below the TLV and is a good warning property. Polymerizes readily.
1,2-Dichloroethylene (1,2-dichloroethene, acetylene dichloride [CAS: 540-59-0]): Vapors mildly irritating to respiratory tract. A CNS depressant at high levels; once used as an anesthetic agent. May cause cardiac arrhythmias. Low hepatotoxicity.	200 ppm	4000 ppm	2	3	2	Colorless liquid with a slightly acrid, etherlike or chloroformlike odor. Vapor pressure is about 220 mm Hg at 20 °C (68 °F). Thermal breakdown products include hydrogen chloride and phosgene.
Dichloroethyl ether (bis[2-chloroethyl] ether, dichloroethyl oxide [CAS: 111-44-4]): Irritating upon direct contact; corneal injury may result. Vapors highly irritating to respiratory tract. A CNS depressant at high levels. Dermal absorption occurs. Animal studies suggest the liver and kidneys are also target organs at high exposures. Limited evidence for carcinogenicity in test animals.	5 ppm, S	250 ppm	2	2	0	Colorless liquid. Obnoxious, chlorinated solvent odor occurs at the TLV and is a good warning property. Flammable. Breaks down on contact with water. Thermal breakdown products include hydrogen chloride.
Dichlorofluoromethane (fluorocarbon 21, Freon 21, Halon 112 [CAS: 75-43-4]): Animal studies suggest much greater hepatotoxicity than most common chlorofluorocarbons. Causes CNS depression, respiratory irritation, and cardiac arrhythmias at very high air levels (eg, 100,000 ppm). Evidence for adverse effects on fetal development (preimplantation losses) in test animals at high levels. See also p 175.	10 ppm	50,000 ppm	2			Colorless liquid or gas with a faint etherlike odor. Thermal breakdown products include hydrogen chloride, hydrogen fluoride, and phosgene.

1,1-Dichloro-1-nitroethane [CAS: 594-72-9]): Based on animal studies, highly irritating upon direct contact. Vapors highly irritating to eyes, skin, and respiratory tract; pulmonary edema may result. In test animals, lethal doses also injured the liver, heart, and kidneys. — 2 ppm — 150 ppm — 2 2 3 — Colorless liquid. Obnoxious odor and tearing occur only at dangerous levels and are poor warning properties. Vapor pressure is 15 mm Hg at 20 °C (68 °F).

2,4-Dichlorophenoxyacetic acid (2,4-D [CAS: 94-75-9]): Direct skin contact can produce a rash. Overexposed workers have rarely experienced peripheral neuropathy. Severe rhabdomyolysis and minor liver and kidney injury may occur. Adverse effects on fetal development at high doses in test animals. There are weak epidemiologic associations of phenoxy herbicides with soft tissue sarcomas. See also p 133. — 10 mg/m³ — 500 mg/m³ —   — White to yellow crystals. Appearance and some hazardous properties vary with the formulation. Odorless. Vapor pressure is negligible at 20 °C (68 °F). Thermal breakdown products include hydrogen chloride and phosgene.

1,3-Dichloropropene (1,3-dichloropropylene, Telone [CAS: 542-75-6]): Based on animal studies, irritating upon direct contact. Well absorbed dermally. Vapors irritating to eyes and respiratory tract. In test animals, moderate doses caused severe injuries to the liver, pancreas, and kidneys. A carcinogen in test animals (IARC 2B). — 1 ppm, S — 1 ppm — 2 3 0 — Colorless or straw-colored liquid. Sharp, chloroformlike odor. Polymerizes readily. Vapor pressure is 28 mm Hg at 25 °C (77 °F). Thermal breakdown products include hydrogen chloride and phosgene.

2,2-Dichloropropionic acid (CAS: 75-99-0): Corrosive upon direct contact with concentrate; severe burns may result. Vapors mildly irritating to eyes and respiratory tract. — 1 ppm —   —   — Colorless liquid. The sodium salt is a solid.

Dichlorotetrafluoroethane (fluorocarbon 114, Freon 114 [CAS: 76-14-2]): Vapors may sensitize the myocardium to arrhythmogenic effects of epinephrine at modestly high air levels (25,000 ppm). Other effects at higher levels (100,000–200,000 ppm) include respiratory irritation and CNS depression. See also p 175. — 1000 ppm — 50,000 ppm —   — Colorless gas with a mild etherlike odor. Thermal breakdown products include hydrogen chloride, hydrogen fluoride, and phosgene.

Dichlorvos (DDVP, 2,2-dichlorovinyl dimethyl phosphate [CAS: 62-73-7]): An organophosphate-type cholinesterase inhibitor (see p 240). Extremely well absorbed through skin. Evidence of carcinogenicity in test animals (IARC 2B). — 0.1 ppm, S — 200 mg/m³ —   — Colorless to amber liquid with a slight chemical odor. Vapor pressure is 0.032 mm Hg at 32 °C (90 °F).

(C) = ceiling air concentration (TLV-C); S = skin absorption can be significant; A1 = ACGIH-confirmed human carcinogen; A2 = ACGIH-suspected human carcinogen; NFPA Hazard Codes: H = health, F = fire, R = reactivity, Ox = oxidizer, W = water-reactive. 0 (none) <—> 4 (severe). ERPG = Emergency Response Planning Guideline. See p 402 for explanation of definitions.

continued

TABLE IV–13. HEALTH HAZARD SUMMARIES FOR INDUSTRIAL AND OCCUPATIONAL CHEMICALS (Continued)

Health Hazard Summaries	ACGIH TLV	IDLH	NFPA Codes H F R			Comments
Dicrotophos (dimethyl cis-2-dimethylcarbamoyl-1-methylvinyl phosphate, Bidrin [CAS: 141-66-2]): An organophosphate cholinesterase inhibitor (see p 240). Dermal absorption occurs.	0.25 mg/m³, S					Brown liquid with a mild ester odor.
Dieldrin (CAS: 60-57-1): Minor skin irritant. Potent convulsant and hepatotoxin. Dermal absorption is a major route of systemic poisoning. Overexposures produce headache, dizziness, twitching, and convulsions. Limited evidence for adverse effects on fetal development and carcinogenicity in test animals (IARC 3). See also p 129.	0.25 mg/m³, S NIOSH CA	450 mg/m³				Light brown solid flakes with a mild chemical odor. Appearance and some hazardous properties vary with the formulation. Vapor pressure is 0.0000002 mm Hg at 32 °C (90 °F). Not combustible.
Diethylamine (CAS: 109-89-7): Corrosive. Highly irritating upon direct contact; severe burns may result. Vapors highly irritating to eyes and respiratory tract; pulmonary edema may occur. Subacute animal studies suggest liver and heart may be target organs.	10 ppm [proposed: 5 ppm, S]	2000 ppm	2	3	0	Colorless liquid. Fishy, ammonialike odor occurs below the TLV and is a good warning property. Vapor pressure is 195 mm Hg at 20 °C (68 °F). Highly flammable. Thermal breakdown products include oxides of nitrogen.
2-Diethylaminoethanol (N,N-diethylethanolamine, DEAE [CAS: 100-37-8]): Based on animal studies, highly irritating upon direct contact and a skin sensitizer. Vapors likely irritating to eyes, skin, and respiratory tract. Reports of nausea and vomiting after a momentary exposure to 100 ppm.	10 ppm, S	500 ppm	3	2	0	Colorless liquid. Weak to nauseating ammonia odor. Flammable. Thermal breakdown products include oxides of nitrogen.
Diethylenetriamine (DETA [CAS: 111-40-0]): Corrosive; highly irritating upon direct contact; severe burns may result. Vapors highly irritating to eyes and respiratory tract. Dermal and respiratory sensitization can occur.	1 ppm, S		3	1	0	Viscous yellow liquid with an ammonialike odor. Vapor pressure is 0.37 mm Hg at 20 °C (68 °F). Combustible. Thermal breakdown products include oxides of nitrogen.
Diethyl ketone (3-pentanone [CAS: 96-22-0]): Mildly irritating upon direct contact. Vapors mildly irritating to eyes and respiratory tract.	200 ppm		1	3	0	Colorless liquid with an acetonelike odor. Flammable.

Chemical	TLV	H	F	R	Comments
Difluorodibromomethane (dibromodifluoromethane, Freon 12B2 [CAS: 75-61-6]): Based on animal tests, vapors irritate the respiratory tract. A CNS depressant. By analogy to other freons, may cause cardiac arrhythmias. In test animals, high-level chronic exposures caused lung, liver, and CNS injury. See also p 175.	100 ppm				Heavy, volatile, colorless liquid with an obnoxious, distinctive odor. Vapor pressure is 620 mm Hg at 20 °C (68 °F). Not combustible. Thermal breakdown products include hydrogen bromide and hydrogen fluoride.
	2500 ppm				
Diglycidyl ether (dil2,3-epoxypropyl)-ether, DGE [CAS: 2238-07-5]): Extremely irritating upon direct contact; severe burns result. Vapors highly irritating to eyes and respiratory tract; pulmonary edema may result. Testicular atrophy and adverse effects on the hematopoietic system at low doses in test animals. CNS depression also noted. An alkylating agent and a carcinogen in test animals.	0.1 ppm NIOSH CA				Colorless liquid with a very irritating odor. Vapor pressure is 0.09 mm Hg at 25 °C (77 °F).
	25 ppm				
Diisobutyl ketone (2,6-dimethyl-4-heptanone [CAS: 108-83-8]): Mildly irritating upon direct contact. Vapors mildly irritate eyes and respiratory tract at high levels.	25 ppm	1	2	0	Colorless liquid with a weak, etherlike odor. Vapor pressure is 1.7 mm Hg at 20 °C (68 °F).
	2000 ppm				
Diisopropylamine (CAS: 108-18-9): Corrosive. Highly irritating upon direct contact; severe burns may result. Vapors very irritating to eyes and respiratory tract. Workers exposed to levels of 25–50 ppm have complained of hazy vision, nausea, and headache.	5 ppm, S	3	3	0	Colorless liquid with an ammonialike odor. Vapor pressure is 60 mm Hg at 20 °C (68 °F). Flammable. Thermal breakdown products include oxides of nitrogen.
	1000 ppm				
Dimethyl acetamide (DMAC [CAS: 127-19-5]): Potent hepatotoxin. Inhalation and skin contact are major routes of absorption. Limited evidence for adverse effects on fetal development in test animals at high doses.	10 ppm, S	2	2	0	Colorless liquid with a weak ammonialike odor. Vapor pressure is 1.5 mm Hg at 20 °C (68 °F). Combustible. Thermal breakdown products include oxides of nitrogen.
	400 ppm				
Dimethylamine (DMA [CAS: 124-40-3]): Corrosive upon direct contact; severe burns may result. Vapors extremely irritating to eyes and respiratory tract. Animal studies suggest liver is a target organ.	5 ppm	3	4	0	Colorless liquid or gas. Fishy or ammonialike odor far below TLV is a good warning property. Flammable. Thermal breakdown products include oxides of nitrogen.
	2000 ppm ERPG-1: 1 ppm ERPG-2: 100 ppm ERPG-3: 500 ppm				

(C) = ceiling air concentration (TLV-C); S = skin absorption can be significant; A1 = ACGIH-confirmed human carcinogen; A2 = ACGIH-suspected human carcinogen; NFPA Hazard Codes: H = health, F = fire, R = reactivity, Ox = oxidizer, W = water-reactive, 0 (none) <—> 4 (severe), ERPG = Emergency Response Planning Guideline. See p 402 for explanation of definitions.

continued

TABLE IV–13. HEALTH HAZARD SUMMARIES FOR INDUSTRIAL AND OCCUPATIONAL CHEMICALS (Continued)

Health Hazard Summaries	ACGIH TLV	IDLH	NFPA Codes H	F	R	Comments
N,N-Dimethylaniline (CAS: 121-69-7): Causes methemoglobinemia (see p 217). A CNS depressant. Well absorbed dermally. Limited evidence for carcinogenicity in test animals.	5 ppm, S	100 ppm	3	2	0	Straw- to brown-colored liquid with an aminelike odor. Vapor pressure is less than 1 mm Hg at 20 °C (68 °F). Combustible. Thermal breakdown products include oxides of nitrogen.
Dimethylcarbamoyl chloride (CAS: 79-44-7): Rapidly hydrolyzed by moisture to dimethylamine, carbon dioxide, and hydrochloric acid (see p 126). Expected to be extremely irritating upon direct contact or by inhalation. A carcinogen in test animals (IARC 2A).	A2					Liquid. Rapidly reacts with moisture to yield dimethylamine and hydrogen chloride.
N,N-Dimethylformamide (DMF [CAS: 68-12-2]): Dermally well absorbed. Symptoms of overexposure include abdominal pain, nausea, and vomiting. This chemical is a potent hepatotoxin in humans. Interferes with ethanol to cause disulfiramlike reactions (see p 155). Limited epidemiologic association with an increased risk of testicular cancer (IARC 2B). Limited evidence for adverse effects on fetal development in animals.	10 ppm, S	3500 ppm	1	2	0	Colorless to pale yellow liquid. Faint ammonialike odor is a poor warning property. Vapor pressure is 2.7 mm Hg at 20 °C (68 °F). Flammable. Thermal breakdown products include oxides of nitrogen.
1,1-Dimethylhydrazine (DMH, UDMH [CAS: 57-14-7]): Corrosive upon direct contact; severe burns may result. Vapors extremely irritating to eyes and respiratory tract; pulmonary edema may occur. Well absorbed through the skin. May cause methemoglobinemia (see p 217); may cause hemolysis. A potent hepatotoxin and carcinogen in test animals (IARC 2B).	0.5 ppm, S, A2 [proposed: 0.01 ppm, S, A2] NIOSH CA	50 ppm	3	3	1	Colorless liquid with yellow fumes. Amine odor. Vapor pressure is 103 mm Hg at 20 °C (68 °F). Thermal breakdown products include oxides of nitrogen.
Dimethyl sulfate (CAS: 77-78-1): Powerful vesicant action; hydrolyzes to sulfuric acid (see p 126) and methanol. Extremely irritating upon direct contact; severe burns have resulted. Vapors irritating to eyes and respiratory tract; delayed pulmonary edema may result. Skin absorption is rapid. Evidence for adverse effects on fetal development in test animals (IARC 2A).	0.1 ppm, S, A2	10 ppm	4	2	0	Colorless, oily liquid. Very mild onion odor is barely perceptible and is a poor warning property. Vapor pressure is 0.5 mm Hg at 20 °C (68 °F). Combustible. Thermal breakdown products include sulfur oxides.

Dinitrobenzene: May stain tissues yellow upon direct contact. Vapors are irritating to respiratory tract. Potent inducer of methemoglobinemia (see p 217). Chronic exposures may result in anemia and liver damage. Injures testes in test animals. Very well absorbed through the skin.

0.15 ppm, S — 200 mg/m³ — 3 1 4 — Pale yellow crystals. Explosive; detonated by heat or shock. Vapor pressure is much less than 1 mm Hg at 20 °C (68 °F). Thermal breakdown products include oxides of nitrogen.

Dinitro-o-cresol (2-methyl-4,6-dinitrophenol [CAS: 534-52-1]): Highly toxic; uncouples oxidative phosphorylation in mitochondria, increasing metabolic rate and leading to fatigue, sweating, rapid breathing, tachycardia, and fever. Liver and kidney injury may occur. Symptoms may last for days, as it is very slowly excreted. May induce methemoglobinemia (see p 217). Poisonings may result from dermal exposure. Yellow-stained skin may mark exposure. See also p 246.

0.2 mg/m³, S — 5 mg/m³ — Yellow solid crystals. Odorless. Dust is explosive. Vapor pressure is 0.00005 mm Hg at 20 °C (68 °F). Thermal breakdown products include oxides of nitrogen.

2,4-Dinitrophenol (CAS: 25550-58-7): Potent uncoupler of oxidative phosphorylation. Initial findings include hypertension, fever, dyspnea, and tachypnea. May cause methemoglobinemia and harm liver and kidneys. May stain skin at point of contact. Limited evidence for adverse effects on fetal development. See also p 246.

2,4-Dinitrotoluene (DNT [CAS: 25321-14-6]): May cause methemoglobinemia (see p 217). Uncouples oxidative phosphorylation, leading to increased metabolic rate and hyperthermia, tachycardia, and fatigue. A hepatotoxin. May cause vasodilation; headache and drop in blood pressure are common. Cessation of exposure may precipitate angina pectoris in pharmacologically dependent workers. Well absorbed by all routes. May stain skin yellow. Injures testes in test animals and possibly, exposed workers. A carcinogen in test animals.

0.15 mg/m³, A2, S NIOSH CA — 200 mg/m³ — 3 1 3 — Orange-yellow solid (pure) or oily liquid with a characteristic odor. Explosive. Thermal breakdown products include oxides of nitrogen. Vapor pressure is 1 mm Hg at 20 °C (68 °F).

1,4-Dioxane (1,4-diethylene dioxide [CAS: 123-91-1]): Vapors irritating to eyes and respiratory tract. Inhalation or dermal exposures may cause gastrointestinal upset and liver and kidney injury. A carcinogen in test animals (IARC 2B).

25 ppm, S NIOSH CA — 2000 ppm — 2 3 1 — Colorless liquid. Mild etherlike odor occurs only at dangerous levels and is a poor warning property. Vapor pressure is 29 mm Hg at 20 °C (68 °F). Flammable.

continued

(C) = ceiling air concentration (TLV-C); S = skin absorption can be significant; A1 = ACGIH-confirmed human carcinogen; A2 = ACGIH-suspected human carcinogen; NFPA Hazard Codes: H = health, F = fire, R = reactivity, Ox = oxidizer, W = water-reactive, 0 (none) <—> 4 (severe). ERPG = Emergency Response Planning Guideline. See p 402 for explanation of definitions.

TABLE IV–13. HEALTH HAZARD SUMMARIES FOR INDUSTRIAL AND OCCUPATIONAL CHEMICALS (Continued)

Health Hazard Summaries	ACGIH TLV	IDLH	NFPA Codes H	Comments
Dioxathion (2,3-*p*-dioxanedithiol *S,S*-bis[*O,O*-diethyl phosphorodithioate) [CAS: 78-34-2]): An organophosphate-type cholinesterase inhibitor (see p 240). Well absorbed dermally.	0.2 mg/m³, S			Amber liquid. Vapor pressure is negligible at 20 °C (68 °F). Thermal breakdown products include oxides of sulfur.
Dipropylene glycol methyl ether (DPGME [CAS: 34590-94-8]): Mildly irritating to eyes upon direct contact. A CNS depressant at very high levels.	100 ppm, S			Colorless liquid with a mild etherlike odor. Nasal irritation is a good warning property. Vapor pressure is 0.3 mm Hg at 20 °C (68 °F). Combustible.
Diquat (1,1-ethylene-2,2'-dipyridinium dibromide, Reglone, Dextrone [CAS: 85-00-7]): Corrosive in high concentrations. Acute renal failure and reversible liver injury may occur. Chronic feeding studies caused cataracts in test animals. Although pulmonary edema might occur, unlike paraquat, pulmonary fibrosis has not been shown with human diquat exposures. See also p 245.	0.5 mg/m³ [proposed: 0.5 mg/m³ (total dust) 0.1 mg/m³ (respirable dust), S]		0 2 0	Yellow solid crystals. Appearance and some hazardous properties vary with the formulation.
Disulfiram (tetraethylthiuram disulfide, Antabuse [CAS: 97-77-8]): Inhibits aldehyde dehydrogenase, an enzyme involved in ethanol metabolism. Exposure to disulfiram and alcohol will produce flushing, headache, and hypotension. Disulfiram may also interact with other industrial solvents that share metabolic pathways with ethanol. Limited evidence for adverse effects on fetal development in test animals. See also p 155.	2 mg/m³			Crystalline solid. Thermal breakdown products include oxides of sulfur.
Disulfoton (*O,O*-diethyl-*S*-ethylmercapto-ethyl dithiophosphate) [CAS: 298-04-4]): An organophosphate-type cholinesterase inhibitor (see p 240). Dermally well absorbed.	0.1 mg/m³			Vapor pressure is 0.00018 mm Hg at 20 °C (68 °F). Thermal breakdown products include oxides of sulfur.
Divinylbenzene (DVB, vinylstyrene [CAS: 1321-74-0]): Mildly irritating upon direct contact. Vapors mildly irritating to eyes and respiratory tract.	10 ppm		2 2 2	Pale yellow liquid. Combustible. Must contain inhibitor to prevent explosive polymerization.

Chemical	Air concentration	ERPG	NFPA (H F R)	Comments
Emery (corundum, impure aluminum oxide [CAS: 112-62-9]): An abrasive, nuisance dust causing physical irritation to eyes, skin, and respiratory tract.	10 mg/m³			Solid crystals of aluminum oxide. Often used for its abrasive properties (eg, emery cloth, emery wheel).
Endosulfan [CAS: 115-29-7]: Inhalation and skin absorption are major routes of exposure. Symptoms include nausea, confusion, excitement, twitching, and convulsions. Animal studies suggest liver and kidney injury from very high exposures. Limited evidence for adverse effects on male reproduction and fetal development in animal studies. See also p 129.	0.1 mg/m³, S			Chlorinated hydrocarbon insecticide. Tan, waxy solid with a mild sulfur dioxide odor. Thermal breakdown products include oxides of sulfur and hydrogen chloride.
Endrin [CAS: 72-20-8]: Endrin is the stereoisomer of dieldrin, and its toxicity is very similar. Well absorbed through skin. Overexposure may produce headache, dizziness, nausea, confusion, twitching, and convulsions. Adverse effects on fetal development in test animals. See also p 129.	0.1 mg/m³, S			Colorless, white, or tan solid. A stereoisomer of dieldrin. A mild chemical odor and negligible vapor pressure of 0.0000002 mm Hg at 20 °C (68 °F). Not combustible. Thermal breakdown products include hydrogen chloride.
Epichlorohydrin (chloropropylene oxide) [CAS: 106-89-8]: Extremely irritating upon direct contact; severe burns may result. Vapors highly irritating to eyes and respiratory tract; pulmonary edema has been reported. Other effects include nausea, vomiting, and abdominal pain. Sensitization has been occasionally reported. Animal studies suggest a potential for liver and kidney injury. High doses reduce fertility in test animals. A carcinogen in test animals (IARC 2B).	2 ppm, S [proposed: 0.1 ppm, S, A2] NIOSH CA	ERPG-1: 2 ppm ERPG-2: 20 ppm ERPG-3: 100 ppm	3 2 2	Colorless liquid. The irritating, chloroformlike odor is detectable only at extremely high exposures and is a poor warning property. Vapor pressure is 13 mm Hg at 20 °C (68 °F). Flammable. Thermal breakdown products include hydrogen chloride and phosgene.
EPN (O-ethyl O-p-nitrophenyl phenylphosphonothioate [CAS: 2104-64-5]): An organophosphate-type cholinesterase inhibitor (see p 240).	0.5 mg/m³, S		...	Yellow solid or brown liquid. Vapor pressure is 0.0003 mm Hg at 100 °C (212 °F).

(C) = ceiling air concentration (TLV-C); S = skin absorption can be significant; A1 = ACGIH-confirmed human carcinogen; A2 = ACGIH-suspected human carcinogen; NFPA Hazard Codes: H = health, F = fire, R = reactivity, Ox = oxidizer, W = water-reactive, 0 (none) <—> 4 (severe). ERPG = Emergency Response Planning Guideline. See p 402 for explanation of definitions.

continued

TABLE IV–13. HEALTH HAZARD SUMMARIES FOR INDUSTRIAL AND OCCUPATIONAL CHEMICALS (Continued)

Health Hazard Summaries	ACGIH TLV	IDLH	NFPA Codes H F R	Comments
Ethanolamine (2-aminoethanol) [CAS: 141-43-5]: Highly irritating upon direct contact; severe burns may result. Prolonged contact with skin is irritating. Animal studies suggest that, at high levels, vapors are irritating to eyes and respiratory tract and liver and kidney injury may occur. Limited evidence for adverse effects on fetal development in animal studies.	3 ppm	1000 ppm	2 2 0	Colorless liquid. A mild ammonialike odor occurs at the TLV and is an adequate warning property. Vapor pressure is less than 1 mm Hg at 20 °C (68 °F). Combustible. Thermal breakdown products include oxides of nitrogen.
Ethion (phosphorodithioic acid [CAS: 563-12-2]): An organophosphate-type cholinesterase inhibitor (see p 240). Well absorbed dermally.	0.4 mg/m³, S			Colorless, odorless liquid when pure. Technical products have an objectionable odor. Vapor pressure is 0.000002 mm Hg at 20 °C (68 °F). Thermal breakdown products include oxides of sulfur.
2-Ethoxyethanol (ethylene glycol monoethyl ether, EGEE, Cellosolve [CAS: 110-80-5]): Mildly irritating on direct contact. Skin contact is a major route of absorption. Overexposures may reduce sperm counts in men. A potent teratogen in both rats and rabbits. Large doses cause lung, liver, testes, kidney, and spleen injury in test animals. See also p 163.	5 ppm, S	6000 ppm	2 2 0	OSHA is in the process of greatly lowering its permissible exposure limit (proposed value 0.1 ppm) to provide some protection against the reproductive toxicity of this agent. Colorless liquid. Very mild, sweet odor occurs only at very high levels and is a poor warning property. Vapor pressure is 4 mm Hg at 20 °C (68 °F).
2-Ethoxyethyl acetate (ethylene glycol monoethyl ether acetate, Cellosolve acetate [CAS: 111-15-9]): Mildly irritating upon direct contact. May produce CNS depression and kidney injury. Skin contact is a major route of absorption. Metabolized to 2-ethoxyethanol. Adverse effects on fertility and fetal development in animals. See also p 163.	5 ppm, S	2500 ppm	2 2 0	OSHA is in the process of greatly lowering its permissible exposure limit (proposed value 0.1 ppm) to provide some protection against the reproductive toxicity of this agent. Colorless liquid. Mild etherlike odor occurs at the TLV and is a good warning property. Flammable.
Ethyl acetate [CAS: 141-78-6]: Slightly irritating to eyes and skin. Vapors irritating to eyes and respiratory tract. A CNS depressant at very high levels. Metabolized to ethanol and acetic acid, so may have some of the fetotoxic potential of ethanol.	400 ppm	10,000 ppm	1 3 0	Colorless liquid. Fruity odor occurs at the TLV and is a good warning property. Vapor pressure is 76 mm Hg at 20 °C (68 °F). Flammable.

Chemical	TLV	ERPG	H	F	R	Comments
Ethyl acrylate (CAS: 140-88-5): Extremely irritating upon direct contact; severe burns may result. A skin sensitizer. Vapors highly irritating to eyes and respiratory tract. In animal tests, heart, liver, and kidney damage was observed at high doses. A carcinogen in test animals (IARC 2B).	5 ppm, A2	2000 ppm	2	3	2	Colorless liquid. Acrid odor occurs below the TLV and is a good warning property. Vapor pressure is 29.5 mm Hg at 20 °C (68 °F). Flammable. Contains an inhibitor to prevent dangerous self-polymerization.
Ethyl alcohol (alcohol, grain alcohol, ethanol, EtOH [CAS: 64-17-5]): At high levels, vapors irritating to eyes and respiratory tract. A CNS depressant at high levels of exposure. Strong evidence for adverse effects on fetal development in test animals and humans with chronic ingestion (fetal alcohol syndrome). See also p 160.	1000 ppm		0	3	0	Colorless liquid with a mild, sweet odor. Vapor pressure is 43 mm Hg at 20 °C (68 °F). Flammable.
Ethylamine (CAS: 75-04-7): Corrosive upon direct contact; severe burns may result. Vapors highly irritating to eyes, skin, and respiratory tract; delayed pulmonary edema may result. Animal studies suggest potential for liver and kidney injury at moderate doses.	10 ppm [proposed: 5 ppm]	4000 ppm	3	4	0	Colorless liquid or gas with an ammonialike odor. Highly flammable. Thermal breakdown products include oxides of nitrogen.
Ethyl amyl ketone (5-methyl-3-heptanone [CAS: 541-85-5]): Irritating to eyes upon direct contact. Vapors irritating to eyes and respiratory tract. A CNS depressant at high levels.	25 ppm					Colorless liquid with a strong, distinctive odor. Flammable.
Ethylbenzene (CAS: 100-41-4): Mildly irritating to eyes upon direct contact. May cause skin burns upon prolonged contact. Dermally well absorbed. Vapors irritating to eyes and respiratory tract. A CNS depressant at high levels of exposure.	100 ppm	2000 ppm	2	3	0	Colorless liquid. Aromatic odor and irritation occur at levels close to the TLV and are adequate warning properties. Vapor pressure is 7.1 mm Hg at 20 °C (68 °F). Flammable.
Ethyl bromide (CAS: 74-96-4): Irritating to skin upon direct contact. A CNS depressant at high levels, and may cause cardiac arrhythmias. Former use as an anesthetic agent was discontinued because of fatal liver, kidney, and myocardial injury. Evidence for carcinogenicity in test animals.	200 ppm [proposed: 5 ppm, S, A2]	3500 ppm	2	1	0	Colorless to yellow liquid. Etherlike odor detectable only at high, dangerous levels. Vapor pressure is 375 mm Hg at 20 °C (68 °F). Highly flammable. Thermal breakdown products include hydrogen bromide and bromine gas.

(C) = ceiling air concentration (TLV-C); S = skin absorption can be significant; A1 = ACGIH-confirmed human carcinogen; A2 = ACGIH-suspected human carcinogen; NFPA Hazard Codes: H = health, F = fire, R = reactivity, Ox = oxidizer, W = water-reactive, 0 (none) <—> 4 (severe). ERPG = Emergency Response Planning Guideline. See p 402 for explanation of definitions.

continued

TABLE IV–13. HEALTH HAZARD SUMMARIES FOR INDUSTRIAL AND OCCUPATIONAL CHEMICALS (Continued)

Health Hazard Summaries	ACGIH TLV	IDLH	NFPA Codes H F R			Comments
Ethyl butyl ketone (3-heptanone [CAS: 106-35-4]): Mildly irritating to eyes upon direct contact. Vapors irritating to eyes and respiratory tract. A CNS depressant at high levels.	50 ppm	3000 ppm	1	2	0	Colorless liquid. Fruity odor is a good warning property. Vapor pressure is 4 mm Hg at 20 °C (68 °F). Flammable.
Ethyl chloride (CAS: 75-00-3): Mildly irritating to eyes and respiratory tract. A CNS depressant at high levels; has caused cardiac arrhythmias at anesthetic doses. Animal studies suggest the kidneys and liver are target organs at high doses. Structurally similar to the carcinogenic chloroethanes.	1000 ppm	20,000 ppm	2	4	0	Colorless liquid or gas with a pungent, etherlike odor. Highly flammable. Thermal breakdown products include hydrogen chloride and phosgene.
Ethylene chlorohydrin (2-chloroethanol [CAS: 107-07-3]): Irritating to eyes upon direct contact. Skin contact is extremely hazardous because it is not irritating and absorption is rapid. Vapors irritating to eyes and respiratory tract; pulmonary edema has been reported. Systemic effects include CNS depression, myocardiopathy, shock, and liver and kidney damage.	1 ppm (C), S	10 ppm	3	2	0	Colorless liquid with a weak etherlike odor. Vapor pressure is 5 mm Hg at 20 °C (68 °F). Combustible. Thermal breakdown products include hydrogen chloride and phosgene.
Ethylenediamine (CAS: 107-15-3): Highly irritating upon direct contact; burns result. Respiratory and dermal sensitization may occur. Vapors irritating to eyes and respiratory tract. Animal studies suggest potential for kidney injury at high doses.	10 ppm	2000 ppm	3	2	0	Colorless viscous liquid or solid. Ammonialike odor occurs at the PEL and is an adequate warning property. Vapor pressure is 10 mm Hg at 20 °C (68 °F). Flammable. Thermal breakdown products include oxides of nitrogen.
Ethylene dibromide (1,2-dibromoethane, EDB [CAS: 106-93-4]): Highly irritating upon direct contact; severe burns result. Highly toxic by all routes. Vapors highly irritating to eyes and respiratory tract. Severe liver and kidney injury may occur. A CNS depressant. Adverse effects on the testes in test animals and, possibly, humans. A carcinogen in test animals (IARC 2A). See p 162.	S, A2 NIOSH CA	400 ppm	3	0	0	Colorless liquid or solid. Mild, sweet odor is a poor warning property. Vapor pressure is 11 mm Hg at 20 °C (68 °F). Not combustible. Thermal breakdown products include hydrogen bromide and bromine gas. Fumigant and chemical intermediate used in organic synthesis.

Substance	TLV	IDLH	H	F	R	Comments
Ethylene glycol (antifreeze [CAS: 107-21-1]): A CNS depressant. Metabolized to oxalic and other acids; severe acidosis may result. Precipitation of calcium oxalate crystals in tissues can cause extensive injury. Adversely affects fetal development in animal studies at very high doses. Not well absorbed dermally. See also p 163.	50 ppm (C)		1	1	0	Colorless viscous liquid. Odorless with a very low vapor pressure.
Ethylene glycol dinitrate (EGDN [CAS: 628-96-6]): Causes vasodilation similar to other nitrite compounds. Headache, hypotension, flushing, palpitation, delirium, and CNS depression may occur. Well absorbed by all routes. Tolerance and dependence may develop to vasodilatory effects; cessation after repeated exposures may cause angina pectoris. Weak inducer of methemoglobinemia (see p 217).	0.05 ppm, S	80 ppm				Yellow oily liquid. Vapor pressure is 0.05 mm Hg at 20 °C (68 °F). Explosive.
Ethyleneimine [CAS: 151-56-4]: Strong caustic. Highly irritating upon direct contact; severe burns may result. Vapors irritating to eyes and respiratory tract; delayed-onset pulmonary edema may occur. Overexposures have resulted in nausea, vomiting, headache, and dizziness. Well absorbed dermally. A carcinogen in animals.	0.5 ppm, S OSHA CA NIOSH CA		3	3	2	Colorless liquid with an aminelike odor. Vapor pressure is 160 mm Hg at 20 °C (68 °F). Flammable. Contains inhibitor to prevent explosive self-polymerization.
Ethylene oxide [CAS: 75-21-8]: Highly irritating upon direct contact. Vapors irritating to eyes and respiratory tract; delayed pulmonary edema has been reported. A CNS depressant at very high levels. Chronic overexposures can cause peripheral neuropathy and possible permanent CNS impairment. Adverse effects on fetal development and fertility in test animals and limited evidence in humans. A carcinogen in animal studies. Limited evidence of carcinogenicity in humans (IARC 2A). See also p 167.	1 ppm, A2 OSHA CA NIOSH CA	800 ppm	2	4	3	Colorless. Highly flammable. Etherlike odor is a poor warning property. Important source of exposures is sterilization operations in health care industry.
Ethyl ether (diethyl ether [CAS: 60-29-7]): Vapors irritating to eyes and respiratory tract. A CNS depressant and anesthetic agent; tolerance may develop to this effect. Overexposure produces nausea, headache, dizziness, anesthesia, and respiratory arrest. Evidence for adverse effects on fetal development in test animals.	400 ppm	19,000 ppm	2	4	1	Colorless liquid. Etherlike odor occurs at low levels and is a good warning property. Vapor pressure is 439 mm Hg at 20 °C (68 °F). Highly flammable.

continued

(C) = ceiling air concentration (TLV-C); S = skin absorption can be significant; A1 = ACGIH-confirmed human carcinogen; A2 = ACGIH-suspected human carcinogen; NFPA Hazard Codes: H = health, F = fire, R = reactivity, Ox = oxidizer, W = water-reactive, 0 (none) <—> 4 (severe). ERPG = Emergency Response Planning Guideline. See p 402 for explanation of definitions.

TABLE IV–13. HEALTH HAZARD SUMMARIES FOR INDUSTRIAL AND OCCUPATIONAL CHEMICALS (Continued)

Health Hazard Summaries	ACGIH TLV	IDLH	NFPA Codes H F R	Comments
Ethyl formate (CAS: 109-94-4): Slightly irritating to the skin upon direct contact. Vapors mildly irritating to eyes and upper respiratory tract. In test animals, very high levels caused rapid narcosis and pulmonary edema.	100 ppm	8000 ppm	2 3 0	Colorless liquid. Fruity odor and irritation occur near the TLV and are good warning properties. Vapor pressure is 194 mm Hg at 20 °C (68 °F). Highly flammable.
Ethyl mercaptan (ethanethiol [CAS: 75-08-1]): Vapors mildly irritating to eyes and respiratory tract. Respiratory paralysis and CNS depression at very high levels. Headache, nausea, and vomiting likely owing to strong odor.	0.5 ppm	2500 ppm	2 4 0	Colorless liquid. Penetrating, offensive, mercaptanlike odor. Vapor pressure is 442 mm Hg at 20 °C (68 °F).
N-Ethylmorpholine (CAS: 100-74-3): Irritating to eyes upon direct contact. Vapors irritating to eyes and respiratory tract. Workers exposed to levels near the TLV reported drowsiness and temporary visual disturbances, including corneal edema. Animal testing suggests potential for skin absorption.	5 ppm, S	2000 ppm	2 3 0	Colorless liquid with ammonialike odor. Vapor pressure is 5 mm Hg at 20 °C (68 °F). Flammable. Thermal breakdown products include oxides of nitrogen.
Ethyl silicate (tetraethyl orthosilicate, tetraethoxysilane [CAS: 78-10-4]): Irritating upon direct contact. Vapors irritating to eyes and respiratory tract. All human effects noted at vapor exposures above the odor threshold. In subchronic animal testing, high vapor levels produced liver, lung, and kidney damage, and delayed-onset pulmonary edema.	10 ppm	1000 ppm	2 2 0	Colorless liquid. Faint alcohollike odor and irritation are good warning properties. Vapor pressure is 2 mm Hg at 20 °C (68 °F). Flammable.
Fenamiphos (ethyl 3-methyl-4-(methylthio)-phenyl[1-methylethyl]phosphoramide [CAS: 22224-92-6]): An organophosphate-type cholinesterase inhibitor (see p 240). Well absorbed dermally.	0.1 mg/m³, S			Tan, waxy solid. Vapor pressure is 0.000001 mm Hg at 30 °C (86 °F).
Fensulfothion (O,O-diethyl O-[4-(methyl-sulfinyl)phenyl]phosphorothioate [CAS: 115-90-2]): An organophosphate-type cholinesterase inhibitor (see p 240).	0.1 mg/m³			Brown liquid.

Fenthion (O,O-dimethyl O-[3-methyl-4-(methylthio)phenyl] phosphorothioate [CAS: 55-38-9]): An organophosphate-type cholinesterase inhibitor (see p 240). Highly lipid soluble; toxicity may be prolonged. Dermal absorption is rapid.

0.2 mg/m³, S

Yellow to tan viscous liquid with a mild garliclike odor. Vapor pressure is 0.00003 mm Hg at 20 °C (68 °F).

Ferbam (ferric dimethyldithiocarbamate [CAS: 14484-64-1]): Thiocarbamates do not act through cholinesterase inhibition. Dusts irritating upon direct contact; causes dermatitis in persons sensitized to sulfur. Dusts are mild respiratory tract irritants. Limited evidence for adverse effects on fetal development in test animals.

10 mg/m³

Odorless, black solid. Vapor pressure is negligible at 20 °C (68 °F). Thermal breakdown products include oxides of nitrogen and sulfur. Used as a fungicide.

Ferrovanadium dust (CAS: 12604-58-9): Mild irritant of eyes and respiratory tract.

1 mg/m³

Odorless, dark-colored powders.

Fibrous glass dust: Human exposures have not clearly produced any effects other than dermatitis and respiratory irritation at high concentrations. Limited experimental and epidemiologic evidence for carcinogenicity.

10 mg/m³

Continuous fibers or woollike batts.

Fluoride dust (as fluoride): Irritating to eyes and respiratory tract. Workers exposed to levels 10 mg/m³ suffered nasal irritation and bleeding. Lower level exposures have produced nausea and eye and respiratory tract irritation. Chronic overexposures may result in skin rashes. Fluorosis, a bone disease with chronic high-level fluoride ingestion, is not associated with occupational dust inhalation. See also p 168.

2.5 mg/m³ (as F)

500 mg/m³

Appearance varies with the compound. Sodium fluoride is a colorless to blue solid.

Fluorine (CAS: 7782-41-4): Rapidly reacts with moisture to form ozone and hydrofluoric acid. The gas is a severe eye, skin, and respiratory tract irritant; severe penetrating burns and pulmonary edema have resulted. Systemic hypocalcemia can occur with fluorine or hydrogen fluoride exposure. See also p 180.

1 ppm

25 ppm

4 0 3
W
Ox

Pale yellow gas. Sharp odor is a poor warning property. Highly reactive; will ignite many oxidizable materials. Uses include rocket fuel oxidizer.

(C) = ceiling air concentration (TLV-C); S = skin absorption can be significant; A1 = ACGIH-confirmed human carcinogen; A2 = ACGIH-suspected human carcinogen; NFPA Hazard Codes: H = health, F = fire, R = reactivity, Ox = oxidizer, W = water-reactive, 0 (none) <—> 4 (severe), ERPG = Emergency Response Planning Guideline. See p 402 for explanation of definitions.

continued

TABLE IV–13. HEALTH HAZARD SUMMARIES FOR INDUSTRIAL AND OCCUPATIONAL CHEMICALS (Continued)

Health Hazard Summaries	ACGIH TLV	IDLH	NFPA Codes H	Comments
Fonofos (*O*-ethyl *S*-phenyl ethylphosphono-thiolothionate, Dyfonate [CAS: 944-22-9]): An organophosphate-type cholinesterase inhibitor (see p 240). Highly toxic; oral toxicity in test animals ranged from 3 to 13 mg/kg for rats, and rabbits died after eye instillation.	0.1 mg/m³, S			Vapor pressure is 0.00021 mm Hg at 20 °C (68 °F). Thermal breakdown products include oxides of sulfur.
Formaldehyde (formic aldehyde, methanal, HCHO, formalin [CAS: 50-00-0]): Highly irritating to eyes upon direct contact; severe burns result. Irritating to skin; may cause a sensitization dermatitis. Vapors highly irritating to eyes and respiratory tract. Sensitization may occur. A carcinogen in test animals (IARC 2A). See also p 174.	0.3 ppm (C), A2 OSHA CA NIOSH CA	30 ppm ERPG-1: 1 ppm ERPG-2: 10 ppm ERPG-3: 25 ppm	2 4 0 (gas) 2 2 0 (formalin)	Colorless gas with a suffocating odor. Combustible. Formalin (15% methanol) solutions are flammable.
Formamide (methanamide [CAS: 75-12-7]): In animal tests, mildly irritating upon direct contact. Adverse effects on fetal development in test animals at very high doses.	10 ppm, S		2 1	Clear, viscous liquid. Odorless. Vapor pressure is 2 mm Hg at 70 °C (158 °F). Combustible. Thermal breakdown products include oxides of nitrogen.
Formic acid (CAS: 64-18-6): Acid is corrosive; severe burns may result from contact of eyes and skin with concentrated acid. Vapors highly irritating to eyes and respiratory tract. Ingestion may produce severe metabolic acidosis and blindness (see methanol, p 215).	5 ppm	100 ppm	3 2 0	Colorless liquid. Pungent odor and irritation occur near the TLV and are adequate warning properties. Vapor pressure is 30 mm Hg at 20 °C (68 °F). Combustible.
Furfural (bran oil [CAS: 98-01-1]): Highly irritating upon direct contact; burns may result. Vapors highly irritating to eyes and respiratory tract; pulmonary edema may result. Animal studies indicate the liver is a target organ. Hyperreflexia and convulsions occur at large doses in test animals.	2 ppm, S	250 ppm	2 2 0	Colorless to light brown liquid. Almondlike odor occurs below the TLV and is a good warning property. Vapor pressure is 2 mm Hg at 20 °C (68 °F). Combustible. Thermal breakdown products include oxides of nitrogen.
Furfuryl alcohol (CAS: 98-00-0): Dermal absorption occurs. Vapors irritating to eyes and respiratory tract. A CNS depressant at high air levels.	10 ppm, S	250 ppm	1 2 1	Clear, colorless liquid. Upon exposure to light and air, changes color to red or brown. Vapor pressure is 0.53 mm Hg at 20 °C (68 °F). Combustible.

Gasoline (CAS: 8006-61-9): Although exact composition varies, the acute toxicity of all gasolines is similar. Vapors irritating to eyes and respiratory tract at high levels. A CNS depressant; symptoms include incoordination, dizziness, headaches, and nausea. Benzene (generally < 1%) is one significant chronic health hazard. Other additives such as ethylene dibromide and tetraethyl and tetramethyl lead are present in low amounts and may be absorbed through the skin. Very limited evidence for carcinogenicity in test animals. See also p 178 — 300 ppm — Clear to amber liquid with a characteristic odor. Highly flammable. Gasoline is sometimes inappropriately used as a solvent. Substance abuse via inhalation has been reported.

Germanium tetrahydride (CAS: 7782-65-2): A hemolytic agent with effects similar to but less potent than arsine in animals. Symptoms include abdominal pain, hematuria, anemia, and jaundice. — 0.2 ppm — Colorless gas. Highly flammable.

Glutaraldehyde (1,5-pentandial (CAS: 111-30-8)): The purity and therefore the toxicity of glutaraldehyde varies widely. Allergic dermatitis may occur. Highly irritating on contact; severe burns may result. Vapors highly irritating to eyes and respiratory tract; respiratory sensitization may occur. In animal studies, the liver is a target organ at high doses. — 0.2 ppm (C) — Colorless solid crystals. Vapor pressure is 0.0152 mm Hg at 20 °C (68 °F). Can undergo hazardous self-polymerization. Commonly used as a sterilizing agent in medical settings.

Glycidol (2,3-epoxy-1-propanol (CAS: 556-52-5)): Highly irritating to eyes on contact; burns may result. Moderately irritating to skin and respiratory tract. Evidence for carcinogenicity and testicular toxicity in test animals. — 25 ppm — 500 ppm — Colorless liquid. Vapor pressure is 0.9 mm Hg at 25 °C (77 °F). Combustible.

Hafnium (CAS: 7440-58-6): Based on animal studies, dusts are mildly irritating to eyes and skin. Liver injury may occur at very high doses. — 0.5 mg/m³ — 250 mg/m³ — The metal is a gray solid. Other compounds vary in appearance.

Heptachlor (CAS: 76-44-8): CNS convulsant. Skin absorption is rapid and has caused convulsions and death. Hepatotoxic. Stored in fatty tissues. Limited evidence for adverse effects on fetal development in test animals at high doses. See also p 129. — 0.5 mg/m³, S [proposed: 0.05 mg/m³, S, A2] — 100 mg/m³ — White or light tan, waxy solid with a camphorlike odor. Vapor pressure is 0.0003 mm Hg at 20 °C (68 °F). Thermal breakdown products include hydrogen chloride. Not combustible.

(C) = ceiling air concentration (TLV-C); S = skin absorption can be significant; A1 = ACGIH-confirmed human carcinogen; A2 = ACGIH-suspected human carcinogen; NFPA Hazard Codes: H = health, F = fire, R = reactivity, Ox = oxidizer, W = water-reactive, 0 (none) <—> 4 (severe). ERPG = Emergency Response Planning Guideline. See p 402 for explanation of definitions.

continued

TABLE IV-13. HEALTH HAZARD SUMMARIES FOR INDUSTRIAL AND OCCUPATIONAL CHEMICALS (Continued)

Health Hazard Summaries	ACGIH TLV	IDLH	NFPA Codes H F R	Comments
n-Heptane (CAS: 142-82-5): Vapors only slightly irritating to eyes and respiratory tract. May cause euphoria, vertigo, CNS depression, and cardiac arrhythmias at high levels.	400 ppm	5000 ppm	1 3 0	Colorless clear liquid. Mild gasolinelike odor occurs below the TLV and is a good warning property. Vapor pressure is 40 mm Hg at 20 °C (68 °F). Flammable.
Hexachlorobutadiene (CAS: 87-68-3): Based on animal studies, rapid dermal absorption is expected. The kidney is the major target organ. A carcinogen in test animals (IARC 3).	0.02 ppm, S, A2	ERPG-1: 3 ppm ERPG-2: 10 ppm ERPG-3: 30 ppm	2 1 1	Heavy, colorless liquid. Thermal breakdown products include hydrogen chloride and phosgene.
Hexachlorocyclopentadiene (CAS: 77-47-4): Vapors extremely irritating to eyes and respiratory tract; lacrimation, salivation. In animal studies, a potent kidney and liver toxin. At higher levels the brain, heart, and adrenal glands were affected. Tremors occurred at high doses.	0.01 ppm			Yellow to amber liquid with a pungent odor. Vapor pressure is 0.08 mm Hg at 20 °C (68 °F). Not combustible.
Hexachloroethane (perchloroethane) (CAS: 67-72-1): Hot fumes irritating to eyes, skin, and mucous membranes. Based on animal studies, causes CNS depression and kidney and liver injury at high doses. Limited evidence of carcinogenicity in test animals (IARC 3).	1 ppm, S, A2 NIOSH CA	300 ppm		White solid with a camphorlike odor. Vapor pressure is 0.22 mm Hg at 20 °C (68 °F). Not combustible. Thermal breakdown products include phosgene, chlorine gas, and hydrogen chloride.
Hexachloronaphthalene (Halowax 1014 [CAS: 1335-87-1]): Based on workplace experience, a potent toxin causing severe chloracne and severe, occasionally fatal, liver injury. Skin absorption can occur.	0.2 mg/m³, S	2 mg/m³		Light yellow solid with an aromatic odor. Vapor pressure is less than 1 mm Hg at 20 °C (68 °F). Not combustible.
Hexamethylphosphoramide (CAS: 680-31-9): Low-level exposures produced nasal cavity cancer in rats (IARC 2B). Adverse effects on the testes in test animals.	S, A2			Colorless liquid with an aromatic odor. Vapor pressure is 0.07 mm Hg at 20 °C (68 °F). Thermal breakdown products include oxides of nitrogen.

Substance	TLV	H	F	R	Comments
n-Hexane (normal hexane [CAS: 110-54-3]): Vapors mildly irritating to eyes and respiratory tract. A CNS depressant at high levels, producing headache, dizziness, and gastrointestinal upset. Occupational overexposures have resulted in peripheral neuropathies. Methyl ethyl ketone potentiates this toxicity. Testicular toxicity in animal studies.	50 ppm	1	3	0	Colorless, clear liquid with a mild gasoline odor. Vapor pressure is 124 mm Hg at 20 °C (68 °F). Highly flammable.
Hexane isomers (other than n-hexane, isohexane, 2,3-dimethylbutane): Vapors mildly irritating to eyes and respiratory tract. A CNS depressant at high levels, producing headache, dizziness, and gastrointestinal upset.	500 ppm				Colorless liquids with a mild petroleum odor. Vapor pressures are high at 20 °C (68 °F). Highly flammable.
sec-Hexyl acetate (1,3-dimethylbutyl acetate [CAS: 108-84-9]): At low levels, vapors irritating to eyes and respiratory tract. Based on animal studies, a CNS depressant at high levels.	50 ppm	1	2	0	Colorless liquid. Unpleasant fruity odor and irritation are both good warning properties. Vapor pressure is 4 mm Hg at 20 °C (68 °F). Flammable.
Hexylene glycol (2-methyl-2,4-pentanediol [CAS: 107-41-5]): Irritating upon direct contact; vapors irritating to eyes and respiratory tract. A CNS depressant at very high doses in animal studies.	25 ppm (C)	1	1	0	Liquid with a faint sweet odor. Vapor pressure is 0.05 mm Hg at 20 °C (68 °F). Combustible.
Hydrazine (diamine [CAS: 302-01-2]): Corrosive upon direct contact; severe burns result. Vapors extremely irritating to eyes and respiratory tract; pulmonary edema may occur. Highly hepatotoxic. A convulsant and hemolytic agent. Kidneys are also target organs. Well absorbed by all routes. A carcinogen in test animals (IARC 2B).	0.1 ppm, S, A2 [proposed: 0.01 ppm, S, A2] NIOSH CA	3	3	2 (vapors explosive)	Colorless, fuming, viscous liquid with an amine odor. Vapor pressure is 10 mm Hg at 20 °C (68 °F). Flammable. Thermal breakdown products include oxides of nitrogen. Used as rocket fuel.
Hydrogen bromide (HBr [CAS: 10035-10-6]): Direct contact with concentrated solutions may cause corrosive acid burns. Vapors highly irritating to eyes and respiratory tract; pulmonary edema may result.	3 ppm (C)	3	0	0	Colorless gas or pressurized liquid. Acrid odor and irritation occur near the TLV and are adequate warning properties. Not combustible.
Hydrogen chloride (muriatic acid, HCl [CAS: 7647-01-0]): Direct contact with concentrated solutions may cause corrosive acid burns. Vapors highly irritating to eyes and respiratory tract; pulmonary edema has resulted.	5 ppm (C) ERPG-1: 3 ppm ERPG-2: 20 ppm ERPG-3: 100 ppm	3	0	0	Colorless gas with a pungent, choking odor. Irritation occurs near the TLV and is a good warning property. Not combustible.

continued

(C) = ceiling air concentration (TLV-C); S = skin absorption can be significant; A1 = ACGIH-confirmed human carcinogen; A2 = ACGIH-suspected human carcinogen; NFPA Hazard Codes: H = health, F = fire, R = reactivity, Ox = oxidizer, W = water-reactive, 0 (none) <—> 4 (severe). ERPG = Emergency Response Planning Guideline. See p 402 for explanation of definitions.

TABLE IV–13. HEALTH HAZARD SUMMARIES FOR INDUSTRIAL AND OCCUPATIONAL CHEMICALS (Continued)

Health Hazard Summaries	ACGIH TLV	IDLH	NFPA Codes H	Comments
Hydrogen cyanide (hydrocyanic acid, prussic acid, HCN [CAS: 74-90-8]): A rapidly acting, potent metabolic asphyxiant that inhibits cytochrome oxidase and stops cellular respiration. See also p 145.	10 ppm (C), S	50 mg/m³	4 4 2 (vapors extremely toxic)	Colorless to pale blue liquid or colorless gas with a sweet, bitter almond smell that is an inadequate warning property even for those sensitive to it. Vapor pressure is 620 mm Hg at 20 °C (68 °F). Cyanide salts will release HCN gas with exposure to acids or heat.
Hydrogen fluoride (hydrofluoric acid, HF [CAS: 7664-39-3]): Produces severe, penetrating burns to eyes, skin, and deeper tissues upon direct contact with solutions. Onset of pain and erythema may be delayed as much as 12–16 hours. As a gas, highly irritating to the eyes and respiratory tract; pulmonary edema has resulted. Severe hypocalcemia may occur with overexposure. See p 180.	3 ppm (C) (as F)	30 ppm ERPG-1: 5 ppm ERPG-2: 20 ppm ERPG-3: 50 ppm	4 0 0	Colorless fuming liquid or gas. Irritation occurs at levels below the TLV and is an adequate warning property. Vapor pressure is 760 mm Hg at 20 °C (68 °F). Not combustible. Commercial rust-removing products may contain HF, but generally at lower concentrations (< 10%).
Hydrogen peroxide (CAS: 7722-84-1): A strong oxidizing agent. Direct contact with concentrated solutions can produce severe eye damage and skin irritation, including erythema and vesicle formation. Vapors irritating to eyes, skin, mucous membranes, and respiratory tract.	1 ppm	75 ppm	2 0 3 (52% or greater) 2 0 1 (35–52%)	Colorless liquid with a slightly sharp, distinctive odor. Vapor pressure is 5 mm Hg at 30 °C (86 °F). Because of instability, usually found in aqueous solutions. Not combustible but a very powerful oxidizing agent.
Hydrogen selenide (CAS: 7783-07-5): Vapors extremely irritating to eyes and respiratory tract. Systemic symptoms from low-level exposure include nausea and vomiting, fatigue, metallic taste in mouth, and a garlicky breath odor. Animal studies indicate hepatotoxicity.	0.05 ppm	2 ppm	2 0 1	Colorless gas. The strongly offensive odor and irritation occur only at levels far above the TLV and are poor warning properties. Flammable. Water-reactive.
Hydrogen sulfide (sewer gas [CAS: 7783-06-4]): Vapors irritating to eyes and respiratory tract. At higher levels, a potent, rapid systemic toxin causing cellular asphyxia and death. Systemic effects of low-level exposure include headache, cough, nausea, and vomiting. See also p 182.	10 ppm	300 ppm ERPG-1: 0.1 ppm ERPG-2: 30 ppm ERPG-3: 100 ppm	3 4 0	Colorless gas. Although the strong rotten egg odor can be detected at very low levels, olfactory fatigue occurs. Odor is therefore a poor warning property. Flammable. Produced by the decay of organic material as may occur in sewers, manure pits, and fish processing. Fossil fuel production also may generate the gas.

Substance	TLV		H	F	R	Comments
Hydroquinone (1,4-dihydroxybenzene) [CAS: 123-31-9]): Highly irritating to eyes upon direct contact. Chronic occupational exposures may cause partial discoloration and opacification of the cornea. Systemic effects reported result from ingestion and include tinnitus, headache, dizziness, gastrointestinal upset, CNS excitation, and skin depigmentation. May cause methemoglobinemia (see p 217). Limited evidence of carcinogenicity in test animals.	2 mg/m³	200 mg/m³	2	1	0	White solid crystals. Vapor pressure is less than 0.001 mm Hg at 20 °C (68 °F). Combustible.
2-Hydroxypropyl acrylate (HPA [CAS: 999-61-1]): Highly irritating upon direct contact; severe burns may result. Vapors highly irritating to eyes and respiratory tract. Based on structural analogies, compounds containing the acrylate moiety may be carcinogens.	0.5 ppm, S		3	1	1	Combustible liquid.
Indene (CAS: 95-13-6): Repeated direct contact with the skin produced a dry dermatitis but no systemic effects. Vapors likely irritating to eyes and respiratory tract. Based on animal studies, high air levels may cause liver and kidney damage.	10 ppm					Colorless liquid.
Indium (CAS: 7440-74-6): Based on animal studies, the soluble salts are extremely irritating to eyes upon direct contact. Dusts irritating to eyes and respiratory tract. In animal studies, indium compounds are highly toxic parenterally but much less toxic orally.	0.1 mg/m³					Appearance varies with the compound. The elemental metal is a silver-white lustrous solid.
Iodine (CAS: 7553-56-2): Extremely irritating upon direct contact; severe burns result. Vapors extremely irritating and corrosive to eyes and respiratory tract. Rarely, a skin sensitizer. Medicinal use of iodine-containing drugs has been associated with fetal goiter, a potentially life-threatening condition for the fetus or infant. Iodine causes adverse effects on fetal development in test animals. See also p 187.	0.1 ppm (C)	10 ppm				Violet-colored solid crystals. Sharp, characteristic odor is a poor warning property. Vapor pressure is 0.3 mm Hg at 20 °C (68 °F). Not combustible.
Iron oxide fume (CAS: 1309-37-1): Fumes and dusts can produce a benign pneumoconiosis (siderosis) with shadows on chest radiographs.	5 mg/m³ (as Fe)					Red-brown fume with a metallic taste. Vapor pressure is negligible at 20 °C (68 °F).

(C) = ceiling air concentration (TLV-C); S = skin absorption can be significant; A1 = ACGIH-confirmed human carcinogen; A2 = ACGIH-suspected human carcinogen; NFPA Hazard Codes: H = health, F = fire, R = reactivity, Ox = oxidizer, W = water-reactive, 0 (none) <—> 4 (severe). ERPG = Emergency Response Planning Guideline. See p 402 for explanation of definitions.

continued

TABLE IV–13. HEALTH HAZARD SUMMARIES FOR INDUSTRIAL AND OCCUPATIONAL CHEMICALS (Continued)

Health Hazard Summaries	ACGIH TLV	IDLH	NFPA Codes H	Comments
Iron pentacarbonyl (iron carbonyl) [CAS: 13463-40-6]): Acute toxicity resembles that of nickel carbonyl. Inhalation of vapors can cause lung and systemic injury without warning signs. Symptoms of overexposure include headache, nausea and vomiting, and dizziness. Symptoms of severe poisoning are fever, extreme weakness, and pulmonary edema; effects may be delayed for up to 36 hours.	0.1 ppm			Colorless to yellow viscous liquid. Vapor pressure is 40 mm Hg at 30.3 °C (86.5 °F). Highly flammable.
Isoamyl acetate (banana oil, 3-methyl butyl acetate [CAS: 123-92-2]): May be irritating to skin upon prolonged contact. Vapors mildly irritating to eyes and respiratory tract. Symptoms in men exposed to 950 ppm for 0.5 hour included headache, weakness, dyspnea, and irritation of the nose and throat. A CNS depressant at high doses in test animals.	100 ppm	3000 ppm	1 3 0	Colorless liquid. Bananalike odor and irritation occur at low levels and are good warning properties. Vapor pressure is 4 mm Hg at 20 °C (68 °F). Flammable.
Isoamyl alcohol (3-methyl-1-butanol [CAS: 123-51-3]): Vapors irritating to eyes and respiratory tract. A CNS depressant at high levels.	100 ppm	8000 ppm	1 2 0	Colorless liquid. Irritating alcohollike odor and irritation are good warning properties. Vapor pressure is 2 mm Hg at 20 °C (68 °F). Flammable.
Isobutyl acetate (2-methylpropyl acetate [CAS: 110-19-0]): Vapors mildly irritating to eyes and respiratory tract. A CNS depressant at high levels.	150 ppm	7500 ppm	1 3 0	Colorless liquid. Pleasant fruity odor is a good warning property. Vapor pressure is 13 mm Hg at 20 °C (68 °F). Flammable.
Isobutyl alcohol (2-methyl-1-propanol [CAS: 78-83-1]): A CNS depressant at high levels.	50 ppm	8000 ppm	1 3 0	Colorless liquid. Mild characteristic odor is a good warning property. Vapor pressure is 9 mm Hg at 20 °C (68 °F). Flammable.
Isophorone (trimethylcyclohexenone [CAS: 78-59-1]): Vapors irritating to eyes and respiratory tract. Workers exposed to 5–8 ppm complained of fatigue and malaise after 1 month. Higher exposures result in nausea, headache, dizziness, and a feeling of suffocation at 200–400 ppm.	5 ppm (C)	800 ppm	2 2 0	Colorless liquid with a camphorlike odor. Vapor pressure is 0.2 mm Hg at 20 °C (68 °F). Flammable.

Name / Toxicology	TLV	H	F	R	ERPG	Comments
Isophorone diisocyanate (CAS: 4098-71-9): Based on animal studies, extremely irritating upon direct contact; severe burns may result. By analogy with other isocyanates, vapors or mists likely to be potent respiratory sensitizers, causing asthma. See also p 191.	0.005 ppm					Colorless to pale yellow liquid. Vapor pressure is 0.0003 mm Hg at 20 °C (68 °F). Possible thermal breakdown products include oxides of nitrogen and hydrogen cyanide.
2-Isopropoxyethanol (isopropyl Cellosolve, ethylene glycol monoisopropyl ether [CAS: 109-59-1]): Defatting agent causing dermatitis. May cause hemolysis.	25 ppm					Clear colorless liquid with a characteristic odor.
Isopropyl acetate (CAS: 108-21-4): Vapors irritating to the eyes and respiratory tract. A weak CNS depressant.	250 ppm	1	3	0	16,000 ppm	Colorless liquid. Fruity odor and irritation are good warning properties. Vapor pressure is 43 mm Hg at 20 °C (68 °F). Flammable.
Isopropyl alcohol (isopropanol, 2-propanol [CAS: 67-63-0]): Vapors produce mild eye and respiratory tract irritation. High exposures can produce CNS depression. See also p 193.	400 ppm	1	3	0	12,000 ppm	Rubbing alcohol. Sharp odor and irritation are adequate warning properties. Vapor pressure is 33 mm Hg at 20 °C (68 °F). Flammable.
Isopropylamine (2-aminopropane [CAS: 75-31-0]): Corrosive upon direct contact; severe burns may result. Vapors highly irritating to the eyes and respiratory tract. Exposure to vapors can cause transient corneal edema.	5 ppm	3	4	0	4000 ppm	Colorless liquid. Strong ammonia odor and irritation are good warning properties. Vapor pressure is 478 mm Hg at 20 °C (68 °F). Highly flammable. Thermal breakdown products include oxides of nitrogen.
Isopropyl ether (diisopropyl ether [CAS: 108-20-3]): A skin irritant upon prolonged contact with liquid. Vapors mildly irritating to the eyes and respiratory tract. A CNS depressant.	250 ppm	2	3	1	10,000 ppm	Colorless liquid. Offensive and sharp etherlike odor and irritation are good warning properties. Vapor pressure is 119 mm Hg at 20 °C (68 °F). Highly flammable. Contact with air causes formation of explosive peroxides.
Isopropyl glycidyl ether (CAS: 4016-14-2): Irritating upon direct contact. Allergic dermatitis may occur. Vapors irritating to eyes and respiratory tract. In animals, a CNS depressant at high oral doses; chronic exposures produced liver injury. Some glycidyl ethers possess hematopoietic and testicular toxicity.	50 ppm					Flammable. Vapor pressure is 9.4 mm Hg at 25 °C (77 °F).

(C) = ceiling air concentration (TLV-C); S = skin absorption can be significant; A1 = ACGIH-confirmed human carcinogen; A2 = ACGIH-suspected human carcinogen; NFPA Hazard Codes: H = health, F = fire, R = reactivity, Ox = oxidizer, W = water-reactive, 0 (none), <—> 4 (severe). ERPG = Emergency Response Planning Guideline. See p 402 for explanation of definitions.

continued

TABLE IV-13. HEALTH HAZARD SUMMARIES FOR INDUSTRIAL AND OCCUPATIONAL CHEMICALS (Continued)

Health Hazard Summaries	ACGIH TLV	IDLH	NFPA Codes H	Comments
Kepone (chlordecone [CAS: 143-50-0]): Neurotoxin; overexposure causes slurred speech, memory impairment, incoordination, weakness, tremor, and convulsions. Causes infertility in males. Hepatotoxic. Well absorbed by all routes. A carcinogen in test animals. See also p 129.	NIOSH CA			A solid.
Ketene (ethenone [CAS: 463-51-4]): Vapors extremely irritating to the eyes and respiratory tract; pulmonary edema may result and can be delayed for up to 72 hours. Toxicity similar to that of phosgene (see p 256), of which it is the nonchlorinated analog, in both magnitude and time course.	0.5 ppm	25 ppm		Colorless gas with a sharp odor. Polymerizes readily. Acetylating agent. Water-reactive.
Lead (inorganic compounds, dusts, and fumes): Toxic to CNS and peripheral nerves, kidneys, and hematopoietic system. Toxicity may result from acute or chronic exposures. Inhalation and ingestion are the major routes of absorption. Symptoms and signs include abdominal pain, anemia, mood or personality changes, and peripheral neuropathy. Encephalopathy may develop with high blood levels. Adversely affects reproductive functions in men and women. Adverse effects on fetal development in test animals. Some inorganic lead compounds are carcinogenic in animal studies (IARC 2B). See also p 196.	0.15 ppm			The elemental metal is dark gray. Vapor pressure is low, about 2 mm Hg at 1000 °C (1832 °F). Major industrial sources include smelting, battery manufacture, radiator repair, and glass and ceramic processing.
Lead arsenate (CAS: 10102-48-4): Most common acute poisoning symptoms are caused by arsenic, with lead being responsible for chronic toxicity. Symptoms include abdominal pain, headache, vomiting, diarrhea, nausea, itching, and lethargy. Liver and kidney damage may also occur. See both lead and arsenic, pp 196 and 87.	0.15 mg/m³	300 mg/m³	2 0 0	White powder often dyed pink. Not combustible.

Substance	TLV / air conc.		NFPA Hazard Codes (H F R)	Comments
Lead chromate (chrome yellow) [CAS: 7758-97-6]: Toxicity may result from both the chromium and the lead components. Lead chromate is a suspect human carcinogen owing to the carcinogenicity of hexavalent chromium and inorganic lead compounds. See both lead and hexavalent chromium, pp 196 and 135.	0.05 mg/m³ (as Pb) 0.012 mg/m³ (as Cr), A2			Yellow pigment in powder or crystal form.
Lindane (gamma-hexachlorocyclohexane) [CAS: 58-89-9]: A CNS stimulant and convulsant. Vapors irritating to the eyes and mucous membranes and produce severe headaches and nausea. Well absorbed by all routes. Animal feeding studies have resulted in lung, liver, and kidney damage. May injure bone marrow. Equivocal evidence of carcinogenicity in test animals. See also p 129.	0.5 mg/m³, S	1000 mg/m³	2 1 0 (solution) 2 0 0 (solid)	White crystalline substance with a musty odor if impure. Not combustible. Vapor is 0.0000094 mm Hg at 20 °C (68 °F). Although an agricultural chemical, lindane is more commonly found as a pediculocide in dilute solution (Kwell®).
Lithium hydride [CAS: 7580-67-8]: Strong vesicant and alkaline corrosive. Extremely irritating upon direct contact; severe burns result. Dusts extremely irritating to eyes and respiratory tract; pulmonary edema may develop. Symptoms of systemic toxicity include nausea, tremors, confusion, blurring of vision, and coma.	0.025 mg/m³	50 mg/m³	3 4 2 W	Off-white, translucent solid powder that darkens on exposure. Odorless. Very water-reactive, yielding highly flammable hydrogen gas and caustic lithium hydroxide. Finely dispersed powder may ignite spontaneously.
LPG (liquified petroleum gas [CAS: 68476-85-7]): A simple asphyxiant and possible CNS depressant. Flammability dangers greatly outweigh toxicity concerns. See also hydrocarbons, p 178.	1000 ppm	19,000 ppm		Colorless gas. An odorant is usually added as the pure product is odorless. Highly flammable.
Magnesium oxide fume (CAS: 1309-48-4): Slightly irritating to eyes and upper respiratory tract. May cause syndrome like metal fume fever (see p 214).	10 mg/m³			White fume.
Malathion (O,O-dimethyl dithiophosphate of diethyl mercaptosuccinate [CAS: 121-75-5]): An organophosphate-type cholinesterase inhibitor (see p 240). May cause skin sensitization. Absorbed dermally.	10 mg/m³, S	5000 mg/m³		Colorless to brown liquid with mild skunklike odor. Vapor pressure is 0.00004 mm Hg at 20 °C (68 °F). Thermal breakdown products include oxides of sulfur and phosphorus.

(C) = ceiling air concentration (TLV-C); S = skin absorption can be significant; A1 = ACGIH-confirmed human carcinogen; A2 = ACGIH-suspected human carcinogen; NFPA Hazard Codes: H = health, F = fire, R = reactivity, Ox = oxidizer, W = water-reactive, 0 (none) <—> 4 (severe); ERPG = Emergency Response Planning Guideline. See p 402 for explanation of definitions.

continued

TABLE IV–13. HEALTH HAZARD SUMMARIES FOR INDUSTRIAL AND OCCUPATIONAL CHEMICALS (Continued)

Health Hazard Summaries	ACGIH TLV	IDLH	NFPA Codes H	F	R	Comments
Maleic anhydride (2,5-furandione [CAS: 108-31-6]): Extremely irritating upon direct contact; severe burns may result. Vapors and mists extremely irritating to eyes, skin, and respiratory tract. A skin and respiratory tract sensitizer (asthma).	0.25 ppm		3	1	1	Colorless to white solid. Strong, penetrating odor. Eye irritation occurs at the TLV and is an adequate warning property. Vapor pressure is 0.16 mm Hg at 20 °C (68 °F). Combustible.
Manganese (CAS: 7439-96-5): Chronic overexposure results in a CNS toxicity manifested as psychosis which may be followed by a progressive toxicity similar to parkinsonism (Manganism). See also p 208.	5 mg/m³ (C) (dusts and compounds, as Mn) 1 mg/m³ (fume, as Mn) [proposed: 0.2 mg/m³ (elemental and inorganic compounds, as Mn)]	10,000 mg/m³				Elemental metal is a gray, hard, brittle solid. Other compounds vary in appearance. Exposure occurs in mining and milling of the metal, in ferromanganese steel production, and through electric arc welding.
Mercury (quicksilver [CAS: 7439-97-6]): Acute exposures to high vapor levels reported to cause toxic pneumonitis and pulmonary edema. Well absorbed by inhalation. Skin contact can produce irritation and sensitization dermatitis. Mercury salts but not metallic mercury are primarily toxic to the kidneys by acute ingestion. High acute or chronic overexposures can result in CNS toxicity (erythrism), chronic renal disease, brain injury, and peripheral neuropathies. Some inorganic mercury compounds have adverse effects on fetal development in test animals. See also p 210.	0.05 mg/m³ (metal), S 0.1 mg/m³ (aryl and inorganic compounds as Hg), S	10 mg/m³				Elemental metal is a dense, silvery liquid. Odorless. Vapor pressure is 0.0012 mm Hg at 20 °C (68 °F). Sources of exposure include small-scale gold refining operations by hobbyists and mercury-containing instruments.

Name / Description	TLV	ERPG	H	F	R	Properties
Mercury, alkyl compounds (dimethylmercury, diethyl mercury, ethylmercuric chloride, phenylmercuric acetate): Irritating upon direct contact; some compounds may cause burns. Well absorbed by all routes. Slow excretion may allow accumulation to occur. Readily crosses blood–brain barrier and placenta. High acute or chronic overexposures can cause kidney damage, organic brain disease, and peripheral neuropathy. Methylmercury is teratogenic in humans. See also p 210.	0.01 mg/m³ (alkyl compounds, as Hg), S	10 mg/m³				Colorless liquids or solids. Many alkyl compounds have a disagreeable odor. Inorganic mercury can be converted to alkyl mercury compounds in the environment. Phenylmercuric acetate until recently was used as a fungicide in paints.
Mesityl oxide (4-methyl-3-penten-2-one [CAS: 141-79-7]): Causes dermatitis upon prolonged contact. Vapors very irritating to eyes and respiratory tract. Based on animal tests, a CNS depressant and injures kidney and liver at high levels.	15 ppm	5000 ppm	3	3	0	Colorless viscous liquid with a peppermintlike odor. Irritation is an adequate warning property. Vapor pressure is 8 mm Hg at 20 °C (68 °F). Flammable. Readily forms peroxides.
Methacrylic acid (2-methylpropenoic acid [CAS: 79-41-4]): Corrosive upon direct contact; severe burns result. Vapors highly irritating to eyes and, possibly, respiratory tract. Based on structural analogies, compounds containing the acrylate moiety may be carcinogens.	20 ppm		3	2	2	Liquid with an acrid, disagreeable odor. Vapor pressure is less than 0.1 mm Hg at 20 °C (68 °F). Combustible. Polymerizes above 15 °C (59 °F), emitting toxic gases.
Methomyl (S-methyl N ((methylcarbamoyl)oxy] thioacetimidate, Lannate, Nudrin [CAS: 16752-77-5]): A carbamate-type cholinesterase inhibitor (see p 118).	2.5 mg/m³					A slight sulfur odor. Vapor pressure is 0.00005 mm Hg at 20 °C (68 °F). Thermal breakdown products include oxides of nitrogen and sulfur.
Methoxychlor (dimethoxy-DDT, 2,2-bis(p-methoxyphenol)-1,1,1-trichloroethane [CAS: 72-43-5]): A convulsant at very high doses in test animals. Limited evidence for adverse effects on male reproduction and fetal development in test animals at high doses. See also p 129.	10 mg/m³	7500 mg/m³				Colorless to tan solid with a mild fruity odor. Appearance and some hazardous properties vary with the formulation. Vapor pressure is very low at 20 °C (68 °F).

(C) = ceiling air concentration (TLV-C); S = skin absorption can be significant; A1 = ACGIH-confirmed human carcinogen; A2 = ACGIH-suspected human carcinogen; NFPA Hazard Codes: H = health, F = fire, R = reactivity, Ox = oxidizer, W = water-reactive. 0 (none) <—> 4 (severe). ERPG = Emergency Response Planning Guideline. See p 402 for explanation of definitions.

continued

TABLE IV–13. HEALTH HAZARD SUMMARIES FOR INDUSTRIAL AND OCCUPATIONAL CHEMICALS (Continued)

Health Hazard Summaries	ACGIH TLV	IDLH	NFPA Codes H	F	R	Comments
2-Methoxyethanol (ethylene glycol monomethyl ether, methyl Cellosolve [CAS: 109-86-4]): Workplace overexposures have resulted in depression of the hematopoietic system and encephalopathy. Symptoms include disorientation, lethargy, and anorexia. Well absorbed dermally. Animal testing revealed testicular atrophy and teratogenicity at low doses. Overexposure associated with reduced sperm counts in workers. See also p 163.	5 ppm, S	2000 ppm	2	2	0	Clear, colorless liquid with a faint odor. Vapor pressure is 6 mm Hg at 20 °C (68 °F). Flammable.
2-Methoxyethyl acetate (ethylene glycol monomethyl ether acetate, methyl Cellosolve acetate [CAS: 110-49-6]): Mildly irritating to eyes upon direct contact. Dermally well absorbed. Vapors slightly irritating to the respiratory tract. A CNS depressant at high levels. Based on animal studies, may cause kidney damage, leukopenia, testicular atrophy, and birth defects. See also p 163.	5 ppm, S	4000 ppm	1	2		Colorless liquid with a mild, pleasant odor. Flammable.
Methyl acetate (CAS: 79-20-9): Vapors moderately irritating to the eyes and respiratory tract. A CNS depressant at high levels. Hydrolyzed to methanol in the body with possible consequent toxicity similar to that of methanol (see p 215).	200 ppm	10,000 ppm	1	3	0	Colorless liquid with a pleasant, fruity odor that is a good warning property. Vapor pressure is 173 mm Hg at 20 °C (68 °F). Flammable.
Methyl acetylene (propyne [CAS: 74-99-7]): A CNS depressant and respiratory irritant at very high air concentrations in test animals.	1000 ppm	15,000 ppm	2	4	2	Colorless gas with sweet odor. Flammable.
Methyl acrylate (2-propenoic acid methyl ester [CAS: 96-33-3]): Highly irritating upon direct contact; severe burns may result. A possible skin sensitizer. Vapors highly irritating to the eyes and respiratory tract. Based on structural analogies, compounds containing the acrylate moiety may be carcinogens.	10 ppm, S	1000 ppm	2	3	2	Colorless liquid with a sharp, fruity odor. Vapor pressure is 68.2 mm Hg at 20 °C (68 °F). Inhibitor included to prevent violent polymerization.

Compound	TLV/exposure	IDLH/ERPG	H	F	R	Comments
Methylacrylonitrile (2-methyl-2-pro-penenitrile, methacrylonitrile [CAS: 126-98-7]): Mildly irritating upon direct contact. Well absorbed dermally. Metabolized to cyanide (see p 145). In animal tests, acute inhalation at high levels caused death without signs of irritation, probably by a mechanism similar to that of acrylonitrile. Lower levels produced convulsions and loss of motor control in hind limbs.	1 ppm, S					Liquid. Vapor pressure is 40 mm Hg at 13 °C (55 °F).
Methylal (dimethoxymethane [CAS: 109-87-5]): Mildly irritating to eyes and respiratory tract. A CNS depressant at very high levels. Animal studies suggest a potential to injure heart, liver, kidneys, and lungs at very high levels.	1000 ppm	10,000 ppm	2	3	2	Colorless liquid with pungent, chloroformlike odor. Highly flammable.
Methyl alcohol (methanol, wood alcohol [CAS: 67-56-1]): Mildly irritating to eyes and skin. Systemic toxicity may result from absorption by all routes. Toxic metabolites are formate and formaldehyde. A CNS depressant. Signs and symptoms include headache, nausea, abdominal pain, dizziness, shortness of breath, metabolic acidosis, and coma. Visual disturbances (optic neuropathy) range from blurred vision to blindness. See also p 215.	200 ppm, S	25,000 ppm	1	3	0	Colorless liquid with a distinctive, sharp odor that is a poor warning property. Flammable. Found in windshield fluids and antifreezes.
Methylamine (CAS: 74-89-5): Corrosive. Vapors highly irritating to eyes, skin, and respiratory tract; severe burns and pulmonary edema may result.	5 ppm	100 ppm ERPG-1: 10 ppm ERPG-2: 100 ppm ERPG-3: 500 ppm	3	4	0	Colorless gas with a fishy or ammonialike odor. Odor is a poor warning property owing to olfactory fatigue. Flammable.
Methyl-r-amyl ketone (2-heptanone [CAS: 110-43-0]): Vapors are irritating to eyes and respiratory tract. A CNS depressant.	50 ppm	4000 ppm	1	2	0	Colorless or white liquid with a fruity odor. Vapor pressure is 2.6 mm Hg at 20 °C (68 °F). Flammable.
N-methylaniline (CAS: 100-61-8): A potent inducer of methemoglobinemia (see p 217). Well absorbed by all routes. Animal studies suggest potential for liver and kidney injury.	0.5 ppm, S	100 ppm	3	2	0	Yellow to light brown liquid with a weak ammonialike odor. Vapor pressure is less than 1 mm Hg at 20 °C (68 °F). Thermal breakdown products include oxides of nitrogen.

(C) = ceiling air concentration (TLV-C); S = skin absorption can be significant; A1 = ACGIH-confirmed human carcinogen; A2 = ACGIH-suspected human carcinogen; NFPA Hazard Codes: H = health, F = fire, R = reactivity, Ox = oxidizer, W = water-reactive, 0 (none) <—> 4 (severe). ERPG = Emergency Response Planning Guideline. See p 402 for explanation of definitions.

continued

TABLE IV–13. HEALTH HAZARD SUMMARIES FOR INDUSTRIAL AND OCCUPATIONAL CHEMICALS (Continued)

Health Hazard Summaries	ACGIH TLV	IDLH	NFPA Codes H F R			Comments
Methyl bromide (bromomethane [CAS: 74-83-9]): Causes severe irritation and burns upon direct contact. Vapors irritating to the lung; pulmonary edema may result. The CNS, liver, and kidneys are major target organs; acute poisoning causes nausea, vomiting, delirium, and convulsions. Both inhalation and skin exposure may cause systemic toxicity. Chronic exposures associated with peripheral neuropathy in test animals. Evidence for adverse effects on fetal development in test animals. Limited evidence of carcinogenicity in this table. (IARC 3). See also p 219, and chloropicrin in this table.	5 ppm, S NIOSH CA	2000 ppm	3	1	0	Colorless liquid or gas with a mild chloroformlike odor that is a poor warning property. Chloropicrin, a lacrimator, is often added as a warning agent. Methyl bromide is a widely used fumigant in agriculture and in structural pesticide control.
Methyl n-butyl ketone (MBK, 2-hexanone [CAS: 591-78-6]): Vapors irritating to eyes and respiratory tract at high levels. A CNS depressant at high doses. Causes peripheral neuropathy by a mechanism thought to be the same as that of n-hexane. Well absorbed by all routes. Causes testicular toxicity in animal studies.	5 ppm, S	5000 ppm	2	3	0	Colorless liquid with an acetonelike odor. Vapor pressure is 3.8 mm Hg at 20 °C (68 °F). Flammable. NIOSH recommended exposure limit is 1.0 ppm.
Methyl chloride (CAS: 74-87-3): Once used as an anesthetic. Symptoms include headache, confusion, ataxia, convulsions, and coma. Liver, kidney, and bone marrow are other target organs. Evidence for adverse effects on both the testes and fetal development in test animals at high doses.	50 ppm NIOSH CA	10,000 ppm	2	4	0	Colorless gas with a mild, sweet odor that is a poor warning property. Highly flammable.
Methyl-2-cyanoacrylate (CAS: 137-05-3): Vapors irritating to the eyes and upper respiratory tract. May act as a sensitizer. A strong and fast-acting glue that can fasten body parts to each other or surfaces. Direct contact with the eye may result in mechanical injury if the immediate bonding of the eyelids is followed by forced separation.	2 ppm					Colorless viscous liquid. Commonly, this compound and related ones are known as "super glues."

Substance	TLV	IDLH	H	F	R	Comments
Methylcyclohexane (CAS: 108-87-2): Irritating to eyes and respiratory tract. A CNS depressant at high levels. Based on animal studies, some liver and kidney injury may occur at chronic high doses.	400 ppm	10,000 ppm	2	3	0	Colorless liquid with a faint benzenelike odor. Vapor pressure is 37 mm Hg at 20 °C (68 °F). Highly flammable.
o-Methylcyclohexanone (CAS: 583-60-8): Based on animal studies, irritating upon direct contact. Dermal absorption occurs. Vapors irritating to eyes and respiratory tract. A CNS depressant at high levels.	50 ppm, S	2500 ppm	2	0		Colorless liquid with mild peppermint odor. Irritation is a good warning property. Vapor pressure is about 1 mm Hg at 20 °C (68 °F). Flammable.
Methyl demeton (O,O-dimethyl 2-ethylmercaptoethyl thiophosphate [CAS: 8022-00-2]): An organophosphate-type cholinesterase inhibitor (see p 240).	0.5 mg/m³, S					Colorless to pale yellow liquid with an unpleasant odor. Vapor pressure is 0.00036 mm Hg at 20 °C (68 °F). Thermal breakdown products include oxides of sulfur and phosphorus.
4,4'-Methylene-bis(2-chloroaniline) (MOCA [CAS: 101-14-4]): A carcinogen in test animals (IARC 2A). Dermal absorption occurs.	0.02 ppm, S, A2 [proposed: 0.01 ppm, S, A2] NIOSH CA					Tan solid. Thermal breakdown products include oxides of nitrogen and hydrogen chloride.
Methylene bis(4-cyclohexylisocyanate) [CAS: 5124-30-1]): A strong irritant and skin sensitizer. Based on analogy to other isocyanates, vapors are likely to be potent respiratory tract irritants and sensitizers. See also p 191.	0.005 ppm					White to pale yellow solid flakes. Odorless. Possible thermal breakdown products include oxides of nitrogen and hydrogen cyanide.
Methylene bisphenyl isocyanate (4,4-di-phenylmethane diisocyanate, MDI [CAS: 101-68-8]): Irritating upon direct contact. Vapors and dusts highly irritating to eyes and respiratory tract. Potent respiratory tract sensitizer (asthma). See also p 191.	0.005 ppm	10 ppm				White to pale yellow flakes. Odorless. Vapor pressure is 0.05 mm Hg at 20 °C (68 °F). Possible thermal breakdown products include oxides of nitrogen and hydrogen cyanide. Component of urethanes.

(C) = ceiling air concentration (TLV-C); S = skin absorption can be significant; A1 = ACGIH-confirmed human carcinogen; A2 = ACGIH-suspected human carcinogen; NFPA Hazard Codes: H = health, F = fire, R = reactivity, Ox = oxidizer, W = water-reactive, 0 (none) <—> 4 (severe). ERPG = Emergency Response Planning Guideline. See p 402 for explanation of definitions.

continued

TABLE IV–13. HEALTH HAZARD SUMMARIES FOR INDUSTRIAL AND OCCUPATIONAL CHEMICALS (Continued)

Health Hazard Summaries	ACGIH TLV	IDLH	NFPA Codes H F R	Comments
Methylene chloride (methylene dichloride, dichloromethane [CAS: 75-09-2]): Irritating upon prolonged direct contact. Dermal absorption occurs. Vapors irritating to eyes and respiratory tract. A CNS depressant. May cause cardiac arrhythmias. Liver and kidney injury at high concentrations. Converted to carbon monoxide in the body with resultant carboxyhemoglobin formation. A carcinogen in test animals. See also p 220.	50 ppm, A2 OSHA CA NIOSH CA	5000 ppm	2 1 0	Heavy colorless liquid with a chloroformlike odor that is a poor warning property. Vapor pressure is 350 mm Hg at 20 °C (68 °F). Possible thermal breakdown products include phosgene and hydrogen chloride. Methylene chloride is a solvent with many industrial and commercial uses (eg, furniture strippers, carburetor cleaners).
4,4′-Methylene dianiline (4,4′-diaminodiphenylmethane [CAS: 101-77-9]): Vapors highly irritating to eyes and respiratory tract. Hepatotoxicity (cholestatic jaundice) observed in overexposed workers. Systemic toxicity may result from inhalation, ingestion, or skin contact. Methemoglobinemia (see p 217), kidney injury, retinal injury, and evidence of carcinogenicity in animals (IARC 2B).	0.1 ppm, S, A2 NIOSH CA		3 1 0	Light brown solid crystals with a faint amine odor. Combustible. Thermal breakdown products include oxides of nitrogen.
Methyl ethyl ketone, MEK [CAS: 78-93-3]: Vapors irritating to eyes and respiratory tract. A CNS depressant at high levels. Potentiates neurotoxicity of methyl butyl ketone and *n*-hexane.	200 ppm	3000 ppm	1 3 0	Colorless liquid with a mild acetone odor. Vapor pressure is 77 mm Hg at 20 °C (68 °F). Flammable.
Methyl ethyl ketone peroxide [CAS: 1338-23-4]: Based on chemical reactivity, highly irritating upon direct contact; severe burns may result. Vapors or mists likely to be highly irritating to the eyes and respiratory tract. In animal tests, overexposure resulted in liver, kidney, and lung damage.	0.2 ppm (C)			Colorless liquid with a characteristic odor. Shock sensitive. Breaks down above 50 °C (122 °F). Explodes upon rapid heating. May contain additives such as dimethyl phthalate, cyclohexanone peroxide, or diallylphthalate to add stability.
Methyl formate [CAS: 107-31-3]: Vapors highly irritating to eyes and respiratory tract. A CNS depressant at high levels. Exposure has been associated with visual disturbances, including temporary blindness.	100 ppm	5000 ppm	2 4 0	Colorless liquid with a pleasant odor at high levels. Odor is a poor warning property. Vapor pressure is 476 mm Hg at 20 °C (68 °F). Highly flammable.

Methylhydrazine (monomethylhydrazine [CAS: 60-34-4]): Similar to hydrazine in toxic actions. Vapors likely to be highly irritating to the eyes and respiratory tract. Causes methemoglobinemia (see p 217). Potent hemolysin. Highly hepatotoxic. Causes kidney injury. A convulsant in test animals.

0.2 ppm (C), S, A2 [proposed: 0.01 ppm, S, A2] NIOSH CA

50 ppm

3 3 2

Colorless clear liquid. Vapor pressure is 36 mm Hg at 20 °C (68 °F). Flammable. In addition to potential industrial uses, exposure to methylhydrazine can occur from ingestion of false morel mushrooms.

Methyl iodide: (Iodomethane [CAS: 74-88-4]): An alkylating agent. Based on chemical properties, likely to be highly irritating upon direct contact; severe burns may result. Dermal absorption is likely. Vapors highly irritating to respiratory tract; pulmonary edema has resulted. Neurotoxic; signs and symptoms include nausea, vomiting, dizziness, slurred speech, visual disturbances, ataxia, tremor, irritability, convulsions, and coma. Delusions and hallucinations may last for weeks during recovery. Severe hepatic injury may also occur. Limited evidence of carcinogenicity in test animals (IARC 3).

2 ppm, S, A2 NIOSH CA

800 ppm ERPG-1: 25 ppm ERPG-2: 50 ppm ERPG-3: 125 ppm

Colorless, yellow, red, or brown liquid. Not combustible. Vapor pressure is 375 mm Hg at 20 °C (68 °F). Thermal breakdown products include iodine and hydrogen iodide.

Methyl isoamyl ketone (5-methyl-2-hexanone [CAS: 110-12-3]): By analogy to other aliphatic ketones, vapors are likely to be irritating to eyes and respiratory tract. Likely to be a CNS depressant.

50 ppm

50 ppm

1 2 0

Colorless liquid with a pleasant odor. Vapor pressure is 4.5 mm Hg at 20 °C (68 °F). Flammable.

Methyl isobutyl ketone (4-methyl-2-pentanone, hexone [CAS: 108-10-1]): Irritating to eyes upon direct contact. Vapors irritating to eyes and respiratory tract. Reported systemic symptoms in humans are weakness, dizziness, ataxia, nausea, vomiting, and headache. High-dose studies in animals suggest a potential for liver and kidney injury.

50 ppm

3000 ppm

2 3 0

Colorless liquid with a mild odor. Vapor pressure is 7.5 mm Hg at 25 °C (77 °F). Flammable.

(C) = ceiling air concentration (TLV-C); S = skin absorption can be significant; A1 = ACGIH-confirmed human carcinogen; A2 = ACGIH-suspected human carcinogen; NFPA Hazard Codes: H = health, F = fire, R = reactivity, Ox = oxidizer, W = water-reactive, 0 (none) <—> 4 (severe). ERPG = Emergency Response Planning Guideline. See p 402 for explanation of definitions.

continued

TABLE IV-13. HEALTH HAZARD SUMMARIES FOR INDUSTRIAL AND OCCUPATIONAL CHEMICALS (Continued)

Health Hazard Summaries	ACGIH TLV	IDLH	NFPA Codes H F R	Comments
Methyl isocyanate (MIC [CAS: 624-83-9]): Highly reactive; highly corrosive upon direct contact. Vapors extremely irritating to eyes, skin, and respiratory tract; severe burns and pulmonary edema have resulted. A sensitizing agent. Toxicity is not related to cyanide. Evidence that severe poisonings have adverse effects on fetal development. See also p 191.	0.02 ppm, S	20 ppm	2 3 3 W	Colorless liquid with a sharp, disagreeable odor that is a poor warning property. Vapor pressure is 348 mm Hg at 20 °C (68 °F). Flammable. Reacts with water to release methylamine. Polymerizes upon heating. Thermal breakdown products include hydrogen cyanide and oxides of nitrogen. Used as a chemical intermediate in pesticide synthesis. MIC is not in urethanes.
Methyl mercaptan (CAS: 74-93-1): Causes delayed-onset pulmonary edema. CNS effects include narcosis and convulsions. Reported to have caused methemoglobinemia and hemolysis in a patient with G6PD deficiency (see p 217).	0.5 ppm	400 ppm ERPG-1: 0.005 ppm ERPG-2: 25 ppm ERPG-3: 100 ppm	2 4 0	Colorless liquid with an offensive rotten egg odor. Odor and irritation are good warning properties.
Methyl methacrylate (CAS: 80-62-6): Irritating upon direct contact. Vapors irritating to the eyes, skin, and respiratory tract. A sensitizer (asthma). At very high levels may produce headache, nausea, vomiting, dizziness. Limited evidence for adverse effects on fetal development in animal tests at very high doses.	100 ppm	4000 ppm	2 3 2	Colorless liquid with a pungent, acrid, fruity odor. Vapor pressure is 35 mm Hg at 20 °C (68 °F). Flammable. Contains inhibitors to prevent self-polymerization. Used in resin polymers, including medical applications.
Methyl parathion (O,O-dimethyl O-p-nitro-phenylphosphorothioate [CAS: 298-00-0]): A highly potent organophosphate cholinesterase inhibitor (see p 240).	0.2 mg/m³, S		4 1 2 (solid) 4 3 2 (in xylene)	Tan liquid with a strong garliclike odor. Vapor pressure is 0.5 mm Hg at 20 °C (68 °F). Appearance may vary with formulation.
Methyl propyl ketone (2-pentanone [CAS: 107-87-9]): Vapors irritating to eyes and respiratory tract. Based on animal studies, a CNS depressant at high levels.	200 ppm	5000 ppm	2 3 0	Colorless liquid with a characteristic odor. Vapor pressure is 27 mm Hg at 20 °C (68 °F). Flammable.

Chemical	Exposure	H	F	R	Comments
Methyl silicate (tetramethoxy silane) [CAS: 681-84-5]: Highly reactive; corrosive upon direct contact; severe burns and loss of vision may result. Vapors extremely irritating to eyes and respiratory tract; severe eye burns and pulmonary edema may result.	1 ppm				Colorless crystals. Reacts with water, forming silicic acid and methanol.
α-Methylstyrene [CAS: 98-83-9]: Slightly irritating upon direct contact. Vapors irritating to eyes and respiratory tract. A CNS depressant at high levels.	50 ppm	1	2	1	Colorless liquid with a characteristic odor. Irritation is an adequate warning property. Vapor pressure is 1.9 mm Hg at 20 °C (68 °F). Flammable.
Metribuzin(4-amino-6-[1,1-dimethylethyl]-3-[methylthio]-1,2,4-triazin-5[4H]-one [CAS: 21087-64-9]: Human data available reveal no irritation or sensitization after dermal exposure. In animal testing, was poorly absorbed through the skin and produced no direct skin or eye irritation. Repeated high doses caused CNS depression and liver and thyroid effects.	5 mg/m³				Vapor pressure is 0.00001 mm Hg at 20 °C (68 °F). Thermal breakdown products include oxides of sulfur and nitrogen.
Mevinphos (2-carbomethoxy-1-methylvinyl dimethyl phosphate, phosdrin [CAS: 7786-34-7]): An organophosphate cholinesterase inhibitor (see p 240). Well absorbed by all routes. Repeated exposures to low levels can accumulate to produce symptoms.	0.01 ppm, S				Colorless or yellow liquid with a faint odor. Vapor pressure is 0.0022 mm Hg at 20 °C (68 °F). Combustible. Thermal breakdown products include phosphoric acid mist.
Mica [CAS: 12001-25-2]: Dusts may cause pneumoconiosis upon chronic inhalation.	3 mg/m³ (respirable dust)				Colorless solid flakes or sheets. Odorless. Vapor pressure is negligible at 20 °C (68 °F). Noncombustible.
Monocrotophos (dimethyl 2-methylcarbamoyl-1-methylvinyl phosphate [CAS: 6923-22-4]): An organophosphate-type cholinesterase inhibitor (see p 240). Limited human data indicate it is well absorbed through the skin but is rapidly metabolized and excreted.	0.25 mg/m³, S				Reddish-brown solid with a mild odor.
Morpholine (tetrahydro-1,4-oxazine [CAS: 110-91-8]): Corrosive; extremely irritating upon direct contact; severe burns may result. Well absorbed dermally. Vapors irritating to eyes and respiratory tract. Exposure to vapors has caused transient corneal edema. May cause severe liver and kidney injury.	20 ppm, S	2	3	0	Colorless liquid with mild ammonialike odor. Vapor pressure is 7 mm Hg at 20 °C (68 °F). Flammable. Thermal breakdown products include oxides of nitrogen. Found in some consumer polish and wax products.

continued

(C) = ceiling air concentration (TLV-C); S = skin absorption can be significant; A1 = ACGIH-confirmed human carcinogen; A2 = ACGIH-suspected human carcinogen; NPPA Hazard Codes: H = health, F = fire, R = reactivity, Ox = oxidizer, W = water-reactive, 0 (none) <—> 4 (severe). ERPG = Emergency Response Planning Guideline. See p 402 for explanation of definitions.

TABLE IV–13. HEALTH HAZARD SUMMARIES FOR INDUSTRIAL AND OCCUPATIONAL CHEMICALS (Continued)

Health Hazard Summaries	ACGIH TLV	IDLH	NFPA Codes H F R	Comments
Naphthalene (CAS: 91-20-3): Highly irritating to eyes upon direct contact. Vapors are irritating to eyes and may cause cataracts upon chronic exposure. Dermally well absorbed. May induce methemoglobinemia (see p 217). Symptoms of overexposure include headache and nausea. See also p 226.	10 ppm	500 ppm	2	White to brown solid. The mothball odor and respiratory tract irritation are good warning properties. Current mothball formulations in the US do not contain napthalene. Vapor pressure is 0.05 mm Hg at 20 °C (68 °F). Combustible.
β-Naphthylamine (2-aminonaphthalene [CAS: 91-59-8]): Acute overexposures can cause methemoglobinemia (see p 217) or acute hemorrhagic cystitis. Well absorbed through skin. Known human bladder carcinogen.	A1 OSHA CA NIOSH CA			White to reddish crystals. Vapor pressure is 1 mm Hg at 108 °C (226 °F). Combustible.
Nickel carbonyl (nickel tetracarbonyl [CAS: 13463-39-3]): Inhalation of vapors can cause severe lung and systemic injury without irritant warning signs. Symptoms include headache, nausea, vomiting, fever, and extreme weakness. Based on animal studies, liver and brain damage may occur. Adverse effects on fetal development in test animals. A carcinogen in test animals.	0.05 ppm [proposed: 0.05 mg/m³ (as Ni), A1] NIOSH CA	7 ppm	4 3 3	Colorless liquid or gas. The musty odor is a poor warning property. Vapor pressure is 321 mm Hg at 20 °C (68 °F). Highly flammable. Exposures largely limited to nickel refining.
Nickel metal and soluble inorganic salts (nickel chloride, nickel sulfate, nickel nitrate, nickel oxide): May cause a severe sensitization dermatitis, "nickel itch," upon repeated contact. Fumes highly irritating to the respiratory tract. Some compounds have adverse effects on fetal development in test animals. Some compounds are human nasal and lung carcinogens (IARC 1).	1 mg/m³ (metal) 0.1 mg/m³ (soluble inorganic compounds, as Ni) [proposed: 0.05 mg/m³ (elemental, soluble, and insoluble compounds, as Ni), A1] NIOSH CA			Gray metallic powder or green solids. All forms are odorless.

Name (CAS) and toxicology	TLV	ERPG	NFPA (H F R)	Physical properties
Nicotine (CAS: 54-11-5): A potent nicotinic cholinergic receptor agonist. Well absorbed by all routes of exposure. Symptoms include dizziness, confusion, weakness, nausea and vomiting, tachycardia and hypertension, tremors, convulsions, and muscle paralysis. Death from respiratory paralysis can be very rapid. Adverse effects on fetal development in animal studies. See also p 227.	0.5 mg/m³, S	35 mg/m³	4 1 0	Pale yellow to dark brown viscous liquid with a fishy or aminelike odor. Vapor pressure is 0.0425 mm Hg at 20 °C (68 °F). Combustible. Thermal breakdown products include oxides of nitrogen. Although generally thought of in context of tobacco use and abstinence products, nicotine is a widely used pesticide.
Nitric acid (aqua fortis, engraver's acid [CAS: 7697-37-2]): Concentrated solutions corrosive to eyes and skin; very severe penetrating burns result. Vapors highly irritating to eyes and respiratory tract; pulmonary edema has resulted. Chronic inhalation exposure can produce bronchitis and erosion of the teeth.	2 ppm	100 ppm	3 0 0 Ox	Colorless, yellow, or red fuming liquid with an acrid, suffocating odor. Vapor pressure is approximately 62 mm Hg at 25 °C (77 °F). Not combustible.
Nitric oxide (NO, nitrogen monoxide [CAS: 10102-43-9]): Nitric oxide slowly converts to nitrogen dioxide in air; eye and mucous membrane irritation and pulmonary edema are likely from nitrogen dioxide. Overexposures have been reported to result in acute and chronic obstructive airway disease. Based on animal studies, may cause methemoglobinemia (see p 217). Binds to hemoglobin at the same site as oxygen and this may contribute to the toxicity. See also p 230.	25 ppm	100 ppm	3 0 3	Colorless or brown gas. The sharp, sweet odor occurs below the TLV and is a good warning property.
p-Nitroaniline (CAS: 100-01-6): Irritating to eyes upon direct contact; may injure cornea. Well absorbed by all routes. Overexposure results in headache, weakness, respiratory distress, and methemoglobinemia (see p 217). Liver damage may also occur.	3 mg/m³, S	300 mg/m³	3 1 3	Yellow solid with an ammonialike odor that is a poor warning property. Vapor pressure is much less than 1 mm Hg at 20 °C (68 °F). Combustible. Thermal breakdown products include oxides of nitrogen.
Nitrobenzene (CAS: 98-95-3): Irritating upon direct contact; sensitization dermatitis may occur. Well absorbed by all routes. Causes methemoglobinemia (see p 217). Symptoms include headache, cyanosis, weakness, and gastrointestinal upset. May injure liver. Injures testes in animals. Limited evidence for adverse effects on fetal development in animals.	1 ppm, S	200 ppm	3 2 0	Pale yellow to dark brown viscous liquid. Shoe polish-like odor is a good warning property. Vapor pressure is much less than 1 mm Hg at 20 °C (68 °F). Combustible. Thermal breakdown products include oxides of nitrogen.

(C) = ceiling air concentration (TLV-C); S = skin absorption can be significant; A1 = ACGIH-confirmed human carcinogen; A2 = ACGIH-suspected human carcinogen; NFPA Hazard Codes: H = health, F = fire, R = reactivity, Ox = oxidizer, W = water-reactive, 0 (none) <—> 4 (severe). ERPG = Emergency Response Planning Guideline. See p 402 for explanation of definitions.

continued

TABLE IV–13. HEALTH HAZARD SUMMARIES FOR INDUSTRIAL AND OCCUPATIONAL CHEMICALS (Continued)

Health Hazard Summaries	ACGIH TLV	IDLH	NFPA Codes H F R	Comments
p-Nitrochlorobenzene (CAS: 100-00-5): Irritating upon direct contact; sensitization dermatitis may occur upon repeated exposures. Well absorbed by all routes. Causes methemoglobinemia (see p 217). Symptoms include headache, cyanosis, weakness, and gastrointestinal upset. May cause liver and kidney injury.	0.1 ppm, S	1000 ppm	2 1 3	Yellow solid with a sweet odor. Vapor pressure is 0.009 mm Hg at 25 °C (77 °F). Combustible. Thermal breakdown products include oxides of nitrogen and hydrogen chloride.
4-Nitrodiphenyl (4-nitrobiphenyl [CAS: 92-93-3]): Extremely well absorbed through skin. Produces bladder cancer in dogs and rabbits. Metabolized to 4-aminodiphenyl which is a potent carcinogen in humans.	S, A1 OSHA CA NIOSH CA			White solid with a sweet odor. Thermal breakdown products include oxides of nitrogen.
Nitroethane (CAS: 79-24-3): Based on high-exposure studies in animals, vapors are irritating to the respiratory tract. A CNS depressant. Causes liver injury at high levels of exposure in test animals. A structurally similar compound, 2-nitropropane, is a carcinogen.	100 ppm	1000 ppm	1 3 3 (explodes on heating)	Colorless viscous liquid with a fruity odor that is a poor warning property. Vapor pressure is 15.6 mm Hg at 20 °C (68 °F). Flammable. Thermal breakdown products include oxides of nitrogen.
Nitrogen dioxide (CAS: 10102-44-0): Gases and vapors irritating to eyes and respiratory tract; fatal pulmonary edema has resulted. Initial symptoms include cough and dyspnea. Pulmonary edema may appear after a delay of several hours. The acute phase may be followed by a fatal secondary stage, with fever and chills, dyspnea, cyanosis, and delayed-onset pulmonary edema. See also p 230.	3 ppm	50 ppm		Dark brown fuming liquid or gas. Pungent odor and irritation occur only slightly above the TLV and are adequate warning properties. Vapor pressure is 720 mm Hg at 20 °C (68 °F). Important exposures include structural fires, sillage (silo-filling), and gas-shielded (MIG or TIG) welding.
Nitrogen trifluoride (nitrogen fluoride [CAS: 7783-54-2]): Vapors may cause eye irritation. Based on animal studies, may cause methemoglobinemia (see p 217) and liver and kidney damage.	10 ppm	2000 ppm		Colorless gas with a moldy odor that is a poor warning property. Not combustible. Highly reactive and explosive under a number of conditions.

Substance	TLV	ERPG / other	NFPA (H F R)	Comments
Nitroglycerin (glycerol trinitrate) [CAS: 55-63-0]: Causes vasodilation, including coronary arteries. Headache and drop in blood pressure are common. Tolerance to vasodilation can occur; cessation of exposure may precipitate angina pectoris in pharmacologically dependent workers. See also p 229.	0.05 ppm, S		2 2 4	Pale yellow viscous liquid. Vapor pressure is 0.00026 mm Hg at 20 °C (68 °F). Highly explosive.
Nitromethane (CAS: 75-52-5): Based on high-dose animal studies, causes respiratory tract irritation, liver and kidney injury, and CNS depression with ataxia, weakness, convulsions, and, possibly, methemoglobinemia (see p 217).	100 ppm [proposed: 20 ppm]	1000 ppm	1 3 3	Colorless liquid with a faint fruity odor that is a poor warning property. Vapor pressure is 27.8 mm Hg at 20 °C (68 °F). Thermal breakdown products include oxides of nitrogen.
1-Nitropropane (CAS: 108-03-2): Vapors mildly irritating to eyes and respiratory tract. Liver and kidney injury may occur.	25 ppm	2300 ppm	1 3 1 (may explode on heating)	Colorless liquid with a faint fruity odor that is a poor warning property. Vapor pressure is 7.5 mm Hg at 20 °C (68 °F). Flammable. Thermal breakdown products include oxides of nitrogen.
2-Nitropropane (CAS: 79-46-9): Mildly irritating, CNS depressant at high exposures. Highly hepatotoxic; fatalities have resulted. Renal toxicity also occurs. Well absorbed by all routes. Limited evidence for adverse effects on fetal development in test animals. A carcinogen in test animals (IARC 2B).	10 ppm, A2 NIOSH CA	2300 ppm	2 3 1 (may explode on heating)	Colorless liquid. Vapor pressure is 12.9 mm Hg at 20 °C (68 °F). Flammable. Thermal breakdown products include oxides of nitrogen.
N-Nitrosodimethylamine (dimethylnitrosamine) [CAS: 62-75-9]: Overexposed workers suffered severe liver damage. Based on animal studies, well absorbed by all routes. A potent animal carcinogen producing liver, kidney, and lung cancers (IARC 2A).	A2, S OSHA CA NIOSH CA			Yellow viscous liquid. Combustible.

(C) = ceiling air concentration (TLV-C); S = skin absorption can be significant; A1 = ACGIH-confirmed human carcinogen; A2 = ACGIH-suspected human carcinogen; NFPA Hazard Codes: H = health, F = fire, R = reactivity, Ox = oxidizer (TLV-C); S = skin absorption can be significant; A1 = ACGIH-confirmed human carcinogen; A2 = ACGIH-suspected human carcinogen; NFPA Hazard Codes: H = health, F = fire, R = reactivity, Ox = oxidizer, W = water-reactive, 0 (none) <—> 4 (severe). ERPG = Emergency Response Planning Guideline. See p 402 for explanation of definitions.

continued

TABLE IV–13. HEALTH HAZARD SUMMARIES FOR INDUSTRIAL AND OCCUPATIONAL CHEMICALS (Continued)

Health Hazard Summaries	ACGIH TLV	IDLH	NFPA Codes H F R	Comments
Nitrotoluene (o-, m-, p-nitrotoluene [CAS: 99-08-1]): Weak inducer of methemoglobinemia (see p 217). By analogy to structurally similar compounds, dermal absorption is likely.	2 ppm, S	200 ppm	3 1 0 (*para* isomer) 2 1 4 (*ortho* and *meta* isomers)	*Ortho* and *meta*, yellow liquid or solid. *Para*, yellow solid. All isomers have a weak, aromatic odor. Vapor pressure is approximately 0.15 mm Hg at 20 °C (68 °F). Thermal breakdown products include oxides of nitrogen. Intermediate in synthesis of dye-stuffs and explosives.
Nitrous oxide (CAS: 10024-97-2): A CNS depressant. Hematopoietic effects from chronic exposure include megaloblastic anemia. Substance abuse has resulted in neuropathies. May have an adverse effect on human fertility and fetal development. See also p 233.	50 ppm			Colorless gas. Sweet odor. Not combustible. Widely used in dentistry.
Octachloronaphthalene (Halowax 1051 [CAS: 2234-13-1]): By analogy to other chlorinated naphthalenes, workers overexposed by inhalation or skin contact may experience chloracne and liver damage.	0.1 mg/m³, S	200 mg/m³		Pale yellow solid with an aromatic odor. Vapor pressure is less than 1 mm Hg at 20 °C (68 °F). Not combustible. Thermal breakdown products include hydrogen chloride.
Octane (CAS: 111-65-9): Vapors mildly irritating to eyes and respiratory tract. A CNS depressant at very high concentrations.	300 ppm	5000 ppm	0 3 0	Colorless liquid. Gasolinelike odor and irritation are good warning properties. Vapor pressure is 11 mm Hg at 20 °C (68 °F). Flammable.
Osmium tetroxide (osmic acid [CAS: 20816-12-0]): Corrosive upon direct contact; severe burns may result. Fumes are highly irritating to eyes and respiratory tract. Based on high-dose animal studies, bone marrow injury and kidney damage may occur.	0.0002 ppm	1 mg/m³		Colorless to pale yellow solid with a sharp and irritating odor like chlorine. Vapor pressure is 7 mm Hg at 20 °C (68 °F). Not combustible. Catalyst and laboratory reagent.

Substance			NFPA	Comments
Oxalic acid (ethanedioic acid [CAS: 144-62-7]): A strong acid; corrosive to eyes and to skin upon direct contact (see p 126). Fumes irritating to respiratory tract. Highly toxic upon ingestion; precipitation of calcium oxalate crystals can cause hypocalcemia and renal damage. See also p 243.	1 mg/m³	500 mg/m³	1 1 0 (nonfire) 2 1 0 (fire)	Colorless or white solid. Odorless. Vapor pressure is less than 0.001 mm Hg at 20 °C (68 °F).
Oxygen difluoride (oxygen fluoride, fluorine monoxide [CAS: 7783-41-7]): Extremely irritating to the eyes, skin, and respiratory tract. Effects similar to hydrofluoric acid (see p 180). Based on animal studies, may also injure kidney, internal genitalia, and other organs. Workers have complained of severe headaches after low-level exposures.	0.05 ppm (C)	0.5 ppm		Colorless gas with a strong and foul odor. Olfactory fatigue is common, so odor is a poor warning property. A strong oxidizing agent.
Ozone (triatomic oxygen [CAS: 10028-15-6]): Irritating to eyes and respiratory tract. Pulmonary edema has been reported. See also p 176.	0.1 ppm (C)	10 ppm		Colorless or bluish gas. Sharp, distinctive odor is an adequate warning property. A strong oxidizing agent. Gas-shielded and specialty welding are potential sources of exposure.
Paraquat (1,1'-dimethyl-4,4'-bipyridinium dichloride [CAS: 4687-14-7]): Extremely irritating upon direct contact; severe corrosive burns may result. Well absorbed through skin. A potent toxin causing acute multiorgan failure as well as progressive fatal pulmonary fibrosis after ingestion. See also p 245.	0.5 mg/m³ (total dust) 0.1 mg/m³ (respirable fraction)	1.5 mg/m³		Odorless white to yellow solid. Vapor pressure is negligible at 20 °C (68 °F). Not combustible. Thermal breakdown products include oxides of nitrogen and sulfur and hydrogen chloride. While widely used as a herbicide, most deaths occur as a result of ingestion.
Parathion (O,O-diethyl O-p-nitrophenyl phosphorothioate [CAS: 56-38-2]): Highly potent organophosphate cholinesterase inhibitor (see p 217). Systemic toxicity has resulted from inhalation, ingestion, and dermal exposures. Evidence for adverse effects on fetal development in test animals at high doses.	0.1 mg/m³, S	20 mg/m³	4 1 2	Yellow to dark brown liquid with garliclike odor. Odor threshold of 0.04 ppm suggests it has good warning properties. Vapor pressure is 0.0004 mm Hg at 20 °C (68 °F). Thermal breakdown products include oxides of sulfur, nitrogen, and phosphorus. In the field, weathering/oxidation can convert parathion to the even more toxic organophosphate, paraoxon.

(C) = ceiling air concentration (TLV-C); S = skin absorption can be significant; A1 = ACGIH-confirmed human carcinogen; A2 = ACGIH-suspected human carcinogen; NFPA Hazard Codes: H = health, F = fire, R = reactivity, Ox = oxidizer, W = water-reactive, 0 (none) <—> 4 (severe). ERPG = Emergency Response Planning Guideline. See p 402 for explanation of definitions.

continued

TABLE IV–13. HEALTH HAZARD SUMMARIES FOR INDUSTRIAL AND OCCUPATIONAL CHEMICALS (Continued)

Health Hazard Summaries	ACGIH TLV	IDLH	NFPA Codes H F R	Comments
Pentaborane [CAS: 19624-22-7]: Highly irritating upon direct contact; severe burns may result. Vapors irritating to the respiratory tract. A potent CNS toxin; symptoms include headache, nausea, weakness, confusion, hyperexcitability, tremors, seizures, and coma. CNS effects may persist. Liver and kidney injury may also occur.	0.005 ppm	3 ppm	3 3 2	Colorless liquid. Vapor pressure is 171 mm Hg at 20 °C (68 °F). The pungent sour-milk odor occurring only at air levels well above the TLV is a poor warning property. May ignite spontaneously. Reacts violently with halogenated extinguishing media. Thermal breakdown products include boron acids.
Pentachloronaphthalene (Halowax 1013 [CAS: 1321-64-8]): Chloracne results from prolonged skin contact or inhalation. May cause severe, potentially fatal liver injury or necrosis by all routes of exposure.	0.5 mg/m³, S			Pale yellow waxy solid with a pleasant aromatic odor. Odor threshold not known. Vapor pressure is less than 1 mm Hg at 20 °C (68 °F). Not combustible. Thermal breakdown products include hydrogen chloride fumes.
Pentachlorophenol (Penta, PCP [CAS: 87-86-5]): Irritating upon direct contact; burns may result. Vapors irritating to eyes and respiratory tract. A potent metabolic poison; uncouples oxidative phosphorylation. Well absorbed by all routes. Evidence for adverse effects on fetal development and carcinogenicity in test animals (IARC 2B). See also p 246.	0.5 mg/m³, S	150 mg/m³	3 2 0 (solutions) 3 0 0 (dry)	Eye and nose irritation occur slightly above the TLV and are good warning properties. Vapor pressure is 0.0002 mm Hg at 20 °C (68 °F). Not combustible. Thermal breakdown products include hydrogen chloride, chlorinated phenols, and octachlorodibenzodioxin. Widely used as a wood preservative.
Pentane (n-pentane [CAS: 109-66-0]): Vapors mildly irritating to eyes and respiratory tract. A CNS depressant at high levels.	600 ppm	5000 ppm	1 4 0	Colorless liquid with a gasolinelike odor that is an adequate warning property. Vapor pressure is 426 mm Hg at 20 °C (68 °F). Flammable.
Petroleum distillates (petroleum naphtha, petroleum ether): Vapors irritating to eyes and respiratory tract. A CNS depressant. If n-hexane, benzene, or other toxic contaminants are present, those hazards should be addressed. See also p 178.	400 ppm	10,000 ppm	1 4 0 (petroleum ether)	Colorless liquid. Kerosenelike odor at levels below the TLV serves as a warning property. Highly flammable. Vapor pressure is about 40 mm Hg at 20 °C (68 °F).

Phenol (carbolic acid, hydroxybenzene [CAS: 108-95-2]): Corrosive acid and protein denaturant. Direct eye or skin contact causes severe tissue damage or blindness. Deep skin burns can occur without warning pain. Systemic toxicity by all routes; percutaneous absorption of vapor occurs. Vapors highly irritating to eyes and respiratory tract. Symptoms include nausea, vomiting, cardiac arrhythmias, circulatory collapse, convulsions, and coma. Toxic to liver and kidney. A tumor promoter. See also p 249.

5 ppm, S

250 ppm
ERPG-1: 10 ppm
ERPG-2: 50 ppm
ERPG-3: 200 ppm

3 2 0

Colorless to pink crystalline solid, or viscous liquid. Its odor has been described as being distinct, acrid, and aromatic or as being sweet and tarry. As the odor is detected at or below the TLV, it is a good warning property. Vapor pressure is 0.36 mm Hg at 20 °C (68 °F). Combustible.

Phenylenediamine (*p*-diaminobenzene, *p*-aminoaniline [CAS: 106-50-3]): Irritating upon direct contact. May cause skin and respiratory tract sensitization (asthma). Inflammatory reactions of larynx and pharynx have often been noted in exposed workers.

0.1 mg/m³, A2

25 mg/m³

White to light purple or brown solid, depending on degree of oxidation. Combustible. Thermal breakdown products include oxides of nitrogen.

Phenyl ether (diphenyl ether [CAS: 101-84-8]): Mildly irritating upon prolonged direct contact. Vapors irritating to eyes and respiratory tract. Based on high-dose experiments in animals, liver and kidney damage may occur after ingestion.

1 ppm

Colorless liquid or solid. Mildly disagreeable odor detected below the TLV serves as a good warning property. Vapor pressure is 0.02 mm Hg at 25 °C (77 °F). Combustible.

Phenyl glycidyl ether (PGE, 1,2-epoxy-3-phenoxypropane [CAS: 122-60-1]): Irritating upon direct contact. A skin sensitizer. Based on animal studies, vapors are very irritating to eyes and respiratory tract. In high-dose animal studies, a CNS depressant producing liver, kidney, spleen, testes, thymus, and hematopoietic system injury. A carcinogen in test animals (IARC 2B).

1 ppm

Colorless liquid with an unpleasant, sweet odor. Vapor pressure is 0.01 mm Hg at 20 °C (68 °F). Combustible. Readily forms peroxides.

Phenylhydrazine [CAS: 100-63-0]: A strong base and corrosive upon direct contact. A potent skin sensitizer. Dermal absorption occurs. Vapors very irritating to eyes and respiratory tract. May cause hemolytic anemia with secondary kidney damage. Limited evidence of carcinogenicity in test animals.

0.1 ppm, S, A2
NIOSH CA

295 ppm

3 2 0

Pale yellow crystals or oily liquid with a weakly aromatic odor. Darkens upon exposure to air and light. Vapor pressure is less than 0.1 mm Hg at 20 °C (68 °F). Combustible. Thermal breakdown products include oxides of nitrogen.

(C) = ceiling air concentration (TLV-C); S = skin absorption can be significant; A1 = ACGIH-confirmed human carcinogen; A2 = ACGIH-suspected human carcinogen; NFPA Hazard Codes: H = health, F = fire, R = reactivity, Ox = oxidizer, W = water-reactive, 0 (none) <—> 4 (severe). ERPG = Emergency Response Planning Guideline. See p 402 for explanation of definitions.

continued

TABLE IV–13. HEALTH HAZARD SUMMARIES FOR INDUSTRIAL AND OCCUPATIONAL CHEMICALS (Continued)

Health Hazard Summaries	ACGIH TLV	IDLH	NFPA Codes H F R			Comments
Phenylphosphine (CAS: 638-21-1): In animals, subchronic inhalation at 2 ppm caused loss of appetite, diarrhea, tremor, hemolytic anemia, dermatitis, and irreversible testicular degeneration.	0.05 ppm (C)					Crystalline solid. Spontaneously combustible at high air concentrations.
Phorate (O,O-diethyl S-(ethylthio)methyl phosphorodithioate, Thimet, Timet [CAS: 298-02-2]): An organophosphate-type cholinesterase inhibitor (see p 240). Well absorbed by all routes.	0.05 mg/m³, S					Clear liquid. Vapor pressure is 0.002 mm Hg at 20 °C (68 °F).
Phosgene (carbonyl chloride, COCl₂ [CAS: 75-44-5]): Extremely irritating to the lower respiratory tract. Exposure can be insidious because irritation and smell are inadequate as warning properties for pulmonary injury. Higher levels cause irritation of the eyes, skin, and mucous membranes. See also p 256.	0.1 ppm	2 ppm ERPG-2: 0.2 ppm ERPG-3: 1 ppm	4	0	0	Colorless gas. Sweet haylike odor at low concentrations; sharp and pungent odor at high concentrations. Dangerous concentrations may not be detected by odor.
Phosphine (hydrogen phosphide [CAS: 7803-51-2]): Extremely irritating to the respiratory tract; fatal pulmonary edema has resulted. A multisystem poison. Symptoms in moderately overexposed workers included diarrhea, nausea, vomiting, cough, headache, and dizziness. See also p 257.	0.3 ppm	200 ppm	3	4	1	Colorless gas. A fishy or garliclike odor detected well below the TLV is considered to be a good warning property. May ignite spontaneously on contact with air. A common fumigant, generated on-site by aluminim phosphide and moisture.
Phosphoric acid (CAS: 7664-38-2): A strong corrosive acid; severe burns may result from direct contact. Mist or vapors irritating to eyes and respiratory tract.	1 mg/m³		2	0	0	Colorless, syrupy, odorless liquid. Solidifies at temperatures below 20 °C (68 °F). Vapor pressure is 0.03 mm Hg at 20 °C (68 °F). Not combustible.
Phosphorus (yellow phosphorus, white phosphorus, P [CAS: 7723-14-0]): Severe, penetrating burns may result upon direct contact. Material may ignite upon contact with skin. Fumes irritating to eyes and respiratory tract; pulmonary edema may occur. Potent hepatotoxin. Systemic symptoms include abdominal pain, jaundice, and garlic odor on the breath. Historically, chronic poisoning caused jaw bone necrosis (phossy jaw). See also p 257.	0.1 mg/m³		3	3	1	White to yellow, waxy or crystalline solid with acrid fumes. Flammable. Vapor pressure is 0.026 mm Hg at 20 °C (68 °F). Ignites spontaneously on contact with air. Thermal breakdown products include phosphoric acid fume. Historical exposures involved the match industry which has long since substituted other forms of phosphorus. Current uses include munitions and pesticides.

Substance	TLV-C	ERPG	NFPA (H F R)	Comments
Phosphorus oxychloride (CAS: 10025-87-3): Reacts with moisture to release phosphoric and hydrochloric acids; highly corrosive upon direct contact. Fumes extremely irritating to eyes and respiratory tract. Systemic effects include headache, dizziness, and dyspnea. Kidney toxicity may occur.	0.1 ppm		3 0 2 W	Clear colorless to pale yellow, fuming liquid possessing a pungent odor. Vapor pressure is 40 mm Hg at 27.3 °C (81 °F). Not combustible.
Phosphorus pentachloride (CAS: 10026-13-8): Reacts with moisture to release phosphoric and hydrochloric acids; highly corrosive upon direct contact. Fumes extremely irritating to eyes and respiratory tract.	0.1 ppm	200 mg/m³		Pale yellow solid with a hydrochloric acidlike odor. Not combustible.
Phosphorus pentasulfide (CAS: 1314-80-3): Rapidly reacts with moisture and moist tissues to form hydrogen sulfide (see p 182) and phosphoric acid. Severe burns may result from prolonged contact with tissues. Dusts or fumes extremely irritating to eyes and respiratory tract. Systemic toxicology is predominantly caused by hydrogen sulfide.	1 mg/m³	750 mg/m³		Greenish-yellow solid with odor of rotten eggs. Olfactory fatigue reduces value of smell as a warning property. Thermal breakdown products include sulfur dioxide, hydrogen sulfide, phosphorus pentoxide, and phosphoric acid fumes. Ignites spontaneously in the presence of moisture.
Phosphorus trichloride (CAS: 7719-12-2): Reacts with moisture to release phosphoric and hydrochloric acids; highly corrosive upon direct contact. Fumes extremely irritating to eyes and respiratory tract.	0.2 ppm	50 ppm	3 0 2 W	Fuming colorless to yellow liquid. Irritation provides a good warning property. Vapor pressure is 100 mm Hg at 20 °C (68 °F). Not combustible.
Phthalic anhydride (phthalic acid anhydride [CAS: 85-44-9]): Extremely irritating upon direct contact; chemical burns occur after prolonged contact. Dusts and vapors extremely irritating to respiratory tract. A potent skin and respiratory tract sensitizer (asthma).	1 ppm	10,000 ppm	2 1 0	White crystalline solid with choking odor at very high air concentrations. Vapor pressure is 0.05 mm Hg at 20 °C (68 °F). Combustible. Thermal breakdown products include phthalic acid fumes.
Picloram (4-amino-3,5,6-trichloropicolinic acid [CAS: 1918-02-1]): Dusts mildly irritating to skin, eyes, and respiratory tract. Has low oral toxicity in test animals. Limited evidence of carcinogenicity in animals.	10 mg/m³			White powder possessing a bleachlike odor. Vapor pressure is 0.0000006 mm Hg at 35 °C (95 °F). Thermal breakdown products include oxides of nitrogen and hydrogen chloride.

(C) = ceiling air concentration (TLV-C); S = skin absorption can be significant; A1 = ACGIH-confirmed human carcinogen; A2 = ACGIH-suspected human carcinogen; NFPA Hazard Codes: H = health, F = fire, R = reactivity, Ox = oxidizer, W = water-reactive, 0 (none) <—> 4 (severe). ERPG = Emergency Response Planning Guideline. See p 402 for explanation of definitions.

continued

TABLE IV–13. HEALTH HAZARD SUMMARIES FOR INDUSTRIAL AND OCCUPATIONAL CHEMICALS (Continued)

Health Hazard Summaries	ACGIH TLV	IDLH	NFPA Codes H F R	Comments
Picric acid (2,4,6-trinitrophenol [CAS: 88-89-1]): Irritating upon direct contact. Dust stains skin yellow and can cause a sensitization dermatitis. Symptoms of low-level exposure are headache, dizziness, and gastrointestinal upset. May induce methemoglobinemia (see p 217). Ingestion of large amounts causes hemolysis, nephritis, and hepatitis. Staining of the conjunctiva and aqueous humor can give vision a yellow hue. A weak uncoupler of oxidative phosphorylation.	0.1 mg/m³	100 mg/m³	2 4 4	Pale yellow crystalline solid or paste. Odorless. Vapor pressure is much less than 1 mm Hg at 20 °C (68 °F). Decomposes explosively above 120 °C (248 °F). May detonate when shocked. Contact with metals, ammonia, or calcium compounds can form salts that are much more sensitive to shock detonation.
Pindone (Pival, 2-pivaloyl-1,3-indanedione [CAS: 83-26-1]): A vitamin K antagonist anticoagulant (see p 143).	0.1 mg/m³	200 mg/m³		Bright yellow crystalline substance.
Piperazine dihydrochloride (CAS: 142-64-3): Irritating upon direct contact; burns may result. A moderate skin and respiratory sensitizer. Nausea, vomiting, and diarrhea are side effects of medicinal use. Overdosage has caused confusion, lethargy, coma, and seizures.	5 mg/m³			White crystalline solid with a mild fishy odor.
Piperidine (CAS: 110-89-4): Highly irritating upon direct contact; severe burns may result. Vapors irritating to eyes and respiratory tract. Small doses initially stimulate autonomic ganglia; larger doses depress them. A 30–60 mg/kg dose may produce symptoms in humans.			2 3 3	Flammable.
Platinum—soluble salts (sodium chloroplatinate; ammonium chloroplatinate, platinum tetrachloride): Sensitizers causing asthma and dermatitis. Metallic platinum does not share these effects. Soluble platinum compounds are also highly irritating to eyes, mucous membranes, and respiratory tract.	0.002 mg/m³ (as Pt)			Appearance varies with the compound. Thermal breakdown products of some chloride salts include chlorine gas. Used as industrial catalysts and in specialized photographic applications.

Substance	Exposure limit	H	F	R	Comments
Polychlorinated biphenyls (chlorodiphenyls, Aroclor 1242, PCBs): Exposure to high concentrations is irritating to eyes, nose, and throat. Chronically overexposed workers suffer from chloracne and liver injury. Reported symptoms are anorexia, gastrointestinal upset, and peripheral neuropathies. Some health effects may be caused by contaminants or thermal decomposition products. Adverse effects on fetal development and fertility in test animals. A carcinogen in test animals (IARC 2A). See also p 268.	1 mg/m³ (42% chlorine), S NIOSH CA 0.5 mg/m³ (54% chlorine), S NIOSH CA				42% chlorinated: a colorless to dark brown liquid with a slight hydrocarbon odor and a vapor pressure of 0.001 mm Hg at 20 °C (68 °F). 54% chlorinated: light yellow oily liquid with a slight hydrocarbon odor and a vapor pressure of 0.00006 mm Hg at 20 °C (68 °F). Thermal breakdown products include chlorinated dibenzofurans and chlorodibenzodioxins. Although no longer used, old transformers may still contain PCBs.
Polytetrafluoroethylene decomposition products: Overexposures result in polymer fume fever, a disease with flulike symptoms including chills, fever, and cough. See also p 214.					Produced by pyrolysis of Teflon and related materials. Perisofluorobutylene and carbonyl fluoride are among the pyrolysis products.
Polyvinyl chloride decomposition products: Fumes are irritating to the respiratory tract and may cause "meat wrapper's" asthma.					Produced by the high-temperature partial breakdown of polyvinyl chloride plastics.
Portland cement (a mixture of mostly tricalcium silicate and dicalcium silicate with some alumina, calcium aluminate, and iron oxide): Irritant of the eyes, nose, and skin; corrosive burns may occur. Long-term heavy exposure has been associated with dermatitis and bronchitis.	10 mg/m³ (< 1% quartz)				Gray powder. Odorless. Portland cement manufacture is typically associated with sulfur dioxide exposure.
Potassium hydroxide (KOH [CAS: 1310-58-3]): A caustic alkali causing severe burns to tissues upon direct contact. Exposure to dust or mist causes eye, nose, and respiratory tract irritation.	2 mg/m³ (C)	3	0	1	White solid that absorbs moisture. Vapor pressure is negligible at 20 °C (68 °F). Gives off heat and a corrosive mist when in contact with water.
Propane (CAS: 74-98-6): Simple asphyxiant. See also hydrocarbons, p 178.					
Propargyl alcohol (2-propyn-1-ol [CAS: 107-19-7]): Irritating to skin upon direct contact. Dermally well absorbed. A CNS depressant. Causes liver and kidney injury in test animals.	1 ppm, S	3	3	3	Light to straw-colored liquid with a geraniumlike odor. Vapor pressure is 11.6 mm Hg at 20 °C (68 °F). Flammable.

continued

(C) = ceiling air concentration (TLV-C); S = skin absorption can be significant; A1 = ACGIH-confirmed human carcinogen; A2 = ACGIH-suspected human carcinogen; NFPA Hazard Codes: H = health, F = fire, R = reactivity, Ox = oxidizer, W = water-reactive, 0 (none) <—> 4 (severe). ERPG = Emergency Response Planning Guideline. See p 402 for explanation of definitions.

TABLE IV–13. HEALTH HAZARD SUMMARIES FOR INDUSTRIAL AND OCCUPATIONAL CHEMICALS (Continued)

Health Hazard Summaries	ACGIH TLV	IDLH	NFPA Codes H F R			Comments
Propionic acid (CAS: 79-09-4): Irritating to eyes and skin upon direct contact with concentrated solutions; burns may result. Vapors irritating to eyes, skin, and respiratory tract. A food additive of low systemic toxicity.	10 ppm		2	2	0	Colorless oily liquid with a pungent, somewhat rancid odor. Vapor pressure is 10 mm Hg at 39.7 °C (103.5 °F). Flammable.
Propoxur (o-isopropoxyphenyl N-methylcarbamate, DDVP, Baygon [CAS: 114-26-11]: A carbamate anticholinesterase insecticide (see p 118). Limited evidence for adverse effects on fetal development in test animals.	0.5 mg/m³					White crystalline solid with a faint characteristic odor. Vapor pressure is 0.01 mm Hg at 120 °C (248 °F). Common insecticide found in many OTC formulations.
n-Propyl acetate (CAS: 109-60-4): Vapors irritating to eyes and respiratory tract. Excessive inhalation may cause weakness, nausea, and chest tightness. Based on high-exposure studies in test animals, a CNS depressant.	200 ppm	8000 ppm	1	3	0	Colorless liquid. Mild fruity odor and irritant properties provide good warning properties. Vapor pressure is 25 mm Hg at 20 °C (68 °F). Flammable.
Propyl alcohol (1-propanol [CAS: 71-23-8]: Vapors mildly irritating to eyes and respiratory tract. A CNS depressant. See also isopropyl alcohol, p 193.	200 ppm, S	4000 ppm	1	3	0	Colorless volatile liquid. Vapor pressure is 15 mm Hg at 20 °C (68 °F). Mild alcohollike odor is an adequate warning property.
Propylene dichloride (1,2-dichloropropane [CAS: 78-87-5]: Vapors very irritating to eyes and respiratory tract. Causes CNS depression and severe liver and kidney damage at modest doses in animal studies. Testicular toxicity at high doses in test animals.	75 ppm	2000 ppm	2	3	0	Colorless liquid. Chloroformlike odor is considered to be an adequate warning property. Vapor pressure is 40 mm Hg at 20 °C (68 °F). Flammable. Thermal breakdown products include hydrogen chloride. An agricultural nematocide.

Agent	TLV	IDLH	NFPA (H F R)	Comments
Propylene glycol dinitrate (1,2-propylene glycol dinitrate, PGDN [CAS: 6423-43-4]): Mildly irritating upon direct contact. Dermal absorption occurs. Causes vasodilation, including coronary arteries. Headache and drop in blood pressure are common. Well absorbed by all routes. Tolerance to vasodilation can occur; cessation of exposure may precipitate angina pectoris in pharmacologically dependent workers. See also nitrates, p 229.	0.05 ppm, S			Colorless liquid with an unpleasant odor. Thermal breakdown products include oxides of nitrogen.
Propylene glycol monomethyl ether (1-methoxy-2-propanol [CAS: 107-98-2]): Vapors very irritating to the eyes and possibly the respiratory tract. A mild CNS depressant.	100 ppm		0 3 0	Colorless, flammable liquid.
Propylene imine (2-methylaziridine [CAS: 75-55-8]): Very irritating upon direct contact; severe burns may result. Vapors highly irritating to eyes and respiratory tract. May also injure liver and kidneys. Well absorbed dermally. A carcinogen in test animals.	2 ppm, S, A2	100 ppm		A fuming colorless liquid with a strong ammonialike odor. Flammable. Thermal breakdown products include oxides of nitrogen.
Propylene oxide (2-epoxypropane [CAS: 75-56-9]): Highly irritating upon direct contact; severe burns result. Vapors highly irritating to eyes and respiratory tract. Based on high-dose animal studies, may cause CNS depression and peripheral neuropathy. A carcinogen in test animals (IARC 2A).	20 ppm	2000 ppm	2 4 2	Colorless liquid. Its sweet, etherlike odor is considered to be an adequate warning property. Vapor pressure is 442 mm Hg at 20 °C (68 °F). Highly flammable. Polymerizes violently.
n-Propyl nitrate (nitric acid n-propyl ester [CAS: 627-13-4]): Vasodilator causing headaches and hypotension. Causes methemoglobinemia (see p 217). See also nitrates, p 229.	25 ppm	2000 ppm	2 4 3 Ox (may explode on heating)	Pale yellow liquid with an unpleasant sweet odor. Vapor pressure is 18 mm Hg at 20 °C (68 °F). Flammable. Thermal breakdown products include oxides of nitrogen.
Pyrethrum (pyrethrin I or II; cinerin I or II; jasmolin I or II): Dusts cause primary contact dermatitis and skin and respiratory tract sensitization (asthma). Of very low systemic toxicity. See also p 269.	5 mg/m³	5000 mg/m³		Vapor pressure is negligible at 20 °C (68 °F). Combustible. Widely used insecticide.

(C) = ceiling air concentration (TLV-C); S = skin absorption can be significant; A1 = ACGIH-confirmed human carcinogen; A2 = ACGIH-suspected human carcinogen; NFPA Hazard Codes: H = health, F = fire, R = reactivity, Ox = oxidizer, W = water-reactive, 0 (none) <—> 4 (severe). ERPG = Emergency Response Planning Guideline. See p 402 for explanation of definitions.

continued

TABLE IV-13. HEALTH HAZARD SUMMARIES FOR INDUSTRIAL AND OCCUPATIONAL CHEMICALS (Continued)

Health Hazard Summaries	ACGIH TLV	IDLH	NFPA Codes H	F	R	Comments
Pyridine (CAS: 110-86-1): Irritating upon prolonged direct contact; occasional reports of skin sensitization. Vapors irritating to eyes and respiratory tract. A CNS depressant. Induces methemoglobinemia. Chronic ingestion of small amounts has caused fatal liver and kidney injury. Workers exposed to 6–12 ppm have complained of headache, dizziness, and gastrointestinal upset. Dermally well absorbed.	5 ppm	3600 ppm	2	3	0	Colorless or yellow liquid with a nauseating odor and a definite "taste" that serves as a good warning property. Vapor pressure is 18 mm Hg at 20 °C (68 °F). Flammable. Thermal breakdown products include oxides of nitrogen and cyanide.
Pyrogallol (1,2,3-trihydroxybenzene; pyrogallic acid [CAS: 87-66-1]): Highly irritating upon direct contact; severe burns may result. Potent reducing agent and general cellular poison. Causes methemoglobinemia (see p 217). Attacks heart, lungs, liver, kidneys, red blood cells, bone marrow, and muscle. Causes sensitization dermatitis. Deaths have resulted from the topical application of salves containing pyrogallol.						White to gray odorless solid.
Quinone (1,4-cyclohexadienedione, p-benzoquinone [CAS: 106-51-4]): A severe irritant of the eyes and respiratory tract. May induce methemoglobinemia (see p 217). Acute overexposure to dust or vapors can cause conjunctival irritation and discoloration, corneal edema, ulceration, and scarring. Chronic exposures can permanently reduce visual acuity. Skin contact can cause irritation, ulceration, and pigmentation changes.	0.1 ppm	75 ppm	1	2	1	Pale yellow crystalline solid. The acrid odor is not a reliable warning property. Vapor pressure is 0.1 mm Hg at 20 °C (68 °F). Sublimes when heated.
Resorcinol (1,3-dihydroxybenzene [CAS: 108-46-3]): Corrosive acid and protein denaturant; extremely irritating upon direct contact; severe burns result. May cause methemoglobinemia (see p 217). A sensitizer. Dermally well absorbed. See also phenol, p 249.	10 ppm	5000 mg/m³	1	0		White crystalline solid with a faint odor. May turn pink on contact with air. Vapor pressure is 1 mm Hg at 108 °C (226 °F). Combustible.
Ronnel (O,O-dimethyl-O-(2,4,5-trichlorophenyl)phosphorothioate, Fenchlorphos [CAS: 299-84-31]): One of the least toxic organophosphate anticholinesterase insecticides (see p 240).	10 mg/m³	5000 mg/m³				Vapor pressure is 0.0008 mm Hg at 20 °C (68 °F). Not combustible. Unstable above 149 °C (300 °F); harmful gases such as sulfur dioxide, dimethyl sulfide, and trichlorophenol may be released.

Rotenone (tubatoxin, cube root, derris root, derrin [CAS: 83-79-4]): Irritating upon direct contact. Dusts irritate the respiratory tract. A metabolic poison; depresses cellular respiration and inhibits mitotic spindle formation. Ingestion of large doses numbs oral mucosa and causes nausea and vomiting, muscle tremors, and convulsions. Chronic exposure caused liver and kidney damage in animal studies. Limited evidence for adverse effects on fetal development in animals at high doses.

5 mg/m^3 5000 mg/m^3

White to red crystalline solid. Vapor pressure is negligible at 20 °C (68 °F). A natural pesticide extracted from such plants as cube, derris, and timbo. Odorless. Decomposes upon contact with air or light. Unstable to alkali.

Selenium and inorganic compounds (as selenium): Fumes, dusts, and vapors irritating to eyes, skin, and respiratory tract; pulmonary edema may occur. Many compounds are well absorbed dermally. A general cellular poison. Chronic intoxication causes depression, nervousness, dermatitis, gastrointestinal upset, metallic taste in mouth and garlicky odor of breath, excess caries, and loss of fingernails or hair. The liver and kidneys are also target organs. Some selenium compounds have been found to cause birth defects and cancers in test animals. See also p 283.

0.2 mg/m^3 (as Se)   100 mg/m^3

Elemental selenium is a black, gray, or red crystalline or amorphous solid and is odorless.

Selenium dioxide (selenium oxide [CAS: 7446-08-4]): Strong vesicant; severe burns result from direct contact. Converted to selenious acid in the presence of moisture. Well absorbed dermally. Fumes and dusts very irritating to eyes and respiratory tract. See also p 283.

White solid. Reacts with water to form selenious acid.

Selenium hexafluoride (CAS: 7783-79-1): Vesicant. Reacts with moisture to form selenium acids and hydrofluoric acid; severe HF burns may result from direct contact (see p 180). Fumes highly irritating to eyes and respiratory tract; pulmonary edema may result.

0.05 ppm   5 ppm

Colorless gas. Not combustible.

Selenium oxychloride [CAS: 7791-23-3]): Strong vesicant. Direct contact can cause severe burns. Dermally well absorbed. Fumes extremely irritating to eyes and respiratory tract; delayed pulmonary edema may result.

Colorless to yellow liquid. Hydrogen chloride and selenious acid fumes produced on contact with moisture.

(C) = ceiling air concentration (TLV-C); S = skin absorption can be significant; A1 = ACGIH-confirmed human carcinogen; A2 = ACGIH-suspected human carcinogen; NFPA Hazard Codes: H = health, F = fire, R = reactivity, Ox = oxidizer, W = water-reactive, 0 (none) <—> 4 (severe). ERPG = Emergency Response Planning Guideline. See p 402 for explanation of definitions.

continued

TABLE IV–13. HEALTH HAZARD SUMMARIES FOR INDUSTRIAL AND OCCUPATIONAL CHEMICALS (Continued)

Health Hazard Summaries	ACGIH TLV	IDLH	NFPA Codes H F R	Comments
Silica, amorphous (diatomaceous earth, precipitated and gel silica): Possesses little or no potential to cause silicosis. Most sources of amorphous silica contain quartz (see crystalline silica, below). If greater than 1% quartz is present, the quartz hazard must be addressed. When strongly heated (calcined) with limestone, diatomaceous earth becomes crystalline and can cause silicosis. Amorphous silica has been associated with lung fibrosis but the role of crystalline silica contamination remains controversial.	10 mg/m³ (precipitated silica, diatomaceous earth, silica gel) 2 mg/m³ (silica fume, respirable dust)			White to gray powders. Odorless with a negligible vapor pressure. The TLV for dusts is 10 mg/m³ if no asbestos and less than 1% quartz are present.
Silica, crystalline (quartz; fused amorphous silica; cristobolite; tridymite; tripoli [CAS: 14464-46-1]): Inhalation of dusts causes silicosis, a progressive, fibrotic scarring of the lung. Individuals with silicosis are much more susceptible to tuberculosis. Some forms of crystalline silica are carcinogenic (IARC 2A).	0.1 mg/m³ (respirable dust; quartz, fused silica, tripoli) 0.05 mg/m³ (respirable dust; cristobolite; tridymite)			Colorless, odorless solid with a negligible vapor pressure. A component of many mineral dusts.
Silicon (CAS: 7440-21-3): A nuisance dust that does not cause pulmonary fibrosis. Parenteral exposure has been associated with systemic toxicity.	10 mg/m³			Gray to black, lustrous needlelike crystals. Vapor pressure is negligible at 20 °C (68 °F).
Silicon tetrachloride (CAS: 10026-04-7): Generates hydrochloric acid vapor upon contact with moisture; severe burns may result. Extremely irritating to eyes and respiratory tract; pulmonary edema may result.				Not combustible.
Silver (CAS: 7440-22-4): Silver compounds cause argyria, a blue-gray discoloration of tissues, which may be generalized throughout the viscera or localized to the conjunctiva, nasal septum, and gums. Some silver salts are corrosive upon direct contact with tissues.	0.01 mg/m³ (soluble compounds as Ag) 0.1 mg/m³ (metal)			Compounds vary in appearance. Silver nitrate is a strong oxidizer.

Agent and Comments	Exposure Limit		NFPA (H F R)	Physical Description
Sodium azide (hydrazoic acid, sodium salt; NaN₃ [CAS: 26628-22-8]): Potent cellular toxin; inhibits cytochrome oxidase. Eye irritation, bronchitis, headache, hypotension, and collapse have been reported in overexposed workers. See also p 91.	0.11 ppm (C)			White, odorless, crystalline solid.
Sodium bisulfide (NaSH [CAS: 16721-80-5]): Decomposes in the presence of water to form hydrogen sulfide (see p 182) and sodium hydroxide (see p 126). Highly corrosive and irritating to eyes, skin, and respiratory tract.				White crystalline substance with a slight odor of sulfur dioxide.
Sodium bisulfite (sodium hydrogen sulfite, NaHSO₃ [CAS: 7631-90-5]): Irritating to eyes, skin, and respiratory tract. Hypersensitivity reactions (angioedema, bronchospasm, or anaphylaxis) may occur.	5 mg/m³			White crystalline solid with a slight sulfur dioxide odor and disagreeable taste. Widely used as a food additive.
Sodium fluoroacetate (compound 1080 [CAS: 62-74-8]): A highly toxic metabolic poison. Metabolized to fluorocitrate, which prevents the oxidation of acetate in the Krebs cycle. Human lethal oral dose ranges from 2 to 10 mg/kg. See also p 169.	0.05 mg/m³, S	5 mg/m³	3 0 1	Fluffy white solid or a fine white powder. Sometimes dyed black. Hygroscopic. Odorless. Vapor pressure is negligible at 20 °C (68 °F). Not combustible. Thermal breakdown products include hydrogen fluoride. Used as a rodenticide.
Sodium hydroxide (NaOH [CAS: 1310-73-2]): A caustic alkali; may cause severe burns. Fumes or mists are highly irritating to eyes, skin, and respiratory tract. See also p 126.	2 mg/m³ (C)	250 mg/m³		White solid that absorbs moisture. Odorless. Evolves great heat upon solution in water. Soda lye is an aqueous solution.
Sodium metabisulfite (sodium pyrosulfite [CAS: 7681-57-4]): Very irritating to eyes and skin upon direct contact. Dusts irritating to eyes and respiratory tract; pulmonary edema may result. Hypersensitivity reactions may occur.	5 mg/m³			White powder or crystalline material with a slight odor of sulfur dioxide. Reacts to form sulfur dioxide in the presence of moisture.
Stibine (antimony hydride [CAS: 7803-52-3]): A potent hemolytic agent similar to arsine. Gases irritating to the lung; pulmonary edema may occur. Liver and kidney are secondary target organs. See also p 80.	0.1 ppm	40 ppm		Colorless gas. Odor similar to that of hydrogen sulfide but may not be a reliable warning property. Formed when acid solutions of antimony are treated with zinc or strong reducing agents.

(C) = ceiling air concentration (TLV-C); S = skin absorption can be significant; A1 = ACGIH-confirmed human carcinogen; A2 = ACGIH-suspected human carcinogen; NFPA Hazard Codes: H = health, F = fire, R = reactivity, Ox = oxidizer, W = water-reactive, 0 (none) <—> 4 (severe). ERPG = Emergency Response Planning Guideline. See p 402 for explanation of definitions.

continued

TABLE IV–13. HEALTH HAZARD SUMMARIES FOR INDUSTRIAL AND OCCUPATIONAL CHEMICALS (Continued)

Health Hazard Summaries	ACGIH TLV	IDLH	NFPA Codes H	Comments
Stoddard solvent (mineral spirits, a mixture of aliphatic and aromatic hydrocarbons [CAS: 8052-41-3]): Dermal absorption can occur. Vapors irritating to eyes and respiratory tract. A CNS depressant. Chronic overexposures associated with headache, fatigue, bone marrow hypoplasia, and jaundice. May contain a small amount of benzene. See also hydrocarbons, p 178.	100 ppm	5000 ppm		Colorless liquid. Kerosenelike odor and irritation are good warning properties. Vapor pressure is approximately 2 mm Hg at 20 °C (68 °F). Flammable.
Strychnine (CAS: 57-24-9): Neurotoxin binds to inhibitory, postsynaptic glycine receptors, which results in excessive motor neuron activity associated with convulsions and muscular hyperrigidity leading to respiratory impairment or paralysis. See also p 290.	0.15 mg/m³	3 mg/m³		White solid. Odorless. Vapor pressure is negligible at 20 °C (68 °F). Thermal breakdown products include oxides of nitrogen. Street drugs may be adulterated with strychnine.
Styrene monomer (vinylbenzene [CAS: 100-42-5]): Irritating upon direct contact. Dermal absorption occurs. Vapors irritating to respiratory tract. A CNS depressant. Symptoms include headache, nausea, dizziness, and fatigue. Cases of peripheral neuropathy have been reported. Limited evidence for adverse effects on fetal development and cancer in test animals (IARC 2B).	50 ppm, S	5000 ppm	2 3 2	Colorless viscous liquid. Sweet aromatic odor at low concentrations is an adequate warning property. Odor at high levels is acrid. Vapor pressure is 4.5 mm Hg at 20 °C (68 °F). Flammable. Inhibitor must be included to avoid explosive polymerization. Used in SBR, ABS, and SAN polymers.
Subtilisins (proteolytic enzymes of Bacillus subtilis [CAS: 1395-21-7]): Primary skin and respiratory tract irritants. Potent sensitizers causing primary bronchoconstriction and asthma.	0.06 μg/m³ (C)			Light-colored powder. Occupational asthma associated with their introduction into detergent in a powder formulation.
Sulfur dioxide (CAS: 7446-09-5): Forms sulfurous acid upon contact with moisture. Strongly irritating to eyes and skin; burns may result. Extremely irritating to the respiratory tract; irritation of the upper airways has caused obstruction of the upper airways and pulmonary edema. Asthmatics are of documented increased sensitivity to the bronchoconstrictive effects of sulfur dioxide air pollution. See also p 292.	2 ppm	100 ppm ERPG-1: 0.3 ppm ERPG-2: 3 ppm ERPG-3: 15 ppm		Colorless gas. Pungent, suffocating odor with a "taste" and irritative effects that are good warning properties.

Sulfur hexafluoride (CAS: 2551-62-4): Considered to be essentially a nontoxic gas. Asphyxiation by the displacement of air is suggested as the greatest hazard.

1000 ppm

Odorless, colorless dense gas. May be contaminated with other fluorides of sulfur, including the highly toxic sulfur pentafluoride, which release HF or oxyflourides on contact with moisture.

Sulfuric acid (oil of vitriol, H₂SO₄, [CAS: 7664-93-9]): Highly corrosive upon direct contact; severe burns may result. Breakdown may release sulfur dioxide (see p 292). Exposure to the mist can irritate the eyes, skin, and respiratory tract.

1 mg/m³

80 mg/m³
ERPG-1: 2 mg/m³
ERPG-2: 10 mg/m³
ERPG-3: 30 mg/m³

3 0 2
   W

Colorless to dark brown heavy, oily liquid. Odorless. Eye irritation may be an adequate warning property. A strong oxidizer. Addition of water creates strong exothermic reaction. Vapor pressure is less than 0.001 mm Hg at 20 °C (68 °F).

Sulfur monochloride (CAS: 10025-67-9): Forms hydrochloric acid and sulfur dioxide (see p 292) upon contact with water; direct contact can cause burns. Vapors highly irritating to the eyes, skin, and the respiratory tract.

1 ppm (C)

10 ppm

2 1 1

Fuming, amber to red, oily liquid with a pungent, irritating, sickening odor. Eye irritation is a good warning property. Vapor pressure is 6.8 mm Hg at 20 °C (68 °F). Combustible. Breakdown products include hydrogen sulfide, hydrogen chloride, and sulfur dioxide.

Sulfur pentafluoride (disulfur decafluoride [CAS: 5714-22-7]): Vapors are extremely irritating to the lungs; causes pulmonary edema at low levels (0.5 ppm) in test animals.

0.01 ppm (C)

1 ppm

Colorless liquid or vapor with a sulfur dioxidelike odor. Vapor pressure is 561 mm Hg at 20 °C (68 °F). Not combustible. Thermal breakdown products include sulfur dioxide and hydrogen fluoride.

Sulfur tetrafluoride (SF₄, [CAS: 7783-60-0]): Readily hydrolyzed by moisture to form sulfur dioxide (see p 292) and hydrogen fluoride (see p 180). Extremely irritating to the respiratory tract; pulmonary edema may occur. Vapors also highly irritating to eyes and skin.

0.1 ppm (C)

Colorless gas. Reacts with moisture to form sulfur dioxide and hydrogen fluoride.

Sulfuryl fluoride (Vikane, SO₂F₂ [CAS: 2699-79-8]): Irritating to eyes and respiratory tract; fatal pulmonary edema has resulted. Acute high exposure causes tremors and convulsions in test animals. Chronic exposures may cause kidney and liver injury and elevated fluoride. See also p 180.

5 ppm

1000 ppm

Colorless, odorless gas with no warning properties. Chloropicrin, a lacrimator, is often added to provide a warning property. Thermal breakdown products include sulfur dioxide and hydrogen fluoride. A widely used fumigant.

(C) = ceiling air concentration (TLV-C); S = skin absorption can be significant; A1 = ACGIH-confirmed human carcinogen; A2 = ACGIH-suspected human carcinogen; NFPA Hazard Codes: H = health, F = fire, R = reactivity, Ox = oxidizer, 0 (none) <—> 4 (severe). ERPG = Emergency Response Planning Guideline. See p 402 for explanation of definitions.

continued

TABLE IV–13. HEALTH HAZARD SUMMARIES FOR INDUSTRIAL AND OCCUPATIONAL CHEMICALS (Continued)

Health Hazard Summaries	ACGIH TLV	IDLH	NFPA Codes H F R	Comments
Sulprofos (O-ethyl O-[4-(methylthio)phenyl] S-propylphosphorodithioate [CAS: 35400-43-2]): An organophosphate anticholinesterase insecticide (see p 240).	1 mg/m³			Tan-colored liquid with a characteristic sulfide odor.
Talc, containing no asbestos fibers or crystalline silica (CAS: 14807-96-6): A tissue irritant. Pulmonary aspiration may cause serious pneumonitis.	2 mg/m³ (respirable dust; if talc contains asbestos fibers, see asbestos TLV)			
Tantalum compounds (as tantalum): Of low acute toxicity. Dusts mildly irritating to the lungs.	5 mg/m³ (metal and oxide)			Metal is a gray-black solid, platinum-white if polished. Odorless. Tantalum pentoxide is a colorless solid. Used in aerospace and other speciality alloys.
Tellurium and compounds (as tellurium): Complaints of sleepiness, nausea, metallic taste, and garlicky odor on breath and perspiration associated with workplace exposures. Neuropathies have been noted in high-dose studies. Hydrogen telluride causes pulmonary irritation and hemolysis; however, its ready decomposition reduces likelihood of a toxic exposure. Some tellurium compounds are fetotoxic or teratogenic in test animals.	0.1 mg/m³ (as Te)			Metallic tellurium is a solid with a silvery-white or grayish luster.
Tellurium hexafluoride (CAS: 7783-80-4): Slowly hydrolyzes to release hydrofluoric acid (see p 180) and telluric acid. Extremely irritating to the eyes and respiratory tract; pulmonary edema may occur. Has caused headaches, dyspnea, and garlicky odor on the breath of overexposed workers.	0.02 ppm	1 ppm		Colorless gas. Offensive odor. Not combustible. Thermal breakdown products include hydrogen fluoride.

Substance	TLV	IDLH	NFPA (H F R)	Comments
Temephos (Abate, *O,O,O′,O′*-tetramethyl *O,O*-thiodi-*p*-phenylene phosphorothioate [CAS: 3383-96-8]): Primary irritant of eyes, skin, and respiratory tract; a moderately toxic organophosphate-type cholinesterase inhibitor (see p 240). Well absorbed by all routes.	10 mg/m³			
Terphenyls (diphenyl benzenes, triphenyls [CAS: 26140-60-3]): Irritating upon direct contact. Vapors and mists irritating to respiratory tract; pulmonary edema has occurred at very high levels in test animals. Animal studies also suggest a slight potential for liver and kidney injury.	0.53 ppm (C)	3500 mg/m³	0 1 0	White to light yellow crystalline solids. Irritation is a possible warning property. Vapor pressure is very low at 20 °C (68 °F). Combustible. Commercial grades are mixtures of *o-, m-, p*-isomers.
1,1,1,2-Tetrachloro-2,2-difluoroethane (halocarbon 112a; refrigerant 112a [CAS: 76-11-9]): Of low acute toxicity. Very high air levels irritating to the eyes and respiratory tract. A CNS depressant at high levels. By analogy to other freons, may cause cardiac arrhythmias. High-dose studies in animals suggest possible kidney and liver injury. See also p 175.	500 ppm	15,000 ppm		Colorless liquid or solid with a slight etherlike odor. Vapor pressure is 40 mm Hg at 20 °C (68 °F). Not combustible. Thermal breakdown products include hydrogen chloride and hydrogen fluoride.
1,1,2,2-Tetrachloro-1,2-difluoroethane (halocarbon 112; refrigerant 112 [CAS: 76-12-0]): Of low acute toxicity. Once used as an anthelmintic. Very high air levels cause CNS depression. Vapors mildly irritating. By analogy to other freons, may cause cardiac arrhythmias. See also p 175.	500 ppm	15,000 ppm		Colorless liquid or solid with a slight etherlike odor. Odor is of unknown value as a warning property. Vapor pressure is 40 mm Hg at 20 °C (68 °F). Not combustible. Thermal breakdown products include hydrogen chloride and hydrogen fluoride.
1,1,2,2-Tetrachloroethane (acetylene tetrachloride [CAS: 79-34-5]): Dermal absorption may cause systemic toxicity. Vapors irritating to the eyes and respiratory tract. A CNS depressant. By analogy to other chlorinated ethane derivatives, may cause cardiac arrhythmias. May cause hepatic or renal injury. Limited evidence of carcinogenicity in test animals (IARC 3).	1 ppm, S NIOSH CA	150 ppm		Colorless to light yellow liquid. Sweet, suffocating, chloroformlike odor is a good warning property. Vapor pressure is 8 mm Hg at 20 °C (68 °F). Not combustible. Thermal breakdown products include hydrogen chloride and phosgene.

(C) = ceiling air concentration (TLV-C); S = skin absorption can be significant; A1 = ACGIH-confirmed human carcinogen; A2 = ACGIH-suspected human carcinogen; NFPA Hazard Codes: H = health, F = fire, R = reactivity, Ox = oxidizer, W = water-reactive. 0 (none) <—> 4 (severe). ERPG = Emergency Response Planning Guideline. See p 402 for explanation of definitions.

continued

TABLE IV–13. HEALTH HAZARD SUMMARIES FOR INDUSTRIAL AND OCCUPATIONAL CHEMICALS (Continued)

Health Hazard Summaries	ACGIH TLV	IDLH	NFPA Codes H F R	Comments
Tetrachloroethylene (perchloroethylene [CAS: 127-18-4]): Irritating upon prolonged contact; mild burns may result. Vapors irritating to eyes and respiratory tract. A CNS depressant. By analogy to other trichloroethylene and other chlorinated solvents, may cause arrhythmias. Chronic overexposure may cause liver and kidney injury. May cause short-term memory loss and personality changes. Limited evidence for adverse effects on reproductive function in males and fetal development in test animals. Evidence for carcinogenicity in test animals (IARC 2B). See also p 300.	50 ppm [proposed: 25 ppm, A3] NIOSH CA	500 ppm	2 0 0	Colorless liquid. Chloroformlike or etherlike odor and eye irritation are adequate warning properties. Vapor pressure is 14 mm Hg at 20 °C (68 °F). Not combustible. Thermal breakdown products include phosgene and hydrochloric acid. Used in the dry cleaning industry.
Tetrachloronaphthalene (Halowax [CAS: 1335-88-2]): Causes chloracne and jaundice. Stored in body fat. Dermal absorption occurs.	2 mg/m³	20 mg/m³		White to light yellow solid. Aromatic odor of unknown value as a warning property. Vapor pressure is less than 1 mm Hg at 20 °C (68 °F). Thermal breakdown products include hydrogen chloride and phosgene.
Tetraethyl-di-thionopyrophosphate (TEDP, sulfotepp [CAS: 3689-24-5]): An organophosphate anticholinesterase insecticide (see p 240). Well absorbed dermally.		35 mg/m³		Yellow liquid with garlic odor. Not combustible. Thermal breakdown products include sulfur dioxide and phosphoric acid mist.
Tetraethyl lead (CAS: 78-00-2): A potent CNS toxin. Dermally well absorbed. Can cause psychosis, mania, convulsions, and coma. Reports of reduced sperm counts and impotence in overexposed workers. See also p 196.	0.1 mg/m³ (as Pb), S	40 mg/m³ (as Pb)	3 3 3	Colorless liquid. May be dyed blue, red, or orange. Slight musty odor of unknown value as a warning property. Vapor pressure is 0.2 mm Hg at 20 °C (68 °F). Combustible. Decomposes in light. As a gasoline additive, heavy exposure can occur through inappropriate use of gasoline as a solvent and in substance abuse.
Tetraethyl pyrophosphate (TEPP [CAS: 107-49-3]): A potent organophosphate cholinesterase inhibitor (see p 240). Rapidly absorbed through skin.	0.004 ppm, S	10 mg/m³		Colorless to amber liquid with a faint fruity odor. Slowly hydrolyzed in water. Vapor pressure is 1 mm Hg at 140 °C (284 °F). Not combustible. Thermal breakdown products include phosphoric acid mist.

				Comments
Tetrahydrofuran (THF, diethylene oxide [CAS: 109-99-9]): Mildly irritating to eyes and respiratory tract. A CNS depressant at high levels. A liver and kidney toxin at high doses in test animals.	200 ppm	20,000 ppm	2 3 1	Colorless liquid. The etherlike odor is detectable well below the TLV and provides a good warning property. Flammable. Vapor pressure is 145 mm Hg at 20 °C (68 °F).
Tetramethyl lead [CAS: 75-74-1]: A potent CNS toxin thought to be similar to tetraethyl lead. See also p 196.	0.15 mg/m³ (as Pb), S	40 mg/m³ (as Pb)	3 3 3	Colorless liquid. May be dyed red, orange, or blue. Slight musty odor is of unknown value as a warning property. Vapor pressure is 22 mm Hg at 20 °C (68 °F).
Tetramethyl succinonitrile (TMSN [CAS: 3333-52-6]): A potent neurotoxin. Headaches, nausea, dizziness, convulsions, and coma have occurred in overexposed workers.	0.5 ppm, S	5 ppm		Colorless, odorless solid. Thermal breakdown products include oxides of nitrogen.
Tetranitromethane [CAS: 509-14-8]: Highly irritating upon direct contact; mild burns may result. Vapors extremely irritating to eyes and respiratory tract; pulmonary edema has been reported. May cause methemoglobinemia (see p 217). Liver, kidney, and CNS injury in test animals at high doses. Overexposure associated with headaches, fatigue, dyspnea. See also nitrates, p 229.	1 ppm [proposed: 0.005 ppm, A2]	5 ppm		Colorless to light yellow liquid or solid with a pungent, acrid odor. Irritative effects are a good warning property. Vapor pressure is 8.4 mm Hg at 20 °C (68 °F). Not combustible. A weak explosive and oxidizer. Highly explosive in the presence of impurities.
Tetrasodium pyrophosphate [CAS: 7722-88-5]: Alkaline; dusts are mild irritants of eyes, skin, and respiratory tract.	5 mg/m³			White powder. Alkaline in aqueous solution.
Tetryl (nitramine, 2,4,6-trinitrophenylmethylnitramine [CAS: 479-45-8]): Causes severe sensitization dermatitis. Dusts extremely irritating to the eyes and respiratory tract. Stains tissues bright yellow. May injure the liver and kidneys. Overexposures also associated with malaise, headache, nausea, and vomiting.	1.5 mg/m³			White to yellow solid. Odorless. A strong oxidizer. Vapor pressure is much less than 1 mm Hg at 20 °C (68 °F). Explosive used in detonators and primers.

(C) = ceiling air concentration (TLV-C); S = skin absorption can be significant; A1 = ACGIH-confirmed human carcinogen; A2 = ACGIH-suspected human carcinogen; NFPA Hazard Codes: H = health, F = fire, R = reactivity, Ox = oxidizer, W = water-reactive, 0 (none) <—> 4 (severe). ERPG = Emergency Response Planning Guideline. See p 402 for explanation of definitions.

continued

TABLE IV–13. HEALTH HAZARD SUMMARIES FOR INDUSTRIAL AND OCCUPATIONAL CHEMICALS (Continued)

Health Hazard Summaries	ACGIH TLV	IDLH	NFPA Codes H	Comments
Thallium, soluble compounds (thallium sulfate, thallium acetate, thallium nitrate): A potent toxin causing diverse chronic effects including psychosis, peripheral neuropathy, optic neuritis, alopecia, abdominal pain, irritability, and weight loss. Liver and kidney injury may occur. Ingestion causes severe hemorrhagic gastroenteritis. Absorption possible by all routes. See also p 294.	0.1 mg/m³ (as Tl), S	20 mg/m³ (as Tl)		Appearance varies with the compound. The elemental form is a bluish-white, ductile heavy metal with a negligible vapor pressure. Thallium has been used as a rodenticide.
Thioglycolic acid (mercaptoacetic acid [CAS: 68-11-1]): Skin or eye contact with concentrated acid causes severe burns. Vapors irritating to eyes and respiratory tract.	1 ppm, S			Colorless liquid. Unpleasant mercaptanlike odor. Vapor pressure is 10 mm Hg at 18 °C (64 °F). Found in some coldwave and depilatory formulations.
Thiram (tetramethylthiuram disulfide [CAS: 137-26-8]): Dusts mildly irritating to eyes, skin, and respiratory tract. A moderate allergen and a potent skin sensitizer. Has disulfiramlike effects in exposed persons who consume alcohol (see p 155). Experimentally a goitrogen. Adverse effects on fetal development in test animals at very high doses.	1 mg/m³	1500 mg/m³		White to yellow powder with a characteristic odor. May be dyed blue. Vapor pressure is negligible at 20 °C (68 °F). Thermal breakdown products include sulfur dioxide and carbon disulfide. Used in rubber manufacture and as a fungicide.
Tin, metal, and inorganic compounds: Dusts irritating to the eyes, nose, throat, and skin. Prolonged inhalation may cause chest x-ray abnormalities. Some compounds react with water to form acids (tin tetrachloride, stannous chloride, and stannous sulfate) or bases (sodium and potassium stannate).	2 mg/m³ (as Sn)	400 mg/m³ (as Sn)		Metallic tin is odorless with a dull, silvery color.
Tin, organic compounds: Highly irritating upon direct contact; burns may result. Dusts, fumes, or vapors highly irritating to the eyes and respiratory tract. Triethyltin is a potent neurotoxin; triphenyltin acetate is highly hepatotoxic. Trialkyltins are the most toxic, followed in order by the dialkyltins and monoalkyltins. Within each of these classes, the ethyltin compounds are the most toxic. All are well absorbed dermally.	0.1 mg/m³ (as Sn), S	200 mg/m³ (as Sn)		There are many kinds of organotin compounds: mono-, di-, tri-, and tetra-alkyltin and -aryltin compounds exist. Combustible. Organic tin compounds are used in some polymers and paints.

Substance	TLV	Ceiling/other	NFPA (H F R)	Comments
Titanium dioxide [CAS: 13463-67-7]: A mild pulmonary irritant.	10 mg/m³			White odorless powder. Rutile is a common crystalline form. Vapor pressure is negligible.
Tolidine (o-tolidine, 3,3'-dimethylbenzidine [CAS: 119-93-7]): A carcinogen in test animals (IARC 2B).	S, A2 NIOSH CA			White to reddish solid. Oxides of nitrogen are among thermal breakdown products.
Toluene (toluol, methylbenzene [CAS: 108-88-3]): Vapors mildly irritating to eyes and respiratory tract. A CNS depressant; may cause brain, kidney and muscle damage with frequent intentional abuse. May cause cardiac arrhythmias. Liver and kidney injury with heavy exposures. Abusive sniffing during pregnancy associated with birth defects. See also p 298.	50 ppm, S	2000 ppm	2 3 0	Colorless liquid. Aromatic, benzenelike odor detectable at very low levels. Irritation serves as a good warning property. Vapor pressure is 22 mm Hg at 20 °C (68 °F). Flammable.
Toluene 2,4-diisocyanate [CAS: 584-84-9]: A potent respiratory tract sensitizer (asthma) and potent irritant of the eyes, skin, and respiratory tract. Pulmonary edema has resulted with higher exposures. A carcinogen in test animals (IARC 2B). See also p 191.	0.005 ppm	10 ppm	3 1 1 (reacts with water)	Colorless needles or a liquid with a sharp, pungent odor. Vapor pressure is approximately 0.04 mm Hg at 20 °C (68 °F). Combustible.
o-Toluidine (2-methylaniline [CAS: 95-53-4]): A corrosive alkali; can cause severe burns. May cause methemoglobinemia (see p 217). Dermal absorption occurs. A carcinogen in test animals (IARC 2A).	2 ppm, S, A2	100 ppm	3 2 0	Colorless to pale yellow liquid. The weak aromatic odor is thought to be a good warning property. Vapor pressure is less than 1 mm Hg at 20 °C (68 °F).
m-Toluidine (3-methylaniline [CAS: 108-44-1]): A corrosive alkali; can cause severe burns. May cause methemoglobinemia (see p 217). Dermal absorption occurs.	2 ppm, S			Pale yellow liquid. Vapor pressure is less than 1 mm Hg at 20 °C (68 °F).
p-Toluidine (4-methylaniline [CAS: 106-49-0]): A corrosive alkali; can cause severe burns. May cause methemoglobinemia (see p 217). Dermal absorption occurs. A carcinogen in test animals.	2 ppm, S, A2			White solid. Vapor pressure is 1 mm Hg at 20 °C (68 °F).

(C) = ceiling air concentration (TLV-C); S = skin absorption can be significant; A1 = ACGIH-confirmed human carcinogen; A2 = ACGIH-suspected human carcinogen; NFPA Hazard Codes: H = health, F = fire, R = reactivity, Ox = oxidizer, W = water-reactive, 0 (none) <—> 4 (severe). ERPG = Emergency Response Planning Guideline. See p 402 for explanation of definitions.

continued

TABLE IV–13. HEALTH HAZARD SUMMARIES FOR INDUSTRIAL AND OCCUPATIONAL CHEMICALS (Continued)

Health Hazard Summaries	ACGIH TLV	IDLH	NFPA Codes H F R	Comments
Tributyl phosphate (CAS: 126-73-8): Highly irritating upon direct contact; causes severe eye injury and skin irritation. Vapors or mists irritating to the eyes and respiratory tract; high exposure in test animals caused pulmonary edema. Weak anticholinesterase activity. Headache and nausea are reported.	0.2 ppm	1300 mg/m^3	2 1 0	Colorless to pale yellow liquid. Odorless. Vapor pressure is very low at 20 °C (68 °F). Combustible. Thermal breakdown products include phosphoric acid fume.
Trichloroacetic acid (CAS: 76-03-9): A strong acid. A protein denaturant. Corrosive to eyes and skin upon direct contact.	1 ppm			Deliquescent crystalline solid. Vapor pressure is 1 mm Hg at 51 °C (128.3 °F). Thermal breakdown products include hydrochloric acid and phosgene.
1,2,4-Trichlorobenzene (CAS: 120-82-1): Prolonged or repeated contact can cause skin and eye irritation. Vapors irritating to the eyes, skin, and respiratory tract. High-dose animal exposures injure the liver, kidneys, lungs, and CNS. Does not cause chloracne.	5 ppm (C)		2 1 0	A colorless liquid with an unpleasant, mothball-like odor. Vapor pressure is 1 mm Hg at 38.4 °C (101.1 °F). Combustible. Thermal breakdown products include hydrogen chloride and phosgene.
1,1,1-Trichloroethane (methyl chloroform, TCA [CAS: 71-55-6]): Vapors mildly irritating to eyes and respiratory tract. A CNS depressant. May cause cardiac arrhythmias. Some dermal absorption occurs. Liver and kidney injury may occur. See also p 300.	350 ppm	1000 ppm	3 1 1	Colorless liquid. Vapor pressure is 100 mm Hg at 20 °C (68 °F). Not combustible. Thermal breakdown products include hydrogen chloride and phosgene. Widely used chlorinated solvent.
1,1,2-Trichloroethane (CAS: 79-00-5): Dermal absorption may occur. Vapors mildly irritating to eyes and respiratory tract. A CNS depressant. May cause cardiac arrhythmias. Causes liver and kidney injury in test animals. Limited evidence for carcinogenicity in test animals (IARC 3). See also p 300.	10 ppm, S NIOSH CA	500 ppm	3 1 0	Colorless liquid. Sweet, chloroformlike odor is of unknown value as a warning property. Vapor pressure is 19 mm Hg at 20 °C (68 °F). Not combustible. Thermal breakdown products include phosgene and hydrochloric acid.

Chemical	Exposure Limits		NFPA (H F R)	Comments
Trichloroethylene (trichloroethene, TCE [CAS: 79-01-6]): Dermal absorption may occur. Vapors mildly irritating to eyes and respiratory tract. A CNS depressant. May cause cardiac arrhythmias. May cause cranial and peripheral neuropathies and liver damage. Has a disulfiramlike effect, "degreasers' flush" (see p 155. Reported to cause liver and lung cancers in mice (IARC 3). See also p 300.	50 ppm [proposed: 50 ppm, A5] NIOSH CA	1000 ppm	2 1 0	Colorless liquid. Sweet chloroformlike odor. Vapor pressure is 58 mm Hg at 20 °C (68 °F). Not combustible at room temperatures. Decomposition products include hydrogen chloride and phosgene.
Trichlorofluoromethane (Freon 11 [CAS: 75-69-4]): Vapors mildly irritating to eyes and respiratory tract. A CNS depressant. May cause cardiac arrhythmias. See also p 175.	1000 ppm (C)	10,000 ppm		Colorless liquid or gas at room temperature. Vapor pressure is 690 mm Hg at 20 °C (68 °F). Not combustible. Thermal breakdown products include hydrogen chloride and hydrogen fluoride.
Trichloronaphthalene (Halowax [CAS: 1321-65-9]): Causes chloracne. A hepatotoxin at low doses, causing jaundice. Stored in body fat. Systemic toxicity may occur following dermal exposure.	5 mg/m³, S			Colorless to pale yellow solid with an aromatic odor of uncertain value as a warning property. Vapor pressure is less than 1 mm Hg at 20 °C (68 °F). Flammable. Decomposition products include phosgene and hydrogen chloride.
2,4,5-Trichlorophenoxyacetic acid (2,4,5-T [CAS: 93-76-5]): Moderately irritating to eyes, skin, and respiratory tract. Ingestion can cause gastroenteritis and injury to the CNS, muscle, kidney, and liver. A weak uncoupler of oxidative phosphorylation. Polychlorinated dibenzodioxin compounds are contaminants (see p 154). There are reports of sarcomas occurring in applicators. Adverse effects on fetal development in test animals.	10 mg/m³	5000 mg/m³		Colorless to tan solid. Appearance and some hazardous properties vary with the formulation. Odorless. Vapor pressure is negligible at 20 °C (68 °F). Not combustible. Thermal breakdown products include hydrogen chloride and dioxins. A herbicide once widely used as a defoliant in Vietnam, "Agent Orange."
1,1,2-Trichloro-1,2,2-trifluoroethane (Freon 113 [CAS: 76-13-1]): Vapors mildly irritating to eyes and mucous membranes. Very high air levels cause CNS depression and may injure the liver. May cause cardiac arrhythmias at air concentrations as low as 2000 ppm in test animals. See also p 175.	1000 ppm	4500 ppm		Colorless liquid. Sweetish, chloroformlike odor occurs only at very high concentrations and is a poor warning property. Vapor pressure is 284 mm Hg at 20 °C (68 °F). Not combustible. Thermal breakdown products include hydrogen chloride, hydrogen fluoride, and phosgene.

(C) = ceiling air concentration (TLV-C); S = skin absorption can be significant; A1 = ACGIH-confirmed human carcinogen; A2 = ACGIH-suspected human carcinogen; NFPA Hazard Codes: H = health, F = fire, R = reactivity, Ox = oxidizer, W = water-reactive, 0 (none) <—> 4 (severe). ERPG = Emergency Response Planning Guideline. See p 402 for explanation of definitions.

continued

TABLE IV-13. HEALTH HAZARD SUMMARIES FOR INDUSTRIAL AND OCCUPATIONAL CHEMICALS (Continued)

Health Hazard Summaries	ACGIH TLV	IDLH	NFPA Codes H F R			Comments
Triethylamine [CAS: 121-44-8]: An alkaline corrosive; highly irritating to eyes and skin; severe burns may occur. Vapors very irritating to eyes and respiratory tract; pulmonary edema may occur. High doses in animals cause heart, liver, and kidney injury. CNS stimulation possibly resulting from inhibition of monoamine oxidase.	10 ppm	1000 ppm	2	3	0	Colorless liquid with a fishy, ammonialike odor of unknown value as a warning property. Vapor pressure is 54 mm Hg at 20 °C (68 °F). Flammable.
Trifluorobromomethane (Halon 1301; Freon 13B1 [CAS: 75-63-8]): Extremely high air levels (150,000–200,000) can cause CNS depression and cardiac arrhythmias. See also p 175.	1000 ppm	50,000 ppm				Colorless gas with a weak etherlike odor at high levels and poor warning properties. Not combustible.
Trifluoromethane (Freon 23 [CAS: 75-46-7]): Vapors mildly irritating to the eyes and mucous membranes. Very high air levels cause CNS depression and cardiac arrhythmias. See also p 175.						Not combustible.
Trimellitic anhydride (TMAN [CAS: 552-30-7]): Dusts and vapors extremely irritating to eyes, nose, throat, skin, and respiratory tract. Potent respiratory sensitizer (asthma). Can also cause diffuse lung hemorrhage.	0.04 mg/m^3 (C)					Colorless solid. Hydrolyzes to trimellitic acid in aqueous solutions. Vapor pressure is 0.000004 mm Hg at 25 °C (77 °F). TMAN is an important component of certain epoxy coatings.
Trimethylamine [CAS: 75-50-3]: An alkaline corrosive; highly irritating upon direct contact; severe burns may occur. Vapors very irritating to respiratory tract.	5 ppm	ERPG-1: 0.1 ppm ERPG-2: 100 ppm ERPG-3: 500 ppm	2	4	0	Highly flammable gas with a pungent, fishy, ammonialike odor. May be used as a warning agent in natural gas.
Trimethyl phosphite (phosphorous acid trimethylester [CAS: 121-45-9]): Very irritating upon direct contact; severe burns may result. Vapors highly irritating to respiratory tract. Cataracts have developed in test animals exposed to high air levels. Evidence for adverse effects on fetal development in test animals.	2 ppm		0	2	0	Colorless liquid with a characteristic, strong, fishy, or ammonialike odor. Hydrolyzed in water. Vapor pressure is 24 mm Hg at 25 °C (77 °F). Combustible.

	TLV	NFPA H	F	R	Comments
Trinitrotoluene (2,4,6-trinitrotoluene, TNT [CAS: 118-96-7]): Irritating upon direct contact. Stains tissues yellow. Causes sensitization dermatitis. Vapors irritating to the respiratory tract. May cause liver injury, methemoglobinemia (see p 217). Occupational overexposure associated with cataracts. Causes vasodilation, including coronary arteries. Headache and drop in blood pressure are common. Well absorbed by all routes. Tolerance to vasodilation can occur; cessation of exposure may precipitate angina pectoris in pharmacologically dependent workers. See also nitrates, p 229.	0.5 mg/m³, S	2	4	4	White to light yellow crystalline solid. Odorless. Vapor pressure is 0.05 mm Hg at 85 °C (185 °F). Explosive upon heating or shock.
Triorthocresyl phosphate (TOCP [CAS: 78-30-8]): Inhibits acetylcholinesterase (see p 240). Potent neurotoxin causing delayed, partially reversible peripheral neuropathy by all routes.	0.1 mg/m³, S				Colorless viscous liquid. Odorless. Not combustible. Although an anticholinesterase inhibitor, it is widely used as a chemical additive and in chemical synthesis.
Triphenyl phosphate (CAS: 115-86-6): Weak anticholinesterase activity in humans (see p 240). Delayed neuropathy reported in test animals.	3 mg/m³	2	1	0	Colorless solid. Faint phenolic odor. Not combustible. Thermal breakdown products include phosphoric acid fumes.
Tungsten and compounds: Few reports of human toxicity. Some salts may release acid upon contact with moisture. Chronic exposure to tungsten carbide cobalt amalgams in the hard-metals industry may be associated with fibrotic lung disease. See cobalt.	5 mg/m³ (insoluble compounds) 1 mg/m³ (soluble compounds)				Elemental tungsten is a gray, hard, brittle metal. Finely divided powders are flammable.
Turpentine (CAS: 8006-64-2): Irritating to eyes upon direct contact. Dermal absorption occurs. Vapors irritating to respiratory tract. A CNS depressant at high air levels. See also hydrocarbons, p 178.	100 ppm	1	3	0	Colorless to pale yellow liquid with a characteristic paintlike odor that serves as a good warning property. Vapor pressure is 5 mm Hg at 20 °C (68 °F). Flammable.

ERPG: 1900 ppm

(C) = ceiling air concentration (TLV-C); S = skin absorption can be significant; A1 = ACGIH-confirmed human carcinogen; A2 = ACGIH-suspected human carcinogen; NFPA Hazard Codes: H = health, F = fire, R = reactivity, Ox = oxidizer, W = water-reactive, 0 (none) <—> 4 (severe). ERPG = Emergency Response Planning Guideline. See p 402 for explanation of definitions.

continued

TABLE IV–13. HEALTH HAZARD SUMMARIES FOR INDUSTRIAL AND OCCUPATIONAL CHEMICALS (Continued)

Health Hazard Summaries	ACGIH TLV	IDLH	NFPA Codes H			Comments
Uranium compounds: Many salts are irritating to the respiratory tract; soluble salts are potent kidney toxins. Uranium is a weakly radioactive element (alpha emitter); decays to the radionuclide, thorium 230. Uranium has the potential to cause radiation injury to the lungs, tracheobronchial lymph nodes, bone marrow, and skin.	0.2 mg/m³ (insoluble compounds, as U) 0.2 mg/m³ (soluble compounds, as U)	30 mg/m³ 20 mg/m³				Dense, silvery-white, lustrous metal. Finely divided powders are pyrophoric. Radioactive.
Valeraldehyde (pentanal [CAS: 110-62-3]): Very irritating to eyes and skin; severe burns may result. Vapors highly irritating to the eyes and respiratory tract.	50 ppm		1	3	0	Colorless liquid with a fruity odor. Flammable.
Vanadium pentoxide (CAS: 1314-62-1): Dusts or fumes highly irritating to eyes, skin, and respiratory tract. Acute overexposures have been associated with a persistent bronchitis and asthmalike responses, "boilermakers' asthma." Sensitization dermatitis reported. Low-level exposure may cause a greenish discoloration of the tongue, metallic taste, and cough.	0.05 mg/m³	70 mg/m³ (as V)				Yellow-orange to rust-brown crystalline powder or dark gray flakes. Odorless. Not combustible.
Vinyl acetate (CAS: 108-05-4): Highly irritating upon direct contact; severe skin and eye burns may result. Vapors irritating to the eyes and respiratory tract. Mild CNS depressant at high levels. Limited evidence for adverse effects on male reproduction in test animals at high doses.	10 ppm [proposed: 10 ppm, A3]	ERPG-1: 5 ppm ERPG-2: 75 ppm ERPG-3: 500 ppm	2	3	2	Volatile liquid with a pleasant fruity odor at low levels. Vapor pressure is 115 mm Hg at 25 °C (77 °F). Flammable. Polymerizes readily. Must contain inhibitor to prevent polymerization.
Vinyl bromide (CAS: 593-60-2): At high air levels, an eye and respiratory tract irritant and CNS depressant; a kidney and liver toxin. Animal carcinogen (IARC 2A).	5 ppm, A2 NIOSH CA		2	0	1	Colorless, highly flammable gas with a distinctive odor.

Vinyl chloride (CAS: 75-01-4): An eye and respiratory tract irritant at high air levels. Degeneration of distal phalanges with "acroosteolysis," Raynaud's disease, and scleroderma have been associated with heavy workplace overexposures. A CNS depressant at high levels, formerly used as an anesthetic. May cause cardiac arrhythmias. Causes angiosarcoma of the liver in humans (IARC 1).	5 ppm, A1 NIOSH CA			Colorless, highly flammable gas with a sweet etherlike odor. Polymerizes readily. Current potential exposure is limited to vinyl chloride synthesis and polymerization to PVC.
Vinyl cyclohexene dioxide (vinylhexane dioxide [CAS: 106-87-6]): Moderately irritating upon direct contact; severe burns may result. Vapors highly irritating to eyes and respiratory tract. Testicular atrophy, leukemia, and necrosis of the thymus in test animals. Topical application causes skin cancer in animal studies.	10 ppm, S, A2			Colorless liquid. Vapor pressure is 0.1 mm Hg at 20 °C (68 °F).
Vinyl toluene (methylstyrene [CAS: 25013-15-4]): Vapors irritating to eyes and respiratory tract. A CNS depressant at high levels. Hepatic, renal, and hematologic toxicities observed at high doses in test animals. Limited evidence for adverse effects on the developing fetus at high doses.	50 ppm	5000 ppm	2 2 1	Colorless liquid. Strong, unpleasant odor is considered to be an adequate warning property. Vapor pressure is 1.1 mm Hg at 20 °C (68 °F). Flammable. Inhibitor added to prevent explosive polymerization.
VM&P naphtha (varnish makers' and printers' naphtha; ligroin [CAS: 8032-32-4]): Vapors irritating to eyes and respiratory tract. A CNS depressant at high levels. May contain a small amount of benzene. See also p 178.	300 ppm			Colorless volatile liquid.
Warfarin (CAS: 81-81-2): An anticoagulant by ingestion. Medicinal dosages associated with adverse effects on fetal development in test animals and humans. See also p 143.	0.1 mg/m³	200 mg/m³		Colorless crystalline substance. Odorless. Used as a rodenticide. Exposure is typically from inadvertent or deliberate ingestion, rather than through workplace contamination.
Xylene (mixture of o-, m-, p-dimethylbenzenes [CAS: 1330-20-7]): Vapors irritating to eyes and respiratory tract. A CNS depressant. By analogy to toluene and benzene, may cause cardiac arrhythmias. May injure kidneys. Limited evidence for adverse effects on fetal development in test animals at very high doses. See also p 298.	100 ppm	1000 ppm	2 3 0	Colorless liquid or solid. Weak, somewhat sweet, aromatic odor. Irritant effects are adequate warning properties. Vapor pressure is approximately 8 mm Hg at 20 °C (68 °F). Flammable.

(C) = ceiling air concentration (TLV-C); S = skin absorption can be significant; A1 = ACGIH-confirmed human carcinogen; A2 = ACGIH-suspected human carcinogen; NFPA Hazard Codes: H = health, F = fire, R = reactivity, Ox = oxidizer, W = water-reactive, 0 (none) <—> 4 (severe); ERPG = Emergency Response Planning Guideline. See p 402 for explanation of definitions.

continued

TABLE IV–13. HEALTH HAZARD SUMMARIES FOR INDUSTRIAL AND OCCUPATIONAL CHEMICALS (Continued)

Health Hazard Summaries	ACGIH TLV	IDLH	NFPA Codes H F R	Comments
Xylidine (dimethylaniline [CAS: 1300-73-8]): May cause methemoglobinemia (see p 217). Dermal absorption may occur. Liver and kidney damage seen in test animals.	0.5 ppm, S, A2	150 ppm	3 1 0	Pale yellow to brown liquid. Weak, aromatic amine odor is an adequate warning property. Vapor pressure is less than 1 mm Hg at 20 °C (68 °F). Combustible. Thermal breakdown products include oxides of nitrogen.
Yttrium and compounds (yttrium metal; yttrium nitrate hexahydrate; yttrium chloride; yttrium oxide): Dusts may be irritating to the eyes and respiratory tract.	1 mg/m³ (as Y)			Appearance varies with compound.
Zinc chloride (CAS: 7646-85-7): Caustic and highly irritating upon direct contact; severe burns may result. Ulceration of exposed skin from exposure to fumes has been reported. Fumes extremely irritating to respiratory tract; pulmonary edema has resulted.	1 mg/m³	2000 mg/m³		White powder or colorless crystals that absorb moisture. The fume is white and has an acrid odor. Exposure is principally through smoke bombs.
Zinc chromates (basic zinc chromate, ZnCrO₄; zinc potassium chromate, KZn₂(CrO₄)₂(OH); zinc yellow): Contains hexavalent chromium which is associated with lung cancer in workers. See also p 135.	0.01 mg/m³ (as Cr), A1			Basic zinc chromate is a yellow pigment; dichromates are orange.
Zinc oxide (CAS: 1314-13-2): Fumes irritating to the respiratory tract. Causes metal fume fever (see p 214). Symptoms include headache, fever, chills, muscle aches, and vomiting.	5 mg/m³ (fume) 10 mg/m³ (dusts)			A white or yellowish-white powder. Fumes of zinc oxide are formed when elemental zinc is heated. Principal exposure is through brass foundries or welding on galvanized steel.
Zirconium compounds (zirconium oxide, ZrO₂; zirconium oxychloride, ZrOCl; zirconium tetrachloride, ZrCl₄): Zirconium compounds are generally of low toxicity. Some compounds are irritating; zirconium tetrachloride releases HCl upon contact with moisture. Granulomata caused by the use of deodorants containing zirconium have been observed. Dermal sensitization has not been reported.	5 mg/m³ (as Zr)	500 mg/m³		The elemental form is a bluish-black powder or a grayish-white, lustrous metal. The finely divided powder can be flammable.

(C) = ceiling air concentration (TLV-C); S = skin absorption can be significant; A1 = ACGIH-confirmed human carcinogen; A2 = ACGIH-suspected human carcinogen; NFPA Hazard Codes: H = health, F = fire, R = reactivity, Ox = oxidizer, W = water-reactive, 0 (none) <—> 4 (severe). ERPG = Emergency Response Planning Guideline. See p 402 for explanation of definitions.

Subject Index

NOTE: Page numbers in bold face type indicate a major discussion. A *t* following a page number indicates tabular material and an *i* following a page number indicates an illustration. Both proprietary and generic product names are listed in the index. When a proprietary name is used, the reader is encouraged to review the full reference under the generic name for complete information on the product.

Ivory Bar soap, nontoxic exposure to, 236*t*
Ivory Dishwashing Liquid. *See* detergents, **152–153**
Ivy
American, toxicity of, 260*t*
Boston, toxicity of, 260*t*
Devil's, toxicity of, 262*t*
English, toxicity of, 262*t*
glacier, toxicity of, 262*t*
heart, toxicity of, 262*t*
oakleaf, toxicity of, 265*t*
poison, toxicity of, 265*t*
Ivy bush, toxicity of, 263*t*

J wave, 12, 13*i*, **20**
Jack-in-the-pulpit, toxicity of, 263*t*
Jackhammer operators, occupational exposures associated with, 388*t*
Jalap, toxicity of, 263*t*
Jasco Chemical Premium Paint and Epoxy Remover. *See*
methanol, **215–217**
methylene chloride, **220–221**
Jasco Chemical Speedomatic Paint Remover. *See*
methanol, **215–217**
methylene chloride, **220–221**
Jasmolin I or II (pyrethrum, pyrethrins)
hazard summary for, 477*t*
toxicity of, 269–271
Jatropha spp, toxicity of, 260*t*
Jaundice, occupational exposures causing, 392*t*
"Jaw thrust" maneuver, 3, 6*i*
Jellyfish envenomation, **195–196**
Jequirity bean, toxicity of, 263*t*
Jerusalem cherry, toxicity of, 263*t*
Jessamine
Carolina, toxicity of, 263*t*
day or night, toxicity of, 263*t*
toxicity of, 263*t*
yellow, toxicity of, 264*t*
Jetbead, toxicity of, 264*t*
Jetberry bush, toxicity of, 264*t*
Jimmyweed, toxicity of, 264*t*
Jimsonweed, toxicity of, 264*t*
Joint (slang). *See* marijuana, **209–210**
Joy Dishwashing Soap. *See also* detergents, **152–153**
nontoxic exposure to, 236*t*
Jumping spider (*Phidippus*) envenomation, 288–290
Juniper, toxicity of, 264*t*
Juniperus macropoda, toxicity of, 264*t*
Junk (slang). *See* heroin, 239*t*

Kalmia **spp, toxicity of, 263***t*, **265***t*
Kanamycin. *See also* antibiotics, **72–75**
toxicity of, 73*t*
Kantrex. *See* kanamycin, 73*t*
Kaolin, nontoxic exposure to, 236*t*
Karwinskia humboldtiana, toxicity of, 261*t*, 262*t*
Kava-kava, toxicity of, 264*t*

Kayexalate
as binding agent, 49*t*
for hyperkalemia, 35
Keflex. See cephalosporins (cephalexin), 73*t*
Keflin. *See* cephalothin, 73*t*
Keflodin. *See* cephaloridine, 73*t*
Kentucky coffee tree, toxicity of, 264*t*
Kepone. *See also* chlorinated hydrocarbons, **129–130**
hazard summary for, 452*t*
repeat-dose activated charcoal for removal of, 52*t*
toxicity of, 130*t*
Kerlone. *See* betaxolol, 100*t*
Kerosene. *See also* hydrocarbons, **178–180**
toxicity of, 179*t*
Ketamine, dyskinesia caused by, 24*t*
Ketene, hazard summary for, 452*t*
Ketoacidosis, alcoholic, osmolar gap in patients with, 30*t*
Ketoprofen. *See also* nonsteroidal anti-inflammatory drugs, **233–235**
toxicity of, 234*t*
Ketorolac. *See* nonsteroidal anti-inflammatory drugs, **233–235**
KGB (Killer Green Buds) (slang). *See* marijuana, **209–210**
Khat, toxicity of, 264*t*
Kidney failure (renal failure), 36–37
arsine exposure causing, 89
chronic, occupational causes of, 394*t*
without dialysis, osmolar gap in patients with, 30
drugs and toxins causing, 36*t*
hyperkalemia in, 35*t*
hypoglycemia in, 32*t*
Kidneys, occupational exposures affecting, 392, 394*t*
King snake envenomation, 286*t*. *See also* snakebites, **285–288**
Kitacin (IBP). *See also* organophosphates, **240–243**
toxicity of, 241*t*
Kitty litter, nontoxic exposure to, 236*t*
Klonopin. *See* clonazepam, 98*t*
KOH (potassium hydroxide), hazard summary for, 475*t*
Konakion. *See* phytonadione (vitamin K_1), **377–378**
Krait envenomation, 286*t*. *See also* snakebites, **285–288**
"Krystal" (slang). *See* phencyclidine, **248–249**
Kwell Lotion. *See* lindane, 130*t*
$KZn_2(CrO_4)2(OH)$ (zinc potassium chromate), hazard summary for, 496*t*

L-Dopa, monoamine oxidase inhibitor interaction and, 222t
Labetalol, 100*t*, **347–348**. *See also* beta-adrenergic blockers, **99–101**
for monoamine oxidase inhibitor overdose, 223
pharmacology/use of, **347–348**
toxicity of, 100*t*
Labrador tea, toxicity of, 264*t*